# FIFTH EDITION

# CALCULATE

## with *Confidence*

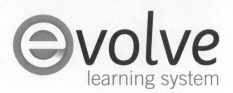

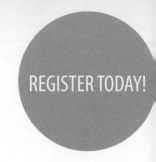
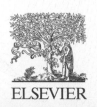
ELSEVIER

# FIFTH EDITION

# CALCULATE
## with *Confidence*

*Deborah Gray Morris*
*RN, BSN, MA, LNC*
Professor of Nursing
Department of Nursing and Allied Health Sciences
Bronx Community College
Bronx, New York

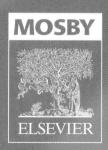
MOSBY
ELSEVIER

3251 Riverport Lane
St. Louis, Missouri 63043

CALCULATE WITH CONFIDENCE                    ISBN: 978-0-323-05629-8
**Copyright © 2010 by Mosby, Inc., an affiliate of Elsevier Inc.**

---

**NOTICE**

Knowledge and best practice in this field are constantly changing. As new research and experience broaden our knowledge, changes in practice, treatment, and drug therapy may become necessary or appropriate. Readers are advised to check the most current information provided (i) on procedures featured or (ii) by the manufacturer of each product to be administered to verify the recommended dose or formula, the method and duration of administration, and contraindications. It is the responsibility of the practitioner, relying on their own experience and knowledge of the patient, to make diagnoses, to determine dosages and the best treatment for each individual patient, and to take all appropriate safety precautions. To the fullest extent of the law, neither the Publisher nor the Author assumes any liability for any injury and/or damage to persons or property arising out of or related to any use of the material contained in this book.

---

**Library of Congress Cataloging-in-Publication Data**

Morris, Deborah Gray.
  Calculate with confidence / Deborah C. Gray Morris. -- 5th ed.
    p. ; cm.
  Includes bibliographical references and index.
  ISBN 978-0-323-05629-8 (pbk. : alk. paper)
  1. Pharmaceutical arithmetic. 2. Nursing--Mathematics. I. Title.
  [DNLM: 1. Drug Dosage Calculations--Problems and Exercises. 2. Nursing Care--methods--Problems and Exercises. 3. Mathematics--Problems and Exercises. 4. Pharmaceutical Preparations--administration & dosage--Problems and Exercises. QV 18.2 M875c 2010]

  RS57.M67 2010
  615'.1401513--dc22

                                                                    2009026162

*Senior Editor:* Yvonne Alexopoulos
*Senior Developmental Editor:* Danielle M. Frazier
*Publishing Services Manager:* Anne Altepeter
*Senior Project Manager:* Doug Turner
*Book Designer:* Charlie Seibel

Printed in Canada

Working together to grow
libraries in developing countries

www.elsevier.com | www.bookaid.org | www.sabre.org

ELSEVIER    BOOK AID International    Sabre Foundation

Last digit is the print number: 9 8 7 6 5 4 3 2 1

*To my family, friends, nursing colleagues, and students past and present,*
*but especially with love to my children, Cameron, Kimberly, Kanin, and Cory.*
*You light up my life and have been proud of whatever I do.*

*To my mother,*
*your guidance and nurturing has made me what I am today.*
*Thanks for always being there to support me.*

*To current practitioners of nursing and future nurses,*
*I hope this book will be valuable in teaching*
*the basic principles of medication administration and*
*will ensure safe administration of medication to all clients regardless of the setting.*

# Reviewers

**Michelle Blackmer, MSN, RNC-OB**
Manager of Education
Trinity Medical Center;
Adjunct Faculty
Trinity College of Nursing
Rock Island, Illinois

**Lou Ann Boose, RN, BSN, MSN**
Associate Professor
Department of Nursing
Harrisburg Area Community College
Harrisburg, Pennsylvania

**Karen Crouse, EdD**
Chair
Department of Nursing
Western Connecticut State University
Danbury, Connecticut

**Kendra S. Seiler, RN, BSN, MSN**
Nursing Instructor
Rio Hondo College
Health Science Division
Whittier, California

**Glenda Shockley, MS, RN**
Director of Nursing
Connors State College
Warner, Oklahoma

**Anne Van Landingham, RN, BSN, MSN**
Nursing Instructor
Orlando Tech Practical Nursing Department
Orlando, Florida

# Preface to the Instructor

The fifth edition of *Calculate with Confidence* was written to meet the needs of current and future practitioners of nursing at any level. This book can be used for in-service education programs and as a reference for the inactive nurse returning to the work force. It is also suitable for courses within nursing curricula whose content reflects the calculation of dosages and solutions. The book can generally be used by any health care professional whose responsibilities include safe administration of medications and solutions to clients in diverse clinical settings.

*Calculate with Confidence* is acknowledged for its simplicity in presenting material relevant to dosage calculation and for enhancing the needs of the learner at different curricular levels. Organized in a progression from simple topics to more complex ones, this book makes content relevant to the needs of the student and uses realistic practice problems to enhance learning and make material clinically applicable. Concepts relating to critical thinking, logical thinking, and nursing process are presented throughout. Numerous illustrations, including full-color medication labels and equipment used in medication administration, continue to be a part of this book. Practice problems are presented in each chapter to test the mastery of the content presented. Shading of syringes continues to be featured in the fifth edition to allow for visualization of dosages. Answers to the practice problems include rationales to enhance understanding of principles and answers related to dosages. Simplified formulas as methods of converting and calculating are presented.

In response to the increased need for competency in basic math as an essential prerequisite for dosage calculation, a pre-test, chapters reviewing basic math, and a post-test are included. The once controversial topic involving the use of calculators is now a more accepted practice, and they are used on many nursing exams, including the NCLEX; however, allowing their use is individualized. The use of calculators has not been encouraged for the basic math review chapters in this book because of the expectation that students should be able to perform calculations proficiently and independently without their use.

Vast technological advances in equipment and methods of medication administration have decreased errors in dosage calculation and medication administration. However, these advances do not completely absolve health care professionals from the responsibility of calculation and thinking critically with regard to both calculation and the administration of medications to ensure client safety. With the increasing focus on providing health care outside the traditional hospital setting, it becomes even more imperative that calculations be precise, performed with thought, and done using critical thinking skills to ensure correct and safe administration of medications to all clients. A working knowledge in the area of dosage calculation is crucial, regardless of the medication system used or the setting involved.

Overall, this edition has maintained a style similar to previous editions. Its revisions are based on feedback from reviewers and instructors. The fifth edition of *Calculate with Confidence* clearly addresses the increasing responsibility of the nurse in medication administration, prioritizes client safety, and reflects the current scope of practice.

## NEW FEATURES TO THE FIFTH EDITION

- New medication labels have been added and outdated medications replaced.
- Common abbreviations used in medication orders have been updated to comply with the standards and recommendations of The Joint Commission (TJC) and the Institute for Safe Medication Practices (ISMP).
- The medication administration chapter has been expanded to direct the learner's attention to the risks and responsibilities in preventing medication errors.
- Increased discussion on preventing medication errors in chapters dealing with dosage calculations such as pediatric calculation, heparin, and insulin.
- The insulin chapter has been updated and expanded to reflect new and current insulins on the market.
- The IV chapter has been divided into two separate chapters to allow mastery of relevant content and calculations.
- Rule boxes are provided to draw the learner's attention to important instructions essential to math calculation.
- Caution boxes have been added to identify issues that may lead to medication errors.
- Tips for Clinical Practice boxes have been included to call attention to information critical to math calculation and patient safety, as well as issues related to practice.
- Critical Thinking boxes have been expanded to reinforce thinking skills and emphasize the importance of accurate dosage calculation and prevention of errors.
- Labels have been enlarged in some instances to ensure legibility and improve readability.

## ANCILLARIES

*Evolve Resources for Calculate with Confidence,* **fifth edition,** is available to enhance student instruction. This online resource can be found at http://evolve.elsevier.com/GrayMorris/; it corresponds with the chapters of the main book and includes the following:

- Instructor's Manual
- Test Bank organized by chapter
- Image Collection
- **NEW!** Drug Label Glossary
- **NEW!** PowerPoint slides
- **NEW!** Answer Key from text
- *Romans & Daugherty Dosages and Solutions CTB, Version III.* This is a generic test bank, available on Evolve at http://evolve.elsevier.com/GrayMorris/. The test bank contains more than 700 questions on general mathematics, converting within the same system of measurements, converting between different systems of measurement, oral dosages, parenteral dosages, flow rates, pediatric dosages, IV calculations, and more.
- *Drug Calculations Companion, Version 4.* A completely updated, interactive student tutorial that includes an extensive menu of various topic areas within drug calculations such as oral, parenteral, pediatric, and intravenous calculations, to name a few. It contains more than 600 practice problems covering ratio and proportion, formula, and dimensional analysis methods and is now available on Evolve at http://evolve.elsevier.com/GrayMorris/.

Finally, it is my hope that this book will be a valuable asset to current and future practitioners. May it help you calculate dosages accurately and with confidence, using calculation and critical-thinking skills to ensure that medications are administered safely to all clients regardless of the setting. This is both a priority and primary responsibility of the nurse.

*Deborah C. Gray Morris*

# Preface to the Student

The nursing profession is undergoing profound changes. Today's nurses face many technological advances, not only in the hospital setting, but also in settings outside of the hospital, such as the community and the home. The nurse has to be competent and able to use critical thinking skills because application of dosage calculations appears in a variety of settings. Accurate calculation of medication dosages is a critical and necessary skill in health care. Serious harm can come to clients from mathematical errors in calculating a medication dosage. Therefore it is a major responsibility of those administering drugs to ensure safe administration of medications by having the ability to accurately calculate a dosage. Remember to always consult appropriate resources when necessary before administering any medication. This text is intended to provide you with the skills to calculate a dosage with accuracy.

Objectives are provided with each chapter to help guide you through the learning process. Each chapter provides you with sufficient practice problems to reinforce concepts and skills learned and to build your confidence in dosage calculation. Full-color labels and syringes provide simulations of the dosages calculated. Key points are summarized and important concepts are highlighted throughout the text. Critical thinking skills are reinforced by emphasizing the need for you to consider the reasonableness of your computation. Remember that many errors in calculation can be avoided if you approach calculation in a systematic fashion. When you perform calculations systematically, you are less likely to make an error. Answers with the solution and rationale are provided in the back of the text. A comprehensive post-test is included at the end of the text to reinforce skills.

Take a look at the following features so that you may familiarize yourself with this text and maximize its value:

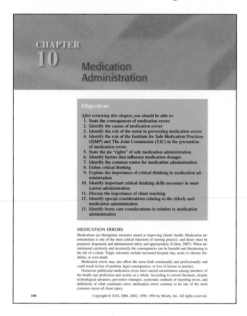

**Objectives** explain what you should accomplish upon completion of each chapter and help guide you through the learning process.

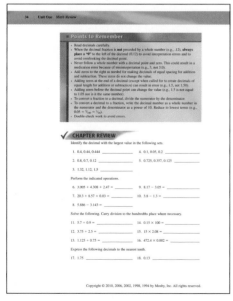

**Points to Remember** boxes highlight pertinent content covered in the chapter and identify important concepts that you should commit to memory.

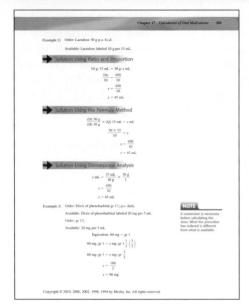

The **Note** feature in the margin makes key information more accessible.

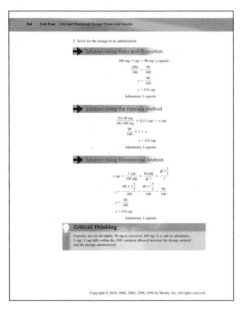

**Critical Thinking** boxes throughout the text present information that should be applied in the clinical setting to avoid drug calculation and administration errors.

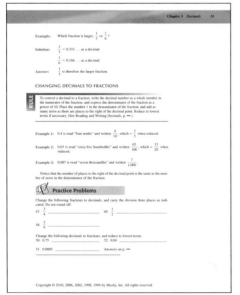

**Rule** boxes present instructions essential to math calculation and familiarize you with information needed to accurately solve medication calculation problems.

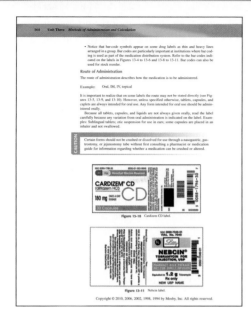

**Caution** boxes identify issues that may lead to medication errors and emphasize actions that must be taken to avoid calculation errors.

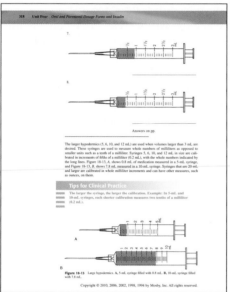

**Tips for Clinical Practice** boxes call attention to information critical to math calculation and patient safety, as well as issues related to practice.

*Drug Calculations Companion, Version 4,* is a completely updated, interactive student tutorial that includes an extensive menu of various topic areas within medication calculations such as oral, parenteral, pediatric, and intravenous calculations, to name a few. It contains more than 600 practice problems covering ratio and proportion, formula, and dimensional analysis methods and is now available on Evolve at http://evolve.elsevier.com/GrayMorris/.

Look for this icon at the end of each chapter. It will refer you to the *Drug Calculations Companion, Version 4,* for additional practice problems and content information.

# Acknowledgments

I wish to extend sincere gratitude and appreciation to my family, friends, and colleagues for their support and encouragement during the writing of the fifth edition. I am indebted to the faculty members from the Department of Nursing and Allied Health Sciences at Bronx Community College for your pertinent suggestions and help in validating and updating the content in this text. Thanks for the problems that you provided from the clinical setting. A special thanks to Professor Lois Augustus, chairperson of the Department of Nursing and Allied Health Sciences, for your encouragement and the inspiration you provided to me. A special thank you to my colleagues Paula Green and Clarence Hodge, who teach Pharmacology Computations with me. Your feedback and suggestions while revising this text were invaluable. Special thanks also to the reviewers of this text; your comments and suggestions were invaluable. Particular thanks to the math reviewers. Thanks to students past and present at Bronx Community College who brought practice problems from the clinical area and helped me to have an appreciation for the problems that students encounter with basic math and calculation of medication dosages. Thanks for your valuable feedback.

I am particularly grateful to former colleagues who provided me with the encouragement and nurturing I needed to consider publication. Who would have thought this book would now be in its fifth edition? Thank you to Professor Germana Glier, former chairperson of Mathematics and Computer Science at Bronx Community College; your help with the aspects of solving for the unknown in the IV chapter and validating mathematical answers was invaluable. Thanks also to the late Dr. Gerald S. Lieblich, former chairperson of the Department of Mathematics at Bronx Community College, who took the time to review and validate content and to make pertinent suggestions for the unit on basic math. To my friend, the late Frank C. Rucker, your encouragement, inspiring words, and admiration for me as an author will always remain with me.

Thanks to St. Barnabas Hospital (Bronx, New York) for permission to reproduce records used in the text.

I am especially grateful to the staff at Elsevier for their support and help in planning, writing, and producing the fifth edition of this text. A special thanks to Danielle M. Frazier for her time, support, patience, and understanding with this revision. Thanks for your encouragement and sincere concern at the times when I needed them most. Thanks to Doug Turner, whose help was invaluable in revising this text.

To Reginald B. Morris, my husband, words cannot begin to express how thankful I am for your help, encouragement, support, and understanding while I revised this text. Thanks for your support, confidence in me, and encouragement during those times when I had doubts that I would meet my deadlines. Thanks for the long and late hours you spent at the computer entering the revisions and doing whatever you could to help me complete this edition. Without your continual support and assistance, this edition could not have been completed.

Anna, my dearest friend who is like a sister, thanks for all of your support, encouragement, and expressions of confidence in me during the times I needed them most.

# Contents

# UNIT One

# Math Review

An essential role of the nurse is providing safe medication administration to all clients. To accurately perform dosage calculations, the nurse must have knowledge of basic math, regardless of the problem-solving method used in calculation. Knowledge of basic math is a necessary component of dosage calculation that nurses need to know to prevent medication errors and ensure the safe administration of medications to all clients, regardless of the setting. Serious harm can result to clients from a mathematical error during calculation and administration of a drug dosage. The nurse must practice and be proficient in the basic math used in dosage calculations. Knowledge of basic math is a prerequisite for the prevention of medication errors and ensures the safe administration of medications.

Although calculators are accessible for basic math operations, the nurse needs to be able to perform the processes involved in basic math. Controversy still exists among educators regarding the use of calculators in dosage calculation. Calculators may indeed be recommended for complex calculations to ensure accuracy and save time; the types of calculations requiring their use are presented later in this text. However, because the basic math required for less complex calculations is often simple and can be done without the use of a calculator, it is a realistic expectation that each practitioner should be competent in the performance of basic math operations without its use. Performing basic math operations enables the nurse to think logically and critically about the dosage ordered and the dosage calculated.

# Pre-Test

This test is designed to evaluate your ability in the basic math areas reviewed in Unit One. The test consists of 55 questions. If you are able to complete the pre-test with 100% accuracy, you may want to bypass Unit One. Any problems answered incorrectly should be used as a basis for what you might need to review. The purposes of this test and the review that follows are to build your confidence in basic math skills and to help you avoid careless mistakes when you begin to perform dosage calculations.

Express the following in Roman numerals.

1. 9 _____

2. 16 _____

3. 23 _____

4. $10\frac{1}{2}$ _____

5. 22 _____

Express the following in Arabic numbers.

6. $\overline{xiss}$ _____

7. $\overline{xii}$ _____

8. $\overline{xviii}$ _____

9. $\overline{xxiv}$ _____

10. $\overline{vi}$ _____

Reduce the following fractions to lowest terms.

11. $\dfrac{14}{21}$ _____

12. $\dfrac{25}{100}$ _____

13. $\dfrac{2}{150}$ _____

14. $\dfrac{24}{30}$ _____

15. $\dfrac{24}{36}$ _____

Perform the indicated operations; reduce to lowest terms where necessary.

16. $\dfrac{2}{3} \div \dfrac{3}{9} =$ _____

17. $4 \div \dfrac{3}{4} =$ _____

18. $\dfrac{2}{5} + \dfrac{1}{9} =$ _____

19. $7\dfrac{1}{7} - 2\dfrac{5}{6} =$ _____

20. $4\dfrac{2}{3} \times 4 =$ _____

Change the following fractions to decimals; express your answer to the nearest tenth.

21. $\dfrac{6}{7}$ _____

22. $\dfrac{6}{20}$ _____

23. $\dfrac{2}{3}$ _____

24. $\dfrac{7}{8}$ _____

Indicate the largest fraction in each group.

25. $\dfrac{3}{4}, \dfrac{4}{5}, \dfrac{7}{8}$ _____

26. $\dfrac{7}{12}, \dfrac{11}{12}, \dfrac{4}{12}$ _____

Perform the indicated operations with decimals. Provide exact answer; do not round off.

27. $20.1 + 67.35 =$ _____     29. $4.6 \times 8.72 =$ _____

28. $0.008 + 5 =$ _____     30. $56.47 - 8.7 =$ _____

Divide the following decimals; express your answer to the nearest tenth.

31. $7.5 \div 0.004 =$ _____     33. $84.7 \div 2.3 =$ _____

32. $45 \div 1.9 =$ _____

Indicate the largest decimal in each group.

34. 0.674, 0.659 _____     36. 0.25, 0.6, 0.175 _____

35. 0.375, 0.37, 0.38 _____

Solve for $x$, the unknown value.

37. $8:2 = 48:x$ _____     39. $\frac{1}{10}:x = \frac{1}{2}:15$ _____

38. $x:300 = 1:150$ _____     40. $0.4:1 = 0.2:x$ _____

Round off to the nearest tenth.

41. 0.43 _____     43. 1.47 _____

42. 0.66 _____

Round off to the nearest hundredth.

44. 0.735 _____     46. 1.227 _____

45. 0.834 _____

Complete the table below, expressing the measures in their equivalents where indicated. Reduce to lowest terms where necessary.

| | Percent | Decimal | Ratio | Fraction |
|---|---|---|---|---|
| 47. | 6% | _____ | _____ | _____ |
| 48. | _____ | _____ | 7:20 | _____ |
| 49. | _____ | _____ | _____ | $5\frac{1}{4}$ |
| 50. | _____ | 0.015 | _____ | _____ |

Find the following percentages. Express answer to the hundredths place as indicated.

51. 5% of 95 _____     54. 20 is what % of 100 _____

52. $\frac{1}{4}$% of 2,000 _____     55. 30 is what % of 164 _____

53. 2 is what % of 600 _____

Answers on p. 600

# Roman Numerals

The Roman numeral system dates back to ancient Roman times and uses letters to designate amounts. Roman numerals are used in the apothecary system of measurement for writing drug dosages.

**Example:**

gr x

Apothecary measure      Roman numeral
(unit of weight)          (Arabic equivalent 10)

Roman numerals are also still used on objects that indicate time (i.e., watches, clocks).

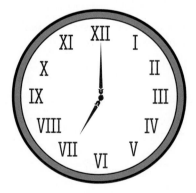

In the Arabic system, numbers, not letters, are used to express amounts. The Arabic system also uses fractions ($\frac{1}{2}$) and decimals (0.5).

Most medication dosages are ordered using metric measurements and Arabic numbers; however, on rare occasions medication orders may include a Roman numeral.

**Example:**     Aspirin gr x, which is correctly interpreted as aspirin 10 grains

     

To calculate drug dosages and assist in the prevention of medication errors, nurses need to know both Roman numerals and Arabic numbers. Lowercase letters are usually used to express Roman numerals in relation to medications. The Roman numerals you will see most often in the calculation of dosages are built on the basic symbols *i, v,* and *x.* To prevent errors in interpretation a line is sometimes drawn over the symbol. If this line is used, the lowercase "i" is dotted above the line, not below.

**Example 1:**   10 grains = gr x

**Example 2:**   2 = ii̇

**CAUTION**

Correctly identifying Roman numerals will assist in preventing medication errors. According to the Institute for Safe Medication Practices (ISMP), abbreviations increase the risk for occurrence of medication errors. Although some health care providers may still use Roman numerals and the apothecary system, the ISMP recommends using the metric system.

**RULE**

As illustrated in the example, with apothecary measures, the label *grains* when abbreviated *(gr)* precedes the Roman numeral. This will be discussed further in Chapter 7.

When the symbol for $\frac{1}{2}$ (ss) is used in conjunction with Roman numerals, the symbol is placed at the end.

**Example 1:**   $3\frac{1}{2}$ = iiiss = iiiss̄

**Example 2:**   $1\frac{1}{2}$ grains = gr iss = gr iss̄

Box 1-1 lists the common Arabic equivalents for Roman numerals (review them if necessary). They are often expressed with lowercase letters. Review this list before proceeding to the rules pertaining to Roman numerals as shown on p. 6. You will most commonly see Roman numerals up to the value of 30 when they are used in relation to medications.

**NOTE**

Larger Roman numerals, such as L(l) = 50, C(c) = 100, and larger, are usually not used in relation to medications.

---

### BOX 1-1   Arabic Equivalents for Roman Numerals

| Arabic Number | Roman Numeral | Arabic Number | Roman Numeral |
|---|---|---|---|
| ½ | ss or s̄s̄ | 7 | vii or v̄iī, VII |
| 1 | i or i̇, I | 8 | viii or v̄iiī, VIII |
| 2 | ii or iī, II | 9 | ix or i̇x̄, IX |
| 3 | iii or iiī, III | 10 | x or x̄, X |
| 4 | iv or i̇v̄, IV | 15 | xv or x̄v̄, XV |
| 5 | v or v̄, V | 20 | xx or x̄x̄, XX |
| 6 | vi or v̄i, VI | 30 | xxx or x̄x̄x̄, XXX |

**RULE**

### Rules Relating to the Roman System of Notation

1. The same Roman numeral is never repeated more than three times.
   a. Example: Convert the Arabic number 4 to a Roman numeral.
      i. Right: 4 = iv
      ii. Wrong: 4 = iiii
   b. Example: Convert the Arabic number 9 to a Roman numeral.
      i. Right: 9 = ix
      ii. Wrong: 9 = viiii
2. When a Roman numeral of a lesser value is placed **after** one of equal or greater value, the numerals are **added.**
   a. Example: Convert the Arabic number 25 to a Roman numeral.
      i. Right: 25 = xxv (10 + 10 + 5 = 25)
   b. Example: Convert the Roman numeral xvi to an Arabic number.
      i. Right: xvi = 16 (10 + 5 + 1 = 16)
3. When a Roman numeral of a lesser value is placed **before** a numeral of greater value, the numerals are **subtracted.**
   a. Example: Convert the Roman numerals ix and xxiv to Arabic numbers.
      i. Right: ix = 9 (10 − 1 = 9)
      ii. Right: xxiv = 24 [10 + 10 + (5 − 1) = 24]
   b. Example: Convert the Arabic numbers 19 and 14 to Roman numerals.
      i. Right: 19 = xix [10 + (10 − 1) = 19]
      ii. Right: 14 = xiv [10 + (5 − 1) = 14]

---

 **Practice Problems**

Write the following as Roman numerals.

1. 15 _____

2. 13 _____

3. 28 _____

4. 11 _____

5. 17 _____

Write the following as Arabic numbers.

6. xiv _____

7. xxix _____

8. iv _____

9. xix _____

10. xxxiv _____

Answers on p. 600

---

 **CHAPTER REVIEW**

Write the following Arabic numbers as Roman numerals.

1. 6 _____

2. 30 _____

3. $1\frac{1}{2}$ _____

4. 27 _____

5. 12 _____

6. 18 _____

7. 20 _____

8. 3 _____

9. 21 _____

10. 26 _____

Write the following Roman numerals as Arabic numbers.

11. $\overline{\text{viiss}}$ _____    16. $\overline{\text{iii}}$ _____

12. $\overline{\text{xix}}$ _____    17. $\overline{\text{xxii}}$ _____

13. $\overline{\text{xv}}$ _____    18. $\overline{\text{xvi}}$ _____

14. $\overline{\text{xxx}}$ _____    19. $\overline{\text{v}}$ _____

15. $\overline{\text{ss}}$ _____    20. $\overline{\text{xxvii}}$ _____

Answers on p. 600

 **For additional practice problems, refer to the Mathematics Review section of Drug Calculations Companion, Version 4, on Evolve.**

# CHAPTER 2

# Fractions

## Objectives

*After reviewing this chapter, you should be able to:*
1. Compare the size of fractions
2. Add fractions
3. Subtract fractions
4. Divide fractions
5. Multiply fractions
6. Reduce fractions to lowest terms

Understanding fractions is necessary for health care professionals. Fractions are seen in medical orders, client records, charting related to care given to clients, and literature related to health care. The nurse often encounters fractions when dealing with apothecary and household measures in dosage calculation.

Fractions may be used occasionally in the writing of a medication order or used by the pharmaceutical manufacturer on a drug label (usually includes the metric equivalent). According to *Medication Errors,* 2nd edition (2007), edited by Michael R. Cohen, president of the Institute for Safe Medication Practices (ISMP), "Occasionally using fractions instead of metric designation could help prevent errors. For example, the dosage embossed on 2.5 mg Coumadin tablets is expressed as '2$\frac{1}{2}$ mg' to prevent confusion with 25 mg."

Coumadin is an anticoagulant. An overdose of Coumadin (example: 25 mg instead of 2$\frac{1}{2}$ mg) can result in a serious adverse effect, such as a severe hemorrhage (Figure 2-1).

As you will see later in the text, some methods of solving dosage calculations rely on expressing relationships in a fraction format. Therefore proficiency with fractions can be beneficial in a variety of situations.

A fraction is a part of a whole number (Figure 2-2). It is a division of a whole into units or parts (Figure 2-3).

**Example:**   $\frac{1}{2}$ is a whole divided into two equal parts.

Fractions are composed of two parts: a **numerator,** which is the top number, and a **denominator,** which is the bottom number.

$$\frac{\text{Numerator}}{\text{Denominator}} : \frac{\text{how many parts of the}}{\text{how many equal parts}}$$
$$\text{the whole is divided into}$$

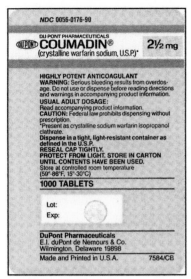

**Figure 2-1**  Coumadin label.

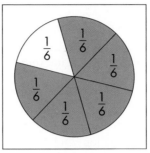

**Figure 2-2**  Diagram representing fractions of a whole. Five parts shaded out of the six parts represent:

$$\frac{5}{6} \quad \frac{\text{Numerator}}{\text{Denominator}}$$

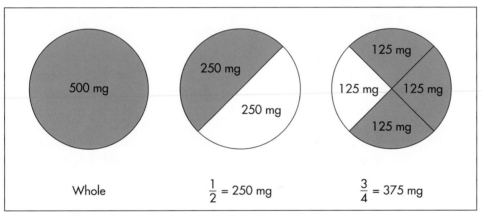

**Figure 2-3**  Fraction pie charts.

**Example:**  In the fraction $\frac{5}{6}$, the whole is divided into 6 equal parts (denominator), and five parts (numerator) are considered.

## TYPES OF FRACTIONS

**Proper Fraction:** Numerator is less than the denominator, and the fraction has a value of less than 1.

**Examples:**  $\frac{1}{8}, \frac{5}{6}, \frac{7}{8}, \frac{1}{150}$

**Improper Fraction:** Numerator is larger than, or equal to, the denominator, and the fraction has a value of 1 or greater than 1.

**Examples:**  $\frac{3}{2}, \frac{7}{5}, \frac{300}{150}, \frac{4}{4}$

**Mixed Number:** Whole number and a fraction with a value greater than 1.

Examples:    $3\dfrac{1}{3}, 5\dfrac{1}{8}, 9\dfrac{1}{6}, 25\dfrac{7}{8}$

**Complex Fraction:** Numerator, denominator, or both are fractions. The value may be less than, greater than, or equal to 1.

Examples:    $\dfrac{3\frac{1}{2}}{2}, \dfrac{\frac{1}{3}}{\frac{1}{2}}, \dfrac{2}{1\frac{1}{4}}, \dfrac{2}{\frac{1}{150}}$

**Whole Numbers:** Have an unexpressed denominator of one (1).

Examples:    $1 = \dfrac{1}{1}, 3 = \dfrac{3}{1}, 6 = \dfrac{6}{1}, 100 = \dfrac{100}{1}$

An improper fraction can be changed to a mixed number or whole number by dividing the numerator by the denominator. If there is a remainder, that number is placed over the denominator and the answer is reduced to lowest terms.

Examples:    $\dfrac{6}{5} = 6 \div 5 = 1\dfrac{1}{5}, \dfrac{100}{25} = 100 \div 25 = 4, \dfrac{10}{8} = 10 \div 8 = 1\dfrac{2}{8} = 1\dfrac{1}{4}$

A mixed number can be changed to an improper fraction by multiplying the whole number by the denominator, adding it to the numerator, and placing the sum over the denominator.

Example:    $5\dfrac{1}{8} = \dfrac{(5 \times 8) + 1}{8} = \dfrac{41}{8}$

Two or more fractions with different denominators can be compared by changing both fractions to fractions with the same denominator (Box 2-1). This is done by finding the lowest common denominator (LCD), or the lowest number evenly divisible by the denominators of the fractions being compared.

---

### BOX 2-1   Rules for Comparing Size of Fractions

Comparing the size of fractions is important in the administration of medications. It helps the new practitioner learn early the value of medication dosages. Here are some basic rules to keep in mind when comparing fractions.

1. If the numerators are the same, the fraction with the smaller denominator has the larger value.

**Example 1:**    $\dfrac{1}{2}$ is larger than $\dfrac{1}{3}$

**Example 2:**    $\dfrac{1}{150}$ is larger than $\dfrac{1}{300}$

2. If the denominators are the same, the fraction with the larger numerator has the larger value.

**Example 1:**    $\dfrac{3}{4}$ is larger than $\dfrac{1}{4}$

**Example 2:**    $\dfrac{3}{100}$ is larger than $\dfrac{1}{100}$

---

**Example:**    Which is larger, $\dfrac{3}{4}$ or $\dfrac{4}{5}$?

**Solution:**    The lowest common denominator is 20, because it is the smallest number that can be divided by both denominators evenly. Change each fraction to the same terms by dividing the lowest common denominator by the denominator and multiplying that answer by the numerator. The answer obtained from this is the new numerator. The numerators are then placed over the lowest common denominator.

**NOTE**

LCD = 20

**For the fraction $\dfrac{3}{4}$:** $20 \div 4 = 5$; $5 \times 3 = 15$; therefore $\dfrac{3}{4}$ becomes $\dfrac{15}{20}$.

**For the fraction $\dfrac{4}{5}$:** $20 \div 5 = 4$; $4 \times 4 = 16$; therefore $\dfrac{4}{5}$ becomes $\dfrac{16}{20}$.

Therefore $\dfrac{4}{5} \left( \dfrac{16}{20} \right)$ is larger than $\dfrac{3}{4} \left( \dfrac{15}{20} \right)$.

Box 2-2 presents fundamental rules of fractions.

### BOX 2-2    Fundamental Rules of Fractions

In working with fractions, there are some fundamental rules that we need to remember.
1. When the numerator and denominator of a fraction are both multiplied or divided by the same number, the value of the fraction remains unchanged.

**Examples:**    $\dfrac{1}{2} = \dfrac{1 \times (2)}{2 \times (2)} = \dfrac{2}{4} = \dfrac{2 \times (25)}{4 \times (25)} = \dfrac{50}{100}$, etc.

$\dfrac{50}{100} = \dfrac{50 \div (10)}{100 \div (10)} = \dfrac{5}{10} = \dfrac{5 \div (5)}{10 \div (5)} = \dfrac{1}{2}$, etc.

As shown in the examples, common fractions can be written in varied forms, provided that the numerator, divided by the denominator, always yields the same number (quotient). The particular form of a fraction that has the smallest possible whole number for its numerator and denominator is called the *fraction in its lowest terms*. In the example, therefore, $^{50}/_{100}$, $^{5}/_{10}$, or $^{2}/_{4}$ is $^{1}/_{2}$ in its lowest terms.
2. To change a fraction to its lowest terms, divide its numerator and its denominator by the largest whole number that will divide both evenly.

**Example:**    Reduce $\dfrac{128}{288}$ to lowest terms.

$$\dfrac{128}{288} = \dfrac{128 \div 32}{288 \div 32} = \dfrac{4}{9}$$

Note: When you do not see at once the largest number that can be divided evenly, the fraction may have to be reduced by using repeated steps.

**Example:**    $\dfrac{128}{288} = \dfrac{128 \div 4}{288 \div 4} = \dfrac{32}{72} = \dfrac{32 \div 8}{72 \div 8} = \dfrac{4}{9}$

Note: If both the numerator and denominator cannot be divided evenly by a whole number, the fraction is in lowest terms. Fractions should always be expressed in their lowest terms.
3. LCD (lowest common denominator) is the smallest whole number that can be divided evenly by all of the denominators within the problem.

**Example:**    $\dfrac{1}{3}$ and $\dfrac{5}{12}$: 12 is evenly divisible by 3; therefore 12 is the LCD.

$\dfrac{3}{7}$, $\dfrac{2}{14}$, and $\dfrac{2}{28}$: 28 is evenly divisible by 7 and 14; therefore 28 is the LCD.

## Practice Problems

Circle the fraction with the lesser value in each of the following sets.

1.  $\dfrac{6}{30}$    $\dfrac{4}{5}$

2.  $\dfrac{5}{4}$    $\dfrac{6}{8}$

3.  $\dfrac{1}{75}$    $\dfrac{1}{100}$    $\dfrac{1}{150}$

4.  $\dfrac{6}{18}$    $\dfrac{7}{18}$    $\dfrac{8}{18}$

5.  $\dfrac{4}{5}$    $\dfrac{7}{5}$    $\dfrac{3}{5}$

6.  $\dfrac{4}{8}$    $\dfrac{1}{8}$    $\dfrac{3}{8}$

7.  $\dfrac{1}{40}$    $\dfrac{1}{10}$    $\dfrac{1}{5}$

8.  $\dfrac{1}{300}$    $\dfrac{1}{200}$    $\dfrac{1}{175}$

9.  $\dfrac{4}{24}$    $\dfrac{5}{24}$    $\dfrac{10}{24}$

10.  $\dfrac{4}{3}$    $\dfrac{1}{2}$    $\dfrac{1}{6}$

Circle the fraction with the higher value in each of the following sets.

11.  $\dfrac{6}{8}$    $\dfrac{5}{9}$

12.  $\dfrac{7}{6}$    $\dfrac{2}{3}$

13.  $\dfrac{1}{72}$    $\dfrac{6}{12}$    $\dfrac{1}{24}$

14.  $\dfrac{1}{10}$    $\dfrac{1}{6}$    $\dfrac{1}{8}$

15.  $\dfrac{1}{75}$    $\dfrac{1}{125}$    $\dfrac{1}{225}$

16.  $\dfrac{2}{5}$    $\dfrac{6}{5}$    $\dfrac{3}{5}$

17.  $\dfrac{1}{8}$    $\dfrac{4}{6}$    $\dfrac{1}{4}$

18.  $\dfrac{7}{9}$    $\dfrac{5}{9}$    $\dfrac{8}{9}$

19.  $\dfrac{1}{10}$    $\dfrac{1}{50}$    $\dfrac{1}{150}$

20.  $\dfrac{2}{15}$    $\dfrac{1}{15}$    $\dfrac{6}{15}$

Answers on p. 601

## REDUCING FRACTIONS

Fractions should always be reduced to their lowest terms.

**RULE**

> To reduce a fraction to its lowest terms, the numerator and denominator are each divided by the largest number by which they are both evenly divisible.

**Example 1:**   Reduce the fraction $\dfrac{6}{20}$.

**Solution:**   Both numerator and denominator are evenly divisible by 2.

$$\frac{6}{20} \div \frac{2}{2} = \frac{3}{10}$$

$$\frac{6}{20} = \frac{3}{10}$$

**Example 2:** Reduce the fraction $\dfrac{75}{100}$.

**Solution:** Both numerator and denominator are evenly divisible by 25.

$$\frac{75}{100} \div \frac{25}{25} = \frac{3}{4}$$

$$\frac{75}{100} = \frac{3}{4}$$

 **Practice Problems**

Reduce the following fractions to their lowest terms.

21. $\dfrac{10}{15} =$ _____

22. $\dfrac{7}{49} =$ _____

23. $\dfrac{64}{128} =$ _____

24. $\dfrac{100}{150} =$ _____

25. $\dfrac{20}{28} =$ _____

26. $\dfrac{14}{98} =$ _____

27. $\dfrac{10}{18} =$ _____

28. $\dfrac{24}{36} =$ _____

29. $\dfrac{10}{50} =$ _____

30. $\dfrac{9}{27} =$ _____

31. $\dfrac{9}{9} =$ _____

32. $\dfrac{15}{45} =$ _____

33. $\dfrac{124}{155} =$ _____

34. $\dfrac{12}{18} =$ _____

35. $\dfrac{36}{64} =$ _____

Answers on p. 601

## ADDING FRACTIONS

**RULE**

To add fractions with the same denominator, add the numerators, place the sum over the denominator, and reduce to lowest terms.

**Example 1:**
$$\frac{1}{6} + \frac{4}{6} = \frac{5}{6}$$

**Example 2:**
$$\frac{1}{6} + \frac{3}{6} + \frac{4}{6} = \frac{8}{6}$$

$$\frac{8}{6} = \frac{4}{3} = 1\frac{1}{3}$$

**NOTE**

In addition to reducing to lowest terms in Example 2, the improper fraction was changed to a mixed number.

To add fractions with different denominators, change fractions to their equivalent fraction with the lowest common denominator, add the numerators, write the sum over the common denominator, and reduce if necessary.

**Example 1:**   $\dfrac{1}{4} + \dfrac{1}{3}$

**Solution:**   The lowest common denominator is 12. Change to equivalent fractions.

$$\dfrac{1}{4} = \dfrac{3}{12}$$
$$+\ \dfrac{1}{3} = \dfrac{4}{12}$$
$$\overline{\qquad\qquad \dfrac{7}{12}}$$

**Example 2:**   $\dfrac{1}{2} + 1\dfrac{1}{3} + \dfrac{2}{4}$

**Solution:**   Change the mixed number $1\dfrac{1}{3}$ to $\dfrac{4}{3}$. Find the lowest common denominator, change fractions to equivalent fractions, add, and reduce if necessary. The lowest common denominator is 12.

$$\dfrac{1}{2} = \dfrac{6}{12}$$
$$\dfrac{4}{3} = \dfrac{16}{12}$$
$$+\ \dfrac{2}{4} = \dfrac{6}{12}$$
$$\overline{\qquad\qquad \dfrac{28}{12} = 2\dfrac{4}{12} = 2\dfrac{1}{3}}$$

## SUBTRACTING FRACTIONS

To subtract fractions with the same denominator, subtract the numerators, and place this amount over the denominator. Reduce to lowest terms if necessary.

**Example 1:**   $\dfrac{5}{4} - \dfrac{3}{4} = \dfrac{2}{4} = \dfrac{1}{2}$

**Example 2:**   $2\dfrac{1}{6} - \dfrac{5}{6}$

**Solution:**   Change the mixed number $2\dfrac{1}{6}$ to $\dfrac{13}{6}$

$$\dfrac{13}{6} - \dfrac{5}{6} = \dfrac{8}{6} = \dfrac{4}{3} = 1\dfrac{1}{3}$$

To subtract fractions with different denominators, find the lowest common denominator, change to equivalent fractions, subtract the numerators, and place the sum over the common denominator. Reduce to lowest terms if necessary.

**Example 3:**   $\dfrac{15}{6} - \dfrac{3}{5}$

**Solution:**   The lowest common denominator is 30. Change to equivalent fractions, and subtract.

$$\dfrac{15}{6} = \dfrac{75}{30}$$

$$-\dfrac{3}{5} = \dfrac{18}{30}$$

$$\dfrac{57}{30} = 1\dfrac{27}{30} = 1\dfrac{9}{10}$$

**Example 4:**   $2\dfrac{1}{5} - \dfrac{4}{3}$

**Solution:**   Change the mixed number $2\dfrac{1}{5}$ to $\dfrac{11}{5}$. Find the lowest common denominator, change to equivalent fractions, subtract, and reduce if necessary. The lowest common denominator is 15.

$$\dfrac{11}{5} = \dfrac{33}{15}$$

$$-\dfrac{4}{3} = \dfrac{20}{15}$$

$$\dfrac{13}{15}$$

## MULTIPLYING FRACTIONS

To multiply fractions, multiply the numerators, multiply the denominators, and reduce if necessary.

**Example 1:**   $\dfrac{3}{\overset{4}{\underset{2}{\cancel{4}}}} \times \dfrac{\overset{1}{\cancel{2}}}{5} = \dfrac{3}{10}$

**NOTE**

If fractions are not in lowest terms, reduction can be done before multiplication.

**Example 2:**   $\dfrac{2}{4} \times \dfrac{3}{4}$

**Solution:**   Reduce $\dfrac{2}{4}$ to $\dfrac{1}{2}$ and then multiply.

$$\dfrac{1}{2} \times \dfrac{3}{4} = \dfrac{3}{8}$$

**NOTE**

The whole number 6 is expressed as a fraction here by placing 1 as the denominator.

**Example 3:**

$$6 \times \frac{5}{6}$$

$$\frac{\cancel{6}^{1}}{1} \times \frac{5}{\cancel{6}_{1}} = 5$$

*or*

$$\frac{6 \times 5}{6} = \frac{30}{6} = 5$$

**Example 4:**

$$3\frac{1}{3} \times 2\frac{1}{2}$$

**Solution:**   Change the mixed numbers to improper fractions. Proceed with multiplication.

$$3\frac{1}{3} = \frac{10}{3}; 2\frac{1}{2} = \frac{5}{2}$$

$$\frac{10}{3} \times \frac{5}{2} = \frac{50}{6} = 8\frac{2}{6} = 8\frac{1}{3}$$

*or*

$$\frac{\cancel{10}^{5}}{3} \times \frac{5}{\cancel{2}_{1}} = \frac{25}{3} = 8\frac{1}{3}$$

## DIVIDING FRACTIONS

**RULE**

To divide fractions, invert (turn upside down) the second fraction (divisor), and multiply. Reduce where necessary.

**Example 1:**

$$\frac{3}{4} \div \frac{2}{3}$$

**Solution:**

$$\frac{3}{4} \times \frac{3}{2} = \frac{9}{8} = 1\frac{1}{8}$$

**Example 2:**

$$1\frac{3}{5} \div 2\frac{1}{10}$$

**Solution:**   Change mixed numbers to improper fractions. Proceed with steps of division.

$$1\frac{3}{5} = \frac{8}{5}; 2\frac{1}{10} = \frac{21}{10}$$

$$\frac{8}{\cancel{5}_{1}} \times \frac{\cancel{10}^{2}}{21} = \frac{16}{21}$$

**Example 3:**

$$5 \div \frac{1}{2}$$

**Solution:**

$$5 \times \frac{2}{1} = \frac{10}{1} = 10$$

*or*

$$\frac{5}{1} \times \frac{2}{1} = \frac{10}{1} = 10$$

When doing dosage calculations that involve division, the fractions may be written as follows: $\dfrac{1/4}{1/2}$. In this case, $\dfrac{1}{4}$ is the numerator and $\dfrac{1}{2}$ is the denominator. Therefore the problem is set up as: $\dfrac{1}{4} \div \dfrac{1}{2}$, which becomes $\dfrac{1}{\underset{2}{\cancel{4}}} \times \dfrac{\cancel{2}}{1} = \dfrac{1}{2}$.

## Practice Problems

Change the following improper fractions to mixed numbers, and reduce to lowest terms.

36. $\dfrac{18}{5} =$ _____

37. $\dfrac{60}{14} =$ _____

38. $\dfrac{13}{8} =$ _____

39. $\dfrac{35}{12} =$ _____

40. $\dfrac{112}{100} =$ _____

Change the following mixed numbers to improper fractions.

41. $1\dfrac{4}{25} =$ _____

42. $4\dfrac{2}{8} =$ _____

43. $4\dfrac{1}{2} =$ _____

44. $3\dfrac{3}{8} =$ _____

45. $15\dfrac{4}{5} =$ _____

Add the following fractions and mixed numbers, and reduce fractions to lowest terms.

46. $\dfrac{2}{3} + \dfrac{5}{6} =$ _____

47. $2\dfrac{1}{8} + \dfrac{2}{3} =$ _____

48. $2\dfrac{3}{10} + 4\dfrac{1}{5} + \dfrac{2}{3} =$ _____

49. $7\dfrac{2}{5} + \dfrac{2}{3} =$ _____

50. $12\dfrac{1}{2} + 10\dfrac{1}{3} =$ _____

Subtract and reduce fractions to lowest terms.

51. $\dfrac{4}{3} - \dfrac{3}{7} =$ _____

52. $3\dfrac{3}{8} - 1\dfrac{3}{5} =$ _____

53. $\dfrac{15}{16} - \dfrac{1}{4} =$ _____

54. $2\dfrac{5}{6} - 2\dfrac{3}{4} =$ _____

55. $\dfrac{1}{8} - \dfrac{1}{12} =$ _____

Multiply the following fractions and mixed numbers, and reduce to lowest terms.

56. $\dfrac{2}{3} \times \dfrac{4}{5} = $ _____

59. $2\dfrac{5}{8} \times 2\dfrac{3}{4} = $ _____

57. $\dfrac{6}{25} \times \dfrac{3}{5} = $ _____

60. $\dfrac{5}{12} \times \dfrac{4}{9} = $ _____

58. $\dfrac{1}{50} \times 3 = $ _____

Divide the following fractions and mixed numbers and reduce to lowest terms.

61. $2\dfrac{6}{8} \div 1\dfrac{2}{3} = $ _____

64. $\dfrac{7}{8} \div \dfrac{7}{8} = $ _____

62. $\dfrac{1}{60} \div \dfrac{1}{2} = $ _____

65. $3\dfrac{1}{3} \div 1\dfrac{7}{12} = $ _____

63. $6 \div \dfrac{2}{5} = $ _____    Answers on p. 601

---

## ✓ CHAPTER REVIEW

Change the following improper fractions to mixed numbers, and reduce to lowest terms.

1. $\dfrac{10}{8} = $ _____

6. $\dfrac{67}{10} = $ _____

2. $\dfrac{30}{4} = $ _____

7. $\dfrac{9}{2} = $ _____

3. $\dfrac{22}{6} = $ _____

8. $\dfrac{11}{5} = $ _____

4. $\dfrac{11}{4} = $ _____

9. $\dfrac{64}{15} = $ _____

5. $\dfrac{59}{14} = $ _____

10. $\dfrac{100}{13} = $ _____

Change the following mixed numbers to improper fractions.

11. $2\dfrac{1}{2} = $ _____

16. $2\dfrac{3}{5} = $ _____

12. $7\dfrac{3}{8} = $ _____

17. $8\dfrac{4}{10} = $ _____

13. $8\dfrac{3}{5} = $ _____

18. $9\dfrac{1}{4} = $ _____

14. $16\dfrac{1}{4} = $ _____

19. $12\dfrac{3}{4} = $ _____

15. $3\dfrac{1}{5} = $ _____

20. $6\dfrac{5}{7} = $ _____

Add the following fractions and mixed numbers. Reduce to lowest terms.

21. $\dfrac{2}{5} + \dfrac{1}{3} + \dfrac{7}{10} =$ _____

22. $\dfrac{1}{4} + \dfrac{1}{6} + \dfrac{1}{8} =$ _____

23. $20\dfrac{1}{2} + \dfrac{1}{4} + \dfrac{5}{4} =$ _____

24. $\dfrac{1}{2} + \dfrac{1}{5} =$ _____

25. $6\dfrac{1}{4} + \dfrac{2}{9} + \dfrac{1}{36} =$ _____

Subtract the following fractions and mixed numbers. Reduce to lowest terms.

26. $\dfrac{4}{9} - \dfrac{3}{9} =$ _____

27. $2\dfrac{1}{4} - 1\dfrac{1}{2} =$ _____

28. $2\dfrac{3}{4} - \dfrac{1}{4} =$ _____

29. $\dfrac{4}{5} - \dfrac{1}{6} =$ _____

30. $\dfrac{6}{4} - \dfrac{1}{2} =$ _____

31. $\dfrac{4}{5} - \dfrac{1}{4} =$ _____

32. $\dfrac{4}{6} - \dfrac{3}{8} =$ _____

33. $4\dfrac{1}{6} - 1\dfrac{1}{3} =$ _____

34. $\dfrac{8}{5} - \dfrac{1}{3} =$ _____

35. $\dfrac{4}{7} - \dfrac{1}{3} =$ _____

Multiply the following fractions and mixed numbers. Reduce to lowest terms.

36. $\dfrac{1}{3} \times \dfrac{4}{12} =$ _____

37. $2\dfrac{7}{8} \times 3\dfrac{1}{4} =$ _____

38. $8 \times 1\dfrac{3}{4} =$ _____

39. $15 \times \dfrac{2}{3} =$ _____

40. $36 \times \dfrac{3}{4} =$ _____

41. $\dfrac{5}{4} \times \dfrac{2}{4} =$ _____

42. $\dfrac{2}{5} \times \dfrac{1}{6} =$ _____

43. $\dfrac{3}{10} \times \dfrac{4}{12} =$ _____

44. $\dfrac{1}{9} \times \dfrac{7}{3} =$ _____

45. $\dfrac{10}{25} \times \dfrac{5}{3} =$ _____

Divide the following fractions and mixed numbers. Reduce to lowest terms.

46. $2\dfrac{1}{3} \div 4\dfrac{1}{6} =$ _____

47. $\dfrac{1}{3} \div \dfrac{1}{2} =$ _____

48. $25 \div 12\dfrac{1}{2} =$ _____

49. $\dfrac{7}{8} \div 2\dfrac{1}{4} =$ _____

50. $\dfrac{6}{2} \div \dfrac{3}{4} =$ _____

51. $\dfrac{4}{6} \div \dfrac{1}{2} =$ _____

52. $\dfrac{3}{10} \div \dfrac{5}{25} = $ _____

54. $\dfrac{15}{30} \div 10 = $ _____

53. $3 \div \dfrac{2}{5} = $ _____

55. $\dfrac{8}{3} \div \dfrac{8}{3} = $ _____

Arrange the following fractions in order from largest to the smallest.

56. $\dfrac{3}{16}, \dfrac{1}{16}, \dfrac{5}{16}, \dfrac{14}{16}, \dfrac{7}{16}$

57. $\dfrac{5}{12}, \dfrac{5}{32}, \dfrac{5}{8}, \dfrac{5}{6}, \dfrac{5}{64}$

58. A client is instructed to drink 20 ounces of water within 1 hour. The client has only been able to drink 12 ounces. What portion of the water remains? (Express your answer as a fraction reduced to lowest terms.) _____

59. A child's oral Motrin Suspension contains 100 mg per teaspoonful. 20 mg represents what part of a dosage? _____

60. A client is receiving 240 mL of Ensure by mouth as a supplement. The client consumes 200 mL. What portion of the Ensure remains? (Express your answer as a fraction reduced to lowest terms.) _____

61. A client takes $1^{1}/_{2}$ tablets of medication four times per day for 4 days. How many tablets will the client have taken at the end of the 4 days? _____

62. A juice glass holds 120 mL. If a client drinks $2^{1}/_{3}$ glasses, how many milliliters did the client consume? _____

63. On admission a client weighed $150^{3}/_{4}$ lb. On discharge the client weighed $148^{1}/_{2}$ lb. How much weight did the client lose? _____

64. How many hours are there in $3^{1}/_{2}$ days? _____

65. A client consumed the following: $2^{1}/_{4}$ ounces of tea, $^{1}/_{3}$ ounce of juice, $1^{1}/_{2}$ ounces of Jello. What is the total number of ounces consumed by the client? _____

Answers on p. 602

 **For additional practice problems, refer to the Mathematics Review section of Drug Calculations Companion, Version 4, on Evolve.**

# CHAPTER 3

# Decimals

## Objectives

*After reviewing this chapter, you should be able to:*
1. Read decimals
2. Write decimals
3. Compare the size of decimals
4. Convert fractions to decimals
5. Convert decimals to fractions
6. Add decimals
7. Subtract decimals
8. Multiply decimals
9. Divide decimals
10. Round decimals to the nearest tenth
11. Round decimals to the nearest hundredth

Medication dosages and other measurements in the health care system use metric measures, which are based on the decimal system. An understanding of decimals is crucial to the calculation of dosages. In the administration of medications, nurses calculate dosages that contain decimals (e.g., levothyroxine 0.075 mg).

Decimal points in dosages have been cited as a major source of medication errors. A misunderstanding of the value of a dosage expressed as a decimal or omission of a decimal point can result in a serious medication error. Decimals should be written with great care to prevent misinterpretation. A clear understanding of the importance of decimal points and their value will assist the nurse in the prevention of medication errors.

**Example 1:** Digoxin 0.125 mg

**Example 2:** Coreg 3.125 mg

A decimal is a fraction that has a denominator that is a multiple of 10. A decimal fraction is written as a decimal by the use of a decimal point (.). The decimal point is used to indicate place value. Some examples are as follows:

| Fraction | Decimal Number |
|---|---|
| $\frac{3}{10}$ | 0.3 |
| $\frac{18}{100}$ | 0.18 |
| $\frac{175}{1000}$ | 0.175 |

The decimal point represents the center. Notice that the numbers written to the right of the decimal point are decimal fractions with a denominator of 10 or a multiple of 10 and represent a value that is less than one (1) or part of one (1). Numbers written to the left of the decimal point are whole numbers, or have a value of one (1) or greater.

The easiest way to understand decimals is to memorize the place values (Box 3-1).

### BOX 3-1    Decimal Place Values

The decimal value is determined by its position to the right of the decimal point.

| Hundred-thousands (100,000) | Ten-thousands (10,000) | Thousands (1000) | Hundreds (100) | Tens (10) | Ones (Units) (1) | Decimal point | Tenths (0.1) | Hundredths (0.01) | Thousandths (0.001) | Ten-thousandths (0.0001) | Hundred-thousandths (0.00001) |
|---|---|---|---|---|---|---|---|---|---|---|---|
| 6 | 5 | 4 | 3 | 2 | 1 | . | 1 | 2 | 3 | 4 | 5 |

**Whole Numbers to the Left**                    **Decimal Numbers to the Right**

The **first** place to the right of the decimal is tenths.
The **second** place to the right of the decimal is hundredths.
The **third** place to the right of the decimal is thousandths.
The **fourth** place to the right of the decimal is ten-thousandths.
In the calculation of medication dosages it is necessary to **consider only three figures after the decimal point (thousandths) (e.g., 0.375 mg).**

**CAUTION**

When there is no whole number before a decimal point, it is important to place a zero (0) to the left of the decimal point to emphasize that the number is a decimal fraction and has a value less than 1. This will emphasize its value and prevent errors in interpretation and avoid errors in dosage calculation. This has been emphasized by the Institute for Safe Medication Practices (ISMP) and is a requirement of The Joint Commission (TJC). The Joint Commission's official "Do Not Use" List (2005) prohibits the writing of a decimal fraction that is less than 1 without a leading zero preceding a decimal point.

**The source of many medication errors is misplacement of a decimal point or incorrect interpretation of a decimal value.**

## READING AND WRITING DECIMALS

Once you understand the place value of decimals, reading and writing them are simple.

**RULE**

To read the decimal numbers, read:
1. The whole number,
2. the decimal point as "and," and
3. the decimal fraction.
Notice that the words for all decimal fractions end in th(s).

**Example 1:**   The number 0.001 is read as "one thousandth."

**Example 2:**   The decimal 4.06 is read as "four and six hundredths."

**Example 3:**   The number 0.4 is read as "four tenths."

> **RULE**
>
> When there is only a zero (0) to the left of the decimal, as in Example 3, the zero is not read aloud.

## Tips for Clinical Practice

An exception to this is in an emergency situation when a nurse must take a verbal order over the phone from a prescriber. When repeating back an order for a medication involving a decimal, the zero should be read aloud to prevent a medication error.

**Example:**   "Zero point 4" would be the verbal interpretation of Example 3. In addition to repeating the order back, the receiver of the order should write down the complete order or enter it into a computer, then read it back, and receive confirmation of the order from the individual giving the order.

> **RULE**
>
> To write a decimal number, write the following:
> 1. The whole number (If there is no whole number, write zero [0].)
> 2. The decimal point to indicate the place value of the rightmost number
> 3. The decimal portion of the number

**Example 1:**   Written, seven and five tenths = 7.5

**Example 2:**   Written, one hundred twenty-five thousandths = 0.125

**Example 3:**   Written, five tenths = 0.5

> **RULE**
>
> When writing decimals, placing a zero after the last digit of a decimal fraction does not change its value.

**Example:**   0.37 mg = 0.370 mg

> **CAUTION**
>
> When writing decimals, unnecessary zeros should not be placed at the end of the number to avoid misinterpretation of a value and the overlooking of a decimal point. This is also a recommendation of the Institute for Safe Medication Practices (ISMP) and is a part of The Joint Commission (TJC) official "Do Not Use" List (2005). TJC forbids the use of trailing zeros for medication orders or other medication-related documentation. Exception: A trailing zero may be used only when required to demonstrate the level of precision of the value being reported, such as for laboratory results, imaging studies that report the size of lesions, or catheter/tube sizes.

Because the last zero does not change the value of the decimal, it is not necessary. The preferred notation, as in the example shown on p. 23, is 0.37 mg, not 0.370 mg, and 30, not 30.0, which could be interpreted as 370 and 300, respectively, if the decimal point is not clear or is missed.

 **Practice Problems**

Write each of the following numbers in word form.

1. 8.35 _____     4. 5.0007 _____

2. 11.001 _____     5. 10.5 _____

3. 4.57 _____     6. 0.163 _____

Write each of the following in decimal form.

7. four tenths _____     10. two and twenty-three hundredths _____

8. eighty-four and seven hundredths _____     11. five hundredths _____

9. seven hundredths _____     12. nine thousandths _____

Answers on p. 602

## COMPARING THE VALUE OF DECIMALS

**RULE**

Zeros added before or after the decimal point of a decimal number change its value.

Example 1:   0.375 mg is not equal to 0.0375 mg

Example 2:   2.025 mg is not equal to 20.025 mg

Example 3:   However, .7 = 0.7 and 12.6250 = 12.625; but you should write 0.7 (with a leading zero) and 12.625 (without a trailing zero).

**CAUTION**

Understanding which decimal is of greater or lesser value is important in the calculation of dosage problems. This helps to prevent errors in dosage and gives the nurse an understanding of the size of a dosage (e.g., 0.5 mg, 0.05 mg). Understanding the value of decimals prevents errors of misinterpretation. There is an appreciable difference between 0.5 mg and 0.05 mg. In fact, 0.5 mg is 10 times larger than 0.05 mg. A misinterpretation of the value of decimals can result in serious consequences in dosage calculations.

**RULE**

When decimal numbers contain whole numbers, the whole numbers are compared to determine which is greater.

Example 1:   4.8 is greater than 2.9

Example 2:   11.5 is greater than 7.5

Example 3:   7.37 is greater than 6.94

**RULE**

If the whole numbers being compared are the **same** (e.g., 5.6 and 5.2) or if there is **no whole number** (e.g., 0.45 and 0.37), then the number in the **tenths** place determines which decimal is greater.

Example 1:   0.45 is greater than 0.37

Example 2:   1.75 is greater than 1.25

**RULE**

If the whole numbers are the same or zero and the numbers in the **tenths place** are the **same,** then the decimal with the higher number in the **hundredths place** has the greater value, and so forth.

Example 1:   0.67 is greater than 0.66

Example 2:   0.17 is greater than 0.14

Example 1:   0.2 is the same as 0.2000, 0.20

Example 2:   4.4 is the same as 4.40, 4.400

 **Practice Problems**

Circle the decimal with the largest value in the following:

| 13. 0.5 | 0.15 | 0.05 | 16. 0.175 | 0.1 | 0.05 |
| 14. 2.66 | 2.36 | 2.87 | 17. 7.02 | 7.15 | 7.35 |
| 15. 0.125 | 0.375 | 0.25 | 18. 0.067 | 0.087 | 0.077 |

Answers on p. 602

## ADDING AND SUBTRACTING DECIMALS

**RULE**

To add or subtract decimals, place the numbers in columns so the decimal points are lined up directly under one another and add or subtract from right to left. Zeros may be added at the end of the decimal fraction, making all decimals of equal length, but unnecessary zeros should be eliminated in the final answer.

**CAUTION**

Eliminate unnecessary zeros in the final answer to avoid confusion and prevent errors of misinterpretation.

**Example 1:**    Add 16.4 + 21.8 + 13.2

$$
\begin{array}{r}
16.4 \\
21.8 \\
+\ 13.2 \\
\hline
51.4 = 51.4
\end{array}
$$

**Example 2:**    Add 2.25 + 1.75

$$
\begin{array}{r}
2.25 \\
+\ 1.75 \\
\hline
4.00 = 4
\end{array}
$$

**Example 3:**    Subtract 2.6 from 18.6

$$
\begin{array}{r}
18.6 \\
-\ 2.6 \\
\hline
16.0 = 16
\end{array}
$$

**Example 4:**    Add 11.2 + 16

$$
\begin{array}{r}
11.2 \\
+\ 16.0 \\
\hline
27.2 = 27.2
\end{array}
$$

**Example 5:**    Subtract 3.78 from 12.84

$$
\begin{array}{r}
12.84 \\
-\ 3.78 \\
\hline
9.06 = 9.06
\end{array}
$$

**Example 6:**    Subtract 0.007 from 0.05

$$
\begin{array}{r}
0.050 \\
-\ 0.007 \\
\hline
0.043 = 0.043
\end{array}
$$

**Example 7:**    Add 6.54 + 2.26

$$
\begin{array}{r}
6.54 \\
+\ 2.26 \\
\hline
8.80 = 8.8
\end{array}
$$

**Example 8:**   Add 0.7 + 0.75 + 0.23 + 2.324

$$
\begin{array}{r}
0.700 \\
0.750 \\
0.230 \\
+\ 2.324 \\
\hline
4.004 = 4.004
\end{array}
$$

**Example 9:**   Subtract 0.2 from 0.375

$$
\begin{array}{r}
0.375 \\
-\ 0.200 \\
\hline
0.175 = 0.175
\end{array}
$$

 **Practice Problems**

Add the following decimals.

19.  4.7 + 5.3 + 8.4 = _____

21.  0.7 + 3.25 = _____

20.  38.52 + 0.029 + 1.90 = _____

22.  2.2 + 1.67 = _____

Subtract the following decimals.

23.  3.67 − 0.75 = _____

25.  0.08 − 0.045 = _____

24.  64.3 − 21.2 = _____

26.  6.75 − 0.87 = _____

Answers on pp. 602-603

## MULTIPLYING DECIMALS

**CAUTION**

When multiplying decimals, be sure the decimal is placed in the correct position in the answer (product). Misplacement of decimal points can lead to a critical medication error.

**RULE**

To multiply decimals, multiply as with whole numbers. In the answer (product), count off from right to left as many decimal places as there are in the numbers being multiplied. Zeros may also be added to the left if necessary.

**Example 1:**                    $1.2 \times 3.2$

$$
\begin{array}{r}
1.2 \\
\times\ 3.2 \\
\hline
24 \\
36 \\
\hline
384.
\end{array}
$$

**Answer:**      3.84

In Example 1, 1.2 has one number after the decimal, and 3.2 also has one. Therefore you will need to place the decimal point two places to the left in the answer (product).

**RULE**

When there are insufficient numbers in the answer for correct placement of the decimal point, add as many zeros as needed to the left of the answer.

**Example 2:**                                $1.35 \times 0.65$

$$\begin{array}{r} 1.35 \\ \times\, 0.65 \\ \hline 675 \\ 810 \\ \hline 8775. \end{array}$$

**Answer:**      0.8775

In Example 2, 1.35 has two numbers after the decimal, and 0.65 also has two. Therefore you will need to place the decimal point four places to the left in the answer (product), and add a zero in front of the decimal point.

**Example 3:**                                $0.11 \times 0.33$

$$\begin{array}{r} 0.11 \\ \times\, 0.33 \\ \hline 33 \\ 33 \\ \hline 0363. \end{array}$$

**Answer:**      0.0363

In Example 3, four decimal places are needed (two numbers after each decimal in 0.11 and 0.33), but there are only three numbers in the product. A zero must be placed to the left of these numbers for correct placement of the decimal point. Place a zero before the decimal point.

**Example 4:**                                $1.6 \times 0.05$

$$\begin{array}{r} 1.6 \\ \times\, 0.05 \\ \hline 080. \end{array}$$

**Answer:**      $0.080 = 0.08$

In Example 4, three decimal places are needed (1.6 has one number after the decimal and 0.05 has two), so a zero has to be placed between the decimal point and 8 to allow for enough places. The unnecessary zero is eliminated in the final answer, and a zero is placed before the decimal point.

## Multiplication by Decimal Movement

**RULE**

This method may be preferred when doing metric conversions because it is based on the decimal system. Multiplying by 10, 100, 1,000, and so forth can be done by moving the decimal point to the right the same number of places as there are zeros in the number by which you are multiplying.

**When multiplying by 10, move the decimal one place to the right; by 100, two places to the right; by 1,000, three places to the right; and so forth.**

**Example 1:**   1.6 × 10 = 16 (decimal moved one place to the right)

**Example 2:**   5.2 × 100 = 520 (decimal moved two places to the right)

**Example 3:**   0.463 × 1,000 = 463 (decimal moved three places to the right)

**Example 4:**   6.64 × 10 = 66.4 (decimal moved one place to the right)

 **Practice Problems**

Multiply the following decimals.

27.  3.15 × 0.015 = _____

28.  3.65 × 0.25 = _____

29.  9.65 × 1,000 = _____

30.  8.9 × 0.2 = _____

31.  14.001 × 7.2 = _____

Answers on p. 603

## DIVIDING DECIMALS

Division of decimals is done in the same manner as division of whole numbers except for placement of the decimal point. Incorrect placement of the decimal point changes the numerical value and can cause errors in calculation. Errors made in the division of decimals are commonly due to improper placement of the decimal point, incorrect placement of numbers in the quotient, and omission of necessary zeros in the quotient.

The parts of a division problem are as follows:

$$\overset{\text{Quotient}}{\text{Divisor}\overline{)\text{Dividend}}}$$

The number being divided is called the **dividend,** the number used to divide by is the **divisor,** and the answer is the **quotient.**

Symbols used to indicate division are as follows:

1. $\overline{)}$

   **Example:**                          9$\overline{)27}$                          Read as 27 divided by 9.

2. ÷

   **Example:**                          27 ÷ 9                          Read as 27 divided by 9.

3. The horizontal bar with the dividend on the top and the divisor on the bottom

   **Example:**                          $\dfrac{27}{9}$                          Read as 27 divided by 9.

4. The slanted bar with the dividend to the left and the divisor to the right

   **Example:**                          $^{27}/_{9}$                          Read as 27 divided by 9.

## Dividing a Decimal by a Whole Number

**RULE**

To divide a decimal by a whole number, place the decimal point in the quotient directly above the decimal point in the dividend. Proceed to divide as with whole numbers.

**Example:**    Divide 17.5 by 5

$$
\begin{array}{r}
3.5 \\
5\overline{)17.5} \\
-15 \phantom{.5} \\
\hline
25 \\
-25 \\
\hline
0
\end{array}
$$

**Answer:**    3.5

## Dividing a Decimal or a Whole Number by a Decimal

**RULE**

To divide by a decimal, the decimal point in the divisor is moved to the right until the number is a whole number. The decimal point in the dividend is moved the same number of places to the right, and zeros are added as necessary. Proceed to divide as with whole numbers.

**Example:**    Divide 6.96 by 0.3

**Step 1:**    $6.96 \div 0.3 = 0.3\overline{)6.9\,6}$

$3\overline{)69.6}$    (after moving decimals in the divisor the same number of places as the dividend)

**Step 2:**

$$
\begin{array}{r}
23.2 \\
3\overline{)69.6} \\
-6 \phantom{9.6} \\
\hline
9 \\
-9 \\
\hline
6 \\
-6 \\
\hline
0
\end{array}
$$

**Answer:**    23.2

## Division by Decimal Movement

**RULE**

To divide a decimal by 10, 100, or 1,000, move the decimal point to the **left** the same number of places as there are zeros in the divisor.

**Example 1:**    $0.46 \div 10 = 0.046$ (The decimal is moved one place to the left.)

**Example 2:**    $0.07 \div 100 = 0.0007$ (The decimal is moved two places to the left.)

**Example 3:**    $0.75 \div 1,000 = 0.00075$ (The decimal is moved three places to the left.)

## ROUNDING OFF DECIMALS

The determination of how many places to carry your division when calculating dosages is based on the equipment being used. Some syringes are marked in **tenths** and some in **hundredths.** As you become familiar with the equipment used in dosage calculation, you will learn how far to carry your division and when to round off. To ensure accuracy, most calculation problems require that you carry your division at least **two decimal places (hundredths place)** and **round off to the nearest tenth.**

**NOTE**

In some instances, such as critical care or pediatrics, it may be necessary to compute decimal calculations to thousandths (three decimal places) and round to hundredths (two decimal places). These areas may require this accuracy.

**RULE**

To express an answer to the nearest tenth, carry the division to the hundredths place (two places after the decimal). If the number in the hundredths place **is 5 or greater, add** one to the tenths place. If the number **is less than 5, drop** the number to the right of the desired decimal place.

Example 1:    Express 4.15 to the nearest tenth.

Answer:        4.2 (The number in the hundredths place is 5, so the number in the tenths place is **increased by one.** 4.1 becomes 4.2.)

Example 2:    Express 1.24 to the nearest tenth.

Answer:        1.2 (The number in the hundredths place is less than 5, so the number in the **tenths place does not change.** The 4 is dropped.)

**RULE**

To express an answer to the nearest hundredth, carry the division to the thousandths place (three places after the decimal). If the number in the thousandths place is 5 or greater, add one to the hundredths place. If the number is less than 5, drop the number to the right of the desired decimal place.

Example 1:    Express 0.176 to the nearest hundredth.

Answer:        0.18 (The number in the thousandths place is 6, so the number in the hundredths place is increased by one. 0.17 becomes 0.18.)

Example 2:    Express 0.554 to the nearest hundredth.

Answer:        0.55 (The number in the thousandths place is less than 5, so the number in the hundredths place does not change.)

**CAUTION**

When rounding for dosage calculations, unnecessary zeros should not be added. Zeros are not necessary to clarify the number.

Example 1:    0.98 (round to tenths) = 1.0 = 1

Example 2:    0.40 (round to hundredths) = 0.4

## Practice Problems

Divide the following decimals. Carry division to the hundredths place where necessary. Do not round off.

32. $2 \div 0.5 =$ _____      35. $39.6 \div 1.3 =$ _____

33. $1.4 \div 1.2 =$ _____      36. $1.9 \div 3.2 =$ _____

34. $63.8 \div 0.9 =$ _____

Express the following decimals to the nearest tenth.

37. 3.57 _____      39. 1.98 _____

38. 0.95 _____

Express the following decimals to the nearest hundredth.

40. 3.550 _____      42. 0.738 _____

41. 0.607 _____

Divide the following decimals.

43. $0.005 \div 10 =$ _____      44. $0.004 \div 100 =$ _____

Multiply the following decimals.

45. $58.4 \times 10 =$ _____      46. $0.5 \times 1,000 =$ _____

Answers on p. 603

## CHANGING FRACTIONS TO DECIMALS

**RULE**

To change a fraction to a decimal, divide the numerator by the denominator and add zeros as needed. If the numerator doesn't divide evenly into the denominator, carry division three places.

**Example 1:**      $\dfrac{2}{5} = 5\overline{)2} = 5\overline{)2.0} \;\; ^{0.4}$

**Example 2:**      $\dfrac{3}{8} = 8\overline{)3} = 8\overline{)3.000} \;\; ^{0.375}$

Changing fractions to decimals can also be a method of comparing fraction size. The fractions being compared are changed to decimals, and the rules relating to comparing decimals are then applied. (See Comparing the Value of Decimals, p. 24.)

**Example:** Which fraction is larger, $\frac{1}{3}$ or $\frac{1}{6}$ ?

**Solution:** $\frac{1}{3} = 0.333\ldots$ as a decimal

$\frac{1}{6} = 0.166\ldots$ as a decimal

**Answer:** $\frac{1}{3}$ is therefore the larger fraction.

## CHANGING DECIMALS TO FRACTIONS

**RULE**

To convert a decimal to a fraction, write the decimal number as a whole number in the numerator of the fraction, and express the denominator of the fraction as a power of 10. Place the number 1 in the denominator of the fraction, and add as many zeros as there are places to the right of the decimal point. Reduce to lowest terms if necessary. (See Reading and Writing Decimals, p. 22.)

**Example 1:** 0.4 is read "four tenths" and written $\frac{4}{10}$, which $= \frac{2}{5}$ when reduced.

**Example 2:** 0.65 is read "sixty-five hundredths" and written $\frac{65}{100}$, which $= \frac{13}{20}$ when reduced.

**Example 3:** 0.007 is read "seven thousandths" and written $\frac{7}{1,000}$.

Notice that the number of places to the right of the decimal point is the same as the number of zeros in the denominator of the fraction.

 **Practice Problems**

Change the following fractions to decimals, and carry the division three places as indicated. Do not round off.

47. $\frac{3}{4}$ _____

49. $\frac{1}{2}$ _____

48. $\frac{5}{9}$ _____

Change the following decimals to fractions, and reduce to lowest terms.

50. 0.75 _____

52. 0.04 _____

51. 0.0005 _____

Answers on p. 603

### ■ Points to Remember

- Read decimals carefully.
- When the decimal fraction is **not** preceded by a whole number (e.g., .12), **always place a "0"** to the left of the decimal (0.12) to avoid interpretation errors and to avoid overlooking the decimal point.
- Never follow a whole number with a decimal point and zero. This could result in a medication error because of misinterpretation (e.g., 3, not 3.0).
- Add zeros to the right as needed for making decimals of equal spacing for addition and subtraction. These zeros do not change the value.
- Adding zeros at the end of a decimal (except when called for to create decimals of equal length for addition or subtraction) can result in error (e.g., 1.5, not 1.50).
- Adding zeros before the decimal point can change the value (e.g., 1.5 is not equal to 1.05 nor is it the same number).
- To convert a fraction to a decimal, divide the numerator by the denominator.
- To convert a decimal to a fraction, write the decimal number as a whole number in the numerator and the denominator as a power of 10. Reduce to lowest terms (e.g., $0.05 = \frac{5}{100} = \frac{1}{20}$).
- Double-check work to avoid errors.

 ## CHAPTER REVIEW

Identify the decimal with the largest value in the following sets.

1. 0.4, 0.44, 0.444 _____    4. 0.1, 0.05, 0.2 _____

2. 0.8, 0.7, 0.12 _____    5. 0.725, 0.357, 0.125 _____

3. 1.32, 1.12, 1.5 _____

Perform the indicated operations. Give exact answers.

6. 3.005 + 4.308 + 2.47 = _____    9. 8.17 − 3.05 = _____

7. 20.3 + 8.57 + 0.03 = _____    10. 3.8 − 1.3 = _____

8. 5.886 − 3.143 = _____

Solve the following. Carry division to the hundredths place where necessary.

11. 5.7 ÷ 0.9 = _____    14. 0.15 × 100 = _____

12. 3.75 ÷ 2.5 = _____    15. 15 × 2.08 = _____

13. 1.125 ÷ 0.75 = _____    16. 472.4 × 0.002 = _____

Express the following decimals to the nearest tenth.

17. 1.75 _____    18. 0.13 _____

Express the following decimals to the nearest hundredth.

19. 1.427 _____    20. 0.147 _____

Change the following fractions to decimals. Carry division three decimal places as necessary.

21. $\dfrac{8}{64}$ _____    23. $6\dfrac{1}{2}$ _____

22. $\dfrac{3}{50}$ _____

Change the following decimals to fractions, and reduce to lowest terms.

24. 1.01 _____    25. 0.065 _____

Add the following decimals.

26. You are to give a client one tablet labeled 0.15 mg and one labeled 0.025 mg. What is the total dosage of these two tablets? _____

27. If you administer two tablets labeled 0.04 mg, what total dosage will you administer? _____

28. You have two tablets, one labeled 0.025 mg and the other 0.1 mg. What is the total dosage of these two tablets? _____

29. You have just administered 3 tablets with dose strength of 1.5 mg each. What was the total dosage? _____

30. If you administer two tablets labeled 0.6 mg, what total dosage will you administer? _____

Multiply the following numbers by moving the decimal.

31. $0.08 \times 10 =$ _____    34. $2.34 \times 10 =$ _____

32. $5.65 \times 100 =$ _____    35. $0.002 \times 100 =$ _____

33. $0.849 \times 1,000 =$ _____

Divide the following numbers, and round to the nearest hundredth.

36. $6.45 \div 10 =$ _____    39. $4 \div 4.1 =$ _____

37. $37.5 \div 100 =$ _____    40. $5 \div 14.3 =$ _____

38. $0.13 \div 0.25 =$ _____

Round the following decimals to the nearest thousandth.

41. 4.2475 _____    44. 7.8393 _____

42. 0.5673 _____    45. 5.8333 _____

43. 2.3249 _____

46. A client's water intake is 1.05 L, 0.65 L, 2.05 L, and 0.8 L. What is the total intake in liters? _____

47. A client's creatinine level on admission was 2.5 mg/dL. By discharge the creatinine level dropped 0.9 mg. What is the client's current creatinine level? _____

48. A baby weighed 4.85 kg at birth and now weighs 7.9 kg. How many kilograms did the baby gain? _____

49. A client is taking $\frac{1}{15}$ of a liquid medication containing 0.375 mg of medication every day. How many milligrams will the client take in 4 days? _____

50. A client's sodium intake at one meal was the following: 0.002 g, 0.35 g. How many grams of sodium did the client consume? _____

51. True or False?  2.4 g = 2.04 g. _____

52. True or False?  5.5 L = 5.500 L. _____

53. 0.7 mg of a medication has been ordered. The recommended maximum dosage of the drug is 0.35 mg and the minimum recommended dosage is 0.175 mg. Is the dosage ordered within the allowable limits? _____

54. Which of the following decimals is largest?  0.125, 0.01, 0.4 _____

55. Which of the following decimals is smallest?  0.855, 0.8, 0.085 _____

Answers on p. 603

 **For additional practice problems, refer to the Mathematics Review section of Drug Calculations Companion, Version 4, on Evolve.**

# CHAPTER 4

# Ratio and Proportion

## Objectives

*After reviewing this chapter, you should be able to:*
1. Define ratio and proportion
2. Define means and extremes
3. Calculate problems for a missing term ($x$) using ratio and proportion

Ratio and proportion is one logical method for calculating medications. It can be used to calculate all types of medication problems. Nurses use ratios to calculate and to check medication dosages. Some medications express the strength of the solution by using a ratio. Example: Epinephrine label may state 1:1,000. Ratios are used in hospitals to determine the client to nurse ratio. Example: If there are 28 clients and 4 nurses on a unit, the ratio of clients to nurses is 28:4 or "28 to 4" or 7:1. As with fractions, ratios should be stated in lowest terms. Like a fraction, which indicates the division of two numbers, a ratio indicates the division of two quantities. The use of ratio and proportion is a logical approach to calculating medication dosages.

## RATIOS

A ratio is used to indicate a relationship between two numbers. These numbers are separated by a colon (:).

**Example:**   3:4

The colon indicates division; therefore a ratio is a fraction.

**RULE**

The numbers or terms of the ratio are the numerator and denominator. The numerator is always to the left of the colon, and the denominator is always to the right of the colon. Like fractions, ratios should be stated in lowest terms.

**Example 1:**   3:4 (3 is the numerator, 4 is the denominator, and the expression can be written as $\frac{3}{4}$)

**Example 2:**   In a nursing class, if there are 25 male students and 75 female students, what is the ratio of male students to female students? 25 male students to 75 female students = 25 male students per 75 female students = $^{25}/_{75} = ^{1}/_{3}$. This is the same as a ratio of 25:75 or 1:3.

### Ratio Measures: in Solutions

Some medications express the strength of the solution by using a ratio. Ratio measures are commonly seen in solutions. Ratios represent parts of medication per parts of solution, for example, 1:10,000 (this means 1 part medication to 10,000 parts solution).

**Example 1:**   A 1:5 solution contains 1 part medication in 5 parts solution.

**Example 2:**   A solution that is 1 part medication in 2 parts solution would be written as 1:2.

Ratio strengths are always expressed in lowest terms.

## Tips for Clinical Practice

The more solution a medication is dissolved in, the less potent the strength becomes. For example, a ratio strength of 1:1,000 (1 part medication to 1,000 parts solution) is more potent than a ratio strength of 1:10,000 (1 part medication in 10,000 parts solution). A misunderstanding of these numbers and what they represent can have serious consequences.

## PROPORTIONS

A proportion is an equation of two ratios of equal value. The terms of the first ratio have a relationship to the terms of the second ratio. A proportion can be written in any of the following formats:

**Example 1:**   3:4 = 6:8 (separated with an equals sign)

**Example 2:**   3:4::6:8 (separated with a double colon)

**Example 3:**   $\dfrac{3}{4} = \dfrac{6}{8}$ (written as a fraction)

*Read as follows:* 3 is to 4 equals 6 is to 8; 3 is to 4 as 6 is to 8; or, as a fraction, three fourths equals six eighths.
  Proving that ratios are equal and that the proportion is true can be done mathematically.

**Example:**                               5:25 = 10:50

*or*

5:25::10:50

The terms in a proportion are called the *means* and *extremes*. Confusion of these terms can result in an incorrect answer. To avoid confusion of terms in proportions, remember **m** for the middle terms (**means**) and **e** for the end terms (**extremes**) of the proportion. Let's refer to our example to identify these terms.
  The extremes are the outer or end numbers (previous example: 5, 50), and the means are the inner or middle numbers (previous example: 25, 10).

**Example:**                               means
                                     ┌─────┐
                              5:25 = 10:50
                              └─extremes ─┘

In a proportion the product of the means equals the product of the extremes.
To find the product of the means and extremes you multiply.

In other words, the answers obtained when you multiply the means and extremes are equal.

**Example:**

$$5:25 = 10:50$$

$$25 \times 10 = 50 \times 5$$

means     extremes

$$250 = 250$$

> **NOTE**
>
> The product of the means, 250, equals the product of the extremes, 250, proving the ratios are equal and the proportion is true.

To verify that the two ratios in a proportion are equal and that the proportion is true, multiply the numerator of each ratio by its opposite denominator. The products should be equal. The numerator of the first fraction and the denominator of the second fraction are the extremes. The numerator of the second fraction and the denominator of the first fraction are the means.

**Example:**

$$5:25 = 10:50$$

$$\frac{5}{25} = \frac{10}{50} \quad \text{(proportion written as a fraction)}$$

$$\frac{5 \text{ (extreme)}}{25 \text{ (mean)}} \times \frac{10 \text{ (mean)}}{50 \text{ (extreme)}}$$

> **NOTE**
>
> When stated as a fraction, the proportion is solved by cross multiplication.
>
> $$5 \times 50 = 25 \times 10$$
>
> $$250 = 250$$

## SOLVING FOR x IN RATIO AND PROPORTION

Because the product of the means always equals the product of the extremes, if three numbers of the two ratios are known, the fourth number can be found. The unknown quantity may be any of the four terms. In a proportion problem, the unknown quantity is represented by $x$. After multiplying the means and extremes, the unknown $x$ is usually placed on the left side of the equation. Begin with the product containing the $x$ that will result in the $x$ being isolated on the **left** and the answer on the **right.**

**Example:**     $12:9 = 8:x$

**Steps:**     $12x = 72$         1. Multiply the extremes and then the means. (This results in $x$ being placed on the left side of the equation.)

$$\frac{12x}{12} = \frac{72}{12}$$

$$x = \frac{72}{12}$$

$$x = 6$$

2. Divide both sides of the equation by the number preceding the $x$, in this instance 12, without changing the relationship. The number used for division should always be the number preceding the unknown ($x$), so that when this step is completed, the unknown ($x$) will stand alone on the left side of the equation.

**Proof:**     Place the answer obtained for $x$ in the equation, and multiply to be certain that the product of the means equals the product of the extremes.

$$12:9 = 8:6$$

$$9 \times 8 = 12 \times 6$$

$$72 = 72$$

Solving for *x* with a proportion in a fraction format can be done by cross multiplication to determine the value of *x*.

**Example:**   $\dfrac{4}{3} = \dfrac{12}{x}$

**Steps:**   $4x = 36$   1. Cross multiply to obtain the product of the means and extremes.

$\dfrac{4x}{4} = \dfrac{36}{4}$   2. Divide both sides by the number preceding *x* (in this example, 4) to obtain the value for *x*.

$x = \dfrac{36}{4}$

$x = 9$

**Proof:**   Place the value obtained for *x* in the equation; the cross products should be equal.

$$\dfrac{4}{3} = \dfrac{12}{9}$$

$$4 \times 9 = 12 \times 3$$

$$36 = 36$$

Solving for *x* in proportions that involve decimals in the equation can be done by the same process.

**Example 1:**   $25:5 = 1.5:x$

**Steps:**   $25x = 5 \times 1.5$   1. Multiply the extremes and then the means. (The *x* will be placed on the left side of the equation.)

$\dfrac{25x}{25} = \dfrac{7.5}{25}$   2. Divide both sides by the number preceding *x* (in this example, 25) to obtain the value for *x*.

$x = \dfrac{7.5}{25}$

$x = 0.3$

**Proof:**   $$25:5 = 1.5:0.3$$

$$25 \times 0.3 = 5 \times 1.5$$

$$7.5 = 7.5$$

**Example 2:**   $\frac{1}{2}:x = \frac{1}{5}:1$

**Steps:**   $\frac{1}{5} \times x = \frac{1}{2} \times 1$   1. Multiply the means and then the extremes. (The *x* will be placed on the left side of the equation.)

$\frac{1}{5}x = \frac{1}{2}$   2. Divide *both* sides by the number preceding *x* (in this example, $\frac{1}{5}$). Division of the two fractions becomes multiplication, and the second fraction is inverted. Multiply numerators and denominators.

$\dfrac{\frac{1}{5}x}{\frac{1}{5}} = \dfrac{\frac{1}{2}}{\frac{1}{5}}$

$x = \frac{1}{2} \div \frac{1}{5}$

$x = \frac{1}{2} \times \frac{5}{1}$

$x = \frac{5}{2} = 2.5$ or $2\frac{1}{2}$   3. Reduce the final fraction to solve for *x*.

**Proof:**

$$\tfrac{1}{2}:2\tfrac{1}{2} = \tfrac{1}{5}:1$$

$$1 \times \tfrac{1}{2} = 2\tfrac{1}{2} \times \tfrac{1}{5} = \tfrac{5}{2} \times \tfrac{1}{5}$$

$$\tfrac{1}{2} = \tfrac{5}{10} = \tfrac{1}{2}$$

$$\tfrac{1}{2} = \tfrac{1}{2}$$

**RULE**

*Note:* If the answer is expressed in fraction format for *x,* it must be reduced to **lowest terms.** Division should be carried **two decimal places** when an answer does not work out evenly and may have to be **rounded to the nearest tenth** to prove the answer correct.

## APPLYING RATIO AND PROPORTION TO DOSAGE CALCULATION

Now that we have reviewed the basic definitions and concepts relating to ratio and proportion, let's look at how this might be applied in dosage calculation.

In dosage calculation, ratio and proportion may be used to represent **the weight of a medication that is in tablet or capsule form.**

**Example 1:** 1 tab:0.125 mg *or* $\dfrac{1 \text{ tab}}{0.125 \text{ mg}}$

This may also be expressed by stating the weight of the medication first:

0.125 mg:1 tab *or* $\dfrac{0.125 \text{ mg}}{1 \text{ tab}}$

This means that 1 tablet contains 0.125 mg or is equal to 0.125 mg of medication.

**Example 2:** If a capsule contains a dosage of 500 mg, this could be represented by a ratio as follows:

1 cap:500 mg *or* $\dfrac{1 \text{ cap}}{500 \text{ mg}}$

This may also be expressed stating the weight of the medication first:

500 mg:1 cap *or* $\dfrac{500 \text{ mg}}{1 \text{ cap}}$

Another use of ratio and proportion in dosage calculation is to express liquid medications used for oral administration and for injection. When stating a dosage of a liquid medication, a ratio expresses the **weight (strength) of a medication in a certain volume of solution.**

**Example 1:** A solution that contains 250 mg of medication in each **1 mL** could be written as:

**250 mg**:1 mL *or* $\dfrac{250 \text{ mg}}{\textbf{1 mL}}$

**1 mL** contains 250 mg of medication

**Example 2:** A solution that contains 80 mg of medication in each **2 mL** would be written as:

80 mg:**2 mL** *or* $\dfrac{80 \text{ mg}}{\textbf{2 mL}}$

**2 mL** contains 80 mg of medication

Proving mathematically that ratios are equal and the proportion is true is important with medications. This can be illustrated by using the previous medication strength examples.

Example 1:                          1 cap : 500 mg = 2 cap : 1,000 mg

If 1 cap contains 500 mg, 2 cap will contain 1,000 mg

extremes

1 cap : 500 mg = 2 cap : 1,000 mg

means

$$500 \times 2 = 1,000 \times 1$$
$$1,000 = 1,000$$

Example 2:                          2 mL : 80 mg = 1 mL : 40 mg
$$80 \times 1 = 2 \times 40$$
$$80 = 80$$

## ■ Points to Remember

- Proportions represent two ratios that are equal and have a relationship to each other.
- When three values are known, the fourth can be easily calculated.
- When solving for the unknown ($x$), regardless of which term of the equation is the unknown, the unknown value ($x$) is usually placed on the left side. Begin with the product containing $x$ so $x$ can be isolated on the left side and the answer on the right side.
- Proportions can be stated using an equal (=) sign, a double colon ( :: ), or a fraction format.
- Ratio can be used to state the amount of medication contained in a volume of solution, tablet, or capsule.
- Proportions are solved by multiplying the means and extremes.
- Ratios are always stated in their lowest terms.
- Double-check work.

 ## Practice Problems

Express the following solution strengths as ratios.
 1.  1 part medication to 100 parts solution _____

 2.  1 part medication to 3 parts solution _____

Identify the strongest solution in each of the following:
 3.  1 : 2, 1 : 20, 1 : 200 _____

 4.  1 : 1,000, 1 : 5,000, 1 : 10,000 _____

 5.  Assume that the ratio of clients to nurses is 15 to 2. Express the ratio in fraction and colon form. _____

Express the following dosages as ratios. Include the unit of weight and the numerical value.

6. An injectable liquid that contains 100 mg in each 0.5 mL _____

7. A tablet that contains 0.25 mg of medication _____

8. An oral liquid that contains 1 g in each 10 mL _____

9. A capsule that contains 500 mg of medication _____

Determine the value for *x* in the following problems. Express your answer to the nearest tenth as indicated.

10. $12.5:5 = 24:x$ _____

11. $1.5:1 = 4.5:x$ _____

12. $750/3 = 600/x$ _____

13. $1/300:3 = 1/120:x$ _____

14. $x:12 = 9:6$ _____

Answers on p. 603

---

 **CHAPTER REVIEW**

Express the following fractions as ratios. Reduce to lowest terms.

1. $\dfrac{2}{3}$ _____

2. $\dfrac{1}{9}$ _____

3. $\dfrac{6}{8}$ _____

4. $\dfrac{1}{5}$ _____

5. $\dfrac{5}{10}$ _____

6. $\dfrac{2}{10}$ _____

Express the following ratios as fractions. Reduce to lowest terms.

7. $3:7$ _____

8. $4:6$ _____

9. $1:7$ _____

10. $8:6$ _____

11. $3:4$ _____

Solve for *x* in the following proportions. Carry division two decimal places as necessary.

12. $20:40 = x:10$ _____

13. $\dfrac{1}{4}:\dfrac{1}{2} = 1:x$ _____

14. $0.12:0.8 = 0.6:x$ _____

15. $\dfrac{1}{250}:2 = \dfrac{1}{150}:x$ _____

16. $x:9 = 5:10$ _____

17. $\dfrac{1}{4}:1.6 = \dfrac{1}{8}:x$ _____

18. $\frac{1}{2}:2 = \frac{1}{3}:x$ _____

22. $15:20 = x:30$ _____

19. $125:0.4 = 50:x$ _____

23. $\frac{2.2}{x} = \frac{8.8}{5}$ _____

20. $x:1 = 0.5:5$ _____

24. $\frac{1}{x} = \frac{10}{6}$ _____

21. $\frac{1}{4}:16 = \frac{1}{8}:x$ _____

25. $0.5:0.15 = 0.3:x$ _____

Express the following dosages as ratios. Be sure to include the units of measure and numerical value.

26. An injectable solution that contains 1,000 units in each mL _____

27. A tablet that contains 0.2 mg of medication _____

28. A capsule that contains 250 mg of medication _____

29. An oral solution that contains 125 mg in each 5 mL _____

30. An injectable solution that contains 40 mg in each mL _____

31. An injectable solution that contains 1,000 mcg in each 2 mL _____

32. An injectable solution that contains 1 g in each 3.6 mL _____

33. A tablet that contains 0.4 mg of medication _____

34. A capsule that contains 1 g of medication _____

35. An oral liquid that contains 0.5 mg in each milliliter _____

Express the following strengths as ratios.

36. 1 part medication to 2,000 parts solution _____

37. 1 part medication to 400 parts solution _____

38. 1 part medication to 50 parts solution _____

Identify the weakest solution in each of the following:

39. 1:50, 1:500, 1:5,000 _____

40. 1:3, 1:6, 1:60 _____

Answers on p. 604

 **For additional practice problems, refer to the Mathematics Review section of Drug Calculations Companion, Version 4, on Evolve.**

# Percentages

*After reviewing this chapter, you should be able to:*
1. Define percent
2. Convert percents to fractions
3. Convert percents to decimals
4. Convert percents to ratios
5. Convert decimals to percents
6. Convert fractions to percents
7. Convert fractions to ratios
8. Determine the percent of numbers

*Percentage* is a commonly used word. Sales tax is a *percentage* of the sale price; a final examination is a certain *percentage* of the final grade; interest on a home mortgage represents a *percentage* of the balance owed; interest on a savings account is expressed as a *percentage*. **Health care professionals see percentages written with medications** (e.g., magnesium sulfate 50%). In addition to its use with medications, *percentage* is also used in the assessment of burns. The size of a burn (percentage of injured skin) is determined by using the rule of nines in an adult (Figure 5-1). The basis of the rule is that the body is divided into anatomical sections, each of which represents 9% or a multiple of 9% of the total body surface area. The total body surface area (BSA) is represented by 100%. Another method used is the age-specific burn diagram or chart. Burn size is expressed as a percentage of the total BSA. In children, age-related charts are used because their body proportions differ from those of an adult and the rule of nines cannot be applied.

Many health care providers use solutions that are expressed in percentages for external as well as internal use (e.g., hydrocortisone cream, lidocaine, and intravenous [IV] solutions).

In current practice, percentage solutions are prepared by the pharmacy, and people can purchase solutions or components of the solutions over the counter. Some institutions require nurses to prepare solutions in house (in the hospital) as well as in home care for clients being cared for at home. Understanding percentages provides the foundation for preparing and calculating dosages for medications that are ordered in percentages.

The term *percent* (%) means parts per hundred. A percentage is the same as a fraction in which the denominator is 100, and the numerator indicates the part of 100 that is being considered.

**Example:** $$4\% = \frac{4}{100} \quad \text{(4 per 100)}$$

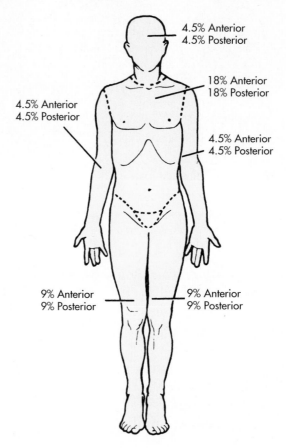

4.5% Anterior
4.5% Posterior

18% Anterior
18% Posterior

4.5% Anterior
4.5% Posterior

4.5% Anterior
4.5% Posterior

9% Anterior
9% Posterior

9% Anterior
9% Posterior

**Figure 5-1**   The rule of nines for estimating burn percentage. (From Ignatavicius D, Winkelman C, Workman M, Hausman K: *Medical-surgical nursing: critical thinking for collaborative care,* ed. 6, St. Louis, 2009, Saunders.)

## PERCENTAGE MEASURES

**IV solutions are ordered in percentage strengths, and nurses need to be familiar with their meaning** (e.g., 1,000 mL 5% dextrose and water). **Percentage solution means the number of grams of solute per 100 mL of diluent.**

**Example 1:**   1,000 mL IV of 5% dextrose and water contains 50 g (grams) of dextrose

$$\% = \text{g per 100 mL; therefore } 5\% = 5 \text{ g per 100 mL}$$

$$5 \text{ g}:100 \text{ mL} = x \text{ g}:1{,}000 \text{ mL}$$

$$x = 50 \text{ g dextrose}$$

**Example 2:**   250 mL IV of 10% dextrose contains 25 g (grams) of dextrose

$$\% = \text{g per 100 mL; therefore } 10\% = 10 \text{ g per 100 mL}$$

$$10 \text{ g}:100 \text{ mL} = x \text{ g}:250 \text{ mL}$$

$$x = 25 \text{ g dextrose}$$

In addition to encountering percentage strengths with IV solutions, the nurse may see percentages used with a variety of other medications, including eye and topical (for external use) ointments and creams. For example, Kenalog cream is available in 0.02%, 0.025%, 0.1%, 0.5%; and pilocarpine hydrochloride ophthalmic solution is available in 0.25%, 0.5%, 1%, 2%, up to 10%.

**CAUTION**

The higher the percentage strength, the stronger the solution or ointment. A misunderstanding of these numbers (%) can have serious consequences.

**Example:** 10% IV solution is more potent than 5%. A solution of 5% is more potent than 0.9%. **Always check the percentage of IV solution prescribed.**

 **Practice Problems**

Determine the number of grams of medication and dextrose as indicated in the following solutions.

1. How many grams of medication will 500 mL of a 10% solution contain?

   _____

2. How many grams of dextrose will 1,000 mL of a 10% solution contain?

   _____

3. How many grams of dextrose will 250 mL of a 5% solution contain?

   _____

4. How many grams of medication will 100 mL of a 50% solution contain?

   _____

5. How many grams of dextrose will 150 mL of a 5% solution contain?

   _____

Identify the strongest solution or ointment in each of the following:

6. Ophthalmic solution 0.1%, 0.5%, 1%    _____

7. Ointment 0.025%, 0.3%, 0.5%    _____

8. Cream 0.02%, 0.025%, 0.25%    _____

Answers on p. 604

## CHANGING PERCENTAGES TO FRACTIONS, DECIMALS, AND RATIOS

The percent sign may be used with a whole number (15%), a fraction (1/2%), a mixed number (14½%), or a decimal (0.6%).

**RULE**

To change a percent to a fraction, drop the percent sign, place the number over 100, and reduce to lowest terms.

**Example 1:**          $8\% = \dfrac{8}{100}$, reduced is $\dfrac{2}{25}$

**Example 2:**          $\dfrac{1}{4}\% = \dfrac{1}{4} \div 100 = \dfrac{1}{4} \times \dfrac{1}{100} = \dfrac{1}{400}$

 **Practice Problems**

Change the following percentages to fractions, and reduce to lowest terms.

9. 1% _____          12. 80% _____

10. 2% _____          13. 3% _____

11. 50% _____

Answers on p. 604

---

**RULE**   To change a percentage to a decimal, drop the percent sign, and move the decimal point two places to the left (add zeros as needed).

---

**Example 1:**                    $25\% = 0.25$

**Example 2:**                    $1.4\% = 0.014$

**NOTE**

Example 3 is an alternative method. Drop the percent sign. Write the remaining number as the numerator. Write "100" as the denominator. Reduce the result to lowest terms. Divide the numerator by the denominator to obtain a decimal.

**Example 3:**   $75\% = \dfrac{75}{100} = \dfrac{3}{4}$   (lowest terms). Divide the numerator of the fraction (3) by the denominator (4).

$$\begin{array}{r} 0.75 \\ 4\overline{)3.00} \end{array}$$

 **Practice Problems**

Change the following percentages to decimals. Round to two decimal places, as indicated.

14. 10% _____          17. 14.2% _____

15. 35% _____          18. $\dfrac{6}{7}\%$ _____

16. 50% _____

Answers on p. 604

---

**RULE**   To change a percentage to a ratio, change it to a fraction, and reduce to lowest terms; then place the numerator as the first term of the ratio and the denominator as the second term. Separate the two terms with a colon (:).

---

**Example:**                    $10\% = \dfrac{10}{100} = \dfrac{1}{10} = 1:10$

**Practice Problems**

Change each of the following percentages to a ratio. Express in lowest terms.

19. 25% _____

20. 11% _____

21. 75% _____

22. 4.5% _____

23. $\frac{2}{5}$% _____

Answers on p. 604

*(handwritten:)*

$$\frac{42}{24} \times \frac{100}{1} = \frac{4200}{24}$$

$$\frac{42}{24}\left(\frac{7}{4} \times \frac{100}{} = \frac{700}{4}\right.$$

## CHANGING FRACTIONS, DECIMALS, AND RATIOS TO PERCENTAGES

**RULE**

To change a fraction to a percentage, multiply the fraction by 100, reduce if necessary, and add the percent sign. This can also be done by changing the fraction to a decimal, multiplying by 100, and adding the percent sign. Multiplying by 100 is the same as moving the decimal point two places to the right.

**Example 1:**   $\frac{3}{4}$ changed to a percent is      *or*      $\frac{3}{4}$ changed to a decimal is

$$\frac{3}{4} \times \frac{100}{1} = \frac{300}{4} = \frac{75}{1} = 75$$

$$4\overline{)3.00} = 0.75$$

$$0.75 \times \frac{100}{1} = 75$$

Add symbol for percent: 75%         Add symbol for percent: 75%

**Example 2:**                $5\frac{1}{2}$ changed to a percent is

Change to an improper fraction: $\frac{11}{2}$      *or*   Change to an improper fraction: $\frac{11}{2}$

$$2\overline{)11.0} = 5.5$$

$$\frac{11}{2} \times \frac{100}{1} = \frac{1,100}{2} = \frac{550}{1} = 550$$

$$5.5 \times \frac{100}{1} = 550$$

Add symbol for percent: 550%         Add symbol for percent: 550%

 **Practice Problems**

Change the following fractions to percentages.

24. $\frac{2}{5}$ _____

25. $\frac{11}{4}$ _____

26. $\frac{1}{2}$ _____

27. $\frac{1}{4}$ _____

28. $\frac{7}{10}$ _____

Answers on p. 604

**RULE**

To change a decimal to a percentage, move the decimal point two places to the right (by multiplying by 100), add zeros if necessary, and add the percent sign.

**Example 1:**   Change 0.45 to %

Move the decimal point two places to the right

Add the symbol for percent: 45%

**Example 2:**   Change 2.35 to %

Move the decimal point two places to the right

Add the symbol for percent: 235%

**RULE**

A decimal may also be changed to a percentage by changing the decimal to a fraction and following the steps to change a fraction to a percentage. If the percentage does not end in a whole number, express the percentage with the remainder as a fraction, to the nearest whole percent, or to the nearest tenth of a percent.

**Example:**     $0.625 = \dfrac{625}{1000} = \dfrac{5}{8} = 62\dfrac{1}{2}\%, 63\%, \text{ or } 62.5\%$

$\dfrac{625}{1000} = \dfrac{5}{8}; \dfrac{5}{8} \times \dfrac{100}{1} = \dfrac{500}{8} = 62.5\%$

**RULE**

To change a ratio to a percentage, change the ratio to a fraction, and proceed with steps for changing a fraction to a percentage. This can also be done by changing the ratio to a fraction, converting the fraction to a decimal, and then converting the decimal to a percentage.

**Example:**    $1:4 = \dfrac{1}{4}, \dfrac{1}{4} \times \dfrac{100}{1} = 25$   *or*        $1:4 = \dfrac{1}{4}$

$4\overline{)1.00}\;^{0.25}$

$0.25 \times \dfrac{100}{1} = 25$

Add symbol for percent: 25%     Add symbol for percent: 25%

 **Practice Problems**

Change the following ratios to percentages.

29.  1:25 _____

30.  3:4 _____

31.  1:10 _____

32.  1:100 _____

33.  1:2 _____

Answers on p. 604

## DETERMINING THE PERCENTAGE OF A QUANTITY

Nurses may find it necessary to determine a given percentage or part of a quantity.

> **RULE**
>
> When determining a given percentage of a number, first change the percentage to a decimal or fraction, and then multiply the decimal or fraction by the number.

Example 1:   A client reports that he drank 25% of his 8-ounce cup of tea. Determine what amount 25% of 8 ounces is.

Solution:   Change the percentage to a decimal:

$$25\% = \frac{25}{100} = .25 = 0.25$$

Multiply the decimal by the number:

$$0.25 \times 8 \text{ ounces} = 2 \text{ ounces}$$

Therefore 25% of 8 ounces = 2 ounces

Example 2:                40% of 90

Solution:          $$40\% = \frac{40}{100} = .40 = 0.4$$

$$0.4 \times 90 = 36$$

Therefore 40% of 90 = 36

## DETERMINING WHAT PERCENTAGE ONE NUMBER IS OF ANOTHER

> **RULE**
>
> To determine what percentage one number is of another, it is necessary to make a fraction with the numbers. The denominator of the fraction is the number following the word "of" in the problem, and the other number is the numerator of the fraction. Convert the fraction to a decimal, and then convert to a percentage.

Example 1:   12 is what percentage of 60? *or* What percentage of 60 is 12?

Solution:   Make a fraction using the two numbers:

$$\frac{12}{60}$$

Convert the fraction to a decimal:

$$60\overline{)12.0}^{\,0.2}$$

Convert the decimal to a percentage:

$$0.2 = 20\%$$

Therefore 12 = 20% of 60 or 20% of 60 = 12

**Example 2:**    1.2 is what percentage of 4.8? *or* What percentage of 4.8 is 1.2?

**Solution:**    Make a fraction using the two numbers:

$$\frac{1.2}{4.8}$$

Convert the fraction to a decimal:

$$4.8\overline{)1.2\underset{\smile}{0}\underset{\smile}{0}}\;{}^{0.25}$$

Convert the decimal to a percentage:

$$0.25 = 25\%$$

Therefore 1.2 = 25% of 4.8 *or* 25% of 4.8 = 1.2

**Example 3:**    $3\frac{1}{2}$ is what percentage of 8.5? *or* What percentage of 8.5 is $3\frac{1}{2}$?

**Solution:**    Make a fraction using the two numbers:

$$\frac{3\frac{1}{2}}{8.5} = \frac{3.5}{8.5}$$

Convert the fraction to a decimal:

$$
\begin{array}{r}
0.411 \\
8.5\overline{)3.5000} \\
-\,340 \\
\hline
100 \\
-\,85 \\
\hline
150
\end{array}
$$

Convert the decimal to a percentage:

$$0.411 = 41.1\%$$

Therefore $3\frac{1}{2}$ = 41.1% of 8.5 or 41.1% of 8.5 = $3\frac{1}{2}$

 **Practice Problems**

Perform the indicated operations. Round decimals to the hundredths place.

34. 60% of 30 _____    40. 0.7% of 60 _____

35. 20% of 75 _____    41. 75% of 165 _____

36. 2 is what percentage of 200? _____    42. 25 is what percentage of 40? _____

37. 50 is what percentage of 500? _____    43. 1.3 is what percentage of 5.2? _____

38. 40 is what percentage of 1,000? _____    44. $\frac{1}{4}$% of 68 _____

39. 3% of 842 _____    45. What percentage of 8.4 is $3\frac{1}{2}$? _____

Answers on p. 604

# ✓ CHAPTER REVIEW

Complete the table below. Express each of the following measures in their equivalents where indicated. Reduce fractions and ratios to lowest terms; round decimals to hundreths.

| | Percent | Ratio | Fraction | Decimal |
|---|---|---|---|---|
| 1. | 52% | _____ | _____ | _____ |
| 2. | 71% | _____ | _____ | _____ |
| 3. | _____ | _____ | $\frac{7}{100}$ | _____ |
| 4. | _____ | 1:50 | _____ | _____ |
| 5. | _____ | _____ | _____ | 0.06 |
| 6. | _____ | _____ | $\frac{3}{8}$ | _____ |
| 7. | _____ | _____ | $\frac{61}{100}$ | _____ |
| 8. | _____ | 7:1,000 | _____ | _____ |
| 9. | 5% | _____ | _____ | _____ |
| 10. | 2.5% | _____ | _____ | _____ |

Perform the indicated operations.

11. A client reports that he drank 40% of his 12 ounce can of ginger ale. How many ounces did the client drink? _____

12. 40% of 140 _____

13. 100 is what percentage of 750? _____

14. $\frac{1}{2}$ is what percentage of 60? _____

15. 15% of 250 _____

16. What percentage of 6.4 is 1.6? _____

17. Which of the following solutions is strongest: 0.0125%, 0.25%, 0.1%? _____

Change each of the following percentages to a ratio, and reduce to lowest terms.

18. 16% _____

19. 45% _____

20. A client is on a 1,000 mL fluid restriction per 24 hours. At breakfast and lunch the client consumed 40% of the fluid allowance. How many milliliters did the client consume? _____

21. A client drank 75% of a 12 ounce can of ginger ale. How many ounces did the client drink? _____

22. A client consumes 55% of a bowl of chicken broth at lunch. The bowl holds 180 mL. How many milliliters did the client consume? _____

23. In a class of 30 students, 6 students did not pass an exam. What percentage of the students did not pass the exam? _____

24. At the first prenatal visit a client weighed 140 pounds. At the second visit the client had a 5% weight increase. How many pounds did the client gain?_____

25. An infant consumed 55% of an 8 ounce bottle of formula. How many ounces of formula did the infant consume? _____

26. In a portion of turkey that is 100 g (grams), there are 23 g of protein and 4 g of fat. What percentage of the portion is protein? _____
What percentage is fat? _____

27. A nursing review test has 130 questions, and you answer 120 correctly. What is your score, as a percentage?_____

28. A client's intake for the day was 2,000 calories, and 600 of the calories came from fat. What percentage of the client's intake came from fat? _____

29. A client began receiving 325 mg (milligrams) of a medication. The prescriber increased the dosage of medication by 10%. What will the new dosage be?
_____ mg

30. The recommended daily allowance (RDA) of a vitamin is 14 mg (milligrams). If a multivitamin provides 55% of the RDA, how many milligrams of the vitamin would the client receive from the multivitamin? _____

Answers on p. 605

 **For additional practice problems, refer to the Mathematics Review section of Drug Calculations Companion, Version 4, on Evolve.**

# Post-Test

After completing Unit One of this text, you should be able to complete this test. The test consists of a total of 60 questions. If you miss any questions in any section, review the chapter relating to that content.

Express the following in Roman numerals.

1. 5 _____     4. 29 _____

2. 17 _____     5. 30 _____

3. 27 _____

Express the following in Arabic numbers.

6. $\overline{\text{viss}}$ _____     9. $\overline{\text{xxv}}$ _____

7. $\overline{\text{xxiv}}$ _____     10. $\overline{\text{xv}}$ _____

8. $\overline{\text{xix}}$ _____

Reduce the following fractions to lowest terms.

11. $\dfrac{8}{6}$ _____     14. $\dfrac{10}{15}$ _____

12. $\dfrac{22}{33}$ _____     15. $\dfrac{16}{10}$ _____

13. $\dfrac{27}{63}$ _____

Perform the indicated operations with fractions; reduce to lowest terms where needed.

16. $\dfrac{5}{6} \div \dfrac{7}{10} =$ _____     19. $5\dfrac{1}{5} - 3\dfrac{4}{7} =$ _____

17. $5\dfrac{1}{2} \div 4\dfrac{1}{2} =$ _____     20. $\dfrac{5}{4} + \dfrac{2}{9} =$ _____

18. $6\dfrac{1}{3} \times 4 =$ _____

Change the following fractions to decimals; express each answer to the nearest tenth.

21. $\dfrac{8}{7}$ _____     23. $\dfrac{1}{15}$ _____

22. $\dfrac{1}{8}$ _____     24. $\dfrac{12}{13}$ _____

Indicate the largest fraction in each group.

25. $\dfrac{1}{2}, \dfrac{2}{3}, \dfrac{5}{9}$ _____     26. $\dfrac{3}{4}, \dfrac{7}{10}, \dfrac{5}{8}$ _____

Perform the indicated operations with decimals. Provide exact answers.

27. $16.7 + 21 =$ _____          29. $10.57 \times 10 =$ _____

28. $0.007 + 17.4 =$ _____          30. $36.8 - 3.86 =$ _____

Divide the following decimals; express each answer to the nearest tenth.

31. $67.8 \div 0.8 =$ _____          33. $5.01 \div 10 =$ _____

32. $9 \div 0.4 =$ _____

Indicate the largest decimal in each group.

34. $0.85, 0.085$ _____          36. $0.478, 0.445, 0.493$ _____

35. $3.002, 0.39, 0.399$ _____

Solve for $x$, the unknown value.

37. $10:20 = x:8$ _____          39. $0.3:x = 1.8:0.6$ _____

38. $500:x = 200:1$ _____          40. $\dfrac{1}{4}:x = \dfrac{1}{8}:2$ _____

Round off to the nearest tenth.

41. $0.57$ _____          43. $1.42$ _____

42. $0.99$ _____

Round off to the nearest hundredth.

44. $0.677$ _____          46. $1.222$ _____

45. $0.832$ _____

Complete the table below. Express each of the measures in their equivalents where indicated. Reduce fractions and ratios to lowest terms; round decimals to hundredths.

| | Percent | Decimal | Ratio | Fraction |
|---|---|---|---|---|
| 47. | _____ | _____ | $1:10$ | _____ |
| 48. | 60% | _____ | _____ | _____ |
| 49. | $66\dfrac{2}{3}\%$ | _____ | _____ | _____ |
| 50. | 25% | _____ | _____ | _____ |

Find the percentage.

51. 9% of 200 _____

52. 2.5% of 750 _____

53. 30 is what percent of 45? _____

54. 5 is what percent of 2,000? _____

55. 25 is what percent of 65? _____

Express the following solution strengths as ratios.

56. 1 part medication to 80 parts solution _____

58. 1 part medication to 300 parts solution _____

57. 1 part medication to 20 parts solution _____

Identify the strongest solution in each of the following:

59. 1:80, 1:800, 1:8,000 _____

60. 1:1,000, 1:2,000, 1:5,000 _____

Answers on p. 605

# UNIT Two

# Systems of Measurement

Three systems of measurement are used to compute medication dosages: metric, apothecary, and household. To be competent in the administration of medications, it is essential that the nurse be familiar with all three systems.

# CHAPTER 6

# Metric System

## Objectives

*After reviewing this chapter, you should be able to:*
1. Express metric measures correctly using rules of the metric system
2. State common equivalents in the metric system
3. Convert measures within the metric system

The metric system is an international decimal system of weights and measures that was introduced in France in the late seventeenth and eighteenth centuries. The system is also referred to as the International System of Units, abbreviated as SI units. SI is the abbreviation taken from the French Système International d'Unités. The metric system is more precise than the apothecary and household systems; therefore it has become the system of choice for the calculation of dosages. The apothecary system is being phased out and gradually being replaced by the metric system. The benefit of the metric system lies in its simplicity and accuracy because it is based on the decimal system, unlike the apothecary system, which is based on fractions and could result in multiple errors. More and more in everyday situations, we are encountering the use of metric measures. For example, soft drinks come in bottles labeled in liters; engine sizes are also expressed in liters.

The metric system has become the system of choice for medications and measurements used in the health care setting. For example, newborn weights are recorded in grams and kilograms, and adult weights are expressed in kilograms, as opposed to pounds and ounces. In obstetrics we express fundal height (upper portion of the uterus) in centimeters. Although a few medications are still prescribed in apothecary and household terms, the nurse will find that the majority of medication calculation and administration skills involve familiarity and accuracy with the metric system to administer medications safely.

## PARTICULARS OF THE METRIC SYSTEM

1. The metric system is based on the decimal system, in which divisions and multiples of 10 are used. Therefore a lot of math can be done by decimal point movement.
2. Three basic units of measure are used:
   a) **Gram**—the basic unit for weight (solid)
   b) **Liter**—the basic unit for volume (liquid)
   c) **Meter**—the basic unit for length

Dosages are calculated by using metric measurements that relate to weight and volume. Meter, which is used for linear (length) measurement, is not used in the calculation of dosages. Linear measurements (meter, centimeter) are commonly used to measure the height of an individual and to determine growth patterns, for serial abdominal girth (the circumference of the abdomen, usually measured at the umbilicus), and for pressure ulcer measurement.

3. Common prefixes in this system denote the numerical value of the unit being discussed. Memorization of these prefixes is necessary for quick and accurate calculations. The prefixes in bold in Table 6-1 are the ones used most often in health care for dosage calculations. However, some of the prefixes may be used to express other values, such as laboratory values. *Kilo* is a common prefix used to identify a measure larger than the basic unit. The other common prefixes used in medication administration are smaller units: *centi, milli,* and *micro.*

Let's look at the following example to see how the prefixes may be used.

**Example:**    67 milligrams

Prefix—*milli*—means measure in thousandths of a unit.
*Gram* is a unit of weight.
Therefore 67 milligrams = 67 thousandths of a gram.

4. Regardless of the size of the unit, the name of the basic unit is incorporated into the measure. This allows easy recognition of the unit of measure.

**Example 1:**    milli**liter**—the word *liter* indicates you are measuring volume (*milli* indicates 1/1,000 of that volume).

**Example 2:**    kilo**gram**—the word *gram* indicates you are measuring weight (*kilo* indicates 1,000 of that weight; 1 kilogram = 1,000 grams).

**Example 3:**    kilo**liter**—the word *liter* indicates you are measuring volume (*kilo* indicates 1,000 of that volume; 1 kiloliter = 1,000 liters).

**Example 4:**    deci**liter**—the word *liter* indicates that you are measuring volume (*deci* indicates 0.1 of that volume [liter], or 100 milliliters). The note, "Female's normal hemoglobin is 12 to 16 g/dL," for example, means there is 12 to 16 grams of hemoglobin contained in 100 milliliters of blood.

**Example 5:**    cubic milli**meter** ($mm^3$)—cubic millimeter is a unit of volume of three-dimensional space (length × width × height). In a normal individual the white blood cell count ranges between 5,000 and 10,000 cells per cubic millimeter of blood. Therefore 1 $mm^3$ of blood contains between 5,000 and 10,000 white blood cells ($5,000/mm^3$ and $10,000/mm^3$).

**CAUTION**

> Do not confuse units of measure in the metric system for weight, volume, and length that have similar names. Milligram is a unit of weight; milliliter is a unit of volume; and millimeter is a unit of length.

**TABLE 6-1**   Common Prefixes Used in Health Care

| Prefix | Numerical Value | Meaning |
|---|---|---|
| **Kilo*** | 1,000 | one thousand times |
| Hecto | 100 | one hundred times |
| Deka | 10 | ten times |
| Deci | 0.1 | one tenth |
| **Centi*** | 0.01 | one hundredth part of |
| **Milli*** | 0.001 | one thousandth part of |
| **Micro*** | 0.000001 | one millionth part of |

*Prefixes used most often in medication administration.

5. The abbreviation for a unit of measure in the metric system is often the first letter of the word. Lowercase letters are used more often than capital letters.

**Example 1:**   g = gram

**Example 2:**   m = meter

The exception to this rule is liter, for which a capital letter is used.

**Example 3:**   liter = L

6. When prefixes are used in combination with the basic unit, the first letter of the prefix and the first letter of the unit of measure are written together in lowercase letters.

**Example 1:**   Milligram—abbreviated as **mg.** The *m* is taken from the prefix *milli* and the *g* from *gram,* the unit of weight.

**Example 2:**   Microgram—abbreviated as **mcg.** Microgram is also written using the symbol μ in combination with the letter *g* from the basic unit *gram* (μg). However, use of the abbreviation μg should be avoided when writing orders. It can be mistaken for "mg" when handwritten and result in an error when orders are transcribed.

**CAUTION**

The abbreviation μg for microgram is listed on the official "Do Not Use" List of TJC (The Joint Commission). Confusion of the symbol used for microgram with the abbreviation for milligram could cause a critical error in dosage calculation. These units differ from each other in value by 1,000.

Although the symbol for microgram is no longer approved for use when writing medication orders, it may be seen on some medication labels (e.g., Lanoxin tablets, Lanoxin injectable, Lanoxin elixir for pediatric use), and you should be familiar with the meaning.

**Example 3:**   Milliliter—abbreviated as **mL.** Note that when *L (liter)* is used in combination with a prefix, it **remains capitalized.**

## Tips for Clinical Practice

You may see gram abbreviated as Gm or gm, liter as lowercase l, or milliliter as ml. These abbreviations are outdated and can lead to misinterpretation. Use only the standardized SI abbreviations. When in doubt about an abbreviation being used, never assume; ask the prescriber for clarification. See Box 6-1 for common metric abbreviations.

### BOX 6-1   Common Metric Abbreviations

gram = g
microgram = mcg
milligram = mg
kilogram = kg
liter = L
*deciliter = dL
milliliter = mL

*Seen in the expression of laboratory values (e.g., hemoglobin, creatinine levels).

It is critical to differentiate between the SI abbreviations for milligram (mg) and milliliter (mL). At a quick glance these abbreviations appear similar; however, confusing these two units can result in lethal consequences for a client.

## RULES OF THE METRIC SYSTEM

Certain rules specific to the metric system are important to remember (Box 6-2). **These rules are critical to the prevention of errors and ensure accurate interpretation of metric notations when used in medication orders.**

---

### BOX 6-2 Metric System Rules

1. Use Arabic numbers to express quantities in this system.

   **Example:**   1, 1,000, 0.5

2. Express parts of a unit or fractions of a unit as decimals.

   **Example:**   0.4 g, 0.5 L $\left(\text{not } \frac{2}{5} \text{ g}, \frac{1}{2} \text{ L}\right)$

3. Always write the quantity, whether in whole numbers or in decimals, before the abbreviation or symbol for a unit of measure.

   **Example:**   1,000 mg, 0.75 mL (not mg 1,000, mL 0.75)

4. Use a full space between the numeral and abbreviation.

   **Example:**   2 mL, 1 L (not 2mL, 1L)

5. Always place a leading zero to the left of the decimal point if there is no whole number. Eliminate trailing zeros to the right of the decimal point.

   **Example:**   0.4 mL, 2 mg (not .4 mL, 2.0 mg)

6. Do not use the abbreviation $\mu g$ for microgram; it might be mistaken for mg. Remember mg is 1,000 times larger.

7. Do not use the abbreviation *cc* for mL. This abbreviation can be misinterpreted as zeros.

   **Example:**   2 mL (not 2 cc)

8. Avoid periods after the abbreviation for a unit of measure to avoid the possibility of it being misread for the number 1 in a poorly handwritten order.

   **Example:**   mg (not mg.)

9. Place commas in values at 1,000 or above. ISMP recommends this to improve readability.

   **Example:**   100,000 units (not 100000 units)

10. Do not add "s" on a unit of measure to make it plural; this could lead to misinterpretation.

    **Example:**   mg (not mgs)

---

**CAUTION**

As part of the National Patient Safety Goals, TJC set up specific guidelines for the use of leading and trailing zeros. This is also a recommendation of ISMP. A zero should always be placed in front of the decimal when the quantity is less than a whole number (leading zero). When the quantity expressed is preceded by a whole number, zeros are not placed after the number (trailing zeros). This rule is critical to preventing misinterpretation and medication errors. Always double-check the placement of decimals and zeros.

**Example 1:**    .52 mL is written as 0.52 mL to **reinforce the decimal** and avoid being misread as 52 mL. Lack of a leading zero before the decimal point could result in the decimal point being missed and cause a critical error in dosage interpretation.

**Example 2:**    2.5 mL is written as 2.5 mL, not 2.50 mL. **Addition of unnecessary zeros can lead to errors in reading;** 2.50 mL may be misread as 250 mL instead of 2.5 mL. Unnecessary zeros can also result in the decimal point being missed and cause a critical error in dosage interpretation.

## UNITS OF MEASURE

Understanding common equivalents in the metric system can assist the nurse in preventing medication errors related to incorrect dosage.

### Weight

The gram is the basic unit of weight. Medications may be ordered in grams or fractions of a gram, such as milligram or microgram.

1. The milligram is 1,000 times smaller than a gram:

$$1 \text{ g} = 1,000 \text{ mg}$$

2. The microgram is 1,000 times smaller than a milligram and 1 million times smaller than a gram. The word *micro* also means tiny or small. Micrograms are tiny parts of a gram (i.e., 1,000 mcg = 1 mg). A milligram is 1,000 times larger than a microgram. It takes 1 million mcg to make 1 g.
3. The kilogram is very large and is not used for measuring medications. A kilogram is 1,000 times larger than a gram (i.e., 1 kg = 1,000 g). This measure is often used to denote weights of clients, on which medication dosages are based. This is the only unit you will see used to identify a unit larger than the basic unit.

Box 6-3 presents the metric units of measure used most often for dosage calculations and measurement of health status. This text will use the standardized abbreviations for metric units throughout.

---

### BOX 6-3    Metric Equivalents to Memorize

**Weight**
1 kilogram (kg) = 1,000 grams (g)
1 gram (g) = 1,000 milligrams (mg)
1 milligram (mg) = 1,000 micrograms (mcg)

**Volume**
1 liter (L) = 1,000 milliliters (mL)
1 milliliter (mL) = 0.001 liter (L)

**Length**
1 meter (m) = 100 centimeters (cm) = 1,000 mm
1 millimeter (mm) = 0.001 meter (m) = 0.1 cm

---

## Volume

1. The **liter** is the basic unit.

$$1 \text{ L} = 1,000 \text{ mL}$$

2. The **milliliter** is 1,000 times smaller than a liter. It is abbreviated as mL.

$$1 \text{ mL} = 0.001 \text{ L}$$

3. The unit of measurement **cubic centimeter** (cc) has been used interchangeably with milliliter (mL). The cubic centimeter is the amount of space that 1 mL of liquid occupies. However, mL is the correct term for volume. The use of cc for mL is currently now prohibited by many health care organizations. TJC has also suggested that institutions prohibit the use of the abbreviation cc and add it to their "Do Not Use" List (TJC, 2005). ISMP also includes cc as an abbreviation that should not be used. (Figure 6-1 shows metric measures that may be seen on a medication cup.)

> Although pint and quart are not metric measures, they have metric equivalents. For example, a quart is approximately the size of a liter: 1 quart ≈ 1,000 mL and 1 pint ≈ 500 mL. Although pint and quart are not measures used in medication administration, you may need them to calculate a solution, especially in home care. For pharmacological purposes the equivalents stated for pint and quart are used.

## CONVERSIONS BETWEEN METRIC UNITS

Because the metric system is based on the decimal system, conversions between one metric system unit and another can be done by moving the decimal point. The number of places to move the decimal point depends on the equivalent. In health care, each unit of measure in common use for purposes of medication administration differs by 1,000. In the metric system the most common terms used are the kilogram, gram, milligram, microgram, liter, milliliter, and centimeter. To **convert** or make a **conversion** means to change from one unit to another. This converting can be simply changing a measure to its equivalent in the same system. Changing from grams to milligrams illustrates a metric measure changed to another metric measure. Each metric unit in common use for *medication administration* differs from the next by a factor of 1,000. Metric conversions can therefore be made by dividing or multiplying by **1,000.** Knowledge of the size of a unit is important when converting by moving the decimal, because this determines whether division or multiplication is necessary to make the conversion.

> Nurses often make conversions within the metric system when administering medications, for example, grams to milligrams.

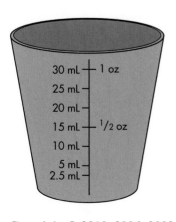

**Figure 6-1**   Medicine cup showing volume measure in milliliters (mL). (From Ogden SJ: *Calculation of drug dosages,* ed. 8, St. Louis, 2007, Mosby.)

To make conversions within the metric system, remember the common conversion factors (1 kg = 1,000 g, 1 g = 1,000 mg, 1 mg = 1,000 mcg, and 1 L = 1,000 mL) and the following rules:

**RULE**

To convert a **smaller** unit to a **larger** one, **divide** by moving the decimal point **three places to the left.**

**Example 1:**   100 mL = ___ L          (conversion factor: 1,000 mL = 1 L)
                     (smaller)     (larger)

100 mL = .100 = 0.1 L   **(Placing zero in front of the decimal is important.)**

**Example 2:**   50 mg = ___ g          (conversion factor: 1,000 mg = 1 g)
                     (smaller)   (larger)

50 mg = .050 = 0.05 g  **(Placing zero in front of the decimal is important.)**

**RULE**

To convert a **larger** unit to a **smaller** one, **multiply** by moving the decimal **three places to the right.**

**Example 1:**   0.75 g = ___ mg          (conversion factor: 1 g = 1,000 mg)
                     (larger)      (smaller)

0.75 g = 0.750 = 750 mg

**NOTE**

Answers to conversions should be labeled with the unit of measure.

**Example 2:**   0.04 kg = ___ g          (conversion factor: 1 kg = 1,000 g)
                     (larger)      (smaller)

0.04 kg = 0.040 = 40 g

 ## Practice Problems

*worksheet*

Convert the following metric measures by moving the decimal.

1. 300 mg = _____ g          11. 529 mg = _____ g

2. 6 mg = _____ mcg          12. 645 mcg = _____ mg

3. 0.7 L = _____ mL          13. 347 L = _____ mL

4. 180 mcg = _____ mg          14. 238 g = _____ mcg

5. 0.02 mg = _____ mcg          15. 3,500 mL = _____ L

6. 4.5 L = _____ mL          16. 0.04 kg = _____ g

7. 4.2 g = _____ mg          17. 658 kg = _____ g

8. 0.9 g = _____ mg          18. 51 mL = _____ L

9. 3,250 mL = _____ L          19. 1.6 mg = _____ mcg

10. 42 g = _____ kg          20. 28 mL = _____ L

Answers on p. 606

## Points to Remember

- The liter and the gram are the basic units used for medication administration.
- Conversion factors must be memorized to do conversions. The common conversion factors in the metric system are 1 kg = 1,000 g, 1 g = 1,000 mg, 1 mg = 1,000 mcg, and 1 L = 1,000 mL (mL is the correct term to use in relation to volume, rather than cc).
- Express answers using the following rules of the metric system:
  1. Fractional metric units are expressed as a decimal.
  2. Place a zero in front of the decimal point when the quantity is less than a whole number to prevent potential dosage error.
  3. Omit trailing zeros to avoid misreading of a value and potential error in dosage.
  4. The abbreviation for a measure is placed after the quantity.
  5. Place a full space between the numeral and abbreviation.
  6. Use standard SI abbreviations.
- Converting common metric units used in medication administration from one unit to another is done by multiplying or dividing by 1,000.
- Answers should be stated with the unit of measure as the label.
- Values at 1,000 or greater than 1,000 should be written with a comma.

 ## CHAPTER REVIEW

1. List the three units of measurement used in the metric system.

   a) _____

   b) _____

   c) _____

2. Which is larger, kilogram or milligram? _____

3. 1 mL = _____ L

4. What units of measure are used in the metric system for:

   a. liquid capacity? _____

   b. weight? _____

5. 1,000 mg = _____ g

6. 1 L = _____ mL

7. 1,000 mcg = _____ mg

8. 1,000 mL = _____ L

9. The abbreviation for liter is _____

10. The abbreviation for microgram is _____

11. The abbreviation for milliliter is _____

12. The abbreviation for gram is _____

13. The abbreviation for kilogram is _____

14. The prefix *kilo* means _____

15. The prefix *milli* means _____

Using abbreviations and the rules of the metric system, express the following quantities correctly.

16. Six tenths of a gram _____

17. Fifty kilograms _____

18. Four tenths of a milligram _____

19. Four hundredths of a liter_____

20. Four and two tenths micrograms _____

21. Five thousandths of a gram _____

22. Six hundredths of a gram _____

23. Two and six tenths milliliters _____

24. One hundred milliliters_____

25. Three hundredths of a milliliter _____

Convert the following metric measures by moving the decimal.

26. 950 mcg = _____ mg

27. 58.5 L = _____ mL

28. 130 mL = _____ L

29. 276 g = _____ mg

30. 550 mL = _____ L

31. 56.5 L = _____ mL

32. 205 g = _____ kg

33. 0.025 kg = _____ g

34. 1 L = _____ mL

35. 0.015 g = _____ mg

36. 250 mcg = _____ mg

37. 8 kg = _____ g

38. 2 kL = _____ L

39. 5 L = _____ mL

40. 0.75 L = _____ mL

41. 0.33 g = _____ mg

42. 750 mg = _____ g

43. 6.28 kg = _____ g

44. 36.5 mg = _____ g

45. 2.2 mg = _____ g

46. 400 g = _____ kg

47. 0.024 L = _____ mL

48. 100 mg = _____ g

49. 150 g = _____ mg

50. 85 mcg = _____ mg     53. 120 mg = _____ g

51. 1.25 L = _____ mL     54. 475 mL = _____ L

52. 0.05 mg = _____ mcg     55. 4.5 g = _____ mg

Which of the following is stated correctly using metric abbreviations and rules?

56. .5 g, 0.5 gm, .5 gm, 0.5 g _____

57. 4 KG, 4.0 Kg, Kg 04, 4 kg _____

58. Lasix 20.0 mg, Lasix 20 mg, Lasix 20 MG, Lasix mg 20 _____

59. Gentamicin $1^1/_2$ mL, gentamicin 1.5 ml, gentamicin 1.5 mL, gentamicin $1^1/_2$ ml _____

60. Ampicillin 500 mg, ampicillin 500.0 mg, ampicillin 500 MG, ampicillin mg 500 _____

Answers on p. 606

 **For additional information, refer to the Introducing Drug Measures section of Drug Calculations Companion, Version 4, on Evolve.**

# CHAPTER 7

# Apothecary and Household Systems

**Objectives**

*After reviewing this chapter, you should be able to:*
1. State the common apothecary equivalents
2. State the common household equivalents
3. State specific rules that relate to the apothecary system
4. State specific rules that relate to the household system
5. Identify symbols and measures in the apothecary system
6. Identify measures in the household system

## APOTHECARY SYSTEM

The apothecary system of measurement is an English system that is considered to be one of the oldest systems of measure. It is also referred to as the *fraction system* because parts of units are expressed by using fractions, with the exception of the fraction one half, which is expressed as ss or $\overline{ss}$. The notations in this system are unusual and can be confusing. The recent trend is to eliminate apothecary measures from use and to use the metric system. The Institute for Safe Medication Practices (ISMP) has recommended that all medications be prescribed and calculated with metric measures. The unusual notations and inclusion of fractions and Roman numerals have caused concern about use of the apothecary system.

**CAUTION**

TJC (2005) published a list of abbreviations, acronyms, and symbols recommended not to use (and for possible future inclusion on the official list). This list included apothecary measures. The Joint Commission does not forbid the use of apothecary measures; it does discourage their use because of confusion with metric use and misinterpretation. For safety and prevention of errors TJC recommends the metric system be used exclusively in relation to medications.

Apothecary measures are now rarely found on medication labels except for labels on older medications that have been in use for many years (e.g., aspirin, phenobarbital, nitroglycerin, atropine). If a medication label does contain an apothecary measure, it is usually in conjunction with the metric equivalent. For example, the label on a bottle of Nitrostat (nitroglycerin) tablets shows that the tablets are labeled in milligrams, which is a metric measure, and also in grains (in parentheses), which is an apothecary measure. Figure 7-1 illustrates the use of metric and apothecary measures on medication labels. However, many of the newer labels do not include apothecary measures.

Although the metric system is the preferred system, apothecary measures, on rare occasions, are still seen on syringes (minim) and medication cups (dram); however, use of these measures has been discouraged. Many of the newer syringes in use today do not have the

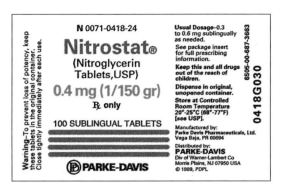

**Figure 7-1** Medication label showing apothecary (gr) and metric (mg) measures. Note: In the apothecary system, the unit of measure precedes the number, although not shown here. Inconsistencies can be seen even in apothecary notation.

minim scale on them because of its inaccuracy. Although the use of the apothecary system is minimal, in the rare circumstances when its use is necessary, those involved in the administration of medications should be familiar with it, because safety in medication administration depends on understanding of the information on medication labels and medication orders. The text focuses on the common apothecary measures used and their metric equivalents. However, apothecary measures should always be converted to metric measures.

## Particulars of the Apothecary System

The notations for the apothecary system are unusual and often inconsistent and the opposite of metric notations. The conversions used in this system are approximations, and caution should be exercised when this system is used because you could place a client at risk. When orders are written with apothecary measures, they should be converted to metric measures by referring to an equivalency table, which is often posted in the medication room. It is wise to check a reference whenever an uncommon measure is used.

The following guidelines should be used to correctly write apothecary notations:

1. The abbreviation or symbol for a unit of measure is written **before** the amount or quantity in lowercase letters.

   **Example:**    six grains. The symbol for grains is gr. Therefore six grains = gr 6, gr vi, or gr $\overline{vi}$.

2. Roman numerals, as well as Arabic numbers, are used. When Roman numerals are used, they are written in lowercase letters. Example: gr v. To prevent errors in interpretation, a line is sometimes drawn over lowercase Roman numerals. A lowercase "i" is dotted above the line.

   **Example:**    $\ddot{ii}$, $\overline{v}$

3. Fractions are used to express quantities that are less than one.

   **Example:**    gr $^3/_4$

4. The symbol "ss" is used for the fraction $^1/_2$, and it can be written ss or $\overline{ss}$. This symbol has been misinterpreted and is discussed for recognition purposes only.

   **Example 1:**    half of a grain, gr ss, gr $\overline{ss}$. The symbol ss can also be used with Roman numerals. When used with Roman numerals, it is placed at the end.

   **Example 2:**    seven and a half grains = gr viiss, gr $\overline{viiss}$. Although the symbol ss can be used for $^1/_2$, the numeral $^1/_2$ can also be used.

5. A combination of Arabic numbers and fractions can also be used to express units of measure.

   **Example:**    gr $7^1/_2$

## Apothecary Units of Measure

Historically, minims and drams, which are units of the apothecary system, were used in medication administration. Their use is now discouraged in medication administration. You only need to be able to recognize them because some syringes may still have a minim scale identified on them and a medicine cup may still have drams indicated on it. Minim is abbreviated with a lowercase "m"; dram is abbreviated as dr, and the symbol is a single-headed Z with a tail (ʒ). A dram is equal to 4 mL.

Some apothecary measures are also used as household measures. Example: pint (pt) and quart (qt). Because the nurse encounters them in everyday situations, you need to know that 1 pint = 16 fluid ounces and 1 quart = 32 fluid ounces or 2 pints.

The common apothecary units used for medication administration are grain (gr) and ounce (℥, oz).

*WEIGHT*   The only one apothecary measure used for weight with which you need to be familiar is grain. The basic unit for weight is the grain.

Grain is abbreviated in lowercase letters as **gr.**

**CAUTION**

> The abbreviation for grain (gr), an apothecary measure, is often confused with gram (g), a metric measure. Remember these two measures are different; when in doubt seek clarification.

Two important metric equivalents to remember are **gr 15 = 1 g** and **60 mg = gr 1.** The equivalent most recognized and used in medication orders is gr 1 = 60 mg. However, some equivalent tables state that gr 1 = 60 to 65 mg. For some common oral medications, 65 mg = gr 1 is the best conversion; the most notable of these are Tylenol, aspirin, and iron (gr x = 650 mg).

Another way to remember common apothecary and metric conversions is to remember the conversion clock. Refer to Figure 7-2 to visualize the relationship of a standard clock to a clock illustrating metric and apothecary conversions.

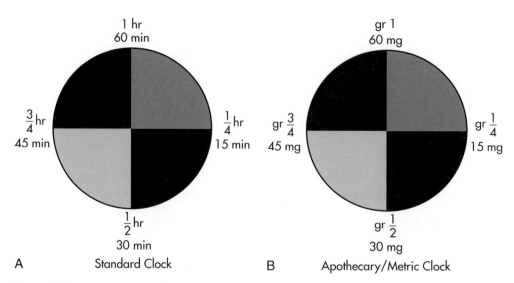

**Figure 7-2   A,** 60 minutes = 1 hour, and fractions of an hour are shown in minutes. **B,** Because 60 mg = gr 1 and there are 60 minutes in 1 hour, you can visualize milligrams as representing minutes on a clock, and the fractions of an hour as grains.

*VOLUME*   The metric equivalent for ounce (1 ounce = 30 mL) is used in medication administration. Medicine cups have a capacity of 1 ounce. Ounce (30 mL—metric equivalent) is also used in keeping a written record of a client's intake and output. (I&O is discussed in a later chapter.)

The symbol for ounce is a **double-headed** Z with a tail (℥). Note: The symbols for dram (ʒ) and ounce (℥) are rarely seen and obsolete. When these measures are indicated on items used in medication administration, such as a medicine cup, the abbreviations are dr for dram and oz for ounce. Therefore the abbreviations will be used in the text as opposed to the symbols.

$$1 \text{ ounce} = 30 \text{ mL}$$

**CAUTION**

Although minim and dram may still appear on syringes and medicine cups, it is important to differentiate them from acceptable units of measure. They should not be used. Always know the institution's policy regarding the use of apothecary notations.

For medication administration it is necessary to be familiar with the apothecary system units shown in Box 7-1.

## HOUSEHOLD SYSTEM

The household system is an old system and the **least accurate** of the three systems of measure. It is a modified system designed for everyday use at home. Nurses need to be familiar with household measures, because clients often use utensils in the home to take prescribed medications. Capacities of utensils such as a teaspoon, a tablespoon, and a cup vary from one house to another; therefore liquid measures are approximate. Because of the increase in nursing care provided at home (home care, visiting nurse), it is imperative that nurses become adept in converting from one system to another. When calculating doses or interpreting the health care provider's instructions for the client at home, the nurse must remember that household measures are used. Consequently the nurse must be able to calculate equivalents for adaptation in the home, even though medication administration spoons, droppers, and medication measuring cups (Figure 7-3) are available.

**BOX 7-1   Units of the Apothecary System**

Weight: grain (gr)

Volume: ounce (oz)

Household/metric

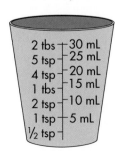

**Figure 7-3**   Medicine cup showing household/metric measurements.

1-Ounce Medicine Cup (30 mL)

**CAUTION**

Using household measures for dosage measurements can place a client at risk. Always advise clients and their families to use the measuring devices or droppers packaged with the medication or provided by the pharmacy.

**NOTE**

Anything less than a teaspoon should be measured in a syringe-type device that has no needle and not in a measuring cup.

Common household measures to memorize are the following:
1 teaspoon (t, tsp) = 5 mL
1 tablespoon (T, tbs) = 15 mL
1 measuring cup = 8 oz

## Tips for Clinical Practice

To ensure accurate dosages at home, utensils used should be marked or calibrated. Determine what kind of measuring devices the client is using at home and teach their proper use. Review the household equivalents and abbreviations, be extremely cautious, and do not confuse the abbreviations for teaspoon (t) and tablespoon (T). 1 teaspoon equals 5 mL, and 1 tablespoon equals 15 mL; confusing the abbreviations and their equivalent could result in a threefold error.

### Particulars of the Household System

1. Some of the units for liquid measures are the same as those in the apothecary system, for example, pint and quart.
2. There are no standard rules for expressing household measures, which accounts for variations in their use.
3. Standard cookbook abbreviations are used in this system.
4. Arabic numerals and fractions are used to express quantities.
5. The smallest unit of measure in the household system is the drop (gtt).

**CAUTION**

Drops should never be used as a measure for medications because the size of drops varies according to the diameter of the utensil and therefore can be inaccurate. When drops are used as a measure for medications, they should be calibrated or used only when associated with a dropper size, as in intravenous (IV) flow rates.

See Box 7-2 for apothecary, household, and metric equivalents.

It is important for the nurse providing care in the home to remember that clients need specific instructions for measuring accurately at home. Sometimes solutions may have to

---

### BOX 7-2   Apothecary/Household/Metric Equivalents

**Volume (Liquid)**
1 ounce (oz) = 30 mL
1 tablespoon (T or tbs) = 15 mL
2 tablespoons (T or tbs) = 1 ounce (oz)
1 teaspoon (t or tsp) = 5 mL
1 cup (standard measuring cup) = 240 mL (8 ounces)
1 pint (pt) = 500 mL (16 ounces)
1 quart (qt) = 1,000 mL (32 ounces)
**Weight**
15 grains (gr) = 1,000 mg = 1 gram (g)
1 grain (gr) = 60 mg
1 pound (lb) = 16 ounces (oz)

---

be made at home with household measures. Some examples illustrating solutions made in the home using household devices are listed.

1. Normal saline solution (0.9%)—2 teaspoons of salt to 4 cups of water
2. Acetic acid solution (0.25%)—3 tablespoons of white vinegar to 4 cups of water for wound/dressing care and cleaning equipment

Household and apothecary measures are most commonly used in the home care setting and less frequently in the clinical setting. With medication errors being one of the most common causes of patient injuries, it is quite possible that these measures may be eliminated in the near future because of the goal within health care to improve medication labeling and recommendations of organizations such as TJC and ISMP regarding abbreviations and use of metric measures in relation to medications to decrease medication errors.

## ■ Points to Remember

- In the apothecary system, the abbreviation or symbol is placed before the quantity. There are inconsistencies in notation rules in the apothecary system.
- Apothecary measures are approximate measures. When converting from apothecary to metric system, equivalents are not exact.
- The apothecary system uses fractions, Roman numerals, and Arabic numerals.
- Know the institution's policy on the use of apothecary notations.
- Teaspoon and tablespoon are common measures used in the household system. For safety, encourage clients to use the measuring device that comes with the medication.
- There are no rules for stating household measures.
- The household system uses fractions and Arabic numerals.
- Conversions between metric, apothecary, and household measures are approximate equivalents.
- Dosages less than a teaspoon should be measured with a syringe-type device that does not have a needle attached.
- When possible, convert apothecary and household measures to metric measures.
- When in doubt about an unfamiliar unit or one that is not used often, consult a reference or an equivalency table.

## Practice Problems

Write the abbreviations for the following measures.

1. ounce _____

3. _____ pint

2. grain _____

Use Box 7-2 to determine the following equivalents.

4. oz $\frac{1}{2}$ = _____ mL

7. $\frac{1}{2}$ pt = oz _____

5. 2 tsp = _____ mL

8. 90 mL = oz _____

6. 45 mL = _____ tbs

Write the following amounts correctly using the correct notation rules for the apothecary system.

9. 10 ounces _____

10. one-half grain _____

11. What household measure might be used to give $\frac{1}{2}$ ounce of cough syrup?

_____

12. The nurse encouraged a client with diarrhea to drink 40 ounces of water per day.

How many cups does this represent? _____

Answers on p. 606

 **CHAPTER REVIEW**

Using the rules of the apothecary system, write the following with the correct abbreviations.

1. Eight and one half grains _____     5. One hundred twenty-fifth of a grain

2. Eight ounces _____     _____

3. Quart _____     6. Two ounces _____

4. Pint _____     7. Five ounces _____

Complete the following:

8. Grain is a unit of _____.     16. The abbreviation t is used for _____

9. gr 15 = _____ g     _____.

10. gr 1 = _____ mg     17. 1 t = _____ mL

11. 1 pt = oz _____     18. 1 oz = _____ mL

12. 1 qt = oz _____     19. 1 cup = _____ ounces

13. gr 15 = _____ mg     20. 1 tbs = _____ mL

14. The abbreviation for drop is _____.     21. 1 pt = _____ ounces

15. T is the abbreviation for _____.     22. 1 qt = _____ ounces

Answers on p. 606

 **For more information, refer to the Introducing Drug Measures section of Drug Calculations Companion, Version 4, on Evolve.**

# CHAPTER 8

# Converting Within and Between Systems

## Objectives

*After reviewing this chapter, you should be able to:*
1. Convert a unit of measure to its equivalent within the same system
2. Convert approximate equivalents among the metric, apothecary, and household systems of measure

## EQUIVALENTS AMONG METRIC, APOTHECARY, AND HOUSEHOLD SYSTEMS

As noted in earlier chapters dealing with the systems of measure, some measures in one system have equivalents in another system; however, equivalents are not exact measures, and there are discrepancies. Several tables have been developed illustrating conversions/equivalents. Sometimes drug companies use different equivalents for a measure. As mentioned previously, a common discrepancy is with grains, which is an apothecary measure. Some sources indicate 60 to 65 mg = gr 1, but remember that **60 mg = gr 1** is used in most medication administration. However, 65 mg = gr 1 is the best conversion factor for some common oral medications, notably aspirin, Tylenol, and iron.

In the health care system it is imperative that nurses be proficient in converting among all three systems of measure (metric, apothecary, household). Nurses are becoming increasingly responsible for administration of medications to clients and teaching clients and family outside of the conventional hospital setting (e.g., home care). Nurses have become more involved in discharge planning and are responsible for ensuring that the client can safely self-administer medications in the correct dosage. Table 8-1 lists some of the equivalents between systems. Memorize these common equivalents!

## CONVERTING

The term *convert* means to change from one form to another. Converting can mean changing a measure to its equivalent in the same system or changing a measurement from one system to another system, which is called *converting between systems*. The measurement obtained when converting between systems is **approximate, not exact.** Thus certain equivalents have been established to ensure continuity.

It is important that nurses be able to make conversions because they are often called on to convert medication dosages among metric, apothecary, and household systems. The nurse therefore must understand the systems of measurement and be able to convert within the same system and from one system to another with accuracy.

Before beginning the actual process of converting, the nurse should remember the following important points that can make converting simple.

**TABLE 8-1**  Approximate Equivalents of Metric, Apothecary, and Household Measures

| Household | Apothecary | Metric |
|---|---|---|
| 1 t, 1 tsp | | 5 mL |
| 1 T, 1 tbs | | 15 mL |
| | gr 15 | 1 g (1,000 mg) |
| | gr i | 60 mg |
| | 1 oz | 30 mL |
| | 1 pt (16 oz) | 500 mL |
| | 1 qt (32 oz) | 1,000 mL, 1 L |
| | 2.2 lb | 1 kg (1,000 g) |
| 1 in | | 2.5 cm |

**NOTE**

Equivalents indicated in this table are those used most often. The accurate and preferred term for liquids is mL.

## Points for Converting

1. Memorization of the equivalents/conversions is essential.
2. Think of memorized equivalents/conversions as essential conversion factors, or as a ratio.

   **Example:**    1,000 mg = 1 g is called a conversion factor.

   1,000 mg : 1 g is a ratio.

3. Follow basic math principles, regardless of the conversion method used.
4. Answers should be expressed by applying specific rules that relate to the system to which you are converting.

   **Example:**    The metric system uses decimals; the apothecary system uses fractions.

5. THINK CRITICALLY—select the appropriate equivalent to make conversions (see Table 8-1).

## METHODS OF CONVERTING

### Moving the Decimal Point

Moving the decimal point is discussed in Chapter 6. Because the metric system is based on the decimal system, conversions within the metric system can be done easily by moving the decimal point. This method cannot be applied in the apothecary or household system because decimal points are not used in either system. **Remember the two rules in moving decimal points:**

**RULE**

To convert a smaller unit to a larger one, divide or move the decimal point to the left.

**Example:**                              350 mg = _____ g

                                            (smaller)   (larger)

**Solution:**    After determining that mg is the smaller unit and you are converting to a larger unit (g), recall the conversion factor that allows you to change milligrams to grams (1 g = 1,000 mg). Therefore 350 is divided by 1,000 by moving the decimal point three places to the left, indicating 350 mg = 0.35 g.

                                    350. mg = 0.35 g

*Note:* The final answer is expressed in decimal form. Remember to always place a zero (0) in front of the decimal point to indicate a value that is less than 1.

To convert a larger unit to a smaller one, multiply or move the decimal point to the right.

---

**Example:**                  0.85 L = _____ mL

                               (larger)     (smaller)

**Solution:** After determining that L is the larger unit and you are converting to a smaller unit (mL), recall the conversion factor that allows you to change liters to milliliters (1 L = 1,000 mL). Therefore 0.85 is multiplied by 1,000 by moving the decimal point three places to the right, indicating 0.85 L = 850 mL.

$$0.850 \text{ L} = 850 \text{ mL}$$

Note the addition of a zero here to allow movement of the decimal point the correct number of places.

 **Practice Problems**

For additional practice in converting by decimal movement, convert the following metric measures to the equivalent units indicated.

1. 600 mL = _____ L      14. 1,700 mL = _____ L

2. 0.016 g = _____ mg      15. 15 kg = _____ g

3. 4 kg = _____ g      16. 3.5 g = _____ mg

4. 3 mcg = _____ mg      17. 0.16 kg = _____ g

5. 0.3 mg = _____ g      18. 0.004 L = _____ mL

6. 0.01 kg = _____ g      19. 1 mL = _____ L

7. 1.9 L = _____ mL      20. 8 mg = _____ g

8. 0.5 g = _____ kg      21. 0.5 g = _____ mg

9. 0.07 mg = _____ mcg      22. 300 g = _____ kg

10. 650 mL = _____ L      23. 25 mg = _____ g

11. 0.04 g = _____ mg      24. 65 kg = _____ g

12. 0.12 g = _____ kg      25. 0.006 mg = _____ mcg

13. 180 mg = _____ g

Answers on p. 607

---

Rather than remembering the right to left rule or left to right rule, you might find it easier to use ratio and proportion as a method of conversion.

80    Unit Two   *Systems of Measurement*

## Using Ratio and Proportion

Using ratio and proportion is one of the easiest ways to make conversions, whether within the same system or between systems. The basics on how to state ratios and proportions and how to solve them when looking for one unknown are presented in Chapter 4. To make conversions using ratio and proportion, a proportion must be set up that expresses a numerical relationship between the two systems. A proportion may be written in colon format or as a fraction when making conversions. Regardless of the format used, there are some basic rules to follow when using this method.

**RULE**

### Rules for Ratio and Proportion

1. State the known equivalent first (memorized equivalent).
2. Add the incomplete ratio on the other side of the equals sign, making sure the units of measurement are written in the same sequence.

   Example:                   mg:g = mg:g

3. Label all terms in the proportion, including $x$. (These labels are not carried when multiplying or dividing.)
4. Solve the problem by using the principles for solving ratios and proportions. (The product of the means equals the product of the extremes.)
5. The final answer for $x$ should be labeled with the appropriate unit of measure or desired unit.

---

When using the method of ratio and proportion to make conversions, as with any method used, the known equivalents must be memorized. Stating the proportion in the fraction format may be a way of avoiding confusion with the terms (means and extremes). However, regardless of the format used, the terms must correspond to each other in value and have a relationship. Division should always be carried at least two decimal places to ensure accuracy.

**Example:**                     8 mg = _____ g

**Solution:**     State the known equivalent first, then add the incomplete ratio, making sure the units are in the same sequence. Label all the terms in the proportion, including $x$.

$$1{,}000 \text{ mg}:1 \text{ g} \quad = \quad 8 \text{ mg}:x \text{ g}$$

(known equivalent)          (unknown)

Read as "1,000 mg is to 1 g as 8 mg is to $x$ g."

**NOTE**

The terms of the proportion are in the same sequence (mg:g = mg:g), and there is a correspondence in the ratio: small:large = small:large.

Once the proportion is stated, solve it by multiplying the means (inner terms) and then the extremes (outer terms). Place the "$x$" product on the left side of the equation.

**Result:**
$$\underbrace{1{,}000 \text{ mg}:\overbrace{1 \text{ g} = 8 \text{ mg}}^{\text{means}}:x \text{ g}}_{\text{extremes}}$$

$$1 \times 8 = 1{,}000 \times x$$

$$\frac{1{,}000\,x}{1{,}000} = \frac{8}{1{,}000}$$

$$x = \frac{8}{1{,}000}$$

$$x = 0.008 \text{ g}$$

Because the measure you are converting to is metric, the fraction is changed to a decimal by dividing 8 by 1,000 to obtain an answer of 0.008 g. However, because the measures are metric in this example, perhaps moving the decimal point would be the preferred method as opposed to actual division.

**Example:**                                 8 mg = _____ g

1. Note that conversion is going from smaller to larger; thus division or moving the decimal point to the left is indicated.
2. Note that the unit is going from milligrams to grams, thus changing by a factor of 1,000.
3. The decimal point will be moved three places to the left to complete this conversion: 8 mg = 0.008 g.

An alternate way of stating the problem illustrated in the previous example would be stating it as a fraction and cross multiplying to solve for $x$.

$$\frac{1,000 \text{ mg}}{1 \text{ g}} \nmid \frac{8 \text{ mg}}{x \text{ g}}$$

$$1,000 \, x = 8$$

$$\frac{1,000 \, x}{1,000} = \frac{8}{1,000}$$

$$x = 0.008 \text{ g}$$

Another way of writing a ratio and proportion to eliminate errors is to set up the conversion problem in a fraction format.

Place the conversion factor first (numerator), and place the problem underneath matching up the units (the denominator); then cross multiply to solve for $x$.

**Example:**                                 8 mg = _____ g

$$\frac{1,000 \text{ mg}}{8 \text{ mg}} \nmid \frac{1 \text{ g}}{x \text{ g}}$$

$$1,000 \, x = 8$$

$$\frac{1,000 \, x}{1,000} = \frac{8}{1,000}$$

$$x = 0.008 \text{ g}$$

> **NOTE**
>
> You have mg under mg, and g under g, ensuring the correct placement of labels.

The remainder of this chapter will show examples of the methods used in converting within the same system and between systems.

## CONVERTING WITHIN THE SAME SYSTEM

Converting within the same system is often seen with metric measures; however, it can be done using the other systems of measurement, such as one apothecary measure being converted to an equivalent within the apothecary system. Any one of the methods discussed can be used, but movement of decimal points is limited to the metric system. Ratio and proportion can be used for all systems.

**Example 1:**                         (metric)     (metric)

                              0.6 mg = _____ mcg

**Solution:**     Equivalent: 1,000 mcg = 1 mg

              A milligram is larger than a microgram; the answer is obtained by moving the decimal point three places to the right (multiply).

**Answer:**     600 mcg

    Alternative: Set up as a proportion, in a fraction, or the colon format.

**Example 2:**                                              (metric)   (metric)

$$40 \text{ g} = \underline{\hspace{2cm}} \text{ kg}$$

**Solution:**      Equivalent: 1 kg = 1,000 g

A gram is smaller than a kilogram; the answer is obtained by moving the decimal three places to the left (divide).

**Answer:**       0.04 kg   (Note the placement of the zero before the decimal point.)

Alternative: Set up in a ratio and proportion using the fraction or colon format.

> The principles presented for solving ratio and proportion problems are used to solve for *x*, when presented in colon format or as a fraction.

*DIMENSIONAL ANALYSIS*   Dimensional analysis is a conversion method that has been used in chemistry and other sciences and will be discussed in more detail in Chapter 16. Dimensional analysis involves manipulation of units to get the desired unit. This method can be used for conversion in all systems. As with other methods discussed, you must know the conversion factor (equivalent).
Steps:
1. Identify the unit you are converting to.
2. Write the conversion factor so that the desired unit is in the denominator, and write the unit in the successive numerator to match the previous unit of measure in the previous denominator.
3. Cancel the alternate denominator/numerator units to leave the unit desired (being calculated).
4. Perform the mathematic process indicated.

**Example:**                                          (metric)    (metric)

$$0.12 \text{ kg}   \text{ to }   \text{ g}$$

**Solution:**      You want to cancel the kilograms and obtain the equivalent amount in grams. Begin by identifying the unknown, in this case, g. Because 1 kg = 1,000 g, the fraction that will allow you to cancel kg is $\dfrac{1,000 \text{ g}}{1 \text{ kg}}$.

$$x \text{ g} = \frac{1,000 \text{ g}}{1 \text{ kg}} \times \frac{0.12 \text{ kg}}{1}$$

*Note:* The unit you want to cancel is always written in the denominator of the fraction. Then proceed by placing as the next numerator the same label as the first denominator, in this case, kg.

*Note:* Placing a 1 under a number does not change its value.

$$\text{Cancel the units } x \text{ g} = \frac{1,000 \text{ g}}{1 \text{ k\!\!\!/g}} \times \frac{0.12 \text{ k\!\!\!/g}}{1}$$

$$1,000 \times 0.12 = 120 \text{ g}$$

$$x = 120 \text{ g}$$

**Answer:**       0.12 kg is equivalent to 120 g.

## Practice Problems

Convert the following measures to the equivalent units indicated.

26. 500 mL = _____ L    34. 600 mg = _____ g

27. 4 kg = _____ g    35. 0.736 mg = _____ mcg

___ = _____ mL    36. 1,600 mL = _____ L

29. 45 mL = _____ oz    37. 0.015 L = _____ mL

30. 4.5 mg = _____ mcg    38. 0.18 g = _____ mg

31. 3½ oz = _____ mL    39. 25 mcg = _____ mg

32. 6.5 L = _____ mL    40. 5.2 g = _____ kg

33. 60 g = _____ kg    Answers on p. 607

## CONVERTING BETWEEN SYSTEMS

The methods presented previously can be used to change a measure in one system to its equivalent in another, or the conversion factor method can be used. This method requires that you consider the size of units. To convert from a larger unit to a smaller unit of measure, you multiply by the conversion factor as shown in Example 1. To convert from a smaller to a larger unit of measure, you must divide by the conversion factor.

**Example 1:**                    (apothecary)  (metric)

$$gr \frac{1}{100} = \underline{\quad} mg$$

(large)      (small)

 Solution Using Conversion Factor Method

Equivalent: gr 1 = 60 mg

Conversion factor is 60.

A grain is larger than a milligram.

Multiply $\frac{1}{100}$ by 60 to obtain $\frac{60}{100}$.

Because the final answer is a metric measure, $^{60}/_{100}$ is changed to a decimal by dividing 100 into 60. The fraction could also be reduced first to its lowest term ($^{3}/_{5}$) and then changed to a decimal by dividing 5 into 3.

**Answer:**    0.6 mg

Alternative: Express the conversion in proportion format and solve for $x$. (One way to remember this method is to remember that it is the known or have : want to know or have.)

 ## Solution Using Ratio and Proportion

$$\text{gr } 1:60 \text{ mg} = \text{gr } \frac{1}{100} : x \text{ mg}$$

$$60 \times \frac{1}{100} = x$$

$$x = 60 \times \frac{1}{100}$$

$$x = \frac{60}{100} = \frac{6}{10}$$

$$x = 0.6 \text{ mg}$$

*or*

$$\frac{\text{gr } 1}{60 \text{ mg}} \times \frac{\text{gr } 1/100}{x \text{ mg}}$$

$$x = \frac{1}{100} \times 60$$

$$x = \frac{60}{100}$$

$$x = 0.6 \text{ mg}$$

**Example 2:**　　　　　　　　(apothecary)　(metric)

$$110 \text{ lb} = \underline{\hspace{1cm}} \text{ kg}$$

 ## Solution Using Conversion Factor Method

Equivalent: 1 kg = 2.2 lb

Conversion factor is 2.2.

A pound is smaller than a kilogram; 110 is divided by 2.2.

**Answer:**　　50 kg

## Solution Using Ratio and Proportion

$$1 \text{ kg}:2.2 \text{ lb} = x \text{ kg}:110 \text{ lb}$$

$$\frac{2.2x}{2.2} = \frac{110}{2.2}$$

$$x = 50 \text{ kg}$$

*or*

$$\frac{1 \text{ kg}}{2.2 \text{ lb}} = \frac{x \text{ kg}}{110 \text{ lb}}$$

*or*

$$\frac{1 \text{ kg}}{x \text{ kg}} = \frac{2.2 \text{ lb}}{110 \text{ lb}}$$

Solution Using Dimensional Analysis

$$x \text{ kg} = \frac{1 \text{ kg}}{2.2 \text{ lb}} \times \frac{110 \text{ lb}}{1}$$

**Example 3:**                    (apothecary)   (metric)

$$\text{gr} \frac{1}{10} = \underline{\hspace{2cm}} \text{ mg}$$

 Solution Using Conversion Factor Method

Equivalent: gr 1 = 60 mg

Conversion factor is 60.

A grain is larger than a milligram.

**Answer:**                    $\text{gr} \dfrac{1}{10} \times 60 = \dfrac{60}{10} = 6 \text{ mg}$

 Solution Using Ratio and Proportion

$$\text{gr } 1 : 60 \text{ mg} = \text{gr} \frac{1}{10} : x \text{ mg}$$

$$60 \times \frac{1}{10} = x$$

$$x = \frac{60}{10}$$

$$x = 6 \text{ mg}$$

*or*

$$\frac{\text{gr } 1}{60 \text{ mg}} = \frac{\text{gr } 1/10}{x \text{ mg}}$$

*or*

$$\frac{\text{gr } 1}{\text{gr } 1/10} = \frac{60 \text{ mg}}{x \text{ mg}}$$

 Solution Using Dimensional Analysis

Here you want to cancel gr to find the equivalent amount in milligrams. Because gr 1 = 60 mg, the fraction you desire so you can cancel gr is:

$$\frac{60 \text{ mg}}{\text{gr } 1}$$

$$\text{Therefore } x \text{ mg} = \frac{60 \text{ mg}}{\text{gr } 1} \times \text{gr} \frac{1}{10}$$

$$60 \times \frac{1}{10} = \frac{60}{10} = 6$$

$$x = 6 \text{ mg}$$

$$6 \text{ mg is equivalent to gr} \frac{1}{10}.$$

# CALCULATING INTAKE AND OUTPUT

The nurse often converts between systems to calculate a client's **intake and output.** Intake and output is abbreviated **I&O.** Intake refers to the monitoring of fluid a client takes orally (p.o.), by feeding tube, or parenterally. Oral intake includes fluids and solids that become liquid at body and room temperature, such as gelatin and Popsicles. Intake also includes water, broth, and juice. Intake does not include solids, such as bread, cereal, or meats. Liquid output refers to fluids that exit the body, such as diarrhea, vomitus, gastric suction, and urine. A client's intake and output are usually recorded on a special form called an intake and output flow sheet (or I&O flow sheet or record) (Figure 8-1), which varies from institution to institution. A variety of clients require I&O monitoring, such as those whose fluids are restricted and those who are receiving diuretic or intravenous (IV) therapy.

Intake and output may still be recorded at some institutions using cubic centimeters or milliliters. The preferred term for volume is milliliters. Milliliters will be used throughout this text. When measuring output, the nurse uses a graduated receptacle calibrated in metric measures (mL), and conversions are not necessary. Oral intake usually must be converted from household measures to metric measures before it can be recorded. Each time a client takes oral liquids, even those administered with medications, the amount and time are recorded on the appropriate form. The total intake and output are recorded at the end of each shift and also totalled for a 24-hour period.

Conversion of a client's intake is usually required when recording measurements such as a bowl or coffee cup. Each agency usually has an I&O sheet with a ledger that indicates the standard measurement for the utensils used in its facility. For example, it may indicate that a standard cup is 6 oz or a coffee cup is 180 mL. A client's oral intake is calculated in the same manner as other conversion problems. After each item is converted, the items are added together for the total intake. Intake and output are based on the conversion factor 1 oz = 30 mL.

| Juice glass | – 180 mL | Jello cup | – 150 mL |
| Water glass | – 210 mL | Ice cream | – 120 mL |
| Coffee cup | – 240 mL | Creamer | – 30 mL |
| Soup bowl | – 180 mL | | |
| Small water cup | – 120 mL | | |

Date __October 30, 2011__

Addressograph with Client Information

| INTAKE | | | | | | OUTPUT | | | | |
| --- | --- | --- | --- | --- | --- | --- | --- | --- | --- | --- |
| ORAL | | | IV | | | | | | OTHER | |
| TIME | TYPE | AMT | TIME | TYPE | AMOUNT ABSORBED | TIME | URINE | STOOL | | |
| 8A | Juice | 60 mL | | | | | | | | |
| | Coffee | 120 mL | | | | | | | | |
| | Milk | 250 mL | | | | | | | | |
| | | | | | | | | | | |
| | | | | | | | | | | |
| | | | | | | | | | | |
| | | | | | | | | | | |
| | | | | | | | | | | |

**Figure 8-1**    Sample I&O flow sheet.

**Example:** Calculate the client's intake for breakfast in milliliters. Assume that the glass holds 6 oz and the cup holds 8 oz. The client had the following for breakfast at 8 AM:

**Items**
⅓ glass of apple juice
2 sausages
1 boiled egg
½ cup of coffee
½ pint of milk

**Conversion Factors**
1 oz = 30 mL
1 pint = 500 mL
1 cup = 8 oz
1 glass = 6 oz

> **NOTE**
>
> Two sausages and one boiled egg are not part of fluid intake.

**Solution:**

1. ⅓ glass of apple juice

$$1 \text{ glass} = 6 \text{ oz}; \frac{1}{3} \text{ of } 6 \text{ oz} = 2 \text{ oz}$$

Therefore 1 oz = 30 mL, 2 oz × 30 mL = 60 mL

*or* 1 oz : 30 mL = 2 oz : *x* mL, *x* = 60 mL

$$x \text{ mL} = \frac{30 \text{ mL}}{1 \text{ o\!\!\!/z}} \times \frac{2 \text{ o\!\!\!/z}}{1}$$

 **Solution Using Dimensional Analysis**

2. ½ cup of coffee

$$1 \text{ cup} = 8 \text{ oz}; \frac{1}{2} \text{ of } 8 \text{ oz} = 4 \text{ oz}$$

Therefore 4 oz × 30 = 120 mL

*or* 1 oz : 30 mL = 4 oz : *x* mL, *x* = 120 mL

$$x \text{ mL} = \frac{30 \text{ mL}}{1 \text{ o\!\!\!/z}} \times \frac{4 \text{ o\!\!\!/z}}{1}$$

 **Solution Using Dimensional Analysis**

3. ½ pint of milk

$$1 \text{ pint} = 500 \text{ mL}; \frac{1}{2} \text{ of } 500 \text{ mL} = 250 \text{ mL}$$

4. Total mL = 60 mL + 120 mL + 250 mL = 430 mL

Another solution would be to total the number of ounces, which in this example is 6 oz, convert that amount to milliliters, and add the half pint of milk (expressed in milliliters).

$$1 \text{ oz} : 30 \text{ mL} = 6 \text{ oz} : x \text{ mL}$$

$$x = 180 \text{ mL}$$

$$180 \text{ mL} + 250 \text{ mL} \left( \frac{1}{2} \text{ pint} \right) = 430 \text{ mL}$$

 **Solution Using Dimensional Analysis**

$$x \text{ mL} = \frac{30 \text{ mL}}{1 \text{ o\!\!\!/z}} \times \frac{6 \text{ o\!\!\!/z}}{1}$$

The conversions are recorded on an I&O flow sheet (or record) next to time ingested. The I&O sheet in Figure 8-1 is filled out with the data for this sample problem.

8:00 AM    juice, 60 mL
           coffee, 120 mL
           milk, 250 mL

In addition to the oral intake, if a client is receiving IV therapy, the amount of IV fluid given is also recorded on the I&O flow sheet (or record). When an IV bottle or bag is hung or added, the nurse indicates the time and the type and amount of fluid in the appropriate column on the I&O flow sheet (or record). When the IV fluid has infused or the IV is changed, the nurse records the actual amount of fluid **infused,** or **absorbed.**

In a situation in which a bag or bottle of IV fluid is not completed by the end of the shift, the nurse beginning the next shift is informed of how much fluid is left in the bag. At some institutions the amount is also indicated on the I&O flow sheet (or record) with the abbreviation LIB (left in bag or bottle).

**Example:**    The nurse hangs a 1,000-mL bag of D5W at 7 AM. At 3 PM 150 mL is left in the bag. The nurse records 850 mL was absorbed and indicates 150 mL is LIB. Refer to the sample I&O form in Figure 8-2 showing how this example is charted.

I&O flow sheets usually have a place for recording p.o. intake, IV intake, and a column or columns for output. Figure 8-3 shows a sample 24-hour I&O flow sheet illustrating the charting of intake.

As discussed, output is also recorded on the I&O form. The most commonly measured output is urine. After a client's output is recorded, sometimes the nurse needs to compute an average. The most important average nurses compute in most health care settings is the hourly urine output. The **hourly** urine output for an adult to maintain proper renal function is 30 mL/hr to 50 mL/hr. Usually the hourly amount is more significant than each voiding. To find the hourly average of urinary output, take the total and divide by the number of hours.

**NOTE**

This amount is above the minimum hourly average (30 mL/hr) for adequate kidney function in the adult.

**Example:**    $\dfrac{400 \text{ mL of urine}}{8 \text{ hr}} = 50$ mL of urine/hr

Juice glass – 180 mL    Small water cup – 120 mL
Water glass – 210 mL    Jello cup – 150 mL
Coffee cup – 240 mL    Ice cream – 120 mL
Soup bowl – 180 mL    Creamer – 30 mL

**Date:** September 21, 2011

Client information

| INTAKE | | | | | OUTPUT | | | | |
|---|---|---|---|---|---|---|---|---|---|
| Time | Type | Amt | Time | IV/ blood type | Amount absorbed | Time | Urine | Stool | Other |
| | | | 7A | D5W 1,000 mL | 850 mL | | | | |
| | | | | | | | | | |
| | | | | | | | | | |
| | | | | | | | | | |
| | | | | | | | | | |
| | | | | | | | | | |
| 8 hr total | | | | | 850 mL | | | | |
| | | | 3P | D5W 150 mL LIB | | | | | |

**Figure 8-2**    Charting IV fluids on an I&O flow sheet. *LIB,* Left in bag.

The charting of I&O varies at each institution. Always check the policies to ensure compliance with a particular institution.

| Juice glass | – 180 mL | Small water cup | – 120 mL |
|---|---|---|---|
| Water glass | – 210 mL | Jello cup | – 150 mL |
| Coffee cup | – 240 mL | Ice cream | – 120 mL |
| Soup bowl | – 180 mL | Creamer | – 30 mL |

**Date:** September 21, 2011

Client information

| INTAKE | | | | | OUTPUT | | | | |
|---|---|---|---|---|---|---|---|---|---|
| Time | Type | Amt | Time | IV/ blood type | Amount absorbed | Time | Urine | Stool | Other |
| 8A | juice | 240 mL | 7A | D5W 1,000 mL | 850 mL | 8A | 300 mL | | |
| | milk | 120 mL | | | | 10A | 200 mL | | |
| | coffee | 200 mL | | | | 1³⁰/P | 425 mL | | |
| 9³⁰/A | water | 60 mL | | | | | | | |
| 12P | broth | 180 mL | | | | | | | |
| | juice | 120 mL | | | | | | | |
| 1P | water | 120 mL | | | | | | | |
| | | | | | | | | | |
| 8 hr total | | 1,040 mL | | | 850 mL | | 925 mL | | |
| 5P | tea | 100 mL | 3P | LIB D5W 150 mL | 150 mL | 4p | 425 mL | | |
| | broth | 360 mL | 5P | D5W 1,000 mL | 750 mL | 7p | 350 mL | | |
| | ice-cream | 120 mL | | | | 9³⁰/P | 200 mL | | |
| 9 P | water | 240 mL | | | | | | | |
| | | | | | | | | | |
| | | | | | | | | | |
| 8 hr total | | 820 mL | | | 900 mL | | 975 mL | | |
| 1A | water | 120 mL | 11P | LIB D5W 250 mL | 250 mL | | | | |
| 5A | tea | 200 mL | 3A | D5W 1,000 mL | 600 mL | 2A | 350 mL | | |
| | | | | | | 5A | 150 mL | | |
| | | | | | | | | | |
| | | | | | | | | | |
| | | | | | | | | | |
| | | | | | | | | | |
| | | | | | | | | | |
| 8 hr total | | 320 mL | | | 850 mL | | 500 mL | | |
| 24 hr total | | 2,180 mL | | | 2,600 mL | | 2,400 mL | | |

Total intake 24 hr: (4,780 mL)   (2,180 mL + 2,600 mL)

Total output 24 hr: (2,400 mL)   (925 mL + 975 mL + 500 mL)

**Figure 8-3**   I&O flow sheet (completed 24 hours). *LIB,* Left in bag.

**Practice Problems**

Convert the following to the equivalent measures indicated.

41. 60 lb = _____ kg

42. 15 mg = gr _____

43. oz 5 = _____ mL

44. gr v = _____ mg

45. 7 oz = _____ mL

46. 250 mL = _____ qt

47. 45 mL = _____ tbs

48. gr 45 = _____ g

49. gr $1\frac{1}{2}$ = _____ mg

50. 20 mL = _____ tsp

51. gr $5\frac{1}{2}$ = _____ mg

52. 4 qt = _____ mL

53. 72 kg = _____ lb

54. gr $\frac{1}{125}$ = _____ mg

55. 2.4 L = _____ mL

Compute how much IV fluid you would document on an I&O form as being absorbed from a 1,000 mL bag if the following amounts remain.

56. 300 mL _____

57. 450 mL _____

58. 100 mL _____

Compute the average hourly urinary output in the following situations (round to nearest whole number).

59. 650 mL in 8 hr _____

60. 250 mL in 8 hr _____

61. 1,000 mL in 24 hr _____

62. 1,240 mL in 24 hr _____

63. A client's output for the 3 to 11 PM shift was as follows:

    325 mL of urine at 4:00 PM
     75 mL of vomitus at 7:00 PM
    225 mL of urine at 8:00 PM
    200 mL of nasogastric (NG) drainage at 11:00 PM
     50 mL of wound drainage at 11:00 PM
    What is the total output in milliliters? _____

64. What is the client's output in liters in question 63? _____

65. If 375 mL of a 500 mL bag of IV solution was absorbed on the 3 to 11 PM shift, the nurse records that 375 mL was absorbed. How many milliliters are recorded as left in bag (LIB)? _____

Answers on p. 607

## ■ Points to Remember

- Regardless of the method used for converting, **memorizing equivalents** is a necessity.
- Answers stated in fraction format should be **reduced** as necessary.
- When more than one equivalent is learned for a unit, use the **most common equivalent** for the measure or use the number that divides equally without a remainder.
- The apothecary system does not convert exactly to metric.
- Division should be carried to the hundredths place or two decimal places to ensure accuracy, and it is not rounded.
- Decimal point movement as a method for converting is limited to the metric system; ratio and proportion, dimensional analysis, and conversion factor method can be used for all systems of measure.
- Oral intake is converted before placing data on an I&O flow sheet (or record). The amount is usually recorded in cubic centimeters at many institutions; however, milliliter is the correct unit for volume. Conversion factor for I&O is 1 oz = 30 mL.
- Always check the policy of the institution regarding I&O and the charting of it.
- The most common units of measure used to calculate dosages are metric units of measurement.

## CHAPTER REVIEW

Convert the following to the equivalent measures indicated.

1. 0.007 g = _____ mg

2. 1 mg = _____ g

3. 6,000 g = _____ kg

4. 5 mL = _____ L

5. 0.45 L = _____ mL

6. 75 mL = oz _____

7. gr $\frac{1}{300}$ = _____ mg

8. 1 mg = gr _____

9. gr ii = _____ mg

10. 1$\frac{1}{2}$ qt = _____ mL

11. 30 mg = gr _____

12. 1.6 L = _____ mL

13. 47 kg = _____ lb

14. 3 mL = _____ L

15. 75 lb = _____ kg

16. 0.008 g = _____ mg

17. 4$\frac{1}{2}$ pt = _____ mL

18. g $\frac{1}{2}$ = _____ mg

19. g $\frac{1}{150}$ = _____ mg

20. 6,172 g = _____ kg

21. 200 mL = _____ tsp

22. 102 lb = _____ kg

23. 204 g = _____ kg

24. 1.5 L = _____ mL

25. 200 mcg = _____ mg

26. 48.6 L = _____ mL

27. 0.7 L = _____ mL

28. 6½ oz = _____ mL

29. 4 tsp = _____ mL

30. gr iv = _____ mg

31. 2 tbs = _____ mL

32. 67.5 mL = _____ t

33. 45 mg = gr _____

34. gr 45 = _____ g

35. 20 oz = _____ mL

36. gr $2\frac{1}{2}$ = _____ mg

37. gr $\frac{3}{8}$ = _____ mg

38. gr x = _____ mg

39. 4 kg = _____ lb

40. 3.25 mg = _____ mcg

41. 10 mL = oz _____

42. gr $\frac{1}{120}$ = _____ mg

43. 6.653 g = _____ mg

44. 4 g = _____ mg

45. 36 mg = _____ g

46. 0.8 g = _____ mg

47. 9 g = gr _____

48. 0.5 mg = gr _____

49. 2 qt = _____ L

Calculate the fluid intake in milliliters. Use the following equivalents for the problems below: 1 cup = 8 oz, 1 glass = 4 oz.

50. Client had the following at lunch:
    4 oz fruit cocktail
    1 tuna fish sandwich
    ½ cup of tea
    ¼ pt of milk

    Total mL = _____

51. Calculate the following individual items and give the total number of milliliters:
    3 Popsicles (3 oz each)
    ½ qt iced tea
    1½ glasses water
    12 oz soft drink

    Total mL = _____

52. Client had the following:
    8 oz milk
    6 oz orange juice
    4 oz water with medication

    Total mL = _____

53. Client had the following:
    10 oz of coffee
    8 oz of water
    6 oz of broth

    Total mL = _____

54. Client had the following:
    ¾ glass of milk
    4 oz water
    2 oz beef broth

    Total mL = _____

55. A client had the following at lunch:
    ¼ glass of apple juice
    8 oz chicken broth
    6 oz gelatin dessert
    1¾ cups of coffee

    Total mL = _____

Convert the following amounts of fluid to milliliters.

56. $3\dfrac{1}{2}$ oz = _____ mL    57. $\dfrac{3}{4}$ C (8 oz cup) = _____ mL

Compute how much IV fluid you would document on an I&O form as being absorbed from a 1,000 mL bag if the following amounts are left in the bag.

58. 275 mL _____    60. 75 mL _____

59. 550 mL _____

Compute the average hourly urinary output in each of the following situations (round to nearest whole number).

61. 500 mL in 8 hr _____    63. 700 mL in 8 hr _____

62. 640 mL in 24 hr _____

Compute how much IV fluid you would document on an I&O form as being absorbed from a 500 mL bag if the following amounts are left in the bag.

64. 125 mL _____

65. 225 mL _____

66. A client received 1,750 mL of IV fluid. How many liters of IV fluid did the client

    receive?_____

67. A client has an order for 125 mcg of digoxin. How many milligrams will you administer to the client? _____

68. The prescriber directs a client to take 15 oz of the laxative agent GoLYTELY. The

    cup holds 6 oz. How many cups will the client have to drink?_____

69. A client has an order for 1,500 mL of water by mouth every 24 hours. How many

    ounces is this?_____

70. A client had an output of 1.1 L. How many milliliters is this? _____

Answers on p. 607

 **For additional practice problems, refer to the Introducing Drug Measures section of Drug Calculations Companion, Version 4, on Evolve.**

# Additional Conversions Useful in the Health Care Setting

## Objectives

*After reviewing this chapter, you should be able to:*
1. Convert between Celsius and Fahrenheit temperature
2. Convert between units of length: inches, centimeters, and millimeters
3. Convert between units of weight: pounds and kilograms, pounds and ounces to kilograms
4. Convert between traditional and military (international) time

## CONVERTING BETWEEN CELSIUS AND FAHRENHEIT

Many health care facilities use electronic digital temperature-taking devices that instantly convert between the two scales; however, such devices do not eliminate the need for the nurse to understand the difference between Celsius and Fahrenheit. In addition, it may be necessary for the nurse to explain to clients or families how to convert from one to the other.

Another factor is the recognition that all persons involved in client care do not have a "universal" measurement for temperature; therefore Fahrenheit or Celsius may be used. Let's look first at some general information that will help you understand the formulas used.

### Differentiating Between Celsius and Fahrenheit

To differentiate which scale is being used (Fahrenheit or Celsius), the temperature reading is followed by an *F* or *C*. *F* indicates Fahrenheit, and *C* indicates Celsius. (*Note:* Celsius was formerly known as *centigrade*.)

**Examples:**     98° F

                 36° C

The freezing point of water on the Fahrenheit scale is **32° F,** and the boiling point is **212° F.** The freezing point of water on the Celsius scale is **0° C,** and the boiling point is **100° C.**

The difference between the freezing and boiling points on the Fahrenheit scale is **180°,** whereas the difference between these points on the Celsius scale is **100°.**

The differences between Fahrenheit and Celsius in relation to the freezing and boiling points led to the development of appropriate conversion formulas. Figure 9-1 shows two thermometers reflecting the relationship of pertinent values between the two scales. Figure 9-2 shows medically important Celsius and Fahrenheit temperature ranges.

The **32° difference** between the freezing point on the scales is used for converting temperature from one scale to the other. There is a **180°** difference between the boiling and freezing points on the Fahrenheit thermometer and **100°** between the boiling and freezing points on the Celsius scale. These differences can be set as a ratio, 180:100. Therefore consider the following:

$$180:100 = \frac{180}{100} = \frac{9}{5}$$

The fraction $\frac{9}{5}$ expressed as a decimal is 1.8; therefore you will see this constant used in temperature conversions.

**Figure 9-1**  Celsius and Fahrenheit temperature scales. (From Clayton BD, Stock YN: *Basic pharmacology for nurses,* ed. 14, St. Louis, 2007, Mosby.) *Note:* Glass thermometers pictured here are for demonstration purposes only. Electronic digital temperature devices are more commonly used in health care settings.

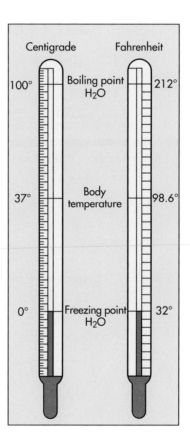

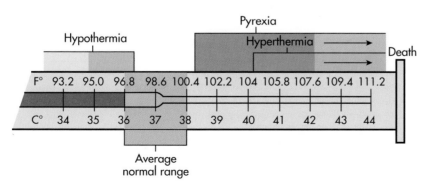

**Figure 9-2**  Ranges of normal temperature values and physiological consequences of abnormal body temperature. (From Potter PA, Perry AG: *Fundamentals of nursing,* ed. 7, St. Louis, 2009, Mosby.)

## FORMULAS FOR CONVERTING BETWEEN FAHRENHEIT AND CELSIUS SCALES

**RULE**

To convert from Celsius to Fahrenheit, multiply by 1.8 and add 32.

**NOTE**

Your preference for one of these formulas is based on whether you find it easier to work with decimals or fractions.

$$^\circ F = 1.8(^\circ C) + 32$$

*or*

$$^\circ F = \frac{9}{5}(^\circ C) + 32$$

**Example:**    Convert 37.5° C to ° F.

$$^\circ F = 1.8(37.5) + 32 \qquad\qquad\qquad ^\circ F = \frac{9}{5}(37.5) + 32$$

$$^\circ F = 67.5 + 32 \qquad\quad or \qquad\quad ^\circ F = 67.5 + 32$$

$$^\circ F = 99.5^\circ \qquad\qquad\qquad\qquad\quad ^\circ F = 99.5^\circ$$

**RULE**

To convert from Fahrenheit to Celsius, subtract 32 and divide by 1.8.

**NOTE**

When converting between Fahrenheit and Celsius, if necessary, carry the math process to hundredths and round to tenths.

$$^\circ C = \frac{^\circ F - 32}{1.8} \qquad or \qquad ^\circ C = (^\circ F - 32) \div \frac{9}{5}$$

**Example:**    Convert 68° F to ° C.

$$^\circ C = \frac{68 - 32}{1.8} \qquad\qquad\qquad ^\circ C = (68 - 32) \div \frac{9}{5}$$

$$^\circ C = \frac{36}{1.8} \qquad\quad or \qquad\quad ^\circ C = 36 \div \frac{9}{5}$$

$$^\circ C = (36) \times \frac{5}{9}$$

$$^\circ C = 20^\circ \qquad\qquad\qquad\qquad ^\circ C = 20^\circ$$

 **Practice Problems**

Convert the following temperatures as indicated (round your answer to tenths).

1. 4° C = _____ ° F    4. 101.3° F = _____ ° C

2. 101° F = _____ ° C    5. 37.5° C = _____ ° F

3. 38.1° C = _____ ° F

Change the given temperatures in the following statements to their corresponding equivalents in ° C or ° F.

6. Store medication at room temperature: 20° to 25 ° C. _____ ° F

7. Notify health care provider for temperature greater than 101° F. _____ ° C

8. Store vaccine serum at 7° F. _____ ° C

9. Normal adult body temperature is 37° C. _____ ° F

10. Do not store IV solutions at less than 46° F. _____ ° C

Answers on p. 607

---

In addition to temperature conversions, other measures that may be encountered in the health care setting relate to linear measurement. As with temperature conversion, even though there are devices that instantly convert these measures, nurses need to understand the process. For the purpose of this chapter, we will focus on millimeters (mm) and centimeters (cm).

## METRIC MEASURES RELATING TO LENGTH

In health care settings metric measures relating to length are used. Diameter of the pupil of the eye may be described in millimeters; the normal diameter of pupils is 3 to 7 mm. Charts may show pupillary size in millimeters. Accommodation of pupils is tested by asking a client to gaze at a distant object (e.g., a far wall) and then at a test object (e.g., a finger or pencil) held by the examiner approximately 10 cm (4 in) from the bridge of the client's nose.

A baby's head and chest circumference are expressed in centimeters. Gauze for dressings is available in different size squares measured in centimeters.

**Example:**  10 × 10 cm (4 × 4 in); 5 × 5 cm (2 × 2 in)

Also, incisions may be expressed in measures such as centimeters (refer to conversions in Box 9-1).

Now let's try some conversions using these equivalents.

**Example 1:**  A client's incision measures 25 mm. How many centimeters is this?

**Conversion factor:**  1 cm = 10 mm

**Solution:**  Think: mm is smaller and cm is larger. Divide by 10, or move the decimal point one place to the left.

$$25 \div 10 = 2.5 \text{ cm } or \; 25. = 2.5 \text{ cm}$$

**Answer:**  2.5 cm

---

### BOX 9-1   Conversions Relating to Length

1 cm = 10 mm
1 in = 2.54 cm*

---

*The approximate conversion of 1 in = 2.5 cm is used for conversions.

In Example 2, you cannot get this answer by decimal movement. You are converting to inches, which is a household measure.

Any of the methods presented in previous chapters may be used for conversion. Remember, however, that decimal movement is limited to conversions from one metric measure to another, and the number of places the decimal is moved is based on the conversion factor. If necessary, review previous chapters relating to converting.

**Example 2:**   Convert 30 cm to inches (in).

**Conversion factor:**   1 in = 2.5 cm

**Solution:**       Think: smaller to larger (divide).

$$30 \div 2.5 = 12 \text{ in}$$

**Answer:**       12 in

**Example 3:**   An infant's head circumference is 35.5 cm. How many millimeters is this?

**Conversion factor:**   1 cm = 10 mm

**Solution:**       Think: larger to smaller (multiply). Multiply by 10, or move the decimal point one place to the right.

$$35.5 \times 10 = 355 \text{ mm } or\ 35.5 = 355 \text{ mm}$$

**Answer:**       355 mm

 **Practice Problems**

Convert the following to the equivalent indicated.

11.  A gauze pad for a dressing is

     10 cm _____ in

12.  A client's incision measures

     45 mm _____ cm

13.  An infant's head circumference is

     37.5 cm _____ mm

14.  A newborn is $20\frac{1}{2}$ in long

     _____ cm

15.  14.8 in = _____ cm

16.  6.5 cm = _____ in

17.  100 in = _____ cm

18.  An infant's chest circumference is

     32 cm _____ in

19.  An infant's head circumference is

     38 cm _____ in

20.  A newborn is 20 in long

     _____ cm

Answers on p. 607

## CONVERSIONS RELATING TO WEIGHT

Determination of body weight is important for calculating dosages in adults, children, and, because of the immaturity of their systems, even more so in infants and neonates. This chapter focuses on converting weights for adults and children. Medications such as heparin are more therapeutic when based on weight in kilograms. The most frequently used calculation method for pediatric medication administration is milligrams per kilogram. Some medications are calculated in micrograms per kilogram.

Because medication dosages in drug references are usually based on kilograms, it is essential to be able to convert from pounds to kilograms. However, the nurse also needs to know how to do the opposite (convert from kilograms to pounds). In addition, because a child's weight may be in pounds and ounces, conversion of these units to kilograms is also important. Knowledge of weight conversions is an important part of general nursing knowledge. The nurse must be able to explain conversions to others to determine and administer medication dosages accurately and safely.

## Converting Pounds to Kilograms

> Equivalent: 2.2 lb = 1 kg
> To convert lb to kg divide by 2.2 (think smaller to larger).
> The answer is rounded to the nearest tenth.

*[handwritten annotation: → put formula on top.]*

**Example 1:** A child weighs 65 lb. Convert to kilograms.

$$65 \div 2.2 = 29.54 = 29.5 \text{ kg}$$

**Example 2:** An adult weighs 135 lb. Convert to kilograms.

$$135 \div 2.2 = 61.36 = 61.4 \text{ kg}$$

## Converting Weight in Pounds and Ounces to Kilograms

*[handwritten annotation: — Add this to form. bx]*

**Step 1:** Convert the ounces to the nearest tenth of a pound, and **add** this to the total pounds.

Equivalent: 16 oz = 1 lb

**Step 2:** Convert the total pounds to kilograms, and round to the nearest tenth.

Equivalent: 2.2 lb = 1 kg

**Example 1:** A child's weight is 10 lb, 2 oz.

Think: smaller to larger.

$$2 \text{ oz} \div 16 = 0.12 = 0.1 \text{ lb}$$

$$10 \text{ lb} + 0.1 \text{ lb} = 10.1 \text{ lb}$$

Think: smaller to larger.

$$10.1 \div 2.2 = 4.59 = 4.6 \text{ kg}$$

**Example 2:** A child's weight is 7 lb, 4 oz.

$$4 \text{ oz} \div 16 = 0.25 = 0.3 \text{ lb}$$

$$7 \text{ lb} + 0.3 \text{ lb} = 7.3 \text{ lb}$$

$$7.3 \div 2.2 = 3.31 = 3.3 \text{ kg}$$

 **Practice Problems**

Convert the following weights to kilograms (round to the nearest tenth).

21. 6 lb, 5 oz _____     23. 10 lb, 4 oz _____

22. 12 lb, 2 oz _____     24. 7 lb, 12 oz _____

Convert the following weights in pounds to kilograms (round to the nearest tenth where indicated).

25.  20 lb = _____ kg    28.  121 lb = _____ kg

26.  64 lb = _____ kg    29.  85 lb = _____ kg

27.  22 lb = _____ kg    Answers on pp. 607-608

---

### Converting Kilograms to Pounds

**RULE**

Equivalent: 2.2 lb = 1 kg
To convert kilograms to pounds, multiply by 2.2. (Think: larger to smaller.)
Answer is expressed to the nearest tenth.

---

**NOTE**

Any of the methods presented in Chapter 8 for converting could also be used to convert from pounds to kilograms and kilograms to pounds, except for decimal movement.

**Example 1:**   A child weighs 24.7 kg. Convert to pounds.

$$(24.7) \times 2.2 = 54.34 = 54.3 \text{ lb}$$

**Example 2:**   An adult weighs 72.2 kg. Convert to pounds.

$$(72.2) \times 2.2 = 158.84 = 158.8 \text{ lb}$$

 **Practice Problems**

**NOTE**

Although a pound is an apothecary measure, a decimal may be used to express weights.

Convert the following weights in kilograms to pounds (round to the nearest tenth where indicated).

30.  20 kg = _____ lb    33.  10.4 kg = _____ lb

31.  46 kg = _____ lb    34.  34.9 kg = _____ lb

32.  98.2 kg = _____ lb    35.  5.8 kg = _____ lb

Answers on p. 608

---

## MILITARY TIME

Another conversion that is necessary for the nurse to know is the conversion of traditional time to military time (international time). Although some watches are manufactured with traditional time and military time visible on the face of the watch to eliminate confusion, learning the conversion of time is the best method for avoiding errors.

Military time (international time) is a 24-hour clock (Figure 9-3). The main advantage of using military time is that it helps prevent errors because numbers are not repeated. The times 7 AM and 7 PM may look very similar if the A and P are not clear. In military time the colon and AM and PM are omitted. Military hours start at 1 AM, or 0100 in the morning and end at 12 midnight, which is 0000 or 2400. The time 0000 is commonly used by the military and read as "zero hundred." Although still referred to as military time, a more accurate term is "computer time." The reason for using the 24-hour clock in computers is that computers cannot understand AM and PM.

Many health care facilities are using military time in documentation such as nursing notes and medical administration records (MARs). Military time is being increasingly used as opposed to traditional time (ante meridiem [AM] and post meridiem [PM]).

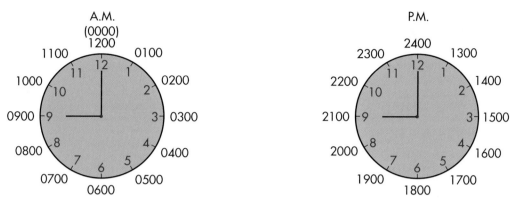

**Figure 9-3** Clocks showing traditional and military time.

## Rules for Conversion to Military Time (Computer Time)

**RULE**

To convert AM time: omit the colon and AM and ensure that a 4-digit number is written, adding a zero in the beginning as needed.

**Example:** 8:45 AM = 0845

**RULE**

To convert PM time: omit the colon and PM; add 1200 to time.

**Example:** 7:50 PM = 750 + 1200 = 1950

## Rules for Converting to Traditional Time

**RULE**

To convert AM time: insert the colon, add AM, and delete any zero in front of number.

**Example:** 0845 = 8:45 AM

**RULE**

To convert PM time: subtract 1200, insert the colon, and add PM.

**Example:** 1950 = 1950 − 1200 = 7:50 PM

## Practice Problems

Convert the following traditional times to military (international) time.

36.  7:30 AM = _____    40.  12:16 AM = _____

37.  10:30 AM = _____    41.  6:20 AM = _____

38.  8:10 PM = _____    42.  1:30 PM = _____

39.  5:45 PM = _____

Convert the following military (international) times to traditional (AM/PM) time.

43.  0207 = _____    46.  0240 = _____

44.  1743 = _____    47.  1259 = _____

45.  0004 = _____    Answers on p. 608

## CALCULATING COMPLETION TIMES

As you will see in Chapter 22 (Basic Intravenous Calcualtions) the nurse can determine the time an IV (intravenous) bag will be completed or empty using military time (international time) or traditional time depending on institutional policy. Now that we have discussed the conversion of time, let's briefly look at how the addition of times (traditional and military) can be used. This will be discussed in more detail in Chapter 22.

### Military (International) Time Calculations

**Example 1:**    An IV started at 0300 is to be completed in 3 hr 30 min. Determine the completion time.

- Add the 3 hr 30 min infusion time to the 0300 start time.

$$
\begin{array}{r}
0300 \\
+\ 330 \\
\hline
0630
\end{array}
$$

- The completion time is 0630.

**Example 2:**    An IV started at 0650 is to be completed in 4 hr 10 min. Determine the completion time.

- Add the 4 hr 10 min infusion time to the 0650 start time.

$$
\begin{array}{r}
0650 \\
+\ 410 \\
\hline
1060
\end{array}
$$

- Change the 60 min to 1 hr, and add to 1000 to equal 1100.

### Traditional Time Calculations

**Example 1:**    An IV medication will infuse in 30 minutes. It is now 6:15 PM. Determine the completion time.

- Add the 30-min infusion time to the 6:15 PM start time.

$$6{:}15 \text{ PM} + 30 \text{ min} = 6{:}45 \text{ PM}$$

- The completion time is 6:45 PM.

**Example 2:**    An IV with an infusion time of 12 hr is started at 2:00 AM. Determine the completion time.

- Add the 12-hr infusion time to the 2:00 AM start time.

$$
\begin{array}{r}
2{:}00 \text{ AM} \\
+\ 12{:}00 \\
\hline
14{:}00
\end{array}
$$

- Subtract 12 hr to make the time 2:00 PM.

 ## Practice Problems

Calculate the following completion times in military (international) time.

48. An IV started at 0215 to infuse in 2 hr 30 min _____

49. An IV started at 0250 to infuse in 5 hr 10 min _____

Calculate the following completion times in traditional time.

50. An IV started at 6:30 AM that has an infusion time of 45 min _____

51. An IV started at 9:00 AM that has an infusion time of 6 hr 30 min _____

Answers on p. 608

## Points to Remember

Use these formulas to convert between Fahrenheit and Celsius temperature.

- To convert from °C to °F: $°F = 1.8\,(°C) + 32 \ or \ \dfrac{9}{5}\,(°C) + 32.$

- To convert from °F to °C: $°C = \dfrac{°F - 32}{1.8} \ or \ (°F - 32) \div \dfrac{9}{5}.$

- When converting between Fahrenheit and Celsius, carry math to hundredths and round to tenths.

### Conversions Relating to Length

- Conversions can be made by using any of the methods presented in the chapter on conversions; however, moving of decimals is limited to converting between metric measures.

$$1 \text{ cm} = 10 \text{ mm}$$
$$1 \text{ inch} = 2.5 \text{ cm}$$

### Conversions Relating to Weight

$$2.2 \text{ lb} = 1 \text{ kg}$$
$$16 \text{ oz} = 1 \text{ lb}$$

- Weight conversion of pounds to kilograms is done most often because many medications are based on kilograms of body weight.
- Body weight is **essential** for determining dosages in infants and neonates.
- To convert pounds to kilograms, divide by 2.2. Round answer to the nearest tenth.
- To convert pounds and ounces to kilograms, convert the ounces to the nearest tenth of a pound; add this to the total pounds. Convert the total pounds to kilograms and round answer to the nearest tenth.
- To convert kilograms to pounds, multiply by 2.2. Round answer to the nearest tenth.

**Conversions Relating to Time**

- Military time is also referred to as international time. A more accurate term is *computer* time.
- To change traditional AM time to military time, omit the colon and AM and make sure that a 4-digit number is written, adding a zero in the beginning as needed.
- To change traditional PM time to military time, omit the colon and PM, and add 1200 to the time.
- To convert military time to traditional AM time, insert a colon and add AM. Delete any zero in front of numbers.
- To convert military time to traditional PM time, subtract 1200, insert the colon, and add PM.
- International time decreases the possibility of error in administering medications or misinterpretation of when a therapy is due or actually was done because no two times are expressed by the same number.

# ✓ CHAPTER REVIEW

For each of the following statements, change the given temperature to its corresponding equivalent in ° C or ° F. (Round to the nearest tenth.)

1. Notify health care provider for temperature greater than 101.4° F. _____ ° C

2. Store medication at room temperature, 77° F. _____ ° C

3. Store medication within temperature range of 15° C to 30° C. _____ ° F

4. An infant has a body temperature of 36.5° C. _____ ° F

5. Store vaccine at 6° C. _____ ° F

6. A nurse reports a temperature of 37.8° C. _____ ° F

7. Do not expose a medication to temperatures greater than 84° F. _____ ° C

8. A medication contains a crystalline substance with a melting point of about 186° C. _____ ° F

9. Store vaccine at 4° C. _____ ° F

10. Do not expose medication to temperatures greater than 88° F. _____ ° C

Convert temperatures as indicated. Round your answer to the nearest tenth.

11. −10° C = _____ ° F     18. 64.4° F = _____ ° C

12. 0° F = _____ ° C     19. 35° C = _____ ° F

13. 102.8° F = _____ ° C     20. 50° F = _____ ° C

14. 29° C = _____ ° F     21. 39.8° C = _____ ° F

15. 106° C = _____ ° F     22. 86° F = _____ ° C

16. 70° F = _____ ° C     23. 41° C = _____ ° F

17. 39.6° C = _____ ° F

Convert the following to the equivalent indicated.

24. 18 in = _____ cm    30. 4 in = _____ cm

25. 31 cm = _____ in    31. 36.6 cm = _____ mm

26. 44.5 cm = _____ mm    32. 6.2 in = _____ cm

27. 32 in = _____ cm    33. 350 mm = _____ in

28. 3 cm = _____ mm    34. 21$^{1}/_{2}$ in = _____ cm

29. 7.9 cm = _____ mm    35. 2 in = _____ mm

Convert the following weights in pounds to kilograms (round to the nearest tenth where indicated).

36. 63 lb = _____ kg    39. 81 lb = _____ kg

37. 150 lb = _____ kg    40. 27 lb = _____ kg

38. 78 lb = _____ kg

Convert the following weights in kilograms to pounds (round to the nearest tenth of a pound).

41. 77.3 kg = _____ lb    44. 9 kg = _____ lb

42. 7 kg = _____ lb    45. 56.1 kg = _____ lb

43. 4.5 kg = _____ lb

46. A child weighs 70 lb during a pediatric clinic visit. How many kilograms does the child weigh? (Round to the nearest tenth.) _____

47. A client's wound measures 41 mm. How many centimeters is this? _____ cm

48. A client weighs 99.2 kg. How many pounds does the client weigh? (Round to the nearest tenth.) _____ lb

49. An infant's head circumference is 40 cm. How many inches is this? _____ in

50. An infant's head circumference is 40.6 cm. How many millimeters is this? _____ mm

Convert the following weights to kilograms. (Round to the nearest tenth.)

51. 7 lb, 1 oz _____    54. 8 lb, 10 oz _____

52. 9 lb, 3 oz _____    55. 5 lb, 5 oz _____

53. 10 lb, 12 oz _____

Convert the following military (international) times to traditional times (AM/PM).

56. 0032 = _____          59. 1345 = _____

57. 0220 = _____          60. 2122 = _____

58. 1650 = _____

Convert the following traditional times to military (international) times.

61. 5:20 AM = _____          64. 4:30 PM = _____

62. 12:00 midnight = _____          65. 1:35 PM = _____

63. 12:05 AM = _____

State whether AM or PM is represented by the following times.

66. 0154 _____

67. 1450 _____

68. If a client had IV therapy for 8 hours, ending at 1100, when on the 24-hour clock

   was the IV started? _____

State the following completion times as indicated.

69. An IV started at 11:50 PM with an infusion time of 3 hr 30 min _____

   (standard time).

70. An IV started at 0025 with an infusion time of 1 hr 15 min _____

   (military time).

Answers on p. 608

 **For additional information, refer to the Introducing Drug
Measures section on Drug Calculations Companion, Version 4,
on Evolve.**

# Methods of Administration and Calculation

Note: The safe and accurate administration of medications to a client is an important and primary responsibility of a nurse. Being able to read and interpret an order correctly and calculate medication dosages is necessary for accurate administration.

# Medication Administration

## Objectives

*After reviewing this chapter, you should be able to:*
1. State the consequences of medication errors
2. Identify the causes of medication errors
3. Identify the role of the nurse in preventing medication errors
4. Identify the role of the Institute for Safe Medication Practices (ISMP) and The Joint Commission (TJC) in the prevention of medication errors
5. State the six "rights" of safe medication administration
6. Identify factors that influence medication dosages
7. Identify the common routes for medication administration
8. Define *critical thinking*
9. Explain the importance of critical thinking in medication administration
10. Identify important critical thinking skills necessary in medication administration
11. Discuss the importance of client teaching
12. Identify special considerations relating to the elderly and medication administration
13. Identify home care considerations in relation to medication administration

## MEDICATION ERRORS

Medications are therapeutic measures aimed at improving clients' health. Medication administration is one of the most critical functions of nursing practice; and doses must be prepared, dispensed, and administered safely and appropriately (Cohen, 2007). When administered carelessly and incorrectly the consequences can be harmful and threatening to the life of a client. Tragic outcomes include increased hospital stay, acute or chronic disability, or even death.

Medication errors may also affect the nurse both emotionally and professionally and could result in loss of position, legal consequences, or loss of license to practice.

Numerous publicized medication errors have caused astonishment among members of the health care profession and society as a whole. According to current literature, despite technological advances, preventive strategies, systematic methods of reporting errors, and definitions of what constitutes error, medication errors continue to be one of the most common causes of client injury.

Hidle (2007-2008) estimated that 44,000 to 98,000 people die each year from medication errors. These errors are most prevalent in infants and children, where medication dosages are calculated by body weight or body surface area. These highly unscientific measures leave children more prone to be victims of medical errors than adults.

Hidle (2007-2008) also refers to medication errors related to clients with underlying diseases, such as impaired renal function, clients in intensive care settings because of complex medical diagnoses, and the large number of medications that nurses must deliver. Medication errors in ambulatory and outpatient settings were reported as related to lack of education concerning over-the-counter drug use and interactions with prescribed medications.

Snyderman (2008), a chief medical editor for a television station, reported that 1 in 15 hospitalized children is harmed each year because of medication errors. She estimated that this translates into 540,000 children each year being given the wrong medication or the wrong dose; and she added that the number might be even higher because community hospitals were not included in the investigation.

Information concerning medication errors has serious implications for health and safety of clients and warrants a collaborative approach with numerous strategies to prevent errors. The central role that nurses play in medication safety is a primary focus of this text and is based on the knowledge and understanding of careful and correct medication administration.

The Institute for Safe Medication Practices (ISMP) and the United States Pharmacopeia are two organizations actively involved in monitoring medication error reports, and they have developed strategies aimed at correcting the problem and educating personnel involved in the administration of medications. The Joint Commission (TJC), which provides accreditation to U.S. hospitals and health care facilities, is also working to achieve high client care standards in the U.S. health care system. One of its goals has been in the area of medication errors. TJC implemented National Patient Safety Goals, one of which is aimed at assisting health care facilities in the prevention of devastating medication errors. Technological advances in terms of medication administration (e.g., use of bar coding, computerized unit dose medication carts) have been instituted in many facilities as a means of preventing and decreasing medication errors; however, computer technology cannot replace human intellect or negate the need to follow various steps in medication administation to ensure client safety.

Medication errors can occur anywhere in the distribution process, and when an error occurs, the cause can involve multiple factors. Michael Cohen, president of ISMP, in the book titled *Medication Errors* (2007), cited some causes of medication errors, such as the following:

- Lack of information about the client (allergies, other medications the client is taking)
- Lack of information about the drug
- Communication and teamwork failures
- Unclear, absent, or look-alike drug labels and packages, and confusing or look-alike or sound-alike drug names
- Unsafe drug standardization, storage, and distribution
- Nonstandard, flawed, or unsafe medication delivery devices

Other causes of medication errors include errors in mathematical calculation of dosages, incomplete orders, failure to observe the six "rights" of medication administration when administering medications, failure to identify a client accurately, and miscommunication of orders.

Miscommunication of medication orders can involve poor handwriting, misuse of zeros and decimal points, confusion of metric and other dosing units, and inappropriate abbreviations.

Other contributing factors to medication errors include failure to educate clients properly about medications they are taking, administration of medications without critical thought, and failure to comply with the required policy or procedure related to medication administration. With the shortage of nursing personnel, factors such as shift changes, floating staff, double shifts, and workload increases have also contributed to errors. Certain medications, referred to as *high-alert medications,* have also been identified as contributing to harmful errors. The medications on this list include concentrated electrolyte solutions, such as potassium chloride. Other medications that are associated with harmful errors include heparin, insulin, morphine, neuromuscular drugs, and chemotherapy drugs.

Although advances in technology such as automatic dispensing cabinets (ADC), computer prescriber order entry (CPOE), and bar-code medication administration have decreased the number of medication errors, it has been stressed that these advances are useful only if they are properly applied and if the systems are effective and efficient.

The reasons for medication errors are not limited to those presented and are not nursing errors alone. The best solution to the problem of medication errors is prevention. To prevent medication errors, personnel involved in the administration of medications must do meticulous planning and implement the task properly, paying close attention to detail.

The administration of medications is more than just giving the medication because it is what the health care provider ordered. The health care provider orders the medication; the nurse should know the action, uses, side effects, expected response, and range of dosage for the medication being administered. Nurses are accountable when administering medications and must understand the activity, indications, and contraindications of the full range of medications they may be called on to administer.

Medication administration involves using the nursing process, which includes assessment, nursing diagnosis, planning, implementation, evaluation, and teaching clients about safe administration.

**CAUTION**

Failure to think about what you are doing and why you are doing it and failure to assess a client can result in errors.

## CRITICAL THINKING AND MEDICATION ADMINISTRATION

There are numerous definitions for *critical thinking*. The best way to define critical thinking is as a process of thinking that includes being reasonable and rational. Thinking is based on reason. Critical thinking is important to all phases of nursing but is particularly relevant in the discussion of medication administration.

Critical thinking encompasses several skills relevant to medication administration. One such skill is the ability to identify an organized approach to the task at hand. For example, in medication administration, calculating dosages in an organized, systematic manner (formula, ratio and proportion, dimensional analysis) decreases the likelihood of errors.

A second skill characteristic of critical thinking is the ability to be an autonomous thinker—for example, challenging a medication order that is written incorrectly rather than passively accepting the order. Critical thinking also involves the ability to distinguish irrelevant information from that which is relevant. For example, when reading a medication label, the nurse is able to decipher from the label the information necessary for calculating the correct dosage. Critical thinking involves reasoning and the application of concepts—for example, choosing the correct type of syringe to administer a dosage, and using concepts learned to decide the appropriateness of a dosage. Critical thinking also involves asking for clarification of what is not understood and not making assumptions. Clarifying a medication order and dosage indicates critical thinking. Checking the accuracy and reliability of information decreases the chance of medication errors. The ability to validate information requires a high level of thinking and decreases the chance of medication errors that could be harmful to the client.

Critical thinking is essential to the safe administration of medications. This process allows a nurse to think before doing, translate knowledge into practice, and make appropriate judgments. To safely administer medication the nurse must base decisions on rational thinking and thorough knowledge of medication administration. Proper medication administration involves evaluation of the client and the medication's effects, which requires critical thinking and skills of assessment. A nurse who administers medication in a routine manner, rather than with thought and reasoning, is not using critical thinking skills.

## Tips for Clinical Practice

Remember that the nurse who administers a medication is legally liable for the medication error regardless of the reason for the error occurrence.

## FACTORS THAT INFLUENCE DRUG DOSAGES AND ACTION

Several factors influence drug dosages and the way they act, including the following:
1. Route of administration
2. Time of administration
3. Age of the client
4. Nutritional status of the client
5. Absorption and excretion of the drug
6. Health status of the client
7. Gender of the client
8. Ethnicity and culture of the client
9. Genetics

All these factors affect how clients react to a medication and the dosage they receive, and all must be considered when medications are prescribed and administered. Because of differences in the actions and types of drugs, clients respond in various ways, and therefore dosages must be individualized. No two clients will respond to a medication in the same manner. Nurses must keep these factors in mind when administering medications. These factors can account for individuals responding differently to the same medication.

## SPECIAL CONSIDERATIONS FOR THE ELDERLY

Elderly individuals can be considered high-risk drug consumers. Approximately two thirds of older adults use both prescription and nonprescription drugs, and one third of all prescriptions are written for older adults. With the number of individuals over the age of 65 rapidly increasing, the use of medications in this age-group will also increase. According to the Administration on Aging (AOA, 2007), the older population (persons 65 years or older) numbered 37.3 million in 2006 (the latest year for which data are available). It is estimated that by the year 2030, there will be approximately 71.5 million older persons, more than twice their number in 2000.

People are now living longer, and older people tend to use health care services more often. As with children (see Chapter 25), special consideration should be given to the client who is over 65 years of age. With the aging process come physiological changes that have a direct effect on medications and their action in the elderly individual. Aging causes the slowing down of the body's functions. Other physiological changes include a decrease in circulation, slower absorption, slower metabolism, a decrease in excretory functions, and a decrease in the ability to respond to stress such as the stress of medications on the system. Other changes with aging include a decrease in body weight, which can affect the dosage of medications, and changes in mental status, possibly caused by the effects of physical illness or physiological changes in the neurological system that can occur with aging. These physiological changes can cause unexpected medication reactions and make the elderly person more sensitive to the effects of many medications.

According to Michael Cohen (*Medication Errors,* 2007) 90% of the elderly take prescription medications and of those who use at least one prescription drug, almost half use five or more medications. An estimated 25% to 30% of hospital admissions of elderly patients are linked to medication-related problems. Because the elderly are often taking more than one medication (polypharmacy), problems such as drug interactions, severe adverse reactions, drug and food interactions, and an increase in medication errors occur. The Beers criteria list medications that should be avoided in clients age 65 years and older and with certain medical disorders and that place the client at unnecessary risk. It is recommended that practitioners be aware of the medications on this list and educate clients regarding prescription and nonprescription medications. As the senior population continues to increase, there is a need to focus on reducing medication errors in this group.

As a rule, the elderly client will require smaller dosages of medications (as dosage size increases, the number of adverse effects and their severity increase), and the dosages should be given farther apart to prevent accumulation of medications and toxic effects. With aging, visual and hearing problems may develop. Special attention must be given when teaching clients about their medications to help prevent medication errors. Develop a relationship with the client; building rapport and trust is important for the elderly. Take time and talk to the elderly, listen to what they say, and never assume they do not know how much or what medications they are taking. Ascertain that all instructions are written as clearly as possible, choosing fonts that are friendly to older eyes. Make sure the client has appropriate measuring devices to facilitate ease and accuracy when measuring (e.g., a dropper or measuring cup with calibrated lines to indicate small dosages [0.2 mg, 0.4 mg, etc.]). To lessen the chance of taking too much medication or forgetting a dosage, try to establish specific times compatible with the client's routine for taking medications. Help the client to recognize pills by the name on the bottle, not by color. If the print on medications is too small for the client to read, encourage the use of a magnifying glass. Other measures might include providing a simple chart that outlines the medications to be taken, times they are to be taken, and special instructions if needed. Such a chart should be geared to the client's visual ability and comprehension level. Encourage the elderly client to request that childproof containers not be used; some older people will have difficulty opening child-resistant containers. Recommend medication aids for the client, such as special medication containers divided into separate compartments for storing daily or weekly medication dosages. (Figure 10-1 shows examples of medication containers.)

When teaching elderly clients, it is important to remember that they are mature adults who are capable of learning; they may need and deserve additional time for learning to take place. Be patient, use simple language, and maintain the independence of the elderly as much as possible. Always allow ample time for processing, individualize the teaching, and remember to always foster feelings of self-worth. Correct teaching can decrease misunderstandings and errors in medication.

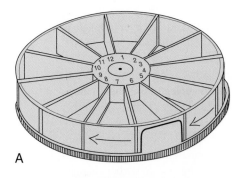

A

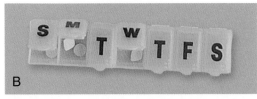

B

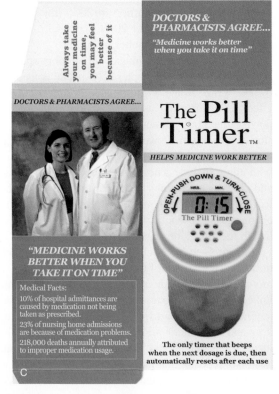

C

**Figure 10-1** **A,** Example of a container that holds a day's medications, stored by hour of administration. **B,** Container that holds a week's medications. **C,** The Pill Timer beeps, flashes, and automatically resets every time it is closed. (**A** From Ogden SG: *Calculation of drug dosages,* ed. 8, St. Louis, 2007, Mosby; **B** From Elkin MK, Perry AG, Potter PA: *Nursing interventions and clinical skills,* ed. 4, St. Louis, 2008, Mosby.)

---

**BOX 10-1   The Six Rights of Medication Administration**

1. The right medication
2. The right dosage
3. The right client

4. The right route
5. The right time
6. The right documentation

---

## THE SIX RIGHTS OF MEDICATION ADMINISTRATION

When the nurse is administering medications to a client, the six rights of medication administration should serve as guidelines. Failure to achieve any of these "rights" constitutes a medication error. The six rights (Box 10-1) should be followed when administering any medication to avoid errors and to ensure client safety.

1. **The right medication**—When medications are ordered, the nurse should compare the MAR (medication administration record) or computer record with the actual order. When administering medications, the nurse should check the label on the medication container against the order. Medications should be checked three times: before preparing, after preparing, and before replacing the container. With unit dosages (each medication dosage is prepared in the prescribed dosage, packaged, labeled, and ready to use), the label should still be checked three times. Remember, regardless of the medication distribution system, the medication label should be checked three times. Errors frequently occur because of similarity in medication names and similar packaging.

**CAUTION**

If the medication name is not clear or the medication does not seem to be appropriate for the client, question the order. Always double-check that you have the correct medication. If you are unfamiliar with a drug, refer to a reference to ensure accuracy and prevent errors.

2. The **right dosage**—Always perform and check calculations carefully, without ignoring decimal points. To ensure the right dose of medication, interpret abbreviations correctly. Factors such as illegible handwriting, miscalculation of the amount, and use of inappropriate abbreviations can result in administration of the wrong dose. Always have someone else check a dosage that causes concern. In some agencies certain medication dosages are required to be checked by two nurses (e.g., insulin, heparin). These medications have been a common source of errors in administration. If a dosage or abbreviation in a written order is not clear, call the prescriber for verification; do not assume. Consult a drug reference to confirm a dosage if in doubt. After dosages are calculated, they should be administered using standard measuring devices, such as calibrated medicine droppers and cups.

3. The **right client**—Always make sure you are administering medications to the right client. Failure to correctly identify the right client has been cited as one of the causes of medication errors. Since 2003, TJC has required that clients be identified with at least two unique client identifiers (e.g., name, birth date, identification number, but not the client's room number). This requirement was initiated as a National Patient Safety Goal; it has been a standard since 2004 and applies to both inpatient and outpatient settings. It is permissible to check the two identifiers with the client's arm band, medication administration record, or chart and ask the client to state his or her name as a third identifier.

## Tips for Clinical Practice

Always verify your client's identity by using the two identifiers designated by your institution each time medications are administered. This will help to ensure you have the right client and avoid an error.

Advanced technology does not eliminate your responsibility to correctly identify a client. Misidentification can result in a client receiving the wrong medication.

4. The **right route**—Medications should be administered by the correct route (e.g., orally or by injection). The route of the medication should be stated on the order. Do not assume which route is appropriate. The nurse should always consult drug references to confirm the route for a medication that is unfamiliar. Orders to administer medications by a feeding tube that should not be crushed (e.g., enteric coated) require that the nurse seek clarification of the order or have the order changed by the prescriber to ensure safe medication administration.

5. **The right time**—Medications should be given at the correct time of day and interval (e.g., three times a day [t.i.d.] or every 6 hours [q6h]). Judgment should be used as to when medications should be given or not given. If several medications are ordered, set priorities and administer medications that must act at a certain time. For example, insulin should be given at an exact time before meals. The right time should also include the right time sequence! For example, a client may be receiving a diuretic b.i.d., and the institution may have b.i.d. as 9:00 AM and 9:00 PM. The nurse will need to know that the diuretic should not be given in the late afternoon, so that the individual is not going to the bathroom all night. This requires critical thinking. The nurse must know whether a time schedule can be altered or requires judgment in determining the proper time to be administered. Know the institutional policy concerning medication times. All medication orders should include the frequency that a medication is to be administered. Administration of a medication at the prescribed time or right time is important to maximize the therapeutic effect and maintain therapeutic blood levels. Errors have occurred in medication administration because of misinterpretation of time and frequency in medication orders. The Joint Commission has taken steps to prevent errors by prohibiting the use of certain abbreviations related to dosing frequency (e.g., qod and qd have been mistaken for each other; instead of qod, write "every other day" and instead of qd write "daily").

6. **The right documentation**—Correct documentation is referred to as the sixth right of medication administration. Medications should be charted accurately as soon as they are given—on the right client's medication record, under the right date, and next to the right time. If a medication is refused, it should be documented as such with a notation on the medication record or in the nurse's notes. Never chart a medication as given before administering it or without documentation as to why it was not given. Follow the policy of the institution when documenting. All documentation should be legible. Unintentional overmedication of a client could result if a nurse fails to document a medication that was given and a nurse on a following shift also gives the medication to the client.

The six rights that have been discussed should always be consistently followed when administering medications. In addition to the six rights, the nurse should always view the client receiving medications as an important and valuable asset in the prevention of medication errors. Always listen to concerns verbalized by the client when administering medications regardless of the checks that you have performed before administration (e.g., "The other nurse just gave me medication," "I have never taken this medication before"). Statements such as these by a client should not be ignored. Always listen carefully and be attentive to the concerns of a client. Consider what the client verbalizes as correct and investigate concerns before administering the medication; this can be valuable in preventing medication errors.

In addition to the six rights of medication administration, a **client has the right to refuse medications.** When this occurs, the nurse needs to document the refusal correctly and make appropriate persons aware of the refusal. The right to refuse may be denied to the client who has a mental illness. A client deemed to be dangerous to self or others can be taken to court and mandated to take medication. Though the client has the right to refuse medication or treatment, the law referred to as Kendra's Law in New York state may provide some exception to a client's right to refuse treatment (e.g., medication). Kendra's Law is legislation designed to protect the public and individuals living with mental illness by ensuring that potentially dangerous mentally ill outpatients are safely and effectively treated.

Kendra's Law is court-ordered assisted outpatient treatment (AOT). It authorizes the courts to issue orders that would require mentally ill persons who are unlikely to survive safely in the community without supervision to accept medications and other needed mental health services. In other words, if a client is in the community and noncompliant with the treatment regimen (e.g., medication), the client can be petitioned to court by an individual (e.g., spouse, parent, adult roommate). The judge can then mandate the client to take medication if he or she is a danger to self or others. It is important to realize, however, that although there is a right to refuse, during an emergency situation, if danger is imminent, the client can be forcibly medicated by order of a judge.

Nurses should always be aware of the state laws, policies, and procedures for their jurisdiction relative to the administration of medications to refusing clients. It is extremely important for nurses to check frequently for side effects related to medications and to listen carefully to client complaints. The reason for the refusal of medications should be carefully analyzed and documented in all cases. Education of the client and a reassuring therapeutic relationship can assist in diminishing a client's refusal.

Another important right has to do with educating the client. **All clients have a right to be educated regarding the medication they are taking.** Clients are more likely to be compliant if they understand why they are taking a medication, and education allows them to make an informed decision.

In addition to some specific mandates mentioned by The Joint Commission to ensure client safety and prevent the occurrence of medication errors, another National Patient Safety Goal focused on medications that clients may be taking, including herbals, vitamins, and nonprescription products. Patients and families may not accurately report all their medications and dosages, as well as home remedies. This can lead to errors in medication administration and adverse effects.

## MEDICATION RECONCILIATION

According to Michael Cohen in the book titled *Medication Errors* (2007), "Poor communication about medications at transition points—admission, transfer, and discharge—is responsible for up to 50% of all medication errors and 20% of adverse drug events in the hospital." In response to this, TJC focused on medication reconciliation as a National Patient Safety Goal to reduce the risk of errors during transition points. This National Patient Safety Goal requires hospitals to reconcile medications across the continuum of care. Medication reconciliation is a requirement for ambulatory care, assisted living, behavioral health, home care, and long-term organizations. Medication reconciliation is to be applied in any setting or service where medications are to be used or the client's response to treatment or service could be affected by medications that the client has been taking.

In the context of the goal, reconciliation is the process of comparing the medications that the client/patient/resident has been taking before the time of admission or entry into a new setting with the medications that the organization is about to provide. The purpose of the reconciliation is to avoid errors of transcription, omission, duplication of therapy, or drug-drug and drug-disease interactions.

Medication reconciliation is an important goal in prevention of medication errors and can assist in obtaining accurate medication histories and ensure continuity of appropriate therapy. This process should begin on admission; discharge orders should be compared and reconciled with the most recent inpatient medication orders and the original list of medications taken at home. Nurses can play a major role in the reconciliation process. This must become an important focus to prevent errors and misunderstanding regarding medications that a client may be taking, especially when discharged. Ensuring client knowledge regarding prehospital medications and posthospital medications may be a step in preventing errors and medication interactions.

## TEACHING THE CLIENT

One of the most important nursing functions is teaching the client. Teaching clients about their medications is imperative in preventing errors and improving the quality of health care. Educating clients regarding medications plays a role in preventing adverse reactions and achieving adherence to prescribed therapy; taking the correct dosage of the right medication at the right time helps prevent problems with medication administration. Remember that clients cannot be expected to follow a medication regimen—taking the correct dosage of the right medication at the right time—if they have not been taught. Not knowing what to do results in noncompliance, inaccurate dosages, and other problems. Nurses are in a unique position to teach clients, and this has been a traditional activity of nursing practice. Teaching should begin in the hospital and be a major part of discharge planning because, once discharged, clients need to have been educated about their medications to continue taking them safely and correctly at home. With today's emphasis on outpatient treatment and early discharge, thorough client education regarding medications is necessary.

When the nurse is teaching a client, it is important to thoroughly assess the needs of the client. Determine what the client knows about the medication prescribed; how to take the medication; and the frequency, time, and dosage. Identify the client's learning needs, including literacy level and language most easily and clearly understood. Identify relevant ethnic, cultural, and socioeconomic factors that may influence medication use; consider factors such as age and physical capabilities. A variety of teaching techniques may have to be used to facilitate and enhance learning. Return demonstrations on proper use of medication equipment and reading dosages, in addition to repeated instructions and directions, may be necessary, especially regarding management at home.

What a client needs to know about a medication varies with that medication. There may be numerous pieces of information clients should learn regarding their medications. The items discussed here relate particularly to dosage administration. To ensure that the client takes the right medication in the right dosage, by the right route at the right time, client education should include the following:

- Both the brand and generic names of the medication or medications being taken
- Clear explanation of the amount of the medication to be taken (e.g., one tablet or 1/2 tablet)
- Clear explanation of when to take the medication (Prepare a chart created with the client's lifestyle in mind. For example, if the medication is to be taken with meals, perhaps the chart can indicate the client's mealtime and the medication scheduled accordingly.)
- Clear demonstration of measuring oral dosages, such as liquids (Encourage the use of measuring devices.)
- Clear explanation of the route of administration (e.g., place under tongue)

In addition to teaching clients about prescription medications they are taking, it is imperative that nurses question clients about any other over-the-counter medications they might be taking at home, including herbal medications. Some herbal medications might interact with medications they are taking (e.g., ephedra can accelerate heart rate, ginkgo and garlic may inhibit blood clotting). Nurses must be alert to any factors that may interfere with client safety.

Though nurses cannot ensure that clients will act on or retain everything they are taught, nurses are responsible for providing information to the client that will prevent error-prone situations and enable safe medication administration. Nurses evaluate retention, provide follow-up, and, if necessary, find alternative ways of dealing with a client who has a "no way" attitude.

## HOME CARE CONSIDERATIONS

Home health nursing has become a large part of the health care delivery system and continues to grow. This is due to factors such as the promotion of cost-effective health care and early discharge. Home care nursing may involve many activities, such as providing treatments, dressing changes, hospice care, client/family teaching, and medication administration. Medication administration involves administration of medications in various ways (e.g., IV, p.o., injection). The increased movement of nursing into the home of the client, which is not a controlled setting, has some important nursing implications. Home health nursing increases the autonomy of practice. The nurse must conduct a thorough assessment, communicate effectively, problem solve, and use expert critical thinking skills. Thinking must be rational, reasonable, and based on knowledge.

The principles regarding medication administration are the same as in a structured setting (e.g., hospital, acute care facility, nursing home). The six rights are still guidelines for the nurse to follow to ensure safe administration. It is imperative that the client be well educated about safe administration. Depending on the client's condition, home nursing services may be provided on a scheduled or intermittent basis to monitor the status of a client. Not all clients have a health aide, family member, or continuous nursing services in the home (around the clock). It is essential that the nurse calculate medication administration in a systematic, organized manner and adhere to the six rights of medication administration. The sixth right—documentation—is essential everywhere, including home health care. Documentation of medications is not just for legal purposes; it plays a significant role in cost reimbursement and payments. Correct interpretation of medication orders and validation are imperative. Proper education of the client concerning the medication, dosage, and route of administration is crucial in order for the client to manage in the home environment. Some may look at it as "the client being totally at your mercy." Clients depend on the nurse to provide direction for them to ensure safe home administration. The nurse must be able to teach the client to use appropriate utensils for measuring dosages and determining the accuracy of the dosage. When possible, encourage clients to use devices that are readily available in many pharmacies, such as calibrated oral syringes or plastic cups with measurements. Use of these devices can help prevent errors that often occur when clients measure their medication with household utensils. (As discussed in the chapters on systems of measure, the nurse must be able to convert dosages among the various systems.) The nurse providing services to the client in the home must be innovative and knowledgeable and demonstrate excellent critical thinking skills. Open communication with the client is essential. It is crucial to know what clients are taking and how. Remember that clients have to be taught. They may not know that they cannot resume previously taken medications or herbal remedies.

## ROUTES OF MEDICATION ADMINISTRATION

**Route refers to how a drug is administered.** Medications come in several forms for administration.

*ORAL (P.O.)*  Oral medication is administered by mouth (e.g., tablets, capsules, caplets, liquid solutions).

*SUBLINGUAL (SL)*  Sublingual medications are placed under the tongue and designed to be readily absorbed through the blood vessels in this area. They should not be swallowed. Nitroglycerin is an example of a medication commonly administered by the sublingual route.

*BUCCAL*  Buccal tablets are placed in the mouth against the mucous membranes of the cheek where the medication will dissolve. The medication is absorbed from the blood vessels of the cheek. Clients should be instructed not to chew or swallow the medication and not to take any liquids with it.

*PARENTERAL*  Parenteral medication is administered by a route other than by mouth or gastrointestinal tract. Parenteral routes include intravenous (IV), intramuscular (IM), subcutaneous (subcut), and intradermal (ID).

*INSERTION*  Medication is placed into a body cavity, where the medication dissolves at body temperature (e.g., suppositories). Vaginal medications, creams, and tablets may also be inserted by using special applicators provided by the manufacturer.

*INSTILLATION*  Medication is introduced in liquid form into a body cavity. It can also include placing an ointment into a body cavity, such as erythromycin eye ointment, which is placed in the conjunctiva of the eye. Nose drops and ear drops are also instillation medications.

*INHALATION*   Medication is administered into the respiratory tract, for example, through nebulizers used by clients for asthma. Bronchodilators and corticosteroids may be administered by inhalation through the mouth using an aerosolized, pressurized metered-dose inhaler (MDI). In some institutions these medications are administered to the client with special equipment, such as positive pressure breathing equipment or the aerosol mask. Other drugs in inhalation form include pentamidine, which is used to treat *Pneumocystis jiroveci,* a type of pneumonia found in clients with acquired immunodeficiency syndrome (AIDS). Devices such as "spacers" or "extenders" have been designed for use with inhalers to allow all of the metered dose to be inhaled, particularly in clients who have difficulty using inhalers.

*INTRANASAL*   A medicated solution is instilled into the nostrils. This method is used to administer corticosteroids, the antidiuretic hormone vasopressin, and a nasal mist influenza vaccine (Flumist).

*TOPICAL*   The medication is applied to the external surface of the skin. It can be in the form of lotion, ointment, or paste.

**Percutaneous.**   Medications are applied to the skin or mucous membranes for absorption. This includes ointments, powders, and lotions for the skin; instillation of solutions onto the mucous membranes of the mouth, ear, nose, or vagina; and inhalation of aerosolized liquids for absorption through the lungs. The primary advantage is that the action of the drug, in general, is localized to the site of application.

**Transdermal.**   Transdermal medication, which is becoming more popular, is contained in a patch or disk and applied topically. The medication is slowly released and absorbed through the skin and enters the systemic circulation. These topical applications may be applied for 24 hours or for as long as 7 days and have systemic effects. Examples include nitroglycerin for chest pain, nicotine transdermal (Nicoderm) for smoking cessation, clonidine for hypertension, fentanyl (Duragesic) for pain, and birth control patches.

Forms of oral medications (tablets, capsules), oral solutions, and routes for parenteral medications are discussed in more detail in later chapters.

## EQUIPMENT USED FOR MEDICATION ADMINISTRATION

*MEDICINE CUP*   Equipment used for oral administration includes a 30-mL or 1-oz medication cup made of plastic, used to measure most liquid medications. The cup has measurements in all three systems of measure (Figure 10-2). By looking at the medicine cup you can see that 30 mL = 1 oz, 5 mL = 1 tsp, and so forth. Remember that any volume less than 1 tsp (5 mL) should be measured with a more accurate device, such as an oral syringe.

*SOUFFLÉ CUP*   A soufflé cup is a small paper or plastic cup used for solid forms of medication, such as tablets and capsules (Figure 10-3).

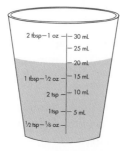

**Figure 10-2**   Medicine cup. (Modified from Brown M, Mulholland JL: *Drug calculations: process and problems for clinical practice,* ed. 8, St. Louis, 2008, Mosby.)

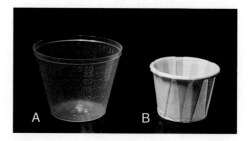

**Figure 10-3**   **A,** Plastic medicine cup. **B,** Soufflé cup. (Courtesy of Chuck Dresner. From Clayton BD, Stock YN, Harroun RD: *Basic pharmacology for nurses,* ed. 14, St. Louis, 2007, Mosby.)

*CALIBRATED DROPPER*    A calibrated dropper may be used to administer small amounts of medication to an adult or child (Figure 10-4). It is usually marked in milliliters. The size of the drops varies and depends on the dropper. Because the size of drops varies, it is important to remember that drops should not be used as a medication measure unless the dropper is calibrated. Droppers used for the administration of eye, nose, and ear medication are designed for that purpose. Certain medications come with a dropper calibrated according to the medication. Examples include children's vitamins and nystatin oral solutions. The calibration allows for accurate dosing, which can be difficult with small dosages unless there is an exact measuring device. Use the calibrated dropper only with the medicine for which it was designed.

*NIPPLE*    An infant feeding nipple with additional holes may be used for administering oral medications to infants (Figure 10-5).

## Critical Thinking

Be safe. THINK! Droppers are accurate when used to measure the specific medication for which they are designed but not for measuring other medications. Using a dropper for the wrong medication could result in a serious medication error.

*ORAL SYRINGE*    An oral syringe may be used to administer liquid medications orally to adults and children. No needle is attached (Figure 10-6).

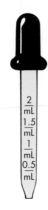

**Figure 10-4**    Medicine dropper. (Modified from Clayton BD, Stock YN Harroun RD: *Basic pharmacology for nurses,* ed. 14, St. Louis, 2007, Mosby.)

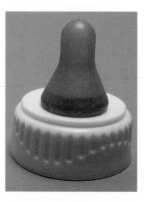

**Figure 10-5**    Nipple. (From Clayton BD, Stock YN, Harroun RD: *Basic pharmacology for nurses,* ed. 14, St. Louis, 2007, Mosby.)

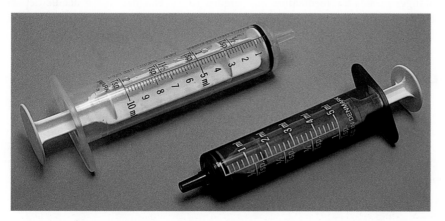

**Figure 10-6**    Oral syringes. (Courtesy of Chuck Dresner. From Clayton BD, Stock YN, Harroun RD: *Basic pharmacology for nurses,* ed. 14, St. Louis, 2007, Mosby.)

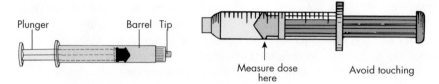

**Figure 10-7**    Parts of a syringe. (From Potter PA, Perry AG: *Fundamentals of nursing,* ed. 7, St. Louis, 2009, Mosby.)

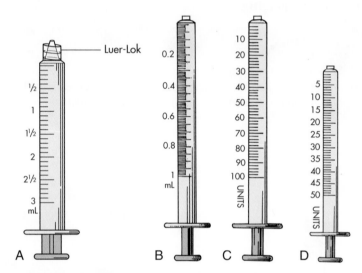

**Figure 10-8**    Types of syringes. **A,** Luer-Lok syringe marked in 0.1 mL (tenths). **B,** Tuberculin syringe marked in 0.01 mL (hundredths) for dosages of less than 1 mL. **C,** Insulin syringe marked in units (100). **D,** Insulin syringe marked in units (50). (From Potter PA, Perry AG: *Fundamentals of nursing,* ed. 7, St. Louis, 2009, Mosby.)

*PARENTERAL SYRINGE*    A parenteral syringe is used for IM, subcut, ID, and IV medications. These syringes come in various sizes and are marked in milliliters or units. The specific types of syringes are discussed in more detail in Chapter 18. The barrel of the syringe holds the medication and has calibrations on it. The needle is attached to the tip. The plunger pushes the medication out (Figure 10-7). The size of the needle depends on how the medication is given (e.g., subcut or IM), the viscosity of the drug, and the size of the client. See Figure 10-8 for samples of the types of syringes.

## EQUIPMENT FOR ADMINISTERING ORAL MEDICATIONS TO A CHILD

Various types of calibrated equipment are on the market for administering medications to children. Most of the available equipment is for oral use. Caregivers should be instructed to always use a calibrated device when administering medications to a child. Household spoons vary in size and are not reliable devices for accurate dosing. Figure 10-9 presents samples of equipment used to administer oral medications to a child.

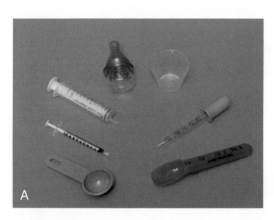 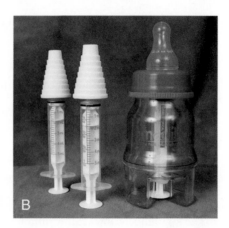

**Figure 10-9**  **A,** Acceptable devices for measuring and administering oral medication to children *(clockwise):* measuring spoon, plastic syringes, calibrated nipple, plastic medicine cup, calibrated dropper, hollow-handled medicine spoon. **B,** Medibottle used to deliver oral medication via a syringe. (**A,** From Hockenberry MJ, Wilson D: *Wong's nursing care of infants and children,* ed. 8, St Louis, 2007, Mosby. **B,** Courtesy Paul Vincent Kuntz, Texas Children's Hospital, Houston.)

 ## Practice Problems

Answer the following questions by filling in the correct word or words to complete the sentence.

1. A medicine cup has _____, _____, and _____ measures on it.

2. The _____ and _____ need special considerations regarding medication dosages.

3. _____ refers to the way in which a drug is administered.

4. Children and the elderly usually require _____ dosages.

5. A _____ cup is used for dispensing solid forms of medication.

6. Application of medication to the external surface of the skin is referred to as the _____ route.

7. Medication administration is a process that requires critical thinking and the nursing process, which includes:

    a. _____

    b. _____

    c. _____

    d. _____

    e. _____

    f. _____

8. Being an autonomous thinker is an example of _____.

9. _____ droppers should be used for medication administration.

10. When medications are placed next to the cheek, they are administered by the

_____ route.

Answers on p. 608

## ■ Points to Remember

- The six rights of medication administration serve as guidelines for nurses when administering medications (the right medication, dosage, client, route, time, and documentation). Client rights include the right to refuse and the right to be educated.
- Medication administration includes using critical thinking and the nursing process.
- There are numerous reasons for medication errors.
- Medication errors can harm clients physically and economically and can be fatal.
- Nurses are accountable for medications administered regardless of the reason for the error.
- Nurses are responsible for ensuring the client's safety when administering medications. This includes ensuring that clients receive the right medication, the right dosage, by the right route, at the right time, with the right documentation.
- Nurses can play a major role in the medication reconciliation process.
- The elderly and children require special considerations with medication administration.
- Home health nursing increase's the autonomy of nursing practice.
- A calibrated dropper should be used when administering medications with a dropper.
- Dosages less than 1 teaspoon should be measured with a device such as a syringe.
- A medication cup has the capacity of 30 mL. A soufflé cup is used to dispense solid forms of medications.
- Medications are administered by various routes.

## ✓ CHAPTER REVIEW

1. Name the six rights of medication administration

Right _____

Right _____

Right _____

Right _____

Right _____

Right _____

2. The Joint Commission requires that clients be identified using _____ client identifiers, neither of which can be the _____.

3. A medication label should be read _____ times.

4. Medications should be charted _____ you have administered them.

5. Name three routes of medication administration. _____

   _____

6. The medicine cup has a _____ capacity.

7. Droppers are calibrated to administer standardized drops regardless of what type of dropper is used. True or False? _____

8. The syringe used to administer a dosage by mouth is referred to as a(an)

   _____.

9. Volume on a syringe is indicated by _____.

10. The medicine cup indicates that 2 tablespoons are approximately _____ mL.

11. Twenty-five to thirty percent of admissions to the hospital for the elderly are because of _____.

12. ISMP is an abbreviation for _____.

13. TJC is an abbreviation for_____.

14. The route by which medicated solutions are instilled into the nostrils is _____.

15. Examples of medications that have been identified as high-alert medications are potassium chloride, _____, _____, and _____.

Answers on p. 608

 **For additional practice problems, refer to the Introducing Drug Measures section of Drug Calculations Companion, Version 4, on Evolve.**

# CHAPTER
# 11
# Understanding and Interpreting Medication Orders

## Objectives

*After reviewing this chapter, you should be able to:*
1. Identify the components of a medication order
2. Identify the meanings of standard abbreviations used in medication administration
3. Interpret a given medication order
4. Identify abbreviations, acronyms, and symbols recommended by the Joint Commission's "Do Not Use" List and ISMP's List of Error-Prone Abbreviations, Symbols, and Dose Designations
5. Read and write correct medical notations.

Before a nurse can administer any medication, there must be a written legal order for it. Medication orders can be written by physicians, dentists, physician's assistants, nurse midwives, or nurse practitioners, depending on state law. Health care providers use medication orders or order sheets to convey the therapeutic plan for a client, which includes medications. Medication orders are written as prescriptions in private practice or in clinics. The medication the health care provider is ordering in these settings is written on a prescription form that usually comes as a pad and is filled by a pharmacist at a drug store (pharmacy) or the hospital. Medication orders are used by health care providers to communicate to the nurse or designated health care worker which medication or medications to administer to a client. Medication orders can be oral or written.

## VERBAL ORDERS

Oral (verbal) and telephone orders should only be accepted in emergencies. The book titled *Medication Errors* (Cohen, 2007) cites reasons for possible errors in verbal orders:
- The order can be misheard
- Various pronunciations
- Accents
- Sound-alike drug names
- Poor cell phone reception

Cohen also points out that errors can occur when verbal orders (spoken) are incomplete and the nurse assumes the prescriber's intention. Recognizing the errors that can occur with verbal orders and wanting to decrease the potential errors when an oral or telephone order is taken, The Joint Commission requires that only "designated qualified staff" may accept verbal or telephone orders. The Joint Commission (2007) requires that the authorized individual receiving a verbal or telephone order first **write it down** in the patient's chart or enter it into the computer, then **read it back** to the prescriber, and then **receive**

**confirmation** from the prescriber who gave the order that it is correct. For the nurse to only repeat back the order is not sufficient to prevent errors and is not allowed by The Joint Commission. Any questions or concerns relating to the order should be clarified with the prescriber during the conversation. A verbal order must contain the same elements as a written order: the date of the order, name and dosage of the medication, route, frequency, any special instructions, and the name of the individual giving the order.

It must be noted that it was an oral or telephone order, and the signature of the nurse taking the order is required. Many institutions require that the order must be signed by the prescriber within 24 hours. Some institutions may require that medication orders written by a person other than a physician be countersigned by designated personnel.

## Tips for Clinical Practice

It is important to be familiar with specific policies regarding medication orders and responsibilities in this regard because they vary according to the institution or health care facility.

The only time in which just a "repeat back" is acceptable to The Joint Commission is in situations where a formal "read back" is not feasible, for example, emergency situations such as a code or in the OR (operating room).

**CAUTION**

Acceptance of a verbal order is a major responsibility and can lead to medication errors. Accept a verbal order only in an emergency situation. If you accept a verbal order follow the policy of The Joint Commission. Always clarify questions about the order during the conversation. If you are unsure of the medication or the spelling, spell it back to the prescriber and get confirmation. NEVER ASSUME.

The medication order indicates the drug treatment plan or medication the health care provider has ordered for a client. Depending on the institution, the medication order may be written on a sheet labeled "physician's order sheet" or "order sheet." After the medication order has been written, the nurse or in some institutions a trained unit clerk transcribes the order. This means the order is written on the medication administration record (MAR). In an instance in which the nurse does not transcribe the order, the nurse is accountable for what is written and for verifying the order, initialing it, and checking it before administering.

At some institutions computers are used for processing medication orders. Medication orders are either electronically transmitted or manually entered directly into the computer from an order form. The use of the computer allows immediate transmission of the order to the pharmacy. The computerized medication record can be seen directly on the computer screen or on a printed copy. Medication orders done by computer entry allow the prescriber to make changes if indicated, and the orders are signed by the prescriber with an assigned electronic code. Once the medication is received on the unit, the medication order is implemented and the client receives the medication.

Computerized physician order entry (CPOE), according to Cohen (2007), "could prevent many problems that occur with written orders as well as clearly communicating medication orders, and avoiding dosing mistakes; it would also help in preventing serious drug interactions and monitoring and documenting adverse events and therapeutic outcomes." In addition, the authors of the 2006 Institute of Medicine (IOM) report *Preventing Medication Errors* call for all health care providers to have plans in place for CPOE by 2008. By 2010, IOM recommends that all prescribers be using electronic prescribing and all pharmacies be capable of accepting electronic prescriptions (Cohen, 2007).

In some institutions fax (facsimile) transmission may be used to avoid telephone orders. Faxed orders, however, may not be clearly legible and can also cause errors in interpretation. Cohen (2007) recommends that faxed orders be reviewed carefully and that the pharmacy verify the order before dispensing the medication or wait for the original.

Despite the advent of technology many institutions still have handwritten orders and nurses must be familiar with transcription of orders.

Before transcribing an order or preparing a dosage, the nurse must be familiar with reading and interpreting an order. To interpret a medication order, the nurse must know the components of a medication order and the standard abbreviations and symbols used in writing a medication order as well as those abbreviations and symbols that should not be used. The nurse therefore must memorize the abbreviations and symbols commonly used in medication orders. The abbreviations include units of measure, route, and frequency for the medication ordered. The common abbreviations and symbols used in medication administration are listed in Tables 11-1 and 11-2 and must be committed to memory. The Joint Commission's "Do Not Use" List is shown in Table 11-3, and ISMP's List of Error-Prone Abbreviations, Symbols, and Dose Designations will be presented later in this chapter.

In writing medication orders, some health care providers may use capital letters, and others may use lowercase letters; some may place a period after an abbreviation or symbol, but others do not. These variations often reflect writing styles.

## Tips for Clinical Practice

The use of abbreviations, acronyms, and symbols in the writing of medication orders can have safety implications, and certain abbreviations can mean more than one thing. For example, AD was used to mean right ear. Imodium A-D refers to an antidiarrheal. OD, which was used to indicate right eye, could also mean overdose. Because of the risk for errors in interpretation that can place clients at risk and to decrease the number of medication errors that occur, TJC created an official "Do Not Use" List and ISMP also came up with an extensive list of abbreviations, symbols, and dose designations that have led to medication errors. ISMP stresses avoiding all items on this list in all forms of communicating medical information, including orders. Care *must* be taken to use only abbreviations, acronyms, and symbols that have been approved. The recommendations of TJC and ISMP are discussed later in this chapter. ***Note:*** OD (right eye), OS (left eye), OU (both eyes), AD (right ear), AS (left ear), and AU (both ears) are also abbreviations that have been recommended to not use by ISMP.

## Critical Thinking

It is important for you to concentrate on understanding what abbreviations or symbols mean in the context of the order.

**TABLE 11-1**    Symbols and Abbreviations for Units of Measure Used in Medication Administration

| Abbreviation/Symbol | Meaning | Abbreviation/Symbol | Meaning |
|---|---|---|---|
| c, C | cup | oz | ounce |
| g | gram | pt | pint |
| gr | grain | qt | quart |
| gtt | drop | T, tbs | tablespoon |
| kg | kilogram | t, tsp | teaspoon |
| L | liter | $\cong$ | approximately |
| mcg | microgram | ↑ | increase |
| mEq* | milliequivalent | ↓ | decrease |
| mg | milligram | Δ | change |
| mL | milliliter | | |

*mEq (milliequivalent) is a drug measure in which electrolytes are measured; it expresses the ionic activity of a drug.

# WRITING A MEDICATION ORDER

The health care provider writes a medication order on a form called the *physician's order sheet*. Order sheets vary from institution to institution. The order sheet should have the client's name on it. A prescription blank is used to write medication orders for clients who are being discharged from the hospital or are seeing the doctor in an outpatient facility. Nurses often have to explain these orders to clients so they understand the dosages and other relevant information relating to their medications to ensure safety.

**TABLE 11-2** Commonly Used Medication Abbreviations

| Abbreviation | Meaning | Abbreviation | Meaning |
|---|---|---|---|
| $\overline{a}$ | before | p.c., pc | after meals |
| aa, $\overline{aa}$ | of each | per | through or by |
| a.c., ac | before meals | pm, PM | evening, before midnight |
| ad lib. | as desired, freely | | |
| am, AM | morning before noon | p.o. | by mouth, oral |
| amp | ampule | p.r. | by rectum |
| aq | aqueous, water | p.r.n., prn | when necessary/required, as needed |
| b.i.d., bid | twice a day | | |
| b.i.w. | twice a week | | |
| $\overline{c}$ | with | q. | every |
| c, C | cup | q.a.m. | every morning |
| cap, caps | capsule | q.h., qh | every hour |
| CD | controlled dose | q2h, q4h, q6h, q8h, q12h | every 2 hours, every 4 hours, every 6 hours, every 8 hours, every 12 hours |
| CR | controlled release | | |
| dil. | dilute | | |
| DS | double strength | | |
| EC | enteric coated | | |
| elix. | elixir | q.i.d., qid | four times a day |
| fl, fld. | fluid | q.s. | a sufficient amount/as much as needed |
| GT | gastrostomy tube | | |
| gtt | drop | rect | rectum |
| h, hr | hour | $\overline{s}$ | without |
| ID | intradermal | sl, SL | sublingual |
| IM | intramuscular | sol, soln | solution |
| IV | intravenous | s.o.s., SOS | may be repeated once if necessary |
| IVPB | intravenous piggyback | SR | sustained release |
| IVSS | intravenous Soluset | S&S | swish and swallow |
| KVO | keep vein open (a very slow infusion rate) | stat, STAT | immediately, at once |
| | | subcut | subcutaneous |
| | | supp | suppository |
| LA | long acting | susp | suspension |
| LOS | length of stay | syp, syr | syrup |
| min | minute | tab | tablet |
| mix | mixture | t.i.d., tid | three times a day |
| NAS | intranasal | tr., tinct | tincture |
| NG, NGT | nasogastric tube | ung., oint | ointment |
| noc, noct | at night | vag, v | vaginally |
| n.p.o., NPO | nothing by mouth | XL | long acting |
| NS, N/S | normal saline | XR | extended release |
| $\overline{p}$ | after | | |

*Note:* Abbreviations identified as "do not use" by TJC have been removed from the abbreviation list, as have dangerous abbreviations identified by the ISMP.

**TABLE 11-3**    The Joint Commission's Official "Do Not Use" List*

| Do Not Use | Potential Problem | Use Instead |
|---|---|---|
| U (unit) | Mistaken for "0" (zero), the number "4" (four), or "cc" | Write "unit" |
| IU (International Unit) | Mistaken for IV (intravenous) | Write "International Unit" |
| Q.D., QD, q.d., qd (daily) | Mistaken for each other | Write "daily" |
| Q.O.D., QOD, q.o.d. qod (every other day) | Period after the Q mistaken for "I" and the "O" mistaken for "I" | Write "every other day" |
| Trailing zero (X.0 mg)† | Decimal point is missed | Write X mg |
| Lack of leading zero (.X mg) | | Write 0.X mg |
| MS | Can mean morphine sulfate or magnesium sulfate | Write "morphine sulfate" |
| MSO4 and MgSO4 | Confused for one another | Write "magnesium sulfate" |

© The Joint Commission, 2008. Reprinted with permission.
*Applies to all orders and all medication-related documentation that is handwritten (including free-text computer entry) or on preprinted forms.
†**Exception:** A "trailing zero" may be used only where required to demonstrate the level of precision of the value being reported, such as for laboratory results, imaging studies that report size of lesions, or catheter/tube sizes. It may not be used in medication orders or other medication-related documentation.

## COMPONENTS OF A MEDICATION ORDER

When a medication order is written, it must contain the following seven important parts or it is considered invalid or incomplete: (1) client's full name, (2) date and time the order was written, (3) name of the medication, (4) dosage of the medication, (5) route of administration, (6) frequency of administration, and (7) signature of the person writing the order. These parts of the medication order are discussed in detail in the following sections.

**CAUTION**

If any of the components of a medication order are missing the order is not complete and not a legal medication order.

*CLIENT'S FULL NAME*    Using the client's full name helps to prevent confusion of one client with another, thereby preventing administration of the wrong medication to a client. Many institutions use a nameplate to imprint the client's name and record number on the order sheet; in addition there is usually a place to indicate allergies. In institutions that use computers, the computer screen may also show identifying information for the client, such as age and known drug allergies.

**NOTE**

A record of the time the order was written is preferred in many institutions, but omission does not invalidate the order. This same information is required in computer entry of medication orders.

*DATE AND TIME THE ORDER WAS WRITTEN*    The date and time of the order include the month, day, year, and the time the order was written. This will help in determining the start and stop of the medication order. In many institutions the health care provider (or person legally authorized to write a medication order) is required to include the length of time the medication is to be given (e.g., 7 days); or he or she may use the abbreviation LOS (length of stay), which means the client is to receive the medication during the entire stay in the hospital. Even when not written as part of the order, LOS is implied unless stated otherwise. The policy regarding indicating the length of time a medication is to be given varies from institution to institution. At some institutions, if there are no specified dosages or days for particular medications, it is assumed to be continued until otherwise stopped by the health care provider or a protocol in place for certain medications, such as controlled substances (narcotics). Some medications have automatic stop times according to the facility (e.g., narcotics, certain antibiotics).

*NAME OF THE MEDICATION*    The medication may be ordered by the generic or brand name (Figures 11-1 and 11-2). To avoid confusion with another medication, the name of the medication should be written clearly and spelled correctly.

**Trade name**—the brand name or proprietary name is the name under which a manufacturer markets the medication. The brand or trade name is followed by the registration symbol, ®. The name either starts with a capital letter or is all in capital letters on the label. It is generally the largest printed information on the label. A medication may have several trade names, according to the manufacturer. It is important to note that some medications may not have trade names.

**Generic name**—proper name, chemical name, or nonproprietary name of the medication. It is usually designated in lowercase letters or a different typeface. Sometimes the generic name is also placed in parentheses. The generic name is usually found under the brand or trade name. Occasionally, only the generic name will appear on the label. Each medication has only one generic name. By law, the generic name must appear on all medication labels. Therefore a medication label must indicate the generic name and some labels may include a trade name. The prescriber may order medications using the generic name.

## Tips for Clinical Practice

Nurses must be familiar with both the generic name and the trade name for a medication. To ensure correct medication identification, nurses should crosscheck trade and generic names as needed with a medication reference.

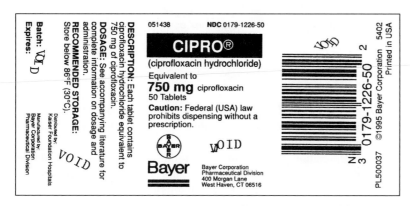

**Figure 11-1**    Cipro label. Notice the two names. The first, *Cipro,* is the trade name, identified by the registration symbol ®. The name in smaller and different print is *ciprofloxacin hydrochloride,* the generic or official name.

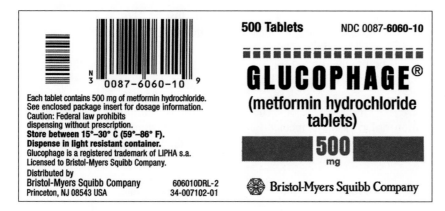

**Figure 11-2**    Glucophage label. Notice the two names. The first, *Glucophage,* is the trade name, identified by the registration symbol ®. The name in smaller and different print is *metformin hydrochloride,* the generic or official name.

Checking the names of medications even when they are generic is essential in preventing errors. Some very different medications have similar generic names, such as pyridostigmine bromide (Mestinon), which is used to treat myasthenia gravis, and pyrimethamine (Daraprim), which is used to treat parasitic disorders, such as toxoplasmosis.

To ensure correct medication information, nurses should crosscheck trade and generic names as needed. When reading the name of a medication, never assume. Sometimes orders may be written with abbreviated medication names. This has been discouraged unless the abbreviation is common and approved. Some abbreviations used for medications can cause confusion with another medication, for example, $MgSO_4$ (intended use: magnesium sulfate) and $MSO_4$ (intended for: morphine sulfate). These two are cited on TJC's "Do Not Use" List because often they have been mistaken for each other.

For example, the acronym AZT may be used. "AZT 100 mg p.o." (intended drug order zidovudine [Retrovir], 100 mg, which is used for HIV) can be misread as azathioprine (Imuran), an immunosuppressant. The use of acronyms in writing medication orders is not recommended by TJC; write the complete medication name to avoid misinterpretation.

## Tips for Clinical Practice

Nurses must be familiar with the names of medications (generic and trade). Many medications on the market have similar names and pronunciations but very different actions. Examples: Glyburide and Glipizide, Procardia and Procardia XL, Percocet and Percodan, quinine and quinidine.

**CAUTION**

A case of mistaken identity with medications can have tragic results.

*DOSAGE OF THE MEDICATION*    The amount and strength of the medication should be written clearly to avoid confusion. Dosage indicates the amount or weight provided in the form (e.g., per tablet, per milliliter).

To avoid misinterpretation, "U," which stands for units, should not be used when insulin, heparin, or any other medication order that uses units is written. The word *units* should be written out. This would also include "mU" (milliunits). Errors have occurred as a result of confusion of "U" with an "O" in a handwritten order. The abbreviation "U" for units is on TJC's Official "Do Not Use" List and on ISMP's List of Error-Prone Abbreviations, Symbols, and Dose Designations.

**NOTE**

The period can cause confusion with "q.i.d." q.d. should not be used when writing medication orders, regardless of form, in upper or lowercase, with or without periods. This abbreviation is on TJC's Official "Do Not Use" List as well as on ISMP's List of Error-Prone Abreviations, Symbols, and Dose Designations.

**Example:**    60 subcut stat of Humulin Regular Insulin. The U is almost completely closed and could be misread as 60 units. The *word units* should be written out. The handwritten letters "q.d.," when used in prescription writing, can be misinterpreted as "q.i.d." if the period is raised and the tail of the "q" interferes. Example: Lasix 40 mg q̶ᵈ.

*ROUTE OF ADMINISTRATION*    The route of administration is a very important part of a medication order, because medications can be administered by several routes. Never assume that you know which route is appropriate. Standard and acceptable abbreviations should be used to indicate the route.

**Examples:**    p.o. (oral, by mouth)         IM (intramuscular)

ID (intradermal)              IV (intravenous)

Administering a medication by a route other than what the form indicates constitutes a medication error. Regardless of the source of an error, if you administer the wrong dosage, or give a medication by a route other than what it is intended for, you have made a medication error and are legally responsible for it.

*TIME AND FREQUENCY OF ADMINISTRATION*  Standard abbreviations should be used to indicate the times a medication is to be given.

**Examples:**  q.i.d. (four times a day), stat (immediately)

The time intervals at which a medication is administered are determined by the institution, and most health care facilities have routine times for administering medications.

**Example:**  t.i.d. (three times a day) may be 9 AM, 1 PM, and 5 PM, or 10 AM, 2 PM, and 6 PM.

Factors such as the purpose of the medication, medication interactions, absorption of the medication, and side effects should be considered when medication times are scheduled. It is important to realize that when abbreviations such as b.i.d. and t.i.d. are used, the amount you calculate is for one dosage and not for the day's total. The frequency indicates the dosage (amount) of medication given at a single time.

*SIGNATURE OF THE PERSON WRITING THE ORDER*  For a medication order to be legal, it must be signed by the health care provider. The health care provider writing the order must include his or her signature on the order, and it should be legible. At some institutions, in addition to the signature of the physician or other person licensed to write orders, to ensure legibility the prescriber must stamp the order with a rubber stamp that has his or her name clearly printed on it after an order has been written. Orders that are done by computer entry require a signature created by using an assigned electronic code or electronic signature. In some institutions, depending on the rank of the physician or the person writing the order, an order may have to be co-signed by a senior physician.

**Example:**  Residents or interns and persons other than a physician writing an order must secure the signature of an attending physician.

In addition to the seven required components of a medication order already discussed, any special instructions or parameters for certain medications need to be clearly written.

**Examples:**  1. Hold if blood pressure (BP) is below 100 systolic.
2. Administer a half hour before meals ($\frac{1}{2}$ hour a.c.).

Medications ordered as needed or whenever necessary (p.r.n.) should indicate the purpose of administration as well. In addition, a frequency must be written to state the minimum time allowed between dosages.

**Examples:**  1. For chest pain
2. Temperature above 101° F
3. For blood pressure (BP) greater than 140 systolic and 90 diastolic

In instances in which specific instructions are not stated, nursing judgment must be used to determine whether it is appropriate to administer a medication.

For dosage calculations, the nurse is usually concerned with the medication name, dosage of the medication, route, and time or frequency of administration. This information is necessary in determining a safe and reasonable dosage for a client.

> NEVER ASSUME WHAT AN ORDER STATES! CLARIFY AN ORDER WHEN IN DOUBT. IF AN ORDER IS NOT CLEAR, OR IF ESSENTIAL COMPONENTS ARE OMITTED, IT IS NOT A LEGAL ORDER AND SHOULD NOT BE IMPLEMENTED. THE NURSE IS ACCOUNTABLE!

## INTERPRETING A MEDICATION ORDER

Medication orders are written in the following order:

1. Name of the medication
2. The dosage, expressed in standard abbreviations or symbols
3. Route
4. Frequency

**Example:**

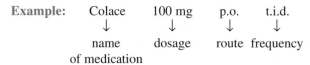

This order means the prescriber wants the client to receive Colace (name of medication), which is a stool softener, 100 milligrams (dosage) by mouth (route), three times a day (frequency). The use of abbreviations in a medication order is a form of shorthand. For the purpose of interpreting orders, it is important for nurses to commit to memory common medical abbreviations as well as abbreviations related to the systems of measure. Refer to Tables 11-1 and 11-2 for medical abbreviations and symbols used in medication administration. Be systematic when interpreting the order to avoid an error. The medication order follows a specific sequence when it is written correctly (the name of the medication first, followed by the dosage, route, and frequency); interpret the order in this manner as well; avoid "scrambling the order."

Orders are transcribed in some institutions where unit dose is used. In some institutions more transcribing may be necessary because the MAR may have the capacity to be used for only a limited period (e.g., 3 days, 5 days). It is therefore necessary to transcribe orders again at the end of the designated period.

In facilities in which computers are used, the medication order is entered into the computer, and a printout lists the currently ordered medications. The computer is able to scan for information such as drug incompatibilities, safe dosage ranges, recommended administration times, and allergies; it can also indicate when a new order for a medication is required.

Computerized order entry and charting do not eliminate the nurse's responsibility for double-checking medication orders before administering. Nurses need to be aware of some of the problems that the use of certain abbreviations and acronyms has created. Use of certain abbreviations has created situations that can be harmful to clients and result in the potential for or actual error in medication administration. Recognize that use of certain abbreviations and symbols in medication orders can be misinterpreted and cause significant harm to clients. TJC and ISMP established a list of abbreviations, acronyms, and symbols to avoid because they are a common source of error and can be easily misinterpreted.

The Joint Commission first published the Official "Do Not Use" List (see Table 11-3) in 2004 (reaffirmed in 2005). It also suggested that there may be other abbreviations and acronyms added to its list in the future (Table 11-4). The Institute for Safe Medication Practices (ISMP, 2006) also published a list of abbreviations, symbols and dose designations that have led to medication errors (Table 11-5). ISMP has recommended that these abbreviations, symbols, and dose designations be strictly prohibited when communicating medical information including medication orders.

A recent abbreviation, "IN", for intranasal route is included on ISMP's List of Error-Prone Abbreviations, Symbols, and Dose Designations (2006). A handwritten IN could be misread as IM or IV. In an oral or telephone order, this may be misheard as IM and result in serious consequences as indicated by Michael Cohen in the book titled *Medication Errors* (2007). Intranasal should be written out as "intranasal" or abbreviated as "NAS."

For the safety of clients and to prevent errors in misinterpretation, prescribers responsible for writing medication orders *must* pay attention to what they write: it could save a life. In addition to knowing correct medication notations, those who administer medications must know the safe dosage and be able to recognize discrepancies in a dosage that can sometimes be caused by misinterpretation of an order.

## Tips for Clinical Practice

Nurses should stay alert to The Joint Commission, ISMP, and their health care institution policies and restrictions regarding abbreviations and medical notations.

**TABLE 11-4** Additional Abbreviations, Acronyms, and Symbols*

| Do Not Use | Potential Problem | Use Instead |
|---|---|---|
| > (greater than) | Misinterpreted as the number "7" (seven) or the letter "L" | Write "greater than" |
| < (less than) | Confused for one another | Write "less than" |
| Abbreviations for drug names | Misinterpreted because of similar abbreviations for multiple drugs | Write drug names in full |
| Apothecary units | Unfamiliar to many practitioners. Confused with metric units | Use metric units |
| @ | Mistaken for the number "2" (two) | Write "at" |
| cc | Mistaken for U (units) when poorly written | Write "mL" or "milliliters" |
| μg | Mistaken for mg (milligrams) resulting in 1,000-fold overdose | Write "mcg" or "micrograms" |

© The Joint Commission, 2008. Reprinted with permission.
*For possible future inclusion in the Official "Do Not Use" List.

**TABLE 11-5** ISMP's List of Error-Prone Abbreviations, Symbols, and Dose Designations

The abbreviations, symbols, and dose designations found in this table have been reported to ISMP through the USP-ISMP Medication Error Reporting Program as being frequently misinterpreted and involved in harmful medication errors. They should NEVER be used when communicating medical information. This includes internal communications, telephone/verbal prescriptions, computer-generated labels, labels for drug storage bins, medication administration records, as well as pharmacy and prescriber computer order entry screens.

The Joint Commission (TJC) has established a National Patient Safety Goal that specifies that certain abbreviations must appear on an accredited organization's do-not-use list; we have highlighted these items with a double asterisk (**). However, we hope that you will consider others beyond the minimum TJC requirements. By using and promoting safe practices and by educating one another about hazards, we can better protect our patients.

*Continued*

**TABLE 11-5**   ISMP's List of Error-Prone Abbreviations, Symbols, and Dose Designations—cont'd

| Abbreviations | Intended Meaning | Misinterpretation | Correction |
|---|---|---|---|
| μg | Microgram | Mistaken as "mg" | Use "mcg" |
| AD, AS, AU | Right ear, left ear, each ear | Mistaken as OD, OS, OU (right eye, left eye, each eye) | Use "right ear," "left ear," or "each ear" |
| OD, OS, OU | Right eye, left eye, each eye | Mistaken as AD, AS, AU (right ear, left ear, each ear) | Use "right eye," "left eye," or "each eye" |
| BT | Bedtime | Mistaken as "BID" (twice daily) | Use "bedtime" |
| cc | Cubic centimeters | Mistaken as "u" (units) | Use "mL" |
| D/C | Discharge or discontinue | Premature discontinuation of medications if D/C (intended to mean "discharge") has been misinterpreted as "discontinued" when followed by a list of discharge medications | Use "discharge" and "discontinue" |
| IJ | Injection | Mistaken as "IV" or "intrajugular" | Use "injection" |
| IN | Intranasal | Mistaken as "IM" or "IV" | Use "intranasal or "NAS" |
| HS | Half-strength | Mistaken as bedtime | Use "half-strength" |
| hs | At bedtime, hours of sleep | Mistaken as half-strength | Use "bedtime" |
| IU** | International unit | Mistaken as IV (intravenous) or 10 (ten) | Use "units" |
| o.d. or OD | Once daily | Mistaken as "right eye" (OD—oculus dexter), leading to oral liquid medications administered in the eye | Use "daily" |
| OJ | Orange juice | Mistaken as OD or OS (right or left eye); drugs meant to be diluted in orange juice may be given in the eye | Use "orange juice" |
| Per os | By mouth, orally | The "os" can be mistaken as "left eye" (OS—oculus sinister) | Use "PO," "by mouth," or "orally" |
| q.d. or QD** | Every day | Mistaken as q.i.d., especially if the period after the "q" or the tail of the "q" is misunderstood as an "i" | Use "daily" |
| qhs | Nightly at bedtime | Mistaken as "qhr" or every hour | Use "nightly" |
| qn | Nightly or at bedtime | Mistaken as "qh" (every hour) | Use "nightly" or "at bedtime" |
| q.o.d. or QOD** | Every other day | Mistaken as "q.d." (daily) or "q.i.d. (four times daily) if the "o" is poorly written | Use "every other day" |
| q1d | Daily | Mistaken as q.i.d. (four times daily) | Use "daily" |
| q6PM, etc. | Every evening at 6 PM | Mistaken as every 6 hours | Use "6 PM nightly" or "6 PM daily" |
| SC, SQ, sub q | Subcutaneous | SC mistaken as SL (sublingual); SQ mistaken as "5 every;" the "q" in "sub q" has been mistaken as "every" (e.g., a heparin dose ordered "sub q 2 hours before surgery" misunderstood as every 2 hours before surgery) | Use "subcut" or "subcutaneously" |

**These abbreviations are included on TJC's "minimum list" of dangerous abbreviations, acronyms, and symbols that must be included on an organization's "do not use" list, effective January 1, 2004. Visit www.jointcommission.org for more information about this TJC requirement.

**TABLE 11-5**   ISMP's List of Error-Prone Abbreviations, Symbols, and Dose Designations—cont'd

| Abbreviations | Intended Meaning | Misinterpretation | Correction |
|---|---|---|---|
| **ss** | Sliding scale (insulin) or ½ (apothecary) | Mistaken as "55" | Spell out "sliding scale", use "one-half" or "1/2" |
| **SSRI** | Sliding scale regular insulin | Mistaken as selective serotonin reuptake inhibitor | Spell out "sliding scale (insulin)" |
| **SSI** | Sliding scale insulin | Mistaken as Strong Solution of Iodine (Lugol's) | Spell out "sliding scale (insulin)" |
| **i/d** | One daily | Mistaken as "tid" | Use "1 daily" |
| **TIW or tiw** | 3 times a week | Mistaken as "3 times a day" or "twice in a week" | Use "3 times weekly" |
| **U or u**\*\* | Unit | Mistaken as the number 0 or 4, causing a 10-fold overdose or greater (e.g., 4U seen as "40" or 4u seen as "44"); mistaken as "cc" so dose given in volume instead of units (e.g., 4u seen as 4cc) | Use "unit" |

| Dose Designations and Other Information | Intended Meaning | Misinterpretation | Correction |
|---|---|---|---|
| **Trailing zero after decimal point (e.g., 1.0 mg)**\*\* | 1 mg | Mistaken as 10 mg if the decimal point is not seen | Do not use trailing zeros for doses expressed in whole numbers |
| **"Naked" decimal point (e.g., .5 mg)**\*\* | 0.5 mg | Mistaken as 5 mg if the decimal point is not seen | Use zero before a decimal point when the dose is less than a whole unit |
| **Drug name and dose run together (especially problematic for drug names that end in "l" such as Inderal40 mg; Tegretol300 mg)** | Inderal 40 mg  Tegretol 300 mg | Mistaken as Inderal 140 mg  Mistaken as Tegretol 1300 mg | Place adequate space between the drug name, dose, and unit of measure |
| **Numerical dose and unit of measure run together (e.g., 10mg, 100mL)** | 10 mg  100 mL | The "m" is sometimes mistaken as a zero or two zeros, risking a 10- to 100-fold overdose | Place adequate space between the dose and unit of measure |
| **Abbreviations such as mg. or mL. with a period following the abbreviation** | mg  mL | The period is unnecessary and could be mistaken as the number 1 if written poorly | Use mg, mL, etc. without a terminal period |
| **Large doses without properly placed commas (e.g., 100000 units; 1000000 units)** | 100,000 units  1,000,000 units | 100000 has been mistaken as 10,000 or 1,000,000; 1000000 has been mistaken as 100,000 | Use commas for dosing units at or above 1,000, or use words such as 100 "thousand" or 1 "million" to improve readability |

*Continued*

**TABLE 11-5**   ISMP's List of Error-Prone Abbreviations, Symbols, and Dose Designations—cont'd

| Drug Name Abbreviations | Intended Meaning | Misinterpretation | Correction |
|---|---|---|---|
| **ARA A** | vidarabine | Mistaken as cytarabine (ARA C) | Use complete drug name |
| **AZT** | zidovudine (Retrovir) | Mistaken as azathioprine or aztreonam | Use complete drug name |
| **CPZ** | Compazine (prochlorperazine) | Mistaken as chlorpromazine | Use complete drug name |
| **DPT** | Demerol-Phenergan-Thorazine | Mistaken as diphtheria-pertussis-tetanus (vaccine) | Use complete drug name |
| **DTO** | Diluted tincture of opium, or deodorized tincture of opium (Paregoric) | Mistaken as tincture of opium | Use complete drug name |
| **HCl** | hydrochloric acid or hydrochloride | Mistaken as potassium chloride (the "H" is misinterpreted as "K") | Use complete drug name unless expressed as a salt of a drug |
| **HCT** | hydrocortisone | Mistaken as hydrochlorothiazide | Use complete drug name |
| **HCTZ** | hydrochlorothiazide | Mistaken as hydrocortisone (seen as HCT250 mg) | Use complete drug name |
| **MgSO4**\*\* | magnesium sulfate | Mistaken as morphine sulfate | Use complete drug name |
| **MS, MS04**\*\* | morphine sulfate | Mistaken as magnesium sulfate | Use complete drug name |
| **MTX** | methotrexate | Mistaken as mitoxantrone | Use complete drug name |
| **PCA** | procainamide | Mistaken as patient-controlled analgesia | Use complete drug name |
| **PTU** | propylthiouracil | Mistaken as mercaptopurine | Use complete drug name |
| **T3** | Tylenol with codeine No. 3 | Mistaken as liothyronine | Use complete drug name |
| **TAC** | triamcinolone | Mistaken as tetracaine, Adrenalin, cocaine | Use complete drug name |
| **TNK** | TNKase | Mistaken as "TPA" | Use complete drug name |
| **ZnSO4** | zinc sulfate | Mistaken as morphine sulfate | Use complete drug name |

| Stemmed Drug Names | Intended Meaning | Misinterpretation | Correction |
|---|---|---|---|
| **"Nitro" drip** | nitroglycerin infusion | Mistaken as sodium nitroprusside infusion | Use complete drug name |
| **"Norflox"** | norfloxacin | Mistaken as Norflex | Use complete drug name |
| **"IV Vanc"** | intravenous vancomycin | Mistaken as Invanz | Use complete drug name |
| **ʒ** | Dram | Symbol for dram mistaken as "3" | Use the metric system |
| **♏** | Minim | Symbol for minim mistaken as "mL" | |
| **x3d** | For three days | Mistaken as "3 doses" | Use "for three days" |
| **> and <** | Greater than and less than | Mistaken as opposite of intended; mistakenly use incorrect symbol; "<10" mistaken as "40" | Use "greater than" or "less than" |
| **/ {slash mark}** | Separates two doses or indicates "per" | Mistaken as the number 1 (e.g., "25 units/10 units" misread as "25 units and 110 units") | Use "per" rather than a slash mark to separate doses |
| **@** | At | Mistaken as "2" | Use "at" |
| **&** | And | Mistaken as "2" | Use "and" |
| **+** | Plus or and | Mistaken as "4" | Use "and" |
| **°** | Hour | Mistaken as a zero (e.g., q2° seen as q 20) | Use "hr," "h," or "hour" |

©ISMP, 2007. Used with permission.

## ■ Points to Remember

- A primary responsibility of the nurse is the safe administration of medications to a client.
- Interpret the order systematically, the way in which it is written (the name of the medication, the dosage, the route, and frequency).
- The seven components of a medication order are as follows:
  1. The full name of the client
  2. Date and time the order was written
  3. Name of the medication to be administered
  4. Dosage of the medication
  5. Route of administration
  6. Time or frequency of administration
  7. Signature of the person writing the order
- All medication orders must be legible, and standard abbreviations and symbols must be used.
- Memorize the meaning of common abbreviations and symbols.
- The nurse needs to be aware of acronyms, symbols, and abbreviations that should not be used. Their use can increase the potential for errors in medication administration.
- Oral (verbal) orders must be written down, read back to the prescriber, and confirmed with the prescriber that the order is correct
- If any of the seven components of a medication order are missing or seem incorrect, the medication order is not legal. Do not assume—clarify the order!
- If you are in doubt as to the meaning of an order, clarify it with the prescriber before administering.
- Always crosscheck medications; misidentification can result in a medication error.

 **Practice Problems**

Interpret the following abbreviations.
  1. p.c. _____

  2. h _____

  3. q12h _____

  4. b.i.d. _____

  5. p.r.n. _____

Interpret the following orders. Use *administer* or *give* at the beginning of the sentence.
  6. Zidovudine 200 mg p.o. q4h. _____

  _____

  7. Procaine penicillin G 400,000 units IV q8h. _____

  _____

  8. Gentamicin sulfate 45 mg IVPB, q12h. _____

  _____

  9. Regular Humulin insulin 5 units subcut, a.c. at 7:30 AM and at bedtime. _____

  _____

10. Vitamin B$_{12}$ 1,000 mcg IM, every other day. _____

_____

11. Prilosec 20 mg p.o. bid. _____

_____

12. Tofranil 75 mg p.o. at bedtime. _____

_____

13. Restoril 30 mg p.o. at bedtime. _____

_____

14. Mylanta 30 mL p.o. q4h p.r.n. _____

_____

15. Synthroid 200 mcg p.o. daily. _____

_____

Answers on p. 609

## ✓ CHAPTER REVIEW

List the seven components of a medication order.

1. _____        5. _____

2. _____        6. _____

3. _____        7. _____

4. _____

Write the meaning of the following abbreviations.

8. b.i.d. _____        14. b.i.w. _____

9. ad. lib. _____        15. elix. _____

10. subcut _____        16. syr _____

11. c̄ _____        17. n.p.o. _____

12. a.c. _____        18. sl _____

13. q.i.d. _____

Give the abbreviations for the following:

19. after meals _____    25. may be repeated once if necessary ___

20. three times a day _____    26. without _____

21. intramuscular _____    27. immediately _____

22. every eight hours _____    28. ointment _____

23. suppository _____    29. milliequivalent _____

24. intravenous _____    30. by rectum _____

Interpret the following orders. Use *administer* or *give* at the beginning of the sentence.

31. Methergine 0.2 mg p.o. q4h for 6 doses. _____

_____

32. digoxin 0.125 mg p.o. once a day. _____

_____

33. Regular Humulin insulin 14 units subcut daily at 7:30 AM. _____

_____

34. Demerol 50 mg IM and atropine 0.4 mg IM on call to the operating room.

_____

35. Ampicillin 500 mg p.o. stat, and then 250 mg p.o. q.i.d. thereafter. _____

_____

36. Lasix 40 mg IM stat. _____

_____

37. Librium 50 mg p.o. q4h p.r.n. for agitation. _____

_____

38. Tylenol 650 mg p.o. q4h p.r.n. for pain._____

_____

39. Mylicon 80 mg p.o. p.c. and bedtime. _____

_____

40. Folic acid 1 mg p.o. every day. _____

_____

41. Nembutal 100 mg p.o. at bedtime p.r.n._____

_____

42. Aspirin gr x p.o. q4h p.r.n. for temperature greater than 101° F. _____

_____

43. Dilantin 100 mg p.o. t.i.d. _____

_____

44. Minipress 2 mg p.o. b.i.d.; hold for systolic BP less than 120._____

_____

45. Compazine 10 mg IM q4h p.r.n. for nausea and vomiting. _____

_____

46. Ampicillin 1 g IVPB q6h for 4 doses. _____

_____

47. Heparin 5,000 units subcut q12h._____

_____

48. Dilantin susp 200 mg by NGT q AM and 300 mg by NGT at bedtime. _____

_____

49. Benadryl 50 mg p.o. stat. _____

_____

50. Vitamin B$_{12}$ 1,000 mcg IM three times a week. _____

_____

51. Milk of magnesia 30 mL p.o. at bedtime p.r.n. for constipation. _____

_____

52. Septra DS tab 1 p.o. daily. _____

_____

53. Neomycin ophthalmic ointment 1% in the right eye t.i.d._____

_____

54. Carafate 1 g via NGT q.i.d. _____

_____

55. Morphine sulfate 15 mg subcut stat and 10 mg subcut q4h p.r.n. for pain. _____

_____

56. Ampicillin 120 mg IVSS q6h for 7 days. _____

_____

57. Prednisone 10 mg p.o. every other day. _____

_____

Identify the missing part from the following medication orders. Assume that the date, time, and signature are included on the orders.

58. Dicloxacillin 250 mg q.i.d. _____

59. Synthroid 0.05 mg p.o. _____

60. Nitrofurantoin p.o. q6h for 10 days. _____

61. 25 mg p.o. q12h, hold if BP less than 100 systolic. _____

62. Solu-Cortef 100 q6h. _____

63. Describe what your action would be if the following order was written:

    Prilosec 20 mg daily. _____

Using the discussion on medication abbreviations, symbols, and acronyms that should not be used, identify the mistake in the following orders and correct each order.

64. Inderal20mg p.o. daily. _____

65. Lasix 10.0 mg p.o. b.i.d. _____

66. Humulin Regular insulin 4U IV stat. _____

67. Haldol .5 mg p.o. t.i.d. _____

Answers on pp. 609-610

 **For additional practice problems, refer to the Safety in Medication Administration section of Drug Calculations Companion, Version 4, on Evolve.**

# CHAPTER 12

# Medication Administration Records and Drug Distribution Systems

## Objectives

*After reviewing this chapter, you should be able to:*
1. Identify the necessary information that must be transcribed to a medication administration record (MAR)
2. Read an MAR and identify medications that are given on a routine basis, including the name of the medication, the dosage, the route of administration, and the time of administration
3. Transcribe medication orders to an MAR
4. Identify the various drug distribution systems used

Documentation is the sixth and last "right of medication administration." Documentation should follow the administration of medication and include not only medications administered but also documentation regarding refusals, delays in administration, and responses to (including adverse effects of) medication administration.

## Tips for Clinical Practice

Document properly and accurately any medications administered to prevent medication errors caused by overmedication or undermedication.

Regardless of the form used to document administration of medications it must be accurate and is considered a legal document.

The medication record system is the most widely used system for medication administration in hospitals. Different forms are used in the home care setting. The medication record is a way of keeping track of medications a client has received and is currently receiving. The name of each medication, as well as the dosage, route, and frequency, is written on the client's medication record. At some institutions a complete schedule is written out for all the administration times for medications given on a continual or routine basis. In some institutions the method of charting medications varies (e.g., some sign for the day and just put in times given). The charting for computerized records also varies. Each time a dosage is given, the nurse initials the record next to the time. In some institutions separate records are maintained for routine, intravenous (IV), and as-needed (prn) medications and for medications administered on a one-time basis, whereas in others these are kept on the same record in a designated area. The medication record system is the same as the medication administration record (MAR).

For medication records and charting, some institutions use a Kardex, an MAR, or a combination of the two.

After a medication order has been verified, the order is transcribed to the official record used at the institution. Each institution has its own medication record. The form may be computer generated or hand written.

> The various medication administration forms used at different institutions represent differences in form only; essential information is common to all.

## ESSENTIAL INFORMATION ON A MEDICATION RECORD

All the information on the medication record must be legible and transcribed carefully to avoid errors. In addition to client information (name, date of birth, medical record number, allergies), the following information is necessary on all medication forms:

1. **Dates.** This information usually includes the date the order was written, the date the medication is to be started (if different from the order date), and when to discontinue it.
2. **Medication Information.** This includes the medication's full name, the dosage, the route, and the frequency. Abbreviations used on the medication record should be standard abbreviations and follow the guidelines and restrictions of The Joint Commission, ISMP, and the health care institution.
3. **Time of Administration.** This will be based on the desired administration schedule stated on the order, such as t.i.d. The desired administration time is placed on the medication record and converted to time periods based on the institution's time intervals for scheduled or routine medications. (Thus t.i.d. may mean 9 AM, 1 PM, and 5 PM at one institution and 10 AM, 2 PM, and 6 PM at another.) A nurse should always become familiar with the hours for medication administration designated by a specific institution. Medication times for p.r.n. and one-time dosages are recorded at the time they are administered. Abbreviations for time and frequency should adhere to The Joint Commission and ISMP guidelines.
4. **Initials.** Most medication records have a place for the initials of the person transcribing the medication to the MAR (Figure 12-1, *A*) and the person administering the medication (Figure 12-1, *B*). The initials are then written under the signature section to identify who gave the medication. Some forms may request the title as well as the signature of the nurse (Figure 12-1, *C*). The policy regarding initialing after each administration varies by institution and by charting system used.
5. **Special Instructions (parameters).** Any special instructions relating to a medication should be indicated on the medication record. For example, "Hold if blood pressure less than 100 systolic" or "p.r.n. for pain."

In addition to the information listed above, some medication records may include legends, as well as an area for charting to indicate when a medication is omitted or a dosage is not given. See Figure 12-1, *D*, for a legend of omitted doses. Other medication records may have an area where the nurse can document the reason for omission of a medication directly on the medication record (Figure 12-1, *E*). Other information may include injection codes so the nurse may indicate the injection site for parenteral medications (Figure 12-1, *F*). In cases in which no injection codes are indicated, the nurse is still expected to indicate the injection site. Space may also be allotted for charting information such as pulse and blood pressure if this information is relevant to the medication.

## Tips for Clinical Practice

The nurse must stay alert to the guidelines of The Joint Commission and ISMP regarding abbreviations and medical notations.

*Text continued p. 147*

## ST. BARNABAS HOSPITAL

BRONX, NY 10457

### DEPARTMENT OF NURSING
MEDICATION ADMINISTRATION RECORD

Addressograph or printed label
with client information

DIAGNOSIS:

| ALLERGIC TO: | DATE: |
|---|---|
| NKDA | 4/2/11 |

D

**LEGEND**
Omitted doses (use red pen):
Document in Medication Omission Record

1. NPO    3. I.V. Out    5. Other
2. Off-Unit    4. Pt. Refused

PAGE _____ OF _____

A

| ORDER DATE / EXP. DATE | REORDER DATE / EXP. DATE | STANDING MEDICATIONS MED-DOSE-FREQ-ROUTE | DATE 2005 TIME | 4/2 INIT. | 4/3 INIT. | 4/4 INIT. | 4/5 INIT. | 4/6 INIT. | 4/7 INIT. | 4/8 INIT. | 4/9 INIT. |
|---|---|---|---|---|---|---|---|---|---|---|---|
| DG 4/2/11 R.N. INIT. | | Keflex 250 mg po | 9A | DG | JN | | | | | | |
| | | qid for 7 days | 1P | DG | JN  B | | | | | | |
| | | | 5P | NN | NN | | | | | | |
| 4/8/11 REORD INIT. | | | 9P | NN | NN | | | | | | |
| DG 4/2/11 R.N. INIT. | | MVI 1 tab po daily | 9A | DG | JN | | | | | | |
| 5/2/11 REORD INIT. | | | | | | | | | | | |
| DG 4/2/11 R.N. INIT. | | Colace 100 mg po bid | 9A | DG | JN | | | | | | |
| | | | 5P | NN | NN | | | | | | |
| 5/2/11 REORD INIT. | | | | | | | | | | | |
| R.N. INIT. | | | | | | | | | | | |
| REORD INIT. | | | | | | | | | | | |
| R.N. INIT. | | | | | | | | | | | |
| REORD INIT | | | | | | | | | | | |

F

**INJECTION CODES:**

| RT = RIGHT THIGH | RA = RIGHT ARM | LU = LEFT UPPER GLUTEAL | ↑ RAB = UPPER RIGHT ABDOMEN | ↑ LAB = UPPER LEFT ABDOMEN |
|---|---|---|---|---|
| LT = LEFT THIGH | LA = LEFT ARM | RU = RIGHT UPPER GLUTEAL | ↓ RAB = LOWER RIGHT ABDOMEN | ↓ LAB = LOWER LEFT ABDOMEN |

**Figure 12-1**    Medication administration record for Practice Exercise 1. (Used with permission of St. Barnabas Hospital, Bronx, New York.)

## ST. BARNABAS HOSPITAL

BRONX, NY 10457

### DEPARTMENT OF NURSING
MEDICATION ADMINISTRATION RECORD

| DIAGNOSIS: |
| --- |
| |
| ALLERGIC TO: | DATE: |

Addressograph or printed label
with client information

| ORDER DATE / EXP. DATE | REORDER DATE / EXP. DATE | P.R.N. MEDICATION MED-DOSE-FREQ-ROUTE | | DOSES GIVEN |
| --- | --- | --- | --- | --- |
| R.N. INIT. / REORD INIT. | | | DATE TIME SITE INIT. | |
| R.N. INIT. / REORD INIT. | | | DATE TIME SITE INIT. | |
| R.N. INIT. / REORD INIT. | | | DATE TIME SITE INIT. | |
| R.N. INIT. / REORD INIT. | | | DATE TIME SITE INIT. | |
| R.N. INIT. / REORD INIT. | | | DATE TIME SITE INIT. | |

C——INITIAL IDENTIFICATION

| | INITIAL | PRINT NAME, TITLE | | INITIAL | PRINT NAME, TITLE | | INITIAL | PRINT NAME, TITLE |
| --- | --- | --- | --- | --- | --- | --- | --- | --- |
| 1 | DG | Deborah Gray RN | 5 | | | 9 | | |
| 2 | NN | Nancy Nurse RN | 6 | | | 10 | | |
| 3 | JN | Jane Nightingale RN | 7 | | | 11 | | |
| 4 | | | 8 | | | 12 | | |

**Figure 12-1, cont'd** Medication administration record for Practice Exercise 1. (Used with permission of St. Barnabas Hospital, Bronx, New York.)

*Continued*

| | | | SINGLE-STAT-PREOP-ORDERS | | | | | | | | |
|---|---|---|---|---|---|---|---|---|---|---|---|
| ORDER DATE | NURSE INIT. | MED-DOSE-ROUTE | TO BE GIVEN | | | ORDER DATE | NURSE INIT. | MED-DOSE-ROUTE | TO BE GIVEN | | |
| | | | DATE | TIME | NURSE INIT. | | | | DATE | TIME | NURSE INIT. |
| | | | | | | | | | | | |
| | | | | | | | | | | | |
| | | | | | | | | | | | |
| | | | | | | | | | | | |
| | | | | | | | | | | | |
| | | | | | | | | | | | |
| | | | | | | | | | | | |
| | | | | | | | | | | | |
| | | | | | | | | | | | |
| | | | | | | | | | | | |
| | | | | | | | | | | | |
| | | | | | | | | | | | |
| | | | | | | | | | | | |
| | | | | | | | | | | | |
| | | | | | | | | | | | |
| | | | | | | | | | | | |
| | | | | | | | | | | | |
| | | | | | | | | | | | |

**MEDICATION OMISSION RECORD**  (Every entry must be dated & signed)

| DATE | HOUR | REMARKS |
|---|---|---|
| | | |
| | | |  ——— E
| | | |
| | | |
| | | |
| | | |
| | | |
| | | |
| | | |
| | | |
| | | |
| | | |
| | | |
| | | |
| | | |
| | | |
| | | |
| | | |
| | | |

**Figure 12-1, cont'd**    Medication administration record for Practice Exercise 1. (Used with permission of St. Barnabas Hospital, Bronx, New York.)

## DOCUMENTATION OF MEDICATIONS ADMINISTERED

MARs include an area for documenting medications administered. After administering the medication, the nurse or other qualified staff member must record his or her initials next to the time the drug was administered. For scheduled medications, a complete schedule is written out, and the initials are recorded next to each given time. As previously mentioned, this practice can vary by institution. With one-time dosages and p.r.n. medication, *the time of administration* is written and again initialed by the person administering it. The medication form has a place for the full name of each person administering medications, along with the identifying initials. This allows for immediate identification of the person's initials if necessary. When medications are not administered, some records have notations, such as an asterisk (*), a circle, or a number corresponding to a legend on the MAR, to indicate this, or there may be an area on the back or at the bottom of the MAR for charting medications not given (see Figure 12-1, *E*). The type of notation used will depend on the institution. In addition to notations made on the MAR, most institutions require documentation in the proper section of the client's chart. (Some institutions have a section designated "nurse's notes." At other institutions nurses may be charting on a progress note and indicate that notation "nurse's notes".

## EXPLANATION OF MEDICATION ADMINISTRATION RECORDS

Many types of MARs are used, and these forms vary among institutions. However, despite the variety of forms, MARs contain essential information that is common to all and to their purpose. The MAR is used to determine what medications are ordered and the dosage, route, and time at which each is to be given. The MAR is also verified with the prescriber's orders. Any MAR requiring transcription of orders should always be checked against the prescriber's orders. In institutions where personnel other than the nurse transcribe orders, the nurse must double-check the transcription to make sure there are no discrepancies. Regardless of the variation in format for MARs, the information common to all is as follows:

1. The name of the client and pertinent data related to the client
2. Medication (dosage, route)
3. Time/frequency desired for administration
4. A place to indicate allergies
5. A place for date, the initials of the person who administers the medication, and a section to identify the name of the person administering the medication

A sample MAR is included in this chapter. As you look at the sample record, it is important to locate and identify the information common to all MARs, with focus on medications that are given on a continual basis.

### Tips for Clinical Practice

Regardless of the type of form used, when medication orders are transcribed to an MAR, the nurse uses the record to check the medication order, prepare the correct dosage, and record the medication administered.

## USE OF COMPUTERS IN MEDICATION ADMINISTRATION

As in other businesses, the use of computers in health care facilities is increasing. As a result of the reported rise in medication errors, many health care facilities have instituted some form of computer-based medication administration. The literature supports the fact that one of the main causes of medication errors is the incorrect transcription of the original prescriber's order. According to Michael Cohen in the book titled *Medication Errors,* (2007), "In transcribed orders, stray marks as well as marks intended as initials, letters, check marks, and so forth can also obscure or change the appearance of a medication order. Handwritten MARs can contribute to errors if they are crowded or illegible or present drug information in an inconsistent manner." Typically, according to Cohen, "orders are transcribed onto the MAR exactly as written; the presentation of information may not be consistent, and error-prone abbreviations and dose expressions may be carried forth from the order."

Many health care facilities have moved away from the written medication order and transcription of orders to the MAR to a computer prescriber order entry (CPOE). This system was designed to eliminate the problem of unclear and ambiguous orders, which was identified as a common reason for medication errors. Medication orders of the prescriber are either electronically transmitted or manually entered into the system. The CPOE system accepts orders in a standard format conforming to strict criteria. Once the order has been entered into the system, it is transmitted to the pharmacy to be processed. Depending on the institution and the sophistication of the software, information such as medication incompatibilities, medication allergies, range of dosages, and recommended medication times may be part of the system. This shows the importance of computers to the safe administration of medication. With the computer used to process medication orders, orders can be viewed on the computer screen or on a printout. A corresponding MAR is available at some institutions based on the computerized order entry. The computerized MAR allows the nurse to enter the charting of medications into the computer, as well as any other essential information relating to medication administration. Each institution generates its own medication record, following a specific format.

At some institutions after the entry of orders into the system, the computer automatically generates a list of all the medications to be given to clients on a unit and the times they are to be given. The computer has become an essential tool for medication administration at some institutions. It is important to note that the use of computers in reference to medication administration times varies from one institution to the next and the sophistication of the computer system depends on the facility and the software purchased.

## MEDICATION DISTRIBUTION SYSTEMS

The medication distribution system varies from one institution to the next. The various distribution systems are discussed in the following sections.

### Unit-Dose System

Many institutions use a system of medication administration referred to as *unit dose*. This system has decreased medication preparation time because the medications are prepared daily in the pharmacy and sent to the unit. Medications are dispensed by the pharmacy in individual dosages as prescribed. Packages provide a single dosage of medication. The package is labeled with generic and trade names (and sometimes manufacturer, lot number, and expiration date). Depending on the distribution system, the individual packages may be labeled with the client's name and bar code. The medications are placed in a client-identified drawer in a large unit-dose cabinet at the nurse's station. "The value of unit dose dispensing in preventing errors should not be underestimated. TJC standards require medications to be dispensed in the most ready-to-administer form possible to minimize opportunities for error" (Cohen, 2007). In *Medication Errors* (2007) Cohen points out that although unit-dose may be used, the system does not extend to all products. (Example: in many institutions nurses are responsible for reconstituting or preparing IV doses from floor stock drugs and no policy exists for double-checking accuracy of calculation, preparation, and labeling.) Errors therefore occur that a fully implemented unit-dose system could have prevented.

Unit dose is also used as part of another medication system in some institutions (e.g., a computerized unit dose medication cart). In the computerized unit-dose system, each dosage for the client is released individually and recorded automatically. This system is used for monitoring controlled substances and other items used in the unit (e.g., medications used by the unit in large volumes). The type of medication form used for this system varies from one institution to another. In some instances this system has decreased the amount of time spent transcribing orders or eliminated the need for transcription. In some institutions, however, transcription of medication orders to the MAR is still required. The prescriber's orders are therefore written on a separate order sheet and sent to the pharmacy. Figure 12-2 illustrates the transcription of orders to the MAR.

At some institutions the prescriber's order is done by computer entry, eliminating the need for transcription. Figure 12-3 shows a unit-dose cabinet.

## ST. BARNABAS HOSPITAL
### BRONX, NY 10457
### DEPARTMENT OF NURSING
MEDICATION ADMINISTRATION RECORD

| DIAGNOSIS: CHF |
|---|

Addressograph or printed label
with client information

| ALLERGIC TO: Aspirin | DATE: 5/1/11 |
|---|---|

**LEGEND**
Omitted doses (use red pen):   1. NPO   3. I.V. Out   5. Other
Document in Medication Omission Record   2. Off-Unit   4. Pt. Refused

PAGE _____ OF _____

| ORDER DATE / EXP. DATE | REORDER DATE / EXP. DATE | STANDING MEDICATIONS MED-DOSE-FREQ-ROUTE | DATE 2005 TIME | 5/1 INIT. | 5/2 INIT. | 5/3 INIT. | 5/4 INIT. | 5/5 INIT. | 5/6 INIT. | 5/7 INIT. | 5/8 INIT. |
|---|---|---|---|---|---|---|---|---|---|---|---|
| NN 5/1/11 R.N. INIT. | | Vasotec 5 mg po daily, | 9A | NN | | | | | | | |
| | | hold for SBP less than 100 | B/P | 130/80 | | | | | | | |
| | | | | | | | | | | | |
| 6/1/11 REORD INIT. | | | | | | | | | | | |
| NN 5/1/11 R.N. INIT. | | Colace 100 mg po tid | 9A | NN | | | | | | | |
| | | | 1P | NN | | | | | | | |
| | | | 5P | JD | | | | | | | |
| 6/1/11 REORD INIT. | | | | | | | | | | | |
| NN 5/1/11 R.N. INIT. | | Digoxin 0.125 mg po daily | 9A | NN | | | | | | | |
| | | | AP | 78 | | | | | | | |
| | | | | | | | | | | | |
| 6/1/11 REORD INIT. | | | | | | | | | | | |
| NN 5/1/11 R.N. INIT. | | Lasix 20 mg po daily, | 9A | NN | | | | | | | |
| | | hold for SBP less than 100 | B/P | 130/80 | | | | | | | |
| | | | | | | | | | | | |
| 6/1/11 REORD INIT. | | | | | | | | | | | |
| NN 5/1/11 R.N. INIT. | | Benadryl 25 mg po hour of sleep for | (9P) | JD | | | | | | | |
| | | 3 nights | | | ① | ② | ③ | | | | |
| | | | | | | | | | | | |
| 5/3/11 REORD INIT | | | | | | | | | | | |

**INJECTION CODES:**
RT = RIGHT THIGH   RA = RIGHT ARM   LU = LEFT UPPER GLUTEAL   ↑ RAB = UPPER RIGHT ABDOMEN   ↑ LAB = UPPER LEFT ABDOMEN
LT = LEFT THIGH   LA = LEFT ARM   RU = RIGHT UPPER GLUTEAL   ↓ RAB = LOWER RIGHT ABDOMEN   ↓ LAB = LOWER LEFT ABDOMEN

**Figure 12-2**  Transcription of medication orders to a medication administration record. (Used with permission of St. Barnabas Hospital, Bronx, New York.)
*Continued*

## ST. BARNABAS HOSPITAL
BRONX, NY 10457
### DEPARTMENT OF NURSING
MEDICATION ADMINISTRATION RECORD

| DIAGNOSIS: |
| --- |
| |

| ALLERGIC TO: | DATE: |
| --- | --- |

Addressograph or printed label
with client information

| ORDER DATE / EXP. DATE | REORDER DATE / EXP. DATE | P.R.N. MEDICATION | | | |
| --- | --- | --- | --- | --- | --- |
| | | **MED-DOSE-FREQ-ROUTE** | | **DOSES GIVEN** | |
| R.N. INIT. / REORD INIT. | | | DATE / TIME / SITE / INIT. | | |
| R.N. INIT. / REORD INIT. | | | DATE / TIME / SITE / INIT. | | |
| R.N. INIT. / REORD INIT. | | | DATE / TIME / SITE / INIT. | | |
| R.N. INIT. / REORD INIT. | | | DATE / TIME / SITE / INIT. | | |
| R.N. INIT. / REORD INIT. | | | DATE / TIME / SITE / INIT. | | |

### INITIAL IDENTIFICATION

| | INITIAL | PRINT NAME, TITLE | | INITIAL | PRINT NAME, TITLE | | INITIAL | PRINT NAME, TITLE |
| --- | --- | --- | --- | --- | --- | --- | --- | --- |
| 1 | NN | Nancy News RN | 5 | | | 9 | | |
| 2 | JD | James Dean RN | 6 | | | 10 | | |
| 3 | | | 7 | | | 11 | | |
| 4 | | | 8 | | | 12 | | |

**Figure 12-2, cont'd** Transcription of medication orders to a medication administration record. (Used with permission of St. Barnabas Hospital, Bronx, New York.)

## Computer-Controlled Dispensing System

The use of automated dispensing cabinets (ADCs) is on the rise in health care facilities. According to the article "Implementing technology to improve medication safety in health care facilities: A literature review" by Ann Hidle (*Journal of the New York State Nurses Association,* Fall/Winter 2007-2008), close to 60% of hospitals have switched to this system. This system is gaining increased popularity in many institutions and health care facilities. The computer-controlled dispensing system is supplied by the pharmacy daily with stock medications. Controlled substances are also kept in the cart, and the system provides a detailed record indicating which controlled substances were used and by whom. The medication order is received by the pharmacy for the client and then entered into the system. To access medications in this system, the nurse uses a security code and password or biometric fingerprint scan.

The three most common dispensing systems are the Pyxis Med Station system (Figure 12-4), the Omnicell Omni Rx and the AcuDose Rx. These systems allow storage of items such as vials and premixed IVs and allow nurses to obtain any medications stored in the device for any client and even to override the system in an emergency. However, overrides eliminate verification of medications by the pharmacy which could result in error. Currently almost 90% of all automated dispensing cabinets are linked to pharmacy information systems, thereby decreasing errors by ensuring that the nurse can only access medications for a specific client.

Some institutions have added bar coding to this process during the administration phase of the medication process. At the client's bedside, the nurse uses a hand-held scanner that records the bar code on the client's wristband and the unit-dose medication packet, linking this information to the client database. If there is an error, the administration process is halted; if the information is correct, the medication is administered and documentation in the MAR occurs automatically. Literature supports that use of ADCs has reduced medication errors by dispensing the correct medication to the administered.

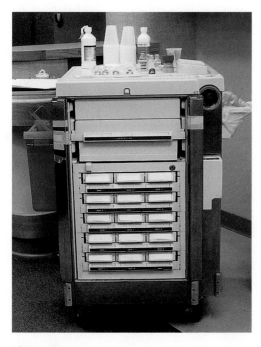

**Figure 12-3**  Unit-dose cabinet. (From Clayton BD, Stock YN, Harroun RD: *Basic pharmacology for nurses,* ed. 14, St. Louis, 2007, Mosby.)

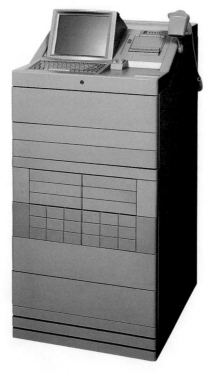

**Figure 12-4**  Pyxis Med Station. (From Clayton BD, Stock YN, Harroun RD: *Basic pharmacology for nurses,* ed. 14, St. Louis, 2007, Mosby.)

## Bar-Code Medication Delivery

Bar-code medication delivery is increasing in some health care facilities. Studies have shown that bar-code medication administration can reduce medication errors by 65% to 86% (Cohen, 2007). It was pioneered by the Veterans Affairs facilities. The basic system of bar coding verifies that a client receives the right dosage of the right medication by the right route at the right time. This system requires that each client wear an ID with a unique bar code to identify the individual. Each medication must therefore have a bar code. Computers installed at the client's bedside and/or hand-held devices enable the nurse to scan the bar code on the client's identification band and the medication to be administered. Once the information has been validated to the client and the client's medication profile, the medication given is documented on an online MAR (see Figure 12-5 showing a bar code for unit medication dose, and Figure 12-6 showing a bar-code reader). Bar coding is being added to some medication distribution systems as mentioned in the discussions of automated dispensing systems and unit-dose systems. Many pharmacists are using the bar-code system to prepare unit-dose medications. Like other systems, bar-code systems with additional features are also available. The complexity or simplicity of the bar-code system depends on the institution. The bar-code medication administration system allows overrides in cases where medications need to be administered in an emergency. However, literature points out that an override bypasses the important step of order verification by the pharmacist.

## Additional Technology in Medication Administration

Additional technology designed to prevent medication errors includes computer-based drug administration (CBDA), a technological software system. The purpose of the software is to automate the medication administration process and improve accuracy and efficiency in documentation. The system comprises the computerized prescriber order system, the bar-code administration system and the electronic medication administration record (eMAR), and the pharmacy information systems.

eMAR is a counterpart to the bar-code medication system that acts as a stringent safeguard to ensure that the right client receives the right medication, the right dose, by the right route, and at the right time. eMAR uses the bar code on the client's arm band and the bar code on the medications supplied by the pharmacy. Before administering medications, bar codes on the client's arm band and the medication are scanned using the bar-code scanner. The computer then checks the medications against the client's history (allergies, medication history) and lab results. The computer verifies and confirms that the nurse is administering the right medications to the right client in the right dosage, by the right route, and at the right time. The computer also alerts the nurse to any conditions that should be checked before administering the medication. The pharmacist and health care provider can access the computerized record to confirm medication delivery. In a study done by Kaplan et al. (2006), this process was shown to reduce the number of medication errors by 34% (Hidle, 2007-2008).

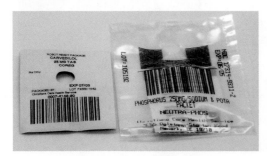

**Figure 12-5**  Bar code for unit drug dose. (From Kee JL, Marshall SM: *Clinical calculations: with applications to general and specialty areas,* ed. 6, St. Louis, 2009, Saunders.)

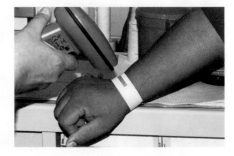

**Figure 12-6**  Bar-code reader. (From Kee JL, Marshall SM: *Clinical calculations: with applications to general and specialty areas,* ed. 6, St. Louis, 2009, Saunders.)

## ADVANTAGES AND DISADVANTAGES OF TECHNOLOGY

The nursing literature supports the belief that technology has decreased the number of medication errors; however, the risks of medication errors with technology have also been discussed. Even though the use of technology in the health care system has increased it has been emphasized that technology as well as medication administration systems are not a total safeguard. Hidle, in an article titled "Implementing technology to improve medication safety in health care facilities: A literature review" in the *Journal of the New York State Nurses Association* (Fall/Winter 2007-2008), points out that "any technology used in health care settings should be considered as additional safety precautions. Additionally, any system implemented in a health care setting should not overshadow the advanced knowledge of providers or decrease basic precautions." The author stresses that basic safety precautions such as the rights of medication administration cannot be eliminated and can help in the reduction of medication errors.

Some of the problems that can result in medication errors have been discussed in this chapter. It is important to remember that technology "can't improve safety unless system design and uses are carefully planned and properly implemented" (Grissinger and Globus, 2004).

In addition to aspects such as being able to override systems, entry errors can occur with computer prescribed order entry when orders are entered by the health care provider. Safeguards on CPOE do not prevent a prescriber from entering an order into the wrong client record or selecting the wrong medication (Grissinger and Globus, 2004), two problems that still exist with the CPOE system. Bar coding, like automated dispensing cabinets, allows overrides in cases where medications need to be administered in an emergency. According to Cohen in the book titled *Medication Errors* (2007), "All caregivers administering medications must understand that using an override bypasses the important step of order verification by a pharmacist." Cohen (2007) recommends that before a health care facility decides to use bar-coding medication administration, "facilities must anticipate failures and develop contingency plans for unexpected results."

It is important to be aware of the technological advances that have been instituted to decrease the occurrence of medication errors and to recognize that although their use has been shown to reduce errors, no system is completely without fault. Regardless of the medication system used, the nurse must recognize the importance of safety first and realize that no system eliminates the need for the nurse to follow the standard administration procedures for medication administration, such as verifying all aspects of the medication order—the right client, right medication, right dosage, right time, right route, and right documentation. In addition, institution of technology into medication administration requires a collaborative approach and commitment by all health care providers who will be affected in the process.

## SCHEDULING MEDICATION TIMES

Many health care facilities have routine schedules for administering medications, which vary from one institution to another. Common abbreviations are used for scheduling and prescribing medications. As previously mentioned in this chapter, the nurse must become familiar with the administration schedule used at a specific institution. Table 12-1 shows some examples of commonly used abbreviations in scheduling of medications. The nurse must be knowledgeable about abbreviations prohibited for use by The Joint Commission related to dosing frequency.

## MILITARY TIME

Many hospitals and health care agencies use military time (international time). Medication orders may include the time of administration in military time when documenting the administration of medications on the medication administration record (MAR). The nurse therefore needs to be familiar with how to convert traditional time to military time. Clinical facilities may use traditional or military (international) time for documentation. As a review,

**TABLE 12-1** Commonly Used Abbreviations for Scheduling Medications

| Abbreviation | Meaning |
|---|---|
| a.c.* | before meals |
| b.i.d | twice a day |
| p.c.* | after meals |
| p.r.n. | as needed (when necessary/required) |
| q.h. | every hour |
| q2h, q3h, q4h | every 2 hours, 3 hours, 4 hours |
| q6h, q8h, q12h, q24h | every 6 hours, 8 hours, 12 hours, 24 hours |
| q.i.d. | four times a day |
| stat | immediately (at once), now |
| t.i.d. | three times a day |

*Based on mealtimes.

military (international) time starts at 1 AM, or 0100 in the morning, and ends at 12 midnight, which is 2400. (0000 is commonly used by the military.) To convert AM, omit the colon and AM and ensure that a 4-digit number is written, adding a zero in the beginning as needed. For each hour beginning with 1 PM standard time, add 12 hours to convert to military.

Example: b.i.d. (twice a day) at a facility could be in standard time, for example, 9 (AM) and 5 (PM) or, in military time, 0900 and 1700.

Review content relating to converting time between traditional and military in Chapter 9 if necessary.

## ■ Points to Remember

- The system used for medication administration plays a role in determining the type of medication record used and whether transcription of orders is necessary.
- Regardless of the type of medication record used at an institution, the nurse should know the data that are essential for the medication record and understand the importance of the accuracy and clarity of medication orders.
- Persons transcribing orders should transcribe them in ink and write legibly to avoid medication errors. All essential notations or instructions should be clearly written on the medication record. Notations used should follow The Joint Commission and ISMP regulations.
- Documentation of medications administered should be done promptly, accurately, and only by the person administering them.
- To avoid errors in administration, always check transcribed orders against the prescriber's orders.
- The use of technology has reduced medication errors.
- Nurses need to be aware of the different distribution systems in use.
- Regardless of the system used, safety is the priority, and the nurse must still use the process in medication administration of verifying the order, administering the medication to the right client, right dosage, right route, right time, and right documentation.
- A facility may use traditional or military (international) time to designate administration times.

**Practice Problems**

1. True or False? Illegible prescribers' handwriting is the most common reason for medication errors on hand-written MARs (medication administration records). _____

2. True or False? The use of technology is a foolproof method to prevent medication errors. _____

3. True or False? Medication administration forms have information that is common to all regardless of the form used. _____

4. "The right _____ must receive the right _____ in the right _____ by the right _____ at the right _____ followed by the right _____."

5. The _____ is responsible for the drug administered regardless of the reason for the error.

6. The Pyxis is an example of _____.

7. The ability to _____ a system eliminates _____ by the pharmacy.

8. True or False? All health care institutions document medications using traditional time. _____

9. What is the last step in medication administration? _____

10. Fill in the blank in the following statement: CPOE is an abbreviation for _____.

Answers on p. 610

 **Practice Problems**

**Exercise 1**

Using the MAR in Figure 12-1, list the medication, dosage, route, and time for the medications given by DG (Deborah C. Gray) on 4/2/11 and by NN (Nancy Nurse) on 4/3/11.

| Date 4/2/11 | Medication | Dosage | Route | Time |
|---|---|---|---|---|
| 1. | _____ | _____ | _____ | _____ |
| 2. | _____ | _____ | _____ | _____ |
| 3. | _____ | _____ | _____ | _____ |
| 4. | _____ | _____ | _____ | _____ |

| Date 4/3/11 | Medication | Dosage | Route | Time |
|---|---|---|---|---|
| 1. | _____ | _____ | _____ | _____ |
| 2. | _____ | _____ | _____ | _____ |
| 3. | _____ | _____ | _____ | _____ |

Answers on p. 610

## ✓ CHAPTER REVIEW

1. Who determines the medication administration times? _____

2. Do b.i.d. and q2h have the same meaning? _____ Explain: _____

   _____

   _____

3. What is the purpose of bar coding? _____

4. The abbreviation *eMAR* stands for _____.

5. Times for medication administration can be indicated in _____or _____.

Answers on p. 610

## ✓ CHAPTER REVIEW

### Exercise 1

**NOTE**

Be sure to include order date and expiration date, complete the initial identification portion on the MAR, and place title as RN (registered nurse), SN (student nurse), or LPN (licensed practical nurse).

Transcribe the following orders to the practice medication sheet (Figure 12-7). When you have completed this, place your initials and signature in the appropriate space on the medication form. Use the times indicated and the date 4/9/11. Indicate client has no known drug allergies (NKDA). Diagnosis: pancreatitis.

1. Norvasc 5 mg p.o. daily, hold for SBP less than 100 (9A), expiration date 5/9/11. Leave space for recording B/P.

2. Thiamine 100 mg p.o. daily (9A), expiration 5/9/11.

3. Heparin 5,000 units subcut q12h 9A, site, 9P, site, expiration 4/16/11.

4. Ferrous sulfate 325 mg p.o. t.i.d. (9A, 1P, 5P), expiration 5/9/11.

Answers on p. 611

## ✓ CHAPTER REVIEW

### Exercise 2

Use Figure 12-8 (prn medication record) for orders 5 and 6. Date ordered is 4/10/11. Be sure to include order, date, and expiration date. Use the same client information provided in Chapter Review Exercise 1.

5. Percocet 2 tabs p.o. q4h p.r.n. for pain for 3 days. Chart that you administered it on 4/10/11 at 2 PM (start date 4/10/11, expiration date 4/13/11).

6. Tylenol 650 mg p.o. q4h p.r.n. temp greater than 101° F. Start date 4/10/11, expiration date 4/17/11.

Answers on p. 612

## ST. BARNABAS HOSPITAL
BRONX, NY 10457
### DEPARTMENT OF NURSING
MEDICATION ADMINISTRATION RECORD

Addressograph or printed label
with client information

| DIAGNOSIS: | |
|---|---|
| ALLERGIC TO: | DATE: |

**LEGEND**
Omitted doses (use red pen):
Document in Medication Omission Record
1. NPO    3. I.V. Out    5. Other
2. Off-Unit    4. Pt. Refused

PAGE _____ OF _____

| ORDER DATE / EXP. DATE | STANDING MEDICATIONS MED-DOSE-FREQ-ROUTE | DATE HOUR | INIT. | INIT. | INIT. | INIT. | INIT. | INIT. | INIT. | INIT. | INIT. |
|---|---|---|---|---|---|---|---|---|---|---|---|
| R.N. INIT. | | | | | | | | | | | |
| R.N. INIT. | | | | | | | | | | | |
| R.N. INIT. | | | | | | | | | | | |
| R.N. INIT. | | | | | | | | | | | |
| R.N. INIT. | | | | | | | | | | | |

**INJECTION CODES:**
RT = RIGHT THIGH    RA = RIGHT ARM    LU = LEFT UPPER GLUTEAL    ↑ RAB = UPPER RIGHT ABDOMEN    ↑ LAB = UPPER LEFT ABDOMEN
LT = LEFT THIGH    LA = LEFT ARM    RU = RIGHT UPPER GLUTEAL    ↓ RAB = LOWER RIGHT ABDOMEN    ↓ LAB = LOWER LEFT ABDOMEN

**Figure 12-7** Medication administration record for Chapter Review Exercise 1. (Used with permission of St. Barnabas Hospital, Bronx, New York.)

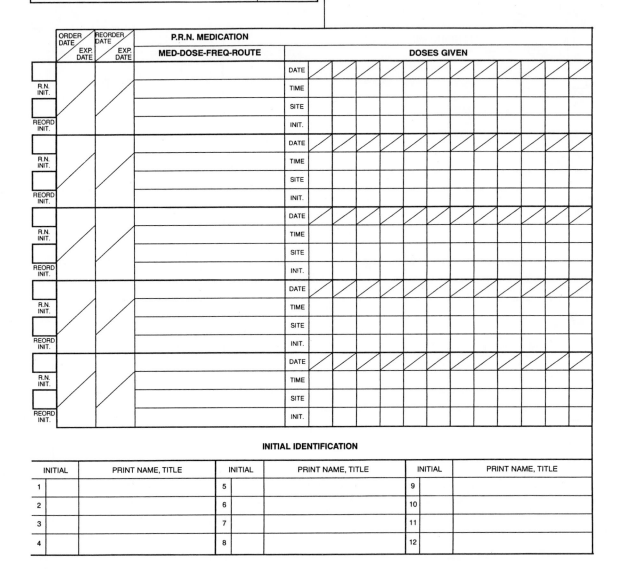

**Figure 12-8**   Medication administration record for Chapter Review Exercise 2. (Used with permission of St. Barnabas Hospital, Bronx, New York.)

 For addditional practice problems, refer to the Safety in Medication Administration section of Drug Calculations Companion, Version 4, on Evolve.

# CHAPTER 13

# Reading Medication Labels

## Objectives

*After reviewing this chapter, you should be able to identify:*
1. The trade and generic names of medications
2. The dosage strength of medications
3. The form in which a medication is supplied
4. The total volume of a medication container where indicated
5. Directions for mixing or preparing a drug where necessary
6. Information on combined-drug labels

To administer medications safely to a client, nurses must be able to read and interpret the information on a medication label. Medication labels indicate the dosage contained in the package. It is important to read the label carefully and recognize essential information.

## READING MEDICATION LABEL

The nurse should be able to recognize the following information on a medication label.

### Generic Name

The generic name is given by the manufacturer that first develops the medication. Medications have only one generic name. Prescribers are ordering medications more often by the generic name, so nurses need to know the generic name as well as the trade name. Pharmacists in many institutions are dispensing medications by generic name to decrease costs. Sometimes only the generic name may appear on a medication label or package. This is common for drugs that have been used for many years, are well known, and do not require marketing under a different trade name.

Examples include morphine, phenobarbital, and atropine (Figure 13-1). Another example of a medication commonly used in the clinical setting and often seen with only the generic name on the label is Demerol. Demerol is the trade or brand name; however, it is often seen with the generic name only (meperidine). Figure 13-2 shows Demerol labels with various strengths. Note that only meperidine is indicated on the label. As stated previously, by law, the generic name must be identified on all medication labels.

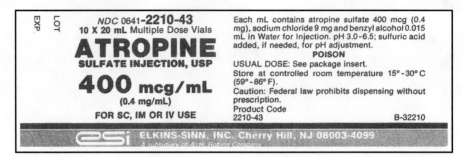

**Figure 13-1**    Atropine label.

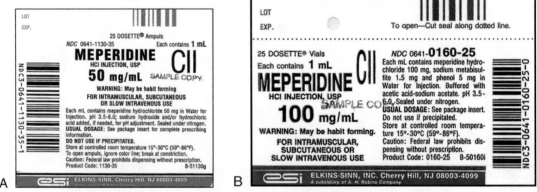

**Figure 13-2**    **A,** Meperidine 50 mg per mL. **B,** Meperidine 100 mg per mL.

## Tips for Clinical Practice

It is important for the nurse to crosscheck all medications, whether just the generic name or both the trade and generic names are indicated on the label, to accurately identify a drug. Failure to crosscheck medications could lead to choosing the wrong medication, a violation of the rights of medication administration (the "right" medication).

Remember that even medications with similar names may have markedly different chemical structures and actions: for example, hydroxyzine (Vistaril), which is an antianxiety medication, and hydralazine (Apresoline), which is used to treat hypertension. Although the names are similar, the action, composition of the medications, and their use are different.

Notice that on all labels shown in Figures 13-1 and 13-2 the acronym *USP* appears after the name of the medication. USP is the acronym for United States Pharmacopoeia, which is one of the two official national listings of medications. The other is the National Formulary, NF. You will see these initials on medication labels. They are placed after the generic name. Do not confuse these abbreviations with other initials that designate a special form of a medication, such as CR, which means controlled release.

**CAUTION**

It is important to avoid confusing these official listings with other initials or abbreviations on a drug label, which may serve to identify additional medications or specific actions of or reactions to a medication. Use caution with medications that have similar spellings.

## Trade Name

The trade name is also referred to as the *brand name* or *proprietary name;* it is the manufacturer's name for the medication. Notice that the brand name is very prominent on the label and is capitalized. It is important to remember that different manufacturers may market a medication under different trade names. The trade name is followed by an ®, which is the registration symbol. Some medications may have the abbreviation ™ after the trade name, which stands for trademark. See Figures 13-3 and 13-4 for the labels for Zyvox oral suspension and Glyset, both manufactured by Pharmacia & Upjohn Company.

Notice the ™ after the names *Zyvox* and *Glyset.* The trade name is the name given to the medication by the manufacturer and therefore cannot be used by any other company. The medication name is a trademark for that company. Once the Patent and Trademark Office formally registers the trademark, the symbol ® then appears on the medication label.

Figure 13-5 shows the label for Zocor. Zocor is a trade name identified by the ® registration symbol. The name underneath in smaller print, Simvastatin, is the generic or official name of the medication.

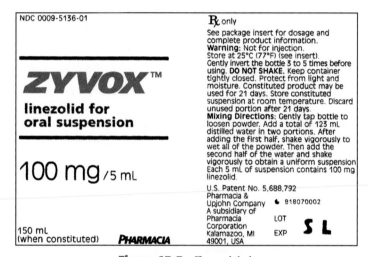

**Figure 13-3** Zyvox label.

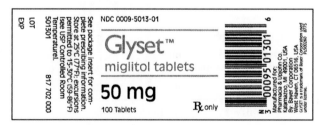

**Figure 13-4** Glyset label.

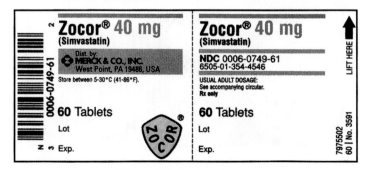

**Figure 13-5** Zocor label.

## Dosage Strength

Dosage strength refers to the weight or amount of the medication provided in a specific unit of measure (the weight per tablet, capsule, milliliter, etc.).

**Example:**    The dosage strength of the Zyvox shown in Figure 13-3 is 100 mg (the weight and specific unit of measurement) per 5 mL. The dosage strength of the Zocor tablets shown in Figure 13-5 is 40 mg per tablet (the weight and specific unit of measurement). Some medications, such as the label for Veetids shown in Figure 13-6, may have two different but equivalent dosage strengths shown on the label. Veetids has a dosage strength of 125 mg (per 5 mL) or 200,000 units (per 5 mL). The prescriber therefore could order the medication in either unit of measurement.

Dosage strength can be expressed in different systems of measure. Some labels may state the dosage strength in apothecary and metric measures (e.g., nitroglycerin). Some oral liquids may state household measures (e.g., each 15 mL [one tablespoon] contains 80 mg). Sometimes you may see solutions expressed (dosage) as a ratio or percentage. Refer to the labels in Figures 13-7 and 13-8; notice that dosage strength is also expressed in milligrams per milliliters.

> **CAUTION**
>
> The Institute for Safe Medication Practices (ISMP) recommends that the slash mark (/) not be used to separate two doses or to indicate *per* because it can be misread and mistaken as the number *1*. Use *per* rather than the slash mark. Example: Use 10 mg per 5 mL rather than 10 mg/5 mL, which could be misread as 10 mg and 15 mL. This will be followed in this text.

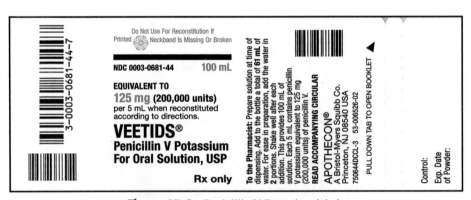

**Figure 13-6**    Penicillin V Potassium label.

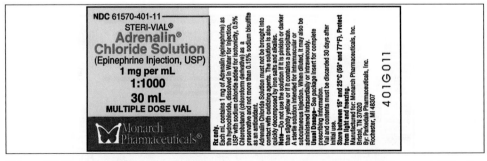

**Figure 13-7**    Adrenalin label. Adrenalin (epinephrine) contains 1 g of medication per 1,000 mL solution (1 : 1,000) and 1 mg per mL.

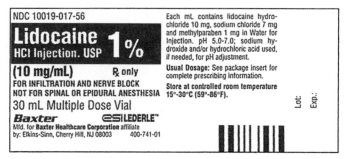

**Figure 13-8**   Lidocaine label. Lidocaine 1% contains 1 g of medication per 100 mL solution and 10 mg per mL.

## Tips for Clinical Practice

Always read a medication label carefully to avoid errors. Medication names can be deceptively similar. Similarity in name does not mean similarity in action. For example, *Inderal* and *Inderide* are similar names, but the action and the contents of the medications are different. Inderal delivers a certain dose of propranolol hydrochloride; Inderide combines two antihypertensive agents (propranolol hydrochloride and hydrochlorothiazide, a diuretic-antihypertensive).

### Form

The form specifies the type of preparation available in the package.
- Examples of forms include tablets, capsules, liquids, suppositories, and ointments. Solutions may be indicated by milliliters (mL) and described as oral suspension or aqueous solution. Some medications are available in powder or granular form or as patches.
- Labels may also indicate abbreviations or words that describe the form of the medication. Examples include CR (controlled release), LA (long acting), DS (double strength), SR (sustained release), and XL (long acting).
- Abbreviations that describe the form of a medication indicate whether the medication has been prepared in a way that allows extended action, or slow release, of the active ingredient. Often, these medications are given less frequently. Examples are Procardia XL, Inderal LA, and verapamil SR. See Figure 13-9 of Calan SR label (verapamil hydrochloride).

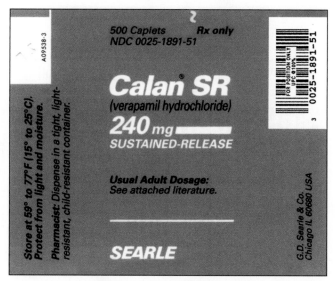

**Figure 13-9**   Calan SR label.

- Notice that bar-code symbols appear on some medication labels as thin and heavy lines arranged in a group. Bar codes are particularly important at institutions where bar coding is used as part of the medication distribution system. Refer to the bar codes indicated on the labels in Figures 13-4 to 13-6 and 13-8 to 13-11. Bar codes can also be used for stock reorder.

## Route of Administration

The route of administration describes how the medication is to be administered.

**Example:**    Oral, IM, IV, topical

It is important to realize that on some labels the route may not be stated directly (see Figures 13-5, 13-9, and 13-10). However, unless specified otherwise, tablets, capsules, and caplets are always intended for oral use. Any form intended for oral use should be administered orally.

Because all tablets, capsules, and liquids are not always given orally, read the label carefully because any variation from oral administration is indicated on the label. Examples: Sublingual tablets; otic suspension for use in ears; some capsules are placed in an inhaler and not swallowed.

**CAUTION**

Certain forms should not be crushed or dissolved for use through a nasogastric, gastrostomy, or jejunostomy tube without first consulting a pharmacist or medication guide for information regarding whether a medication can be crushed or altered.

**Figure 13-10**    Cardizem CD label.

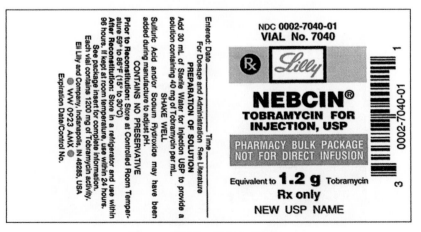

**Figure 13-11**    Nebcin label.

> **CAUTION**
>
> Altering oral medications by crushing may result in an alteration of the drug's action and cause unintended outcomes.

## Total Volume

On labels of solutions for injections or oral liquids, total volume, as well as dosage strength, is stated. Total volume refers to the quantity contained in a bottle, vial, or ampule. For liquids, total volume refers to the total fluid volume.

## Total Amount in Container

For solid forms of medication, such as tablets or capsules, the total amount is the total number of tablets or capsules in the container. The dosage strength, as well as the total amount in the container, is included on labels of solid forms of medication, such as tablets or capsules.

**Examples:**    In Figure 13-5 (Zocor tablets), the total amount of tablets in the container is 60 tablets, whereas the dosage strength is 40 mg per tablet. In Figure 13-9 (Calan SR caplets) the total amount of caplets in the container is 500 caplets, whereas the dosage strength is 240 mg per caplet. On the Zyvox label, shown in Figure 13-3, 150 mL is the total volume when reconstituted (mixed) and the dosage strength is 100 mg per 5 mL. 100 mL is the total volume of the Amoxil once reconstituted (mixed), but the solution or liquid contains 125 mg per 5 mL (Figure 13-12).

> **CAUTION**
>
> It is important to recognize the difference between the amount per milliliter and the total volume to avoid confusion and errors.

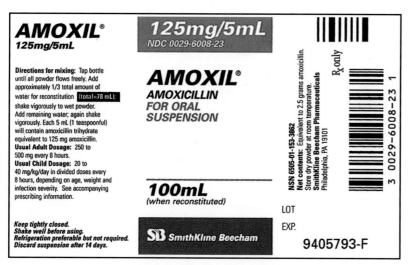

**Figure 13-12**   Amoxil label.

## Directions for Mixing or Reconstituting a Medication

When medication comes in a powdered form, the directions for how to mix or reconstitute it and with what solution are found on the label or package insert. The directions for reconstitution should be followed exactly as stated on the label for accuracy in administration. See the directions on the label in Figure 13-11 for Nebcin; notice that directions are indicated for mixing or reconstituting under Preparation of Solution. In Figure 13-12 (Amoxil label) the directions for mixing Amoxil are shown on the side of the label under Directions for mixing. Reconstitution is discussed in Chapter 19.

## Precautions

Medications may come with warnings, alerts, or precautions that are related to safety, effectiveness, or administration and need to be followed. Storage alerts might also be on the label. These precautions, warnings, and alerts may be printed on the label by the manufacturer or added by the pharmacy that dispenses the medication. Always read precautions or special alerts carefully, and follow the instructions given precisely. Examples of precautions, warnings, or alerts on a label may include the following: shake well, protect from light, may be habit forming. Example: Refer to the lower left side of the Amoxil label in Figure 13-12 (Keep tightly closed. Shake well before using.).

## Expiration Date

Medication labels contain information such as the expiration date (which may be indicated with the abbreviation *Exp*). Expiration dates indicate the last date on which a medication should be used. Typically, the date appears as the month/year. This information can be found on the back or side of a label. Medications requiring reconstitution provide specific expiration instructions. Refer to the Amoxil label in Figure 13-12 ("Discard suspension after 14 days."). In the hospital setting medications that have expired should be returned to the pharmacy. Note the expiration date on the furosemide label (8/2012) in Figure 13-13. *Note:* Expiration dates must always be checked on medications, and expiration dates are always present on actual prescriptions. The labels shown in this text may not all have expiration dates because they are used solely for educational purposes.

## Tips for Clinical Practice

It is imperative that nurses check the expiration dates on medications as a routine habit.

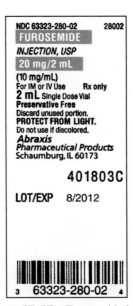

**Figure 13-13**  Furosemide label.

**CAUTION**

Remember to always read the expiration date. After the expiration date, the medication may lose its potency or cause adverse or different effects. Discard expired medications according to agency policy. For some medications, such as narcotics, disposal must be witnessed. Never give expired medications to a client! Clients must be educated in *all* aspects of medication administration, so teach them to check medications for expiration dates.

## Additional Information

Other information on a medication label includes the following:

*Storage Directions*—This section of the medication label provides information as to how a medication should be stored to prevent the medication from losing its potency or effectiveness. Usually information is given on the label relating to temperature for storing the medication. Refer to meperidine label 100 mg per mL (see Figure 13-2, *B*), and Zocor label (see Figure 13-5). When medications come in a powdered form and must be reconstituted, storage information is usually indicated on the label telling how long the medication is effective once it has been reconstituted. Refer to Nebcin label (see Figure 13-11) and Amoxil label (see Figure 13-12).

*Lot/Control Numbers*—Federal law requires that all medication packages be identified by a lot/control number. This number is important in the event that medications have to be recalled. Refer to furosemide label (see Figure 13-13), lot number 401803C.

*National Drug Code (NDC) Number*—This is a number required by federal law to be given to all medications. Each medication has a unique NDC number. The NDC number consists of NDC followed by a group of numbers (example: NDC 0009-5136-01 for Zyvox).

*Manufacturer's Name*—All medication labels contain the name of the company that manufactured the drug (examples: Pharmacia & Upjohn, Lilly). This information can be valuable; if you have questions about the medication refer to the medication labels.

*Abbreviations such as USP (United States Pharmacopoeia), NF (National Formulary)*—USP and NF are the two official national lists of approved medications. Special guidelines are given to the manufacturer related to use and placement of these initials on medication labels. On the Adrenalin label in Figure 13-7 notice that USP follows Epinephrine Injection. Notice the placement of USP in the lidocaine label (see Figure 13-8).

## Tips for Clinical Practice

Do not mistake the abbreviations *USP* and *NF* for initials that designate special forms of the medication, such as XL, which means extended release.

Some medication labels may indicate the usual medication dosage on the label, or the label may say to read the package insert for complete information. The usual dosage tells how much medication is given in a single dose or in a 24-hour period. See Figure 13-2, *B* (meperidine), which refers to the package insert, and Figure 13-12 (Amoxil), which states the usual adult and child dose.

The amount of information found on a medication label varies; however, some information is consistent on all labels (name of medication, dosage, amount in the package, manufacturer's name, expiration date, lot/control number).

## Controlled Medication Labeling

Medications considered controlled substances are classified into schedules that rank them according to their abuse potential and physical and psychological dependence. They are ranked from Schedule I to Schedule V. Medications that have the highest abuse potential are Schedule I, and medications with the lowest or limited abuse potential are Schedule V medications. Refer to the labels for meperidine in Figure 13-2, which state that they are in Schedule II (notice the "C" with II).

## Medication Labels for Combined Drugs

Some medication labels may indicate that a medication contains two or more medications. Combination medications are sometimes ordered by the number of tablets, capsules, or milliliters to be given rather than by the dosage strength. Combined drugs such as Sinemet, which comes in several strengths, cannot be ordered without a specific dosage; the number of tablets alone is insufficient to fill the order. **It must include the dosage!**

Example 1:    The label for Sinemet, which is the trade name for an antiparkinsonian drug, indicates that the medication contains carbidopa and levodopa. The first number specifies the amount of carbidopa, and the second number represents the amount of levodopa. This is further indicated on the bottom of the label. See sample labels in Figures 13-14 and 13-15.

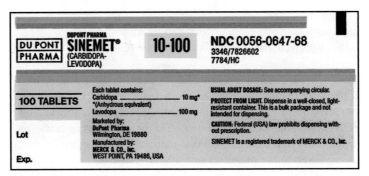

**Figure 13-14**   Sinemet 10-100 label. This label indicates the dosage strength of carbidopa as 10 mg and that of levodopa as 100 mg.

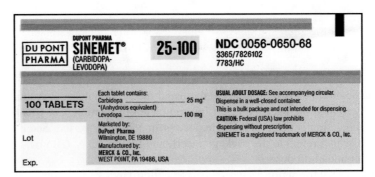

**Figure 13-15**   Sinemet 25-100 label. The dosage strength of carbidopa is 25 mg, and that of levodopa is 100 mg.

**Example 2:** Septra, an antibacterial that is also manufactured under the trade name Bactrim, is a combination of trimethoprim and sulfamethoxazole. For example, a Septra tablet contains 80 mg of trimethoprim and 400 mg of sulfamethoxazole. Septra DS contains 160 mg of trimethoprim and 800 mg of sulfamethoxazole. See the labels for Septra in Figures 13-16 and 13-17.

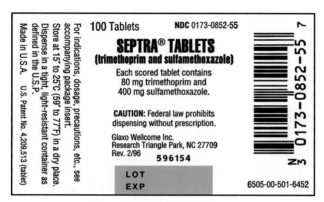

**Figure 13-16** Septra label.

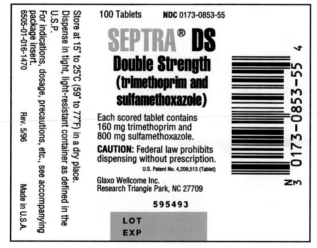

**Figure 13-17** Septra DS label.

**Example 3:** Percocet label. Note the different substances that are combined in each tablet: oxycodone 5 mg, acetaminophen 325 mg (Figure 13-18).

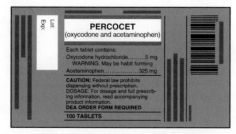

**Figure 13-18** Percocet label. Percocet contains oxycodone (5 mg) and acetaminophen (325 mg).

Remember that extra initials or abbreviations after a medication name identify additional medications in the preparation or a special action. For example, in Figure 13-17, Septra DS is a double-strength tablet.

Although tablets and capsules that contain more than one drug are often ordered by the brand name and number of tablets to be given (e.g., Septra DS 1 tab p.o. b.i.d.), the health care provider may order this medication by another route, for example, intravenous (IV). With the IV order, the nurse calculates the dosage to be given based on the strength of the trimethoprim. The nurse would learn such information described by using appropriate resources, such as a reference medication book (*Physician's Desk Reference [PDR]*), pharmacist, or hospital formulary.

**CAUTION**

Read the label carefully to validate that you have the correct medication and dosage for combined medications.

It is important to remember that some medications may not indicate their strength but are ordered by the number of tablets (e.g., multivitamin tablet 1 p.o. every day, Bactrim DS 1 tablet p.o. b.i.d., Percocet 1 tablet p.o. q4h p.r.n.). This is because these medications are available in one strength only. This is also common with some medications that contain a combination of medications.

Most medications administered in the hospital setting are available in unit dose. The pharmacy provides a 24-hour supply of each medication for the client. In unit dose, the medications will come to the unit in individually wrapped packets that are labeled for an individualized dosage for a specific client. The label on the package includes generic and trade names, manufacturer, lot number, and expiration date. Sometimes the package may only contain the generic name. The strength is indicated on the medication label. The nurse must read the label on unit-dose packages and note that sometimes, even with this method, calculation may be necessary. The pharmacy in some institutions provides the unit with a supply of medications available in multidose containers. These medications may be in unit-dose packaging but are used a great deal by the clients on the unit. Examples include Tylenol and aspirin. Some medications may also be dispensed in bottles—for example, 100 tablets of aspirin 325 mg.

Most hospital units have a combination of unit dose and multidose. However, multidose is rarely seen. Multidose packaging is the packaging of medications in containers that have more than one dose of the medication. The medications may be part of the floor stock. Tablets, capsules, powders, and liquid medications may be supplied in stock bottles for dispensing. Parenteral medications in liquid form or in powder that requires reconstitution may come in multidose vials. Figure 13-19 shows examples of unit-dose packaging.

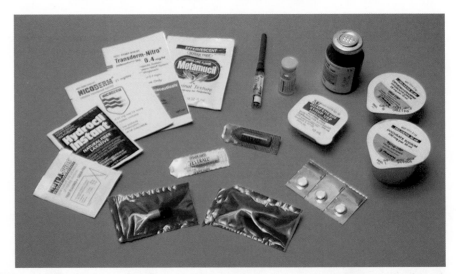

**Figure 13-19**    Unit-dose packages. (From Clayton BD, Stock YN, and Harroun R: *Basic pharmacology for nurses,* ed. 14, St. Louis, 2007, Mosby.)

**CAUTION**

Read labels carefully. Read the total volume on a medication container carefully. Confusing volume with dosage strength can cause a serious medication error.

Let's examine some sample medication labels for review and identify some of the important information on labels.

1. In Figure 13-20, note the following:

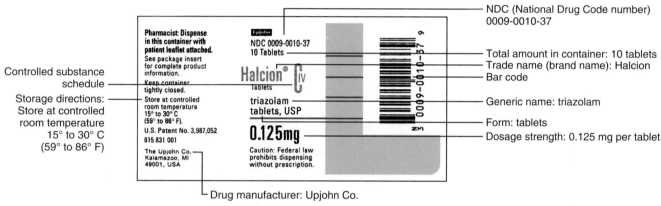

**Figure 13-20** Halcion label.

2. In Figure 13-21, note the following:

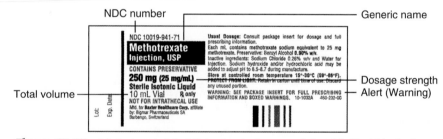

**Figure 13-21** Methotrexate label. Injection is the route; injectable liquid is the form.

3. In Figure 13-22, note the following:

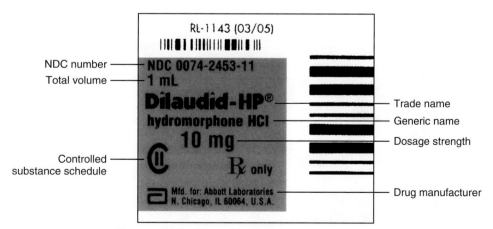

**Figure 13-22** Dilaudid-HP (Dilaudid High Potency)

4. In Figure 13-23, note the following:

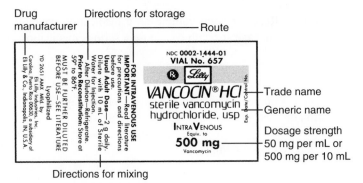

**Figure 13-23** Vancocin HCl label. Form is powder; it must be diluted for use.

5. In Figure 13-24, note the following:

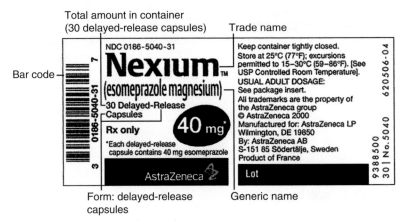

**Figure 13-24** Nexium label.

6. In Figure 13-25, note the following:

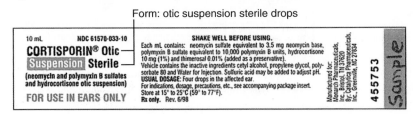

**Figure 13-25** Cortisporin label.

7. In Figure 13-26, note the following:

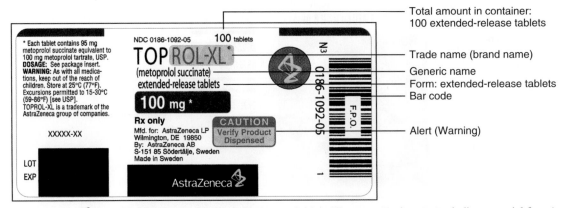

**Figure 13-26** Toprol-XL label (Notice the initials XL next to trade name to indicate special form.)

8. In Figure 13-27, note the following:

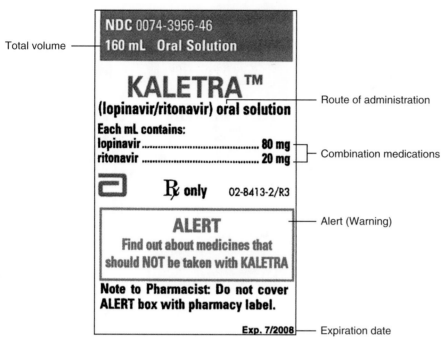

Total volume

NDC 0074-3956-46
160 mL  Oral Solution

KALETRA™
(lopinavir/ritonavir) oral solution

Each mL contains:
lopinavir ............................................. 80 mg
ritonavir ............................................. 20 mg

℞ only     02-8413-2/R3

ALERT
Find out about medicines that
should NOT be taken with KALETRA

Note to Pharmacist: Do not cover
ALERT box with pharmacy label.

Exp. 7/2008

Route of administration

Combination medications

Alert (Warning)

Expiration date

**Figure 13-27**   Kaletra label (combination drug) (lopinavir 80 mg, ritonavir 20 mg).

## ■ Points to Remember

- Read medication labels three times.
- Identify directions for mixing when indicated.
- Read labels carefully, and do not confuse medication names; they are often deceptively similar. When in doubt, check appropriate resources, such as a reference book or the hospital pharmacist. Always cross reference medication names to avoid administering the wrong medication.
- Read the label on combined medications carefully to ascertain whether you are administering the correct medication dosage.
- Extra abbreviations or initials after a medication name may identify additional medications in the preparation or a special action.
- Read labels carefully to identify trade and generic names, dosage strength, form, total amount in container, total volume, and route of administration.
- Do not confuse special forms such as SR (sustained release) and XL (extended release) with USP and NF official listing for medications.
- Read labels carefully, and crosscheck medication with a reference.
- Read directions relating to storage and directions for mixing if indicated.
- Carefully read alerts on medication labels.
- Do not administer expired medications.
- Control medication labels indicate the potential for abuse and are ranked Schedule I to Schedule V.
- When writing dosages, ISMP recommends using *per* instead of a slash (/) because of misinterpretation and being mistaken as the number *1*.

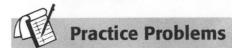

## Practice Problems

Use the labels to identify the information requested.

**AUGMENTIN®**
**125mg/5mL**

**125mg/5mL**
NDC 0029-6085-23

NSN 6505-01-408-8181
**Directions for mixing:**
Tap bottle until all powder flows freely. Add approximately 2/3 of total water for reconstitution **(total = 90 mL);** shake vigorously to wet powder. Add remaining water; again shake vigorously.
**Dosage:** See accompanying prescribing information.

**AUGMENTIN®**
**AMOXICILLIN/**
**CLAVULANATE**
**POTASSIUM**
**FOR ORAL SUSPENSION**

When reconstituted, each 5 mL contains:
**AMOXICILLIN, 125 MG,** as the trihydrate
**CLAVULANIC ACID, 31.25 MG,** as clavulanate potassium

**100mL**
*(when reconstituted)*

Keep tightly closed.
Shake well before using.
Must be refrigerated.
Discard after 10 days.

Use only if inner seal is intact.
**Net contents:** Equivalent to 2.5 g amoxicillin and 0.625 g clavulanic acid.
Store dry powder at room temperature.
**SmithKline Beecham Pharmaceuticals**
Philadelphia, PA 19101

Rx only

3 0029-6085-23 2

LOT

EXP.

**SB** SmithKline Beecham

9405705-D

1. Trade name _____

    Generic name _____

    Form _____

    Dosage strength (when reconstituted)

    _____

    Total volume (when reconstituted)

    _____

FOR INTRAMUSCULAR USE ONLY.
**USUAL ADULT DOSE:** Intramuscularly; 25 - 100 mg stat; repeat every 4 to 6 hours, as needed.
See accompanying prescribing information.
Each mL contains **50 mg** of hydroxyzine hydrochloride, 0.9% benzyl alcohol and sodium hydroxide to adjust to optimum pH.
To avoid discoloration, protect from prolonged exposure to light.
**Rx only**

10 mL        NDC 0049-5460-74
**Vistaril®**
(hydroxyzine hydrochloride)
*Intramuscular Solution*
**50 mg/mL**

*Pfizer* **Roerig**
Division of Pfizer Inc, NY, NY 10017

Store below 86°F (30°C).
PROTECT FROM FREEZING.

PATIENT: _____
ROOM NO.: _____

05-1111-32-4  **9249**
MADE IN USA

2. Trade name _____

    Generic name _____

    Form _____

    Dosage strength _____

    Total volume _____

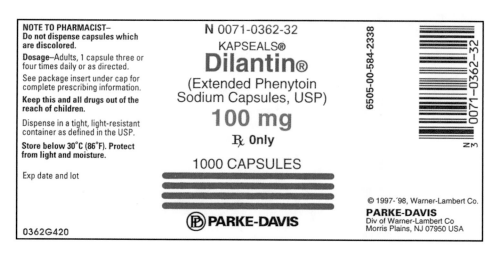

NOTE TO PHARMACIST–
Do not dispense capsules which
are discolored.

**Dosage**–Adults, 1 capsule three or
four times daily or as directed.

See package insert under cap for
complete prescribing information.

**Keep this and all drugs out of the
reach of children.**

Dispense in a tight, light-resistant
container as defined in the USP.

**Store below 30°C (86°F). Protect
from light and moisture.**

Exp date and lot

0362G420

N 0071-0362-32
KAPSEALS®
**Dilantin®**
(Extended Phenytoin
Sodium Capsules, USP)
**100 mg**
℞ Only
1000 CAPSULES

6505-00-584-2338

0071-0362-32

© 1997-'98, Warner-Lambert Co.
**PARKE-DAVIS**
Div of Warner-Lambert Co
Morris Plains, NJ 07950 USA

Ⓟ **PARKE-DAVIS**

3. Dosage strength _____ Total amount in container_____

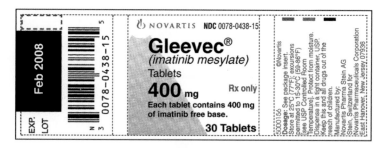

4. Trade name _____ Dosage strength _____

   Generic name _____ Total amount in container_____

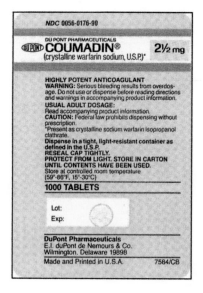

5. Trade name _____ Form _____

   Dosage strength _____ NDC number_____

   Total amount in container_____ Answers on p. 613

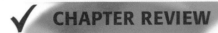

## CHAPTER REVIEW

Read the label, and identify the information requested.

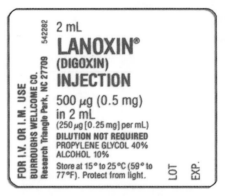

1. Trade name _____   Form _____

     Generic name _____   Dosage strength _____

     Warning _____   Total amount in container _____

2. Trade name _____   Form _____

     Generic name _____   Dosage strength _____

     Total volume _____

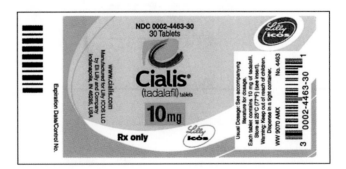

3. Trade name _____   Form _____

     Generic name _____   Dosage strength _____

     Storage directions _____   Total amount in container _____

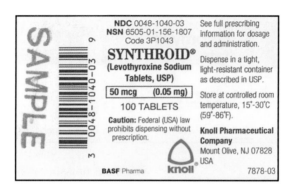

4. Trade name _____     Form _____

   Generic name _____     Dosage strength _____

   Total amount in container _____

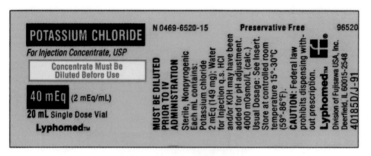

5. Trade name _____     Form _____

   Generic name _____     Dosage strength _____

   Drug manufacturer _____

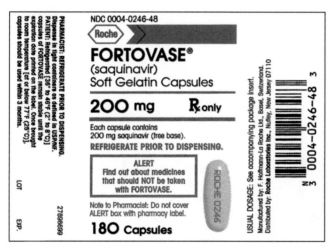

6. Trade name _____     Form _____

   Generic name _____     Dosage strength _____

   Usual dosage_____     Total amount in container_____

   Alert _____

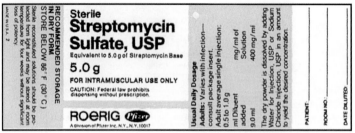

7. Trade name _____

   Generic name _____

   Form _____

   Directions for mixing _____

   Dosage strength after reconstitution

   _____

   Storage instructions _____

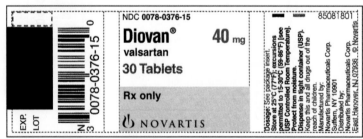

8. Generic name _____

   NDC number _____

   Total volume _____

   Controlled substance schedule _____

   Form _____

   Dosage strength _____

   Warning _____

9. Trade name _____

   Generic name _____

   Storage _____

   Form _____

   Dosage strength _____

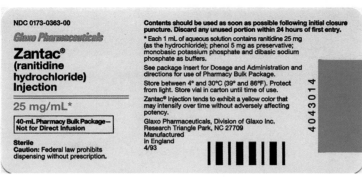

**NDC 0173-0363-00**

*Glaxo Pharmaceuticals*

**Zantac®**
**(ranitidine**
**hydrochloride)**
**Injection**

**25 mg/mL***

**40-mL Pharmacy Bulk Package—**
**Not for Direct Infusion**

**Sterile**
**Caution:** Federal law prohibits
dispensing without prescription.

Contents should be used as soon as possible following initial closure
puncture. Discard any unused portion within 24 hours of first entry.

* Each 1 mL of aqueous solution contains ranitidine 25 mg
(as the hydrochloride); phenol 5 mg as preservative;
monobasic potassium phosphate and dibasic sodium
phosphate as buffers.

See package insert for Dosage and Administration and
directions for use of Pharmacy Bulk Package.

Store between 4° and 30°C (39° and 86°F). Protect
from light. Store vial in carton until time of use.

Zantac® Injection tends to exhibit a yellow color that
may intensify over time without adversely affecting
potency.

Glaxo Pharmaceuticals, Division of Glaxo Inc.
Research Triangle Park, NC 27709
Manufactured
in England
4/93

4043014

10. Trade name _____     Form _____

    Generic name _____     Dosage strength _____

**051438     NDC 0179-1226-50**

**CIPRO®**
**(ciprofloxacin hydrochloride)**
Equivalent to
**750 mg** ciprofloxacin
50 Tablets
**Caution:** Federal (USA) law
prohibits dispensing without a
prescription.

**Bayer**

Bayer Corporation
Pharmaceutical Division
400 Morgan Lane
West Haven, CT 06516

**DESCRIPTION:** Each tablet contains
ciprofloxacin hydrochloride equivalent to
750 mg of ciprofloxacin.
**DOSAGE:** See accompanying literature for
complete information on dosage and
administration.
**RECOMMENDED STORAGE:**
Store below 86°F (30°C).

Batch: VOID
Expires:

Distributed by:
Kaiser Foundation Hospitals

Manufactured by:
Bayer Corporation
Pharmaceutical Division

5402
Printed in USA
©1995 Bayer Corporation
N 3  0179-1226-50  2
PL500037

VOID

11. Trade name _____     Form _____

    Generic name _____     Dosage strength _____

    Total amount in container _____

**50 mg     NDC 0003-0437-30**
**NSN 6505-01-084-9453**
**FUNGIZONE®** Rx only
**INTRAVENOUS**
Amphotericin B for Injection USP
STOP: Verify product name & dosage
if dose exceeds 1.5 mg/kg

For intravenous infusion
in hospitals only
Sterile • See insert
for reconstitution and
dosage information
REFRIGERATE

Manufactured for: APOTHECON®
A Bristol-Myers Squibb Co.
Princeton, NJ 08540 USA
by E. R. Squibb & Sons, Inc.
A Bristol-Myers Squibb Co.
Princeton, NJ 08543 USA
C02176 / 43730

12. Trade name _____     Form _____

    Generic name _____     Drug manufacturer _____

NDC 0009-7376-01
1 mL Single Dose Syringe
Depo-Provera®
Contraceptive Injection
sterile medroxyprogesterone
acetate suspension, USP
**150 mg per mL**
Intramuscular Use Only
**Shake vigorously before use**
816 289 000                    5Q4711/1
The Upjohn Company

Lot:

EXP:

S L

13. Trade name _____    Form _____

Generic name _____    Dosage strength _____

Directions for use _____    NDC number_____

For IM use only.
See package insert for
complete product
information.
Shake vigorously immediately
before each use.
812 224 705
Pharmacia & Upjohn Company
Kalamazoo, MI 49001, USA

NDC 0009-0626-01    2.5 mL Vial
Depo-Provera®
medroxyprogesterone
acetate injectable
suspension, USP
**400 mg /mL**

For IM use only.
See package insert for
complete product
information.
Shake vigorously immediately
before each use.
812 224 705
Pharmacia & Upjohn Company
Kalamazoo, MI 49001, USA

NDC 0009-0626-01    2.5 mL Vial
Depo-Provera®
medroxyprogesterone
acetate injectable
suspension, USP
**400 mg /mL**

14. Trade name _____    Dosage strength _____

Generic name _____    Directions for use _____

NDC 54022-1112-1

**Suggested use:** As a dietary supplement: Adults, one tablet daily; place under the tongue until dissolved, then swallow in order to maximize absorption of Vitamin B-12, or as directed by physician or registered dietitian. Children, as directed by physician.

**High Potency**
**Vitamin B-12**
**2500 mcg**
**Sublingual Tablets**
Dietary Supplement
90 Tablets
▼ VITALINE®
FORMULAS

**Nutrition Facts**
Serving Size 1 Tablet

Amount Per Tablet    % Daily Value

Vitamin B-12  2500 mcg  41,600%
(Cobalamin Concentrate)

OTHER INGREDIENTS: Mannitol, stearic acid, silicon dioxide.

Contains no yeast, wheat, corn, dairy products, soya, animal products, sugar, starch, preservatives, artificial colors or flavorings.

VITALINE CORPORATION
Ashland, Oregon 97520

15. Total amount in container_____    Dosage strength _____

Form _____    Suggested use _____

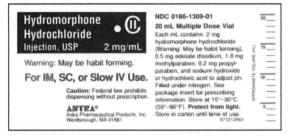

Caution: Federal law prohibits dispensing without prescription. See package insert for complete product information. Store at controlled room temperature (20° to 25° C or 68° to 77° F) [see USP]. Each mL contains: Ibutilide fumarate, 0.1 mg; sodium chloride, 8.90 mg; sodium acetate trihydrate, 0.189 mg; water for injection. When necessary, pH was adjusted with sodium hydroxide and/or hydrochloric acid.

816 416 000

The Upjohn Company
Kalamazoo, MI 49001, USA

NDC 0009-3794-01    10 mL

**Corvert**™

Injection

ibutilide fumarate injection

**0.1 mg per mL**

For IV use only

16.  Trade name _____     Form _____

Generic name _____     Dosage strength _____

Directions for use _____

Hydromorphone Hydrochloride
Injection, USP    2 mg/mL

Warning: May be habit forming.

**For IM, SC, or Slow IV Use.**

Caution: Federal law prohibits dispensing without prescription.

**ASTRA**®
Astra Pharmaceutical Products, Inc.
Westborough, MA 01581

NDC 0186-1309-01

**20 mL Multiple Dose Vial**

Each mL contains: 2 mg hydromorphone hydrochloride (Warning: May be habit forming), 0.5 mg edetate disodium, 1.8 mg methylparaben, 0.2 mg propylparaben, and sodium hydroxide or hydrochloric acid to adjust ph. Filled under nitrogen. See package insert for prescribing information. Store at 15°–30°C (59°–86°F). **Protect from light.** Store in carton until time of use.
071212R01

17.  Trade name _____     Dosage strength _____

Generic name _____     Total volume _____

Directions for use _____     Warning _____

Form _____

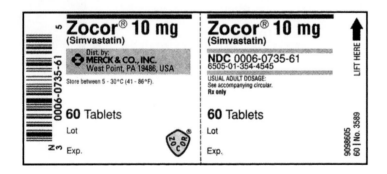

**Zocor**® **10 mg**
(Simvastatin)

Dist. by:
**MERCK & CO., INC.**
West Point, PA 19486, USA

Store between 5 - 30°C (41 - 86°F).

**60** Tablets

Lot

Exp.

**Zocor**® **10 mg**
(Simvastatin)

**NDC 0006-0735-61**
6505-01-354-4545

USUAL ADULT DOSAGE:
See accompanying circular.
**Rx only**

**60** Tablets

Lot

Exp.

18.  Trade name _____     Dosage strength _____

Generic name _____     NDC number _____

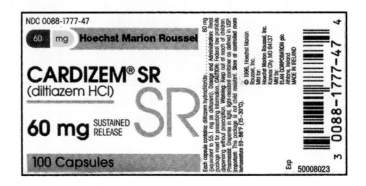

19. Generic name _____    Dosage strength _____

    Form _____

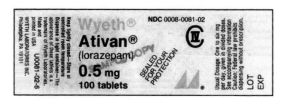

20. Trade name _____    Total amount in container_____

    Dosage strength _____    Controlled substance schedule _____

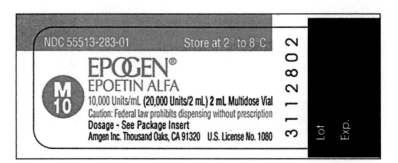

21. Trade name _____    Total volume _____

    Generic name _____    Dosage strength _____

    Storage information _____

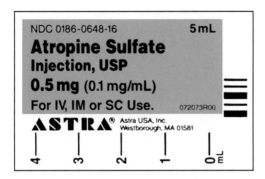

22.  Trade name _____          Dosage strength _____

     Generic name _____          Total volume _____

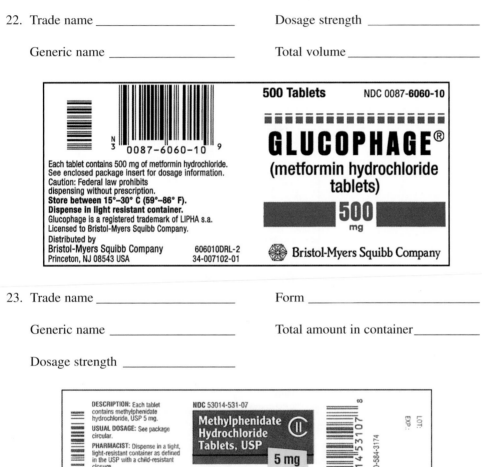

23.  Trade name _____          Form _____

     Generic name _____          Total amount in container_____

     Dosage strength _____

24.  Generic name _____          Dosage strength _____

     Instructions to pharmacist_____

**Easprin®**
(Aspirin Delayed-release
Tablets, USP)
**Enteric Coated**
**15 grain** (975 mg)
**Caution**—Federal law prohibits
dispensing without prescription.
**100 TABLETS**

Ⓟ **PARKE-DAVIS**
People Who Care

25. Trade name _____          Form _____

Total amount in container _____

N 0071-0268-24
**Meclomen®**
(Meclofenamate Sodium
Capsules, USP)
**50 mg**
**Caution**—Federal law prohibits
dispensing without prescription.
**100 CAPSULES**

Ⓟ **PARKE-DAVIS**
People Who Care

26. Trade name _____          Form _____

Generic name _____          Dosage strength _____

NDC 0004-1968-01                                    ITE
ROCHE
**BUMEX®**
(bumetanide)  INJECTION
**0.5 mg / 2 mL**    2 mL Single Use Vials
(0.25 mg per mL)
Sterile. For Intramuscular or Intravenous Use.

27. Trade name _____          Dosage strength _____

Generic name _____          Form _____

Directions for use _____

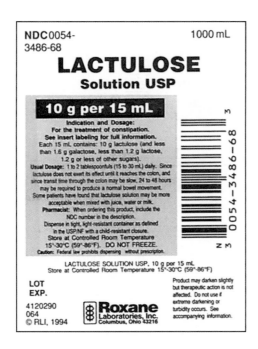

28. Total volume _____     Form _____

    Storage _____     Dosage strength _____

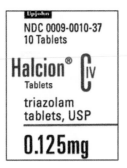

29. Trade name _____     Dosage strength _____

    Generic name _____     Total amount in container_____

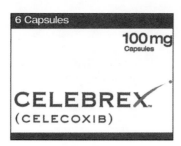

30. Trade name _____     Form _____

    Generic name _____     Dosage strength _____

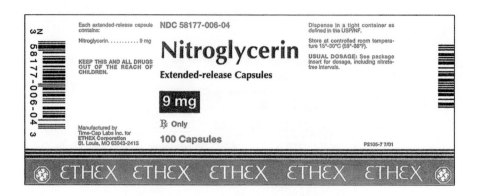

31. Trade name _____      Form _____

    Generic name _____      Dosage strength _____

    Storage information _____

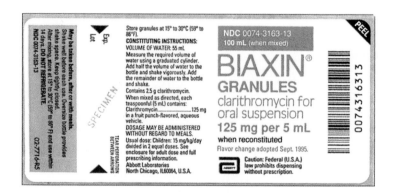

32. Trade name _____      Form _____

    Generic name _____      Dosage strength when reconstituted ____

    Total volume when reconstituted _____

Using the combination drug labels that follow, answer the questions:

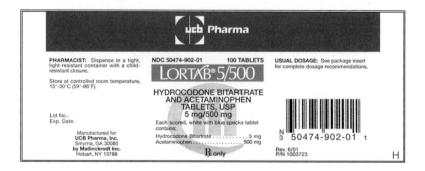

33. The route of administration for this medication would be _____.

34. This medication contains _____ mg of hydrocodone bitartrate and _____ mg
    of acetaminophen.

35. The total amount in the container is _____.

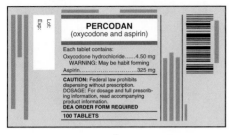
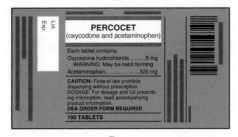

A                    B

36. The prescriber ordered Percocet 1 tab p.o. q4h p.r.n. for pain. The nurse would use which of the medications above to administer the dosage? _____

37. The difference between the medications Percodan and Percocet is that Percodan contains _____ mg of oxycodone hydrochloride and _____ mg of aspirin. Percocet contains _____ mg of oxycodone hydrochloride and _____ mg of acetaminophen.

38. If a client is allergic to aspirin, which medication should the client not be given?

_____

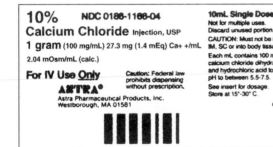

39. The dosage strength of this medication expressed as a percentage is _____.

40. The dosage strength of this medication in milligrams per milliliter is _____.

Answers on pp. 613-615

 **For additional practice problems, refer to the Safety in Medication Administration section on Drug Calculations Companion, Version 4, on Evolve.**

# CHAPTER 14

# Dosage Calculation Using the Ratio and Proportion Method

## Objectives

*After reviewing this chapter, you should be able to:*
1. State a ratio and proportion to solve a given dosage calculation problem
2. Solve simple calculation problems using the ratio and proportion method

Several methods are used for calculating dosages. The most common methods are *ratio and proportion* and *use of a formula.* After presentation of the various methods, students can choose the method they find easiest and most logical to use. First, let's discuss calculating by using ratio and proportion. If necessary, review Chapter 4 on ratio and proportion.

## USE OF RATIO AND PROPORTION IN DOSAGE CALCULATION

Ratio and proportion is useful and easy to use in dosage calculation, because it is often necessary to find only one unknown quantity. Recall that a proportion is a relationship comparing two ratios.

For example, suppose you had a medication with a dosage strength of 50 mg per 1 mL, and the prescriber orders a dosage of 25 mg. A ratio and proportion may be used to determine how many milliliters to administer.

When setting up the ratio and proportion using the fraction format to calculate dosages, the known ratio is what you have available, or the information on the medication label, and is stated first (placed on the left side of the proportion). The desired, or what is ordered to be administered, is the unknown (placed on the right side). Therefore using the example the ratio and proportion would be stated as follows:

**Example 1:**
$$\frac{50 \text{ mg}}{1 \text{ mL}} = \frac{25 \text{ mg}}{x \text{ mL}}$$
(known)  (unknown)

When writing the ratio and proportion using the colons, the known ratio, what you have available or the information on the medication label, is stated first, and the unknown ratio is stated second.

**Example 1:**

50 mg : 1 mL = 25 mg : $x$ mL
(known)        (unknown)

**Solution:** To solve for *x*, use the principles presented in Chapter 4 on ratio and proportion.

$$\frac{50 \text{ mg}}{1 \text{ mL}} = \frac{25 \text{ mg}}{x \text{ mL}}$$
$$\text{(known)} \quad \text{(unknown)}$$

$$\frac{50x}{50} = \frac{25}{50}$$

$$x = 0.5 \text{ mL}$$

Remember that, as shown, the known is stated as the first fraction, and the unknown as the second. When stated in fraction format, solve by cross multiplication.

*or*

$$50 \text{ mg} : 1 \text{ mL} = 25 \text{ mg} : x \text{ mL}$$
$$\text{(known)} \qquad \text{(unknown)}$$

$$50x = \text{product of extremes}$$

$$25 = \text{product of means}$$

$$50x = 25 \text{ is the equation}$$

$$\frac{50x}{50} = \frac{25}{50} \quad \begin{array}{l}\text{(Divide both sides by 50,}\\ \text{the number in front of } x.)\end{array}$$

$$x = 0.5 \text{ mL}$$

**CAUTION**

It is important to remember when stating ratios that the units of measure should be stated in the same sequence (in the examples, $\frac{\text{mg}}{\text{mL}} = \frac{\text{mg}}{\text{mL}}$ or mg:mL = mg : mL). Labeling the terms in the ratios, including *x*, is also essential. These pointers are crucial to preventing calculation errors.

**Example 2:** Order: 40 mg p.o. of a medication.

Available: 20 mg tablets. How many tablets will you administer?

**Solution:**

$$\frac{20 \text{ mg}}{1 \text{ tab}} = \frac{40 \text{ mg}}{x \text{ tab}}$$
$$\text{(known)} \quad \text{(unknown)}$$

$$\frac{20x}{20} = \frac{40}{20}$$

$$x = 2 \text{ tabs}$$

*or*

$$20 \text{ mg} : 1 \text{ tab} = 40 \text{ mg} : x \text{ tab}$$
$$\text{(known)} \qquad \text{(unknown)}$$

$$\frac{20x}{20} = \frac{40}{20}$$

$$x = 2 \text{ tabs}$$

**Example 3:**   Order: 1 g p.o. of an antibiotic

Available: 500 mg capsules. How many capsules will you administer?

**Solution:**   Notice that the dosage ordered is in a different unit from what is available. Proceed first by changing the units of measure so they are the same. As shown in Chapter 8, ratio and proportion can be used for conversion.

After making the conversion, set up the problem and calculate the dosage to be given. In this example the conversion required is within the same system (metric).

In this example grams are converted to milligrams by using the equivalent 1,000 mg = 1 g. After making the conversion of 1 g to 1,000 mg, the ratio is stated as follows:

$$\underset{\text{(known)}\quad\text{(unknown)}}{\frac{500\ \text{mg}}{1\ \text{cap}} = \frac{1,000\ \text{mg}}{x\ \text{caps}}}\ or\ \underset{\text{(known)}\qquad\text{(unknown)}}{500\ \text{mg}:1\ \text{cap} = 1,000\ \text{mg}:x\ \text{caps}}$$

$$x = 2\ \text{caps} \qquad\qquad x = 2\ \text{caps}$$

An alternate method of solving might be to convert milligrams to grams. In doing this, 500 mg would be converted to grams by using the same equivalent: 1,000 mg = 1 g. However, decimals are common when measures are changed from smaller to larger in the metric system: 500 mg = 0.5 g. Even though converting the milligrams to grams would net the same final answer, *conversions that net decimals are often the source of calculation errors.* Therefore if possible, avoid conversions that require their use. As a rule, it is best to convert to the measure stated on the medication label. Doing this consistently can prevent confusion. As with the other examples, this proportion could be stated as a fraction as well.

For the purpose of learning to calculate dosages by using ratio and proportion, this chapter emphasizes the mathematics used to calculate the answer. Determining whether an answer is logical is essential and necessary in the calculation of medication. An answer *must make sense.* Determining whether an answer is logical will be discussed further in later chapters covering the calculation of dosages by various routes.

## ■ Points to Remember

**Important Points When Calculating Dosages Using Ratio and Proportion**
- Make sure all terms are in the same unit and system of measure before calculating. If they are not, a conversion will be necessary before calculating the dosage.
- When conversion of units is required, conversions can be made by converting what is ordered to the units in which the medication is available or by changing what is available to the units in which the medication is ordered. Be consistent as to how you make conversions. It is usual to convert what is ordered to the same unit and system of measure you have the medication available in.
- When stating ratios, the known is stated first. The known ratio is what is available or on hand or the information obtained from the medication label.
- The unknown ratio is stated second. The unknown ratio is the dosage desired, or what the prescriber has ordered.
- The terms of the ratios in a proportion must be written in the same sequence.
  Example: mg : mL = mg : mL *or* $\dfrac{\text{mg}}{\text{mL}} = \dfrac{\text{mg}}{\text{mL}}$.
- Label all terms of the ratios in the proportion, including *x*.

- Before calculating the dosage, make a mental estimate of the approximate and reasonable answer.
- Label the value you obtain for *x* (e.g., mL, tabs). Double-check the label for *x* by referring back to the label of *x* in the original ratio and proportion; it should be the same.
- A proportion can be stated in a horizontal fashion using colons or as a fraction.
- Double-check all work.
- Be consistent in how ratios are stated and conversions are done.
- An error in the setup of the ratio and proportion can cause an error in calculation.

 **Practice Problems**

Answer the following questions by indicating whether you need less than 1 tab or more than 1 tab. Refer to Chapter 4, Ratio and Proportion, if you have difficulty in answering the questions in this area.

1. A client is to receive gr $\frac{1}{300}$ of a medication. The tablets available are gr $\frac{1}{150}$.

    How many tablets do you need? _____

2. A client is to receive 1.25 mg of a medication. The tablets available are 0.625 mg.

    How many tablets do you need? _____

3. A client is to receive gr $\frac{1}{8}$ of a medication. The tablets available are gr $\frac{1}{4}$.

    How many tablets do you need? _____

4. A client is to receive 10 mg of a medication. The tablets available are 20 mg.

    How many tablets do you need? _____

5. A client is to receive 100 mg of a medication. The tablets available are 50 mg.

    How many tablets do you need? _____

Solve the following problems using ratio and proportion. Express your answer in mL to the nearest tenth where indicated, and include the label on the answer.

6. Order: 7.5 mg p.o. of a medication.

    Available: Tablets labeled 5 mg _____

7. Order: gr $\frac{3}{4}$ p.o. of a medication.

    Available: Tablets labeled 30 mg _____

8. Order: gr $1\frac{1}{2}$ p.o. of a medication.

    Available: Capsules labeled 100 mg _____

9. Order: 0.25 mg IM of a medication.

    Available: 0.5 mg per mL _____

10. Order: 100 mg p.o. of a liquid medication.

    Available: 125 mg per 5 mL _____

11. Order: 20 mEq IV of a medication.

    Available: 40 mEq per 10 mL _____

12. Order: 5,000 units subcut of a medication.

    Available: 10,000 units per mL _____

13. Order: 50 mg IM of a medication.

    Available: 80 mg per 2 mL _____

14. Order: 0.5 g p.o. of an antibiotic.

    Available: Capsules labeled 250 mg _____

15. Order: 400 mg p.o. of a liquid medication.

    Available: 125 mg per 5 mL _____

16. Order: 50 mg IM of a medication.

    Available: 80 mg per mL _____

17. Order: gr 1 IM of a medication.

    Available: gr $^1/_2$ per mL _____

18. Order: gr xv of a medication.

    Available: Tablets labeled gr v. _____

19. Order: 0.24 g p.o. of a liquid medication.

    Available: 80 mg per 7.5 mL _____

20. Order: 20 g p.o. of a liquid medication.

    Available: 10 g per 15 mL _____

21. Order: 0.125 mg IM of a medication.

    Available: 0.5 mg per 2 mL _____

22. Order: 0.75 mg IM of a medication.

    Available: 0.25 mg per mL _____

23. Order: 375 mg p.o. of a liquid medication.

    Available: 125 mg per 5 mL _____

24. Order: 10,000 units subcut of a medication.

    Available: 7,500 units per mL _____

25. Order: 0.45 mg p.o. of a medication.

    Available: Tablets labeled 0.3 mg _____

26. Order: 20 mg IM of a medication.

    Available: 25 mg per 1.5 mL _____

27. Order: 150 mg IV of a medication.

    Available: 80 mg per mL _____

28. Order: 2 mg IM of a medication.

    Available: 1.5 mg per 0.5 mL _____

29. Order: 500 mcg IV of a medication.

    Available: 750 mcg per 3 mL _____

30. Order: 0.15 mg IM of a medication.

    Available: 0.2 mg per 1.5 mL _____

31. Order: 1,100 units subcut of a medication.

    Available: 1,000 units per 1.5 mL _____

32. Order: 0.6 g IV of a medication.

    Available: 1 g per 3.6 mL _____

33. Order: 3 g IV of a medication.

    Available: 1.5 g per mL _____

34. Order: 35 mg IM of a medication.

    Available: 40 mg per 2.5 mL _____

35. Order: 0.3 mg subcut of a medication.

    Available: 1,000 mcg per 2 mL _____

36. Order: 200 mg IM of a medication.

    Available: 0.5 g per 2 mL _____

37. Order: 10 mEq IV of a medication.

    Available: 20 mEq per 10 mL _____

38. Order: 165 mg IV of a medication.

    Available: 55 mg per 1.1 mL _____

39. Order: 35 mg subcut of a medication.

    Available: 45 mg per 1.2 mL _____

40. Order: 700 mg IM of a medication.

    Available: 1,000 mg per 2.3 mL _____

Answers on pp. 615-619

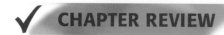

## ✓ CHAPTER REVIEW

### Part I

Read the medication labels where available, and calculate the number of tablets or capsules necessary to provide the dosage ordered. Include the label on your answer.

1.  Order: Phenobarbital gr ¼ p.o. t.i.d.

    Available: Phenobarbital tablets labeled 15 mg _____

2.  Order: Ampicillin 0.25 g p.o. q.i.d.

    Available:

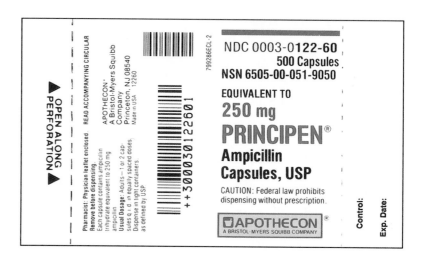

3.  Order: Persantine 50 mg p.o. q.i.d.

    Available:

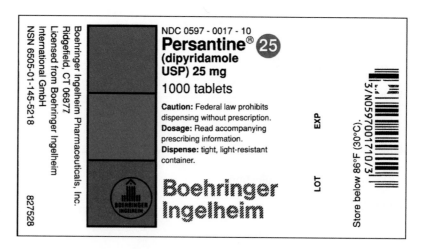

4. Order: Phenobarbital 60 mg p.o. at bedtime.

   Available: Scored phenobarbital tablets (can be broken in half) labeled 30 mg

   _____

5. Order: Baclofen (can be broken in half) 20 mg p.o. t.i.d.

   Available: Scored baclofen tablets (can be broken in half).

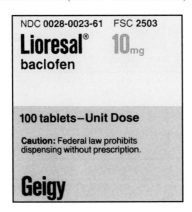

   _____

6. Order: Isosorbide dinitrate 20 mg p.o. t.i.d.

   Available: Scored Isosorbide dinitrate tablets (can be broken in half) labeled 40 mg

   _____

7. Order: Dexamethasone 4 mg p.o. q6h.

   Available:

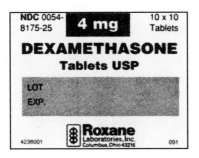

   _____

8. Order: DiaBeta 5 mg p.o. daily.

   Available:

   _____

9. Order: Digoxin 125 mcg p.o. daily.

   Available: Scored digoxin tablets (can be broken in half).

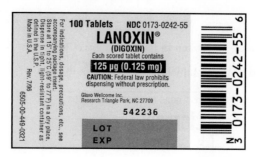

10. Order: Synthroid 0.05 mg p.o. daily.

    Available:

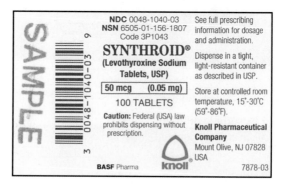

11. Order: Restoril 30 mg p.o. at bedtime p.r.n.

    Available:

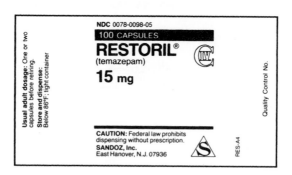

12. Order: Phenobarbital gr 1 p.o. at bedtime.

    Available:

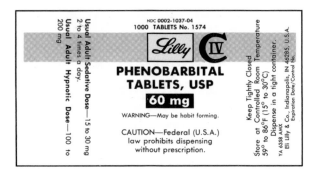

    _____

13. Order: Tigan 200 mg p.o. t.i.d. p.r.n. for nausea.

    Available:

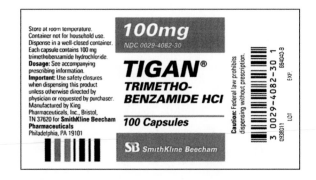

    _____

14. Order: Keflex 0.5 g p.o. q.i.d.

    Available:

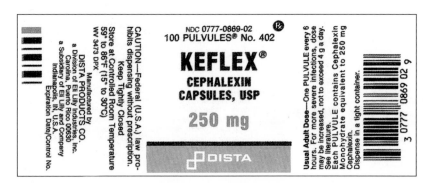

    _____

15. Order: Cogentin 2 mg p.o. b.i.d.

    Available: Cogentin tablets labeled 1 mg    _____

16. Order: Augmentin 0.5 g p.o. q8h.

    Available:

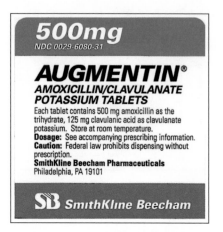

17. Order: Zovirax 400 mg p.o. b.i.d. for 7 days.

    Available:

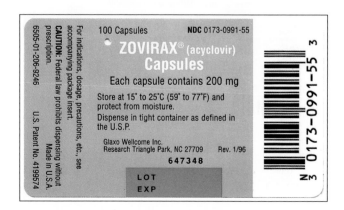

18. Order: Rifampin 0.6 g p.o. daily.

    Available:

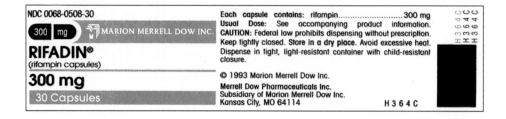

19. Order: Carafate 1,000 mg p.o. b.i.d.

    Available:

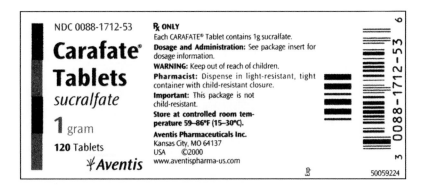

20. Order: Cardizem 240 mg p.o. daily.

    Available:

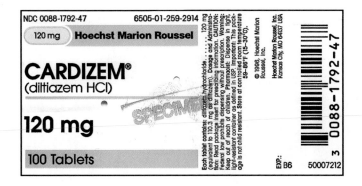

21. Order: Xanax 0.25 mg p.o. b.i.d.

    Available: Scored tablets (can be broken in half)

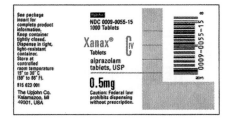

22.  Order: Septra DS 1 tab p.o. daily 3 times per week (Mon, Wed, Fri).

Available:

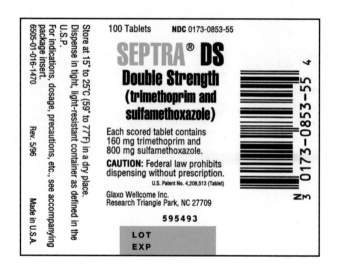

_____

23.  Order: Lotrel 2.5/10  2 caps p.o. daily.

Available:

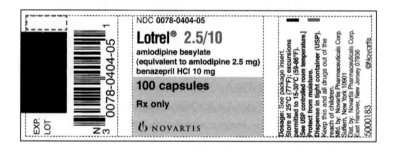

_____

24.  Order: Retrovir 0.2 g p.o. t.i.d.

Available:

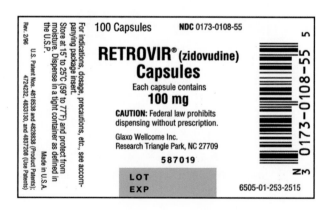

_____

25. Order: Lanoxicaps 0.05 mg p.o. every other day.

    Available:

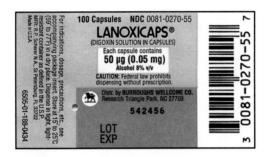

_____

26. Order: Risperdal 3 mg p.o. b.i.d.

    Available: Risperdal scored tablets (can be broken in half) labeled 1 mg.

    _____

27. Order: Flagyl 0.5 g p.o. q8h.

    Available:

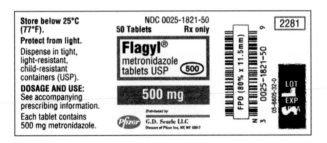

_____

28. Order: Lopressor 100 mg p.o. b.i.d.

    Available:

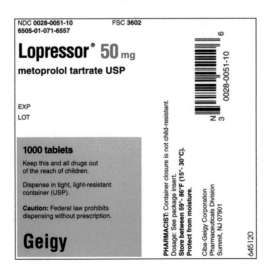

_____

29. Order: Lasix 60 mg p.o. daily.

    Available: Scored tablets (can be broken in half).

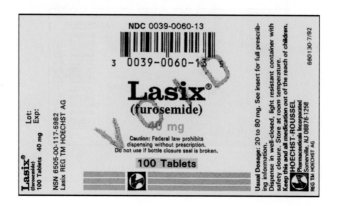

    _____

30. Order: Motrin 600 mg p.o. q6h p.r.n. for pain.

    Available: Motrin tablets labeled 300 mg _____

31. Order: Potassium chloride extended release 30 mEq p.o. daily.

    Available:

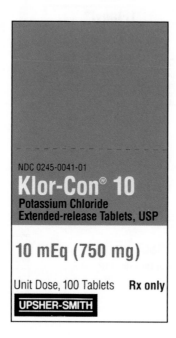

    _____

32. Order: Mevacor 20 mg p.o. daily at 6 PM.

    Available: Mevacor tablets labeled 10 mg _____

33. Order: Effexor 75 mg p.o. b.i.d.

    Available: Scored Effexor tablets (can be broken in half) labeled 37.5 mg _____

34. Order: Nembutal 100 mg p.o. at bedtime.

    Available:

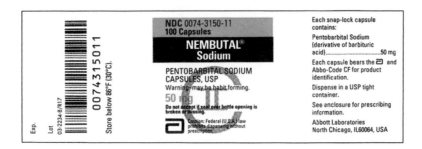

    _____

35. Order: Geodon 40 mg p.o. b.i.d.

    Available:

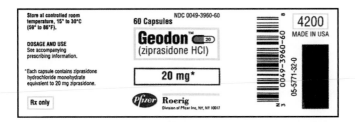

    _____

36. Order: Zarontin 750 mg p.o. b.i.d.

    Available:

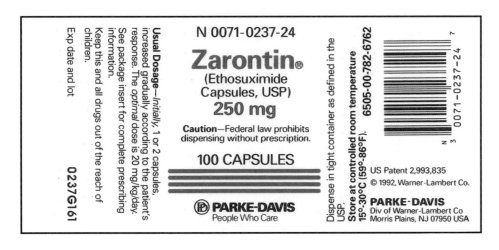

    _____

37. Order: Decadron 0.75 mg p.o. b.i.d.

    Available:

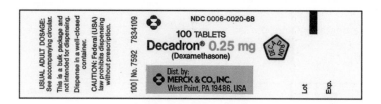

_____

38. Order: Levothroid 150 mcg p.o. every day.

    Available: Scored tablets (can be broken in half).

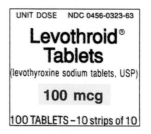

_____

39. Order: Lanoxin 0.125 mg p.o. every day.

    Available: Scored tablets (can be broken in half).

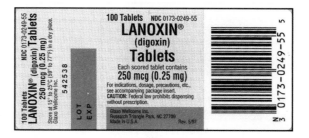

_____

40. Order: Evista 0.06 g p.o. daily.

    Available:

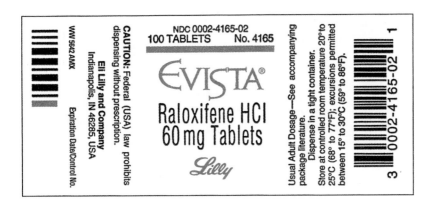

Answers on p. 619

## Part II

Calculate the volume necessary (in milliliters) to provide the dosage ordered, using medication labels where available. Express your answer as a decimal fraction to the nearest tenth where indicated.

41. Order: Dilantin 100 mg by gastrostomy tube t.i.d.

    Available: Dilantin 125 mg per 5 mL    _____

42. Order: Benadryl 50 mg p.o. at bedtime.

    Available: Benadryl elixir 12.5 mg per 5 mL    _____

43. Order: Gentamicin 50 mg IM q8h.

    Available:

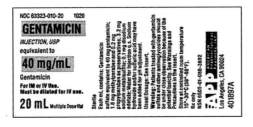

44. Order: Vibramycin 100 mg p.o. q12h.

    Available:

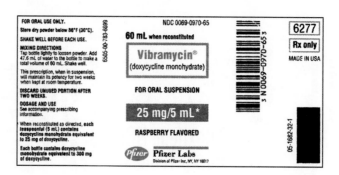

_____

45. Order: Meperidine hydrochloride 50 mg IM q4h p.r.n. for pain.

    Available: Meperidine 75 mg per mL          _____

46. Order: Gentamicin 90 mg IV q8h.

    Available: Gentamicin 40 mg per mL          _____

47. Order: Morphine gr $\frac{1}{4}$ subcut q4h p.r.n. for pain.

    Available:

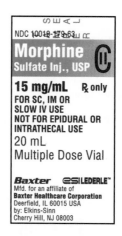

_____

48. Order: Vitamin $B_{12}$ (Cyanocobalamin) 1,000 mcg IM once monthly.

    Available:

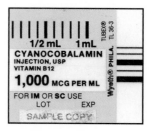

_____

49. Order: Morphine 10 mg subcut stat. (Express answer in hundredths.)

    Available: Morphine 15 mg per mL.  _____

50. Order: Kaon-Cl 20 mEq p.o. daily.

    Available:

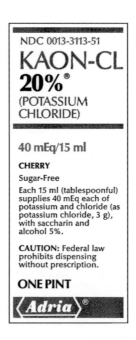

_____

51. Order: Nystatin oral suspension 100,000 units swish and swallow q6h.

    Available:

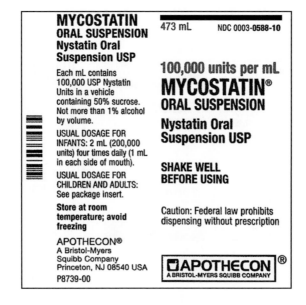

_____

52. Order: Heparin 5,000 units subcut daily.

    Available:

    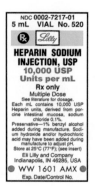

    _____

53. Order: Atropine 0.2 mg subcut stat.

    Available:

    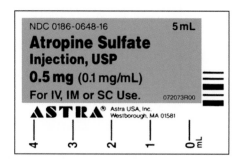

    _____

54. Order: Amoxicillin 500 mg p.o. q6h for 7 days.

    Available:

    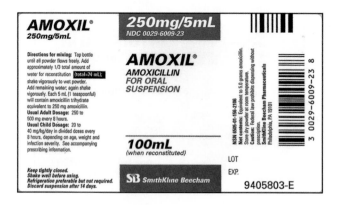

    _____

55. Order: Heparin 7,500 units subcut daily. Express answer in hundredths.

    Available: Heparin 10,000 units per mL    _____

56. Order: Solu-Medrol 70 mg IV daily.

    Available:

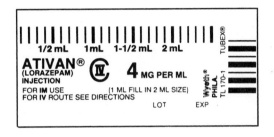

---

57. Order: Ativan 2 mg IM q4h p.r.n. for agitation.

    Available:

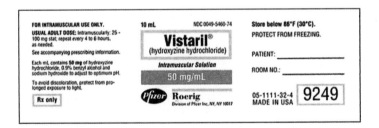

---

58. Order: Vistaril 25 mg IM on call to operating room (OR).

    Available:

---

59. Order: Phenobarbital (Luminal) gr $1^1/_2$ IM stat.

    Available:

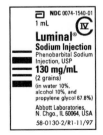

---

60. Order: Aminophylline 100 mg IV q6h.

    Available:

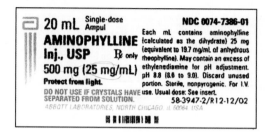

_____

61. Order: Zantac 150 mg IV daily.

    Available:

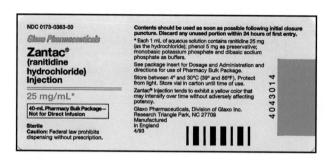

_____

62. Order: Augmentin 0.5 g p.o. q8h.

    Available:

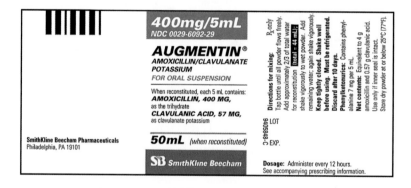

_____

63. Order: Thorazine concentrate 75 mg p.o. daily.

    Available:

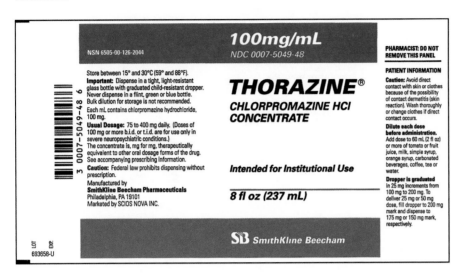

64. Order: Retrovir 200 mg by nasogastric tube t.i.d.

    Available:

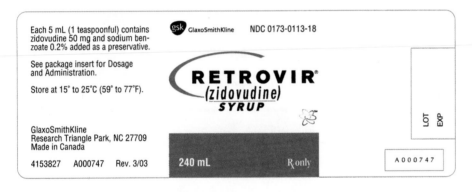

65. Order: Epivir 0.3 g p.o. b.i.d.

    Available:

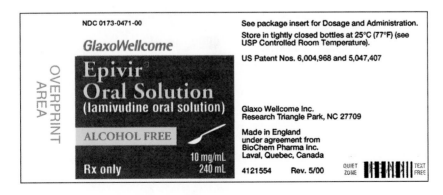

66.  Order: Cipro 0.4 g IV q12h.

Available:

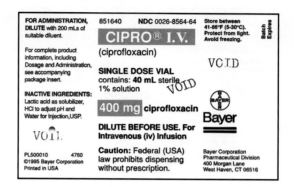

_____

67.  Order: Prozac 40 mg p.o. daily.

Available:

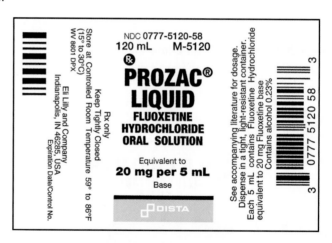

_____

68.  Order: Depo-Provera 0.4 g IM at bedtime once a week on Thursday.

Available:

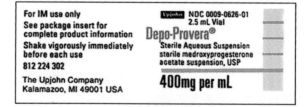

_____

69.  Order: Thorazine concentrate 500 mg p.o. b.i.d.

Available: Thorazine concentrate
labeled 30 mg per mL

_____

70. Order: Lactulose 30 g p.o. t.i.d.

    Available:

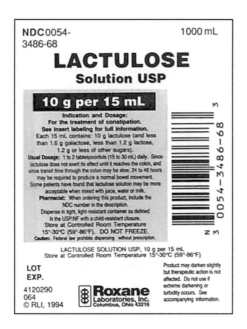

    _____

71. Order: Mellaril 40 mg p.o. b.i.d.

    Available: Mellaril concentrate 30 mg per mL _____

72. Order: Compazine 7 mg IM q4h p.r.n. for vomiting.

    Available:

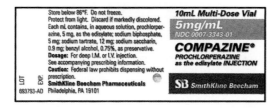

    _____

73. Order: Ceclor 0.5 g p.o. q8h.

    Available:

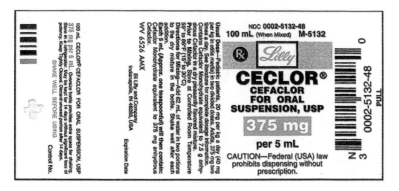

    _____

74.  Order: Dilantin suspension 200 mg per nasogastric tube every day.

Available:

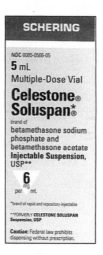

_____

75.  Order: Celestone 7 mg IM stat.

Available:

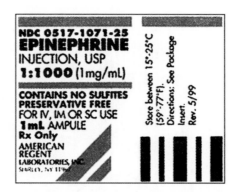

_____

76.  Order: Thiamine hydrochloride 75 mg IM every day.

Available: Thiamine hydrochloride
100 mg per mL                        _____

77.  Order: Epinephrine 0.25 mg IV stat.

Available:

_____

78. Order: Alprazolam 0.25 mg p.o. b.i.d. (Express answer in hundredths.)

    Available:

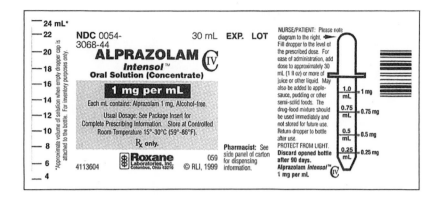

_____

79. Order: Vantin 100 mg p.o. q12h for 10 days.

    Available:

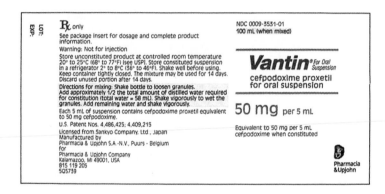

_____

80. Order: Zithromax oral suspension 500 mg p.o. for 1 dose stat then 250 mg daily for 3 days. Determine the amount to administer for the stat dose.

    Available:

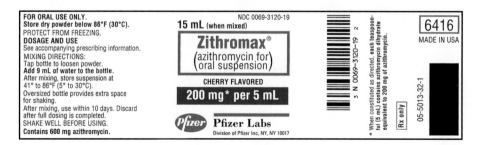

_____

Answers on p. 619

 **For additional practice problems, refer to the Methods of Calculating Dosages section of Drug Calculations Companion, Version 4, on Evolve.**

# CHAPTER 15

# Dosage Calculation Using the Formula Method

## Objectives

*After reviewing this chapter, you should be able to:*
1. Identify the information from a calculation problem to place into the formula given
2. Calculate medication dosages using the formula $\dfrac{D}{H} \times Q = x$
3. Calculate the number of tablets or capsules to administer
4. Calculate the volume to administer for medications in solution

This chapter shows how to use a formula for dosage calculation, which requires substituting information from the problem into the formula. **The nurse should use the formula consistently and in its entirety to avoid calculation errors.**

Errors can be made if you totally rely on a formula to determine a dosage rather than asking yourself whether the answer is reasonable. You will learn, for example, that the maximum number of tablets or capsules for a single dosage is usually three. Anything exceeding that should be a red flag to you, even if the answer is obtained from the use of a formula. Use formulas to validate the dosage you think is reasonable, not the reverse. **Think** before you calculate. Always estimate **before** applying a formula. Thinking first will allow you to detect errors and alert you to try again and question the results you obtained.

## Critical Thinking

### Avoid Dosage Calculation Errors
Do not rely solely on formulas when calculating dosages to be administered. Use critical thinking skills such as considering what the answer should be, reasoning, problem solving, and finding rational justification for your answer. Formulas should be used as tools for validating the dosage you THINK should be given.

## FORMULA FOR CALCULATING DOSAGES

The formula presented in this chapter can be used when calculating dosages in the same system of measurement. When the dosage desired and the dosage on hand are in different systems, convert them to the same system before using the formula, using one of the methods learned for conversion. It is imporant to learn and memorize the following formula:

$$\frac{D}{H} \times Q = x$$

Let's examine the terms in the formula before using it.

D = The dosage desired, or what the prescriber has ordered, including the units of measurement. Examples: mg, g, etc.

H = The dosage strength available, what is on hand, or the weight of the medication on the label, including the unit of measurement. Examples: mg, g, etc.

Q = The quantity or the unit of measure that contains the dosage that is available, in other words, the number of tablets, capsules, milliliters, etc. that contains the available dosage. "Q" is labeled accordingly as tablet, capsule, milliliter, etc.

*x* = The unknown, the dosage you are looking for, the dosage you are going to administer, how many milliliters, tablets, etc. you will give.

> **NOTE**
>
> It is important to note that the unknown "*x*" and "*Q*" will always be stated in the same unit of measure.

When you are solving problems that involve solid forms of medication (tabs, caps), Q is always 1 and can be eliminated from the equation. **For consistency and to avoid chances of error when Q is not 1, always include Q even with tablet and capsule problems.** When you are solving problems for medications in solution, the amount for Q varies and must always be included.

The available dosage on the label for liquid medications may indicate the quantity of medication per 1 milliliter or per multiple milliliters of solution, such as 80 mg per 2 mL, 125 mg per 5 mL. Some liquid medications may also express the quantity in amounts less than a milliliter, such as 2 mg per 0.5 mL. Because the amount for "Q" can vary with liquid medications and is not always 1, **omission of the amount for "Q" can render an error in dosage calculation.**

> **CAUTION**
>
> Label all terms of the formula, including "*x*," as a safeguard to prevent errors in calculation. Think about what is a reasonable amount to administer, and calculate the dosage using the formula.

## STEPS FOR USE OF THE FORMULA

Now that we have reviewed the terms in the formula, let's review the steps for using the formula (Box 15-1) before beginning to calculate dosages using the formula.

---

**BOX 15-1  Steps for Using the Formula**

1. Memorize the formula, or verify the formula from a resource.
2. Place the information from the problem into the formula in the correct position, with all terms in the formula labeled correctly, including "*x*.".
3. Make sure that all measures are in the same units and system of measure; if not, a conversion must be done *before* calculating the dosage.
4. Think logically, and consider what a reasonable amount to administer would be.
5. Calculate your answer, using the formula $\dfrac{D}{H} \times Q = x$.
6. Label all answers—tabs, caps, mL, etc.

---

Now we will look at sample problems illustrating the use of the formula.

**Example 1:** Order: 0.375 mg p.o. of a medication.

Available: Tablets labeled 0.25 mg

**Solution:** The dosage 0.375 mg is desired; the dosage strength available is 0.25 mg per tablet. No conversion is necessary. What is desired is in the same system and unit of measure as what you have on hand.

 Formula Setup

$$\frac{D}{H} \times Q = x$$

The desired (D) is 0.375 mg. You have on hand (H) 0.25 mg per (Q) 1 tablet. The label on *x* is tablet. Notice that the label on *x* is always the same as Q.

$$\frac{\text{(D) 0.375 mg}}{\text{(H) 0.25 mg}} \times \text{(Q) 1 tab} = x \text{ tab}$$

$$x = \frac{0.375}{0.25} \times 1$$

$$x = \frac{0.375}{0.25}$$

$$x = 1.5 = 1\frac{1}{2} \text{ tabs}$$

Therefore *x* = 1.5 tabs, or 1½ tabs. (Because 0.375 mg is larger than 0.25 mg, you will need more than 1 tab to administer 0.375 mg.) *Note:* Although 1.5 tabs is the same as 1½ tabs, for administration purposes, it would be best to state it as 1½ tabs.

**Example 2:** Order: 7,000 units IM of a medication.

Available: 10,000 units in 2 mL

**Solution:**

$$\frac{\text{(D) 7,000 units}}{\text{(H) 10,000 units}} \times \text{(Q) 2 mL} = x \text{ mL}$$

$$x = \frac{7,000 \times 2}{10,000}$$

$$x = \frac{14}{10}$$

$$x = 1.4 \text{ mL}$$

**CAUTION**

Omitting Q here could result in an error. A liquid medication is involved; Q must be included because the amount varies and is not always per 1 mL.

**RULE**

**Rule for Different Units or Systems of Measure**
Whenever the desired amount and the dosage on hand are in different units or systems of measure, follow these steps:
1. Choose the identified equivalent.
2. Convert what is ordered to the same units or system of measure as what is available by using one of the methods presented in the chapter on converting.
3. Use the formula $\frac{D}{H} \times Q = x$ to calculate the dosage to administer.

## Tips for Clinical Practice

When converting before calculating a dosage, convert apothecary and household measurements to their metric equivalents when possible. The metric system is the principal system used in measurement for medications.

**Example 3:** Order: gr $\frac{1}{2}$ p.o.

Available: Tablets labeled 15 mg

**Solution:** Convert gr $\frac{1}{2}$ to mg. The equivalent to use is 60 mg = gr 1. Therefore gr $\frac{1}{2}$ = 30 mg.

Now that you have everything in the same system and units of measure, use the formula presented to calculate the dosage to be administered.

**Solution:**

$$\frac{\text{(D) 30 mg}}{\text{(H) 15 mg}} \times \text{(Q) 1 tab} = x \text{ tab}$$

$$x = \frac{30}{15} \times 1$$

$$x = \frac{30}{15}$$

$$x = 2 \text{ tabs}$$

> **NOTE**
>
> What is desired and what is available must be in the *same units and system of measure.* Remember that it is usual to convert what is desired to what is available. Therefore change gr to mg; this will also eliminate the fraction and decrease the chance of error in calculation.

Therefore $x = 2$ tabs. (Because 30 mg is a larger dosage than 15 mg, it will take more than 1 tab to administer the desired dosage.)

**Example 4:** Order: gr $\frac{1}{6}$ subcutaneous of a medication.

Available: gr $\frac{1}{2}$ per mL (Express the answer to the nearest tenth.)

**Solution:**

$$\frac{\text{(D) gr } \frac{1}{6}}{\text{(H) gr } \frac{1}{2}} \times \text{(Q) 1 mL} = x \text{ mL}$$

$$x = \frac{1}{6} \div \frac{1}{2} \qquad \frac{1}{6} \times \frac{2}{1} = \frac{2}{6} = \frac{1}{3} \qquad x = \frac{1}{3} = 0.33 = 0.3 \text{ mL}$$

Therefore $x = 0.33$ mL = 0.3 mL. (Because $\frac{1}{2}$ is a larger dosage than $\frac{1}{6}$, it will take less than 1 mL to administer the required dosage.)

## Critical Thinking

Always think critically, even when using a formula. It is an essential step in estimating what is reasonable and logical in terms of a dosage. This will help prevent errors in calculation caused by setting up the problem incorrectly or careless math and will remind you to double-check your calculation and identify any error.

> **NOTE**
>
> As you will learn in a later chapter, stating the answer as $\frac{1}{3}$ mL (fraction) would be incorrect. A milliliter is a metric measure and is expressed as a decimal number.

Remember to memorize the formula presented and follow the steps sequentially. Check **FIRST** to see if a conversion is required; if so, convert so that everything is in the same units and system of measure, set up terms into the formula, **THINK** critically as to a reasonable answer, and calculate the dosage using the formula to validate the dosage you anticipated was reasonable.

**CAUTION**

Always double-check your math. Errors can be made in simple calculations because of lack of caution. Always ask yourself whether the answer you have obtained is reasonable and correct.

## ■ Points to Remember

- The formula $\dfrac{D}{H} \times Q = x$ can be used to calculate the dosage to be administered.
- The Q is always 1 for solid forms of medications (tabs, caps, etc.) but varies when medications are in liquid form.
- Before the dosage to be given is calculated, the dosage desired must be in the same units and system of measure as the dosage available or a conversion is necessary.
- Set up the terms in the formula labeled with the units of measure, including "*x*."
- Think about what a reasonable answer would be.
- Calculate the dosage to administer using the formula to validate your answer as to what was reasonable.
- Double-check all your math, and think logically about the answer obtained.
- Label all answers obtained (e.g., tabs, caps, mL).
- The use of a formula does not eliminate the need to think critically.
- Always systematically follow these steps: **Convert** if necessary, set up the terms in the formula, **THINK** about what would be a reasonable answer, **Calculate** the dosage to administer using the formula.

 **Practice Problems**

Calculate the following problems using the formula presented in this chapter. Label answers correctly: tabs, caps.

1. Order: 0.4 mg p.o.

   Available: Tablets labeled 0.2 mg _____

2. Order: 0.75 g p.o.

   Available: Capsules labeled 250 mg _____

3. Order: 90 mg p.o.

   Available: Tablets labeled 60 mg _____

4. Order: 7.5 mg p.o.

   Available: Tablets labeled 2.5 mg _____

5. Order: 0.05 mg p.o.

   Available: Tablets labeled 25 mcg _____

6.  Order: 0.4 mg p.o.

    Available: Tablets labeled 200 mcg _____

7.  Order: 1,000 mg p.o.

    Available: Tablets labeled 500 mg _____

8.  Order: 0.6 g p.o.

    Available: Capsules labeled 600 mg _____

9.  Order: 1.25 mg p.o.

    Available: Tablets labeled 625 mcg _____

Calculate the following in milliliters; round to the nearest tenth where indicated. Label answers mL.

10. Order: 10 mg subcut.

    Available: 15 mg per mL _____

11. Order: 400 mg p.o.

    Available: Oral solution labeled 200 mg per 5 mL _____

12. Order: 15 mEq p.o.

    Available: Oral solution labeled 20 mEq per10 mL _____

13. Order: 125 mg p.o.

    Available: Oral solution labeled 250 mg per 5 mL _____

14. Order: 0.025 mg p.o.

    Available: Oral solution labeled 0.05 mg per 5 mL _____

15. Order: 375 mg p.o.

    Available: Oral solution labeled 125 mg per 5 mL _____

Answers on pp. 620-621

## ✓ CHAPTER REVIEW

Calculate the following dosages using the medication label or information provided. Label answers correctly: tabs, caps, mL. Answers expressed in milliliters should be rounded to the nearest tenth where indicated.

1.  Order: Phenobarbital gr $\frac{1}{2}$ p.o. t.i.d.

    Available: Phenobarbital tablets labeled 30 mg _____

2. Order: Gantrisin 500 mg p.o. q.i.d.

   Available:

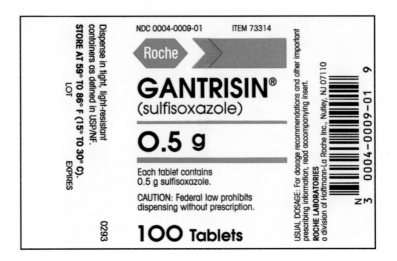

_____

3. Order: Indocin 50 mg p.o. t.i.d.

   Available:

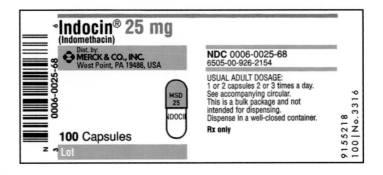

_____

4. Order: Hydrodiuril 50 mg p.o. b.i.d.

   Available:

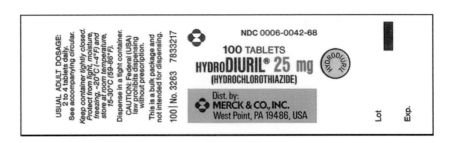

_____

5. Order: Tylenol 650 mg p.o. q4h p.r.n. for pain.

   Available:

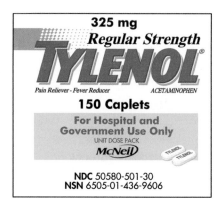

_____

6. Order: Digoxin 0.375 mg p.o. daily.

   Available: Scored tablets (can be broken in half).

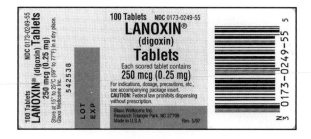

_____

7. Order: Keflex 0.25 g p.o. q6h.

   Available:

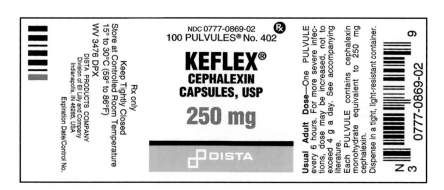

_____

8. Order: Seconal 100 mg p.o. at bedtime.

    Available: Seconal capsules labeled
    100 mg                                            _____

9. Order: Minipress 2 mg p.o. b.i.d. for 2 days.

    Available:

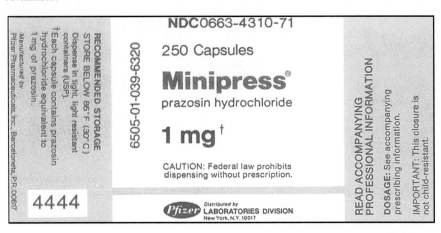

                                                      _____

10. Order: Motrin 0.8 g p.o. q8h p.r.n. for pain.

    Available:

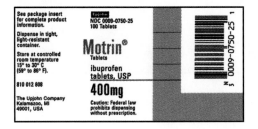

                                                      _____

11. Order: Codeine gr $^3/_4$ p.o. q4h p.r.n. for pain.

    Available: Scored tablets (can be broken in half).

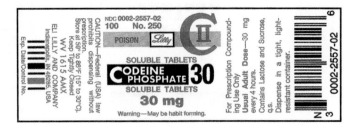

                                                      _____

12. Order: Cephradine 0.5 g p.o. q6h.

    Available: Cephradine 250 mg caps.        _____

13. Order: Cogentin 0.5 mg p.o. at bedtime.

    Available:

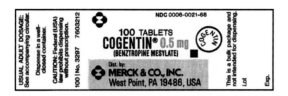

_____

14. Order: Thorazine 75 mg p.o. b.i.d.

    Available:

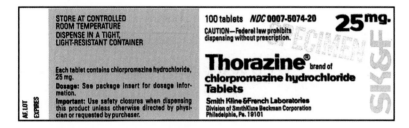

_____

15. Order: Dilantin (extended capsules) 60 mg p.o. b.i.d.

    Available:

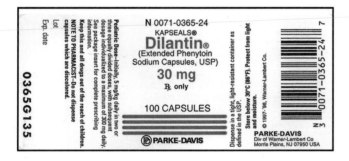

_____

16. Order: Meperidine hydrochloride 50 mg I.M. q4h p.r.n. for pain.

    Available:

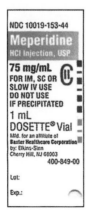

_____

17. Order: Solu-Medrol 60 mg IV daily.

    Available:

    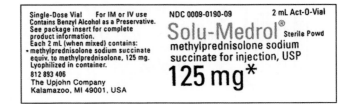

18. Order: Amikacin 90 mg IM q12h.

    Available:

    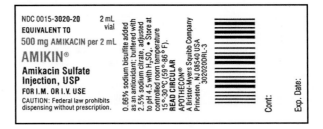

19. Order: Amoxicillin 300 mg p.o. q8h.

    Available:

    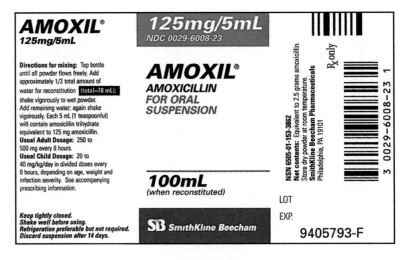

20. Order: Amoxicillin 0.5 g by nasogastric tube q6h.

    Available:

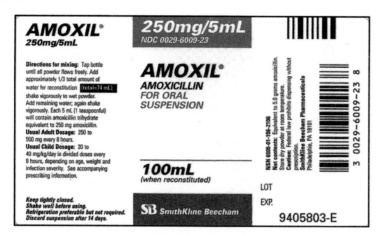

_____

21. Order: Phenobarbital elixir 45 mg p.o. b.i.d.

    Available: Phenobarbital elixir 20 mg per 5 mL _____

22. Order: Heparin 3,000 units subcut b.i.d.

    Available:

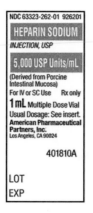

_____

23. Order: Procaine penicillin 600,000 units IM q12h.

    Available:

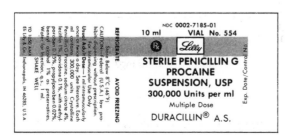

_____

24. Order: Gentamicin 70 mg IV q8h.

    Available:

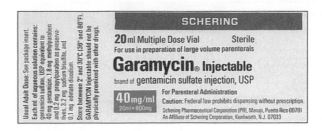

    _____

25. Order: Potassium chloride 20 mEq IV in 1,000 mL 0.9% normal saline.

    Available:

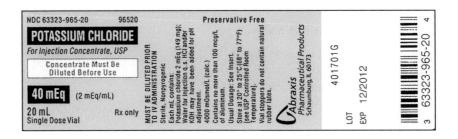

    _____

26. Order: Depo-Medrol 60 mg IM every Monday for 2 weeks.

    Available:

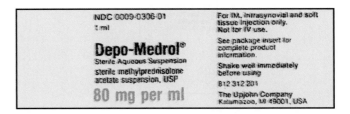

    _____

27. Order: Vistaril 100 mg IM stat.

    Available: Vistaril 50 mg per mL    _____

28.  Order: Morphine sulfate 6 mg subcut q4h p.r.n. for pain.

   Available:

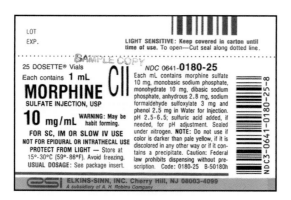

   _____

29.  Order: Atropine 0.3 mg IM stat.

   Available: Atropine 0.4 mg per mL      _____

30.  Order: Stadol 1 mg IM q4h p.r.n. for pain.

   Available:

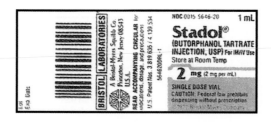

   _____

31.  Order: Ativan 1 mg IM stat.

   Available: Ativan 4 mg per mL      _____

32.  Order: Kanamycin 250 mg IM q6h.

   Available:

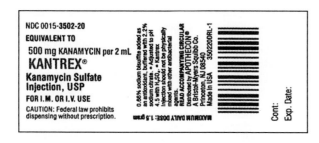

   _____

33. Order: Robinul 0.4 mg IM stat on call to OR.

    Available:

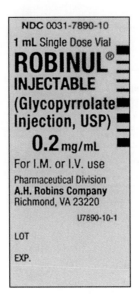

    _____

34. Order: Aminophylline 80 mg IV q6h.

    Available:

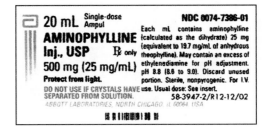

    _____

35. Order: Lithium citrate oral solution 300 mg p.o. t.i.d.

    Available: Lithium citrate 300 mg per 5 mL    _____

36. Order: Sinemet 25-100 p.o. q.i.d.

    Available:

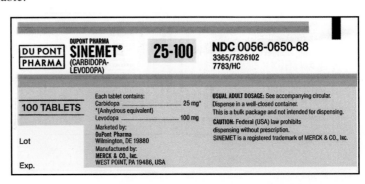

    _____

37. Order: Lopid 0.6 g p.o. b.i.d. 30 minutes before meals.

Available:

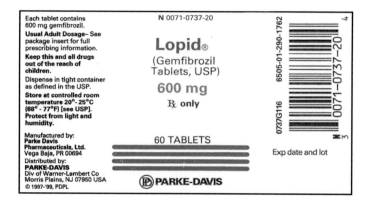

38. Order: Prozac 20 mg p.o. daily.

Available:

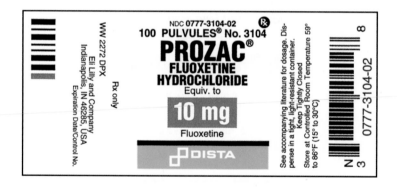

39. Order: Potassium chloride 10 mEq IV in 1,000 mL D5W.

Available:

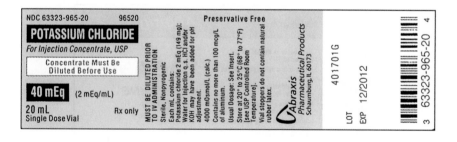

40. Order: Augmentin 0.875 g p.o. q12h.

   Available:

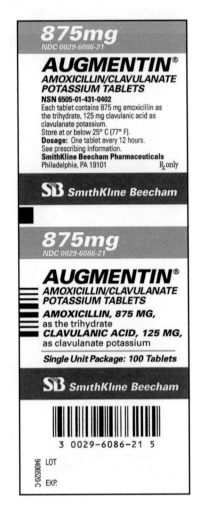

41. Order: Tagamet 800 mg p.o. at bedtime.

   Available:

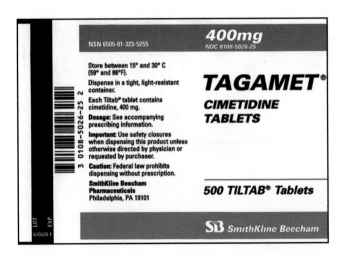

42. Order: Depo-Provera 500 mg IM once a week (on Mondays).

    Available:

    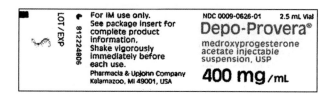

    _____

43. Order: Tagamet 300 mg IV q8h.

    Available:

    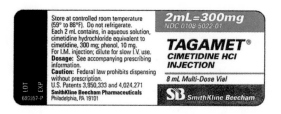

    _____

44. Order: Nembutal 150 mg IM at bedtime p.r.n. for 3 days.

    Available:

    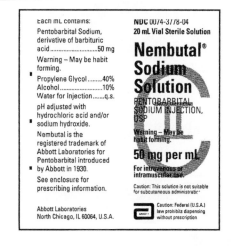

    _____

45. Order: Cipro 1.5 g p.o. q12h.

    Available:

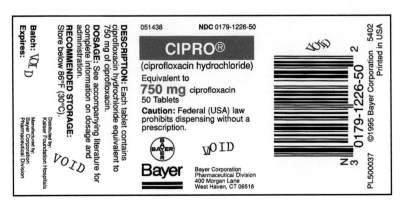

46. Order: Vasotec 5 mg p.o. daily.

    Available:

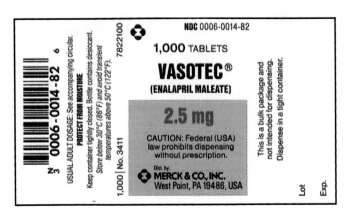

47. Order: Clozaril 50 mg p.o. b.i.d.

    Available:

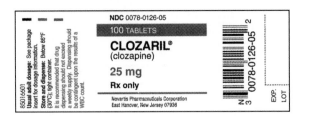

48.  Order: Clindamycin 450 mg p.o. q.i.d. for 5 days.

Available:

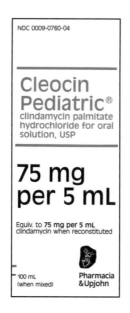

_____

49.  Order: Benadryl 30 mg p.o. t.i.d.

Available: Oral solution labeled
12.5 mg per 5 mL

_____

50.  Order: Primidone 125 mg p.o. daily.

Available: Oral solution labeled
250 mg per 5 mL

_____

51.  Order: Glucophage 0.5 g p.o. b.i.d.

Available:

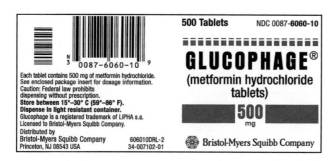

_____

52.  Order: Inderal 40 mg p.o. b.i.d.

Available:

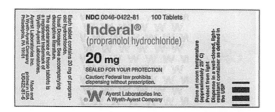

_____

53. Order: Lasix 30 mg p.o. every day at 9 AM.

    Available: Scored tablets (can be broken in half)

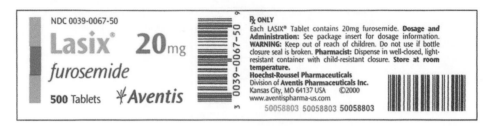

_____

54. Order: Dicloxacillin 0.35 g by nasogastric tube q6h.

    Available:

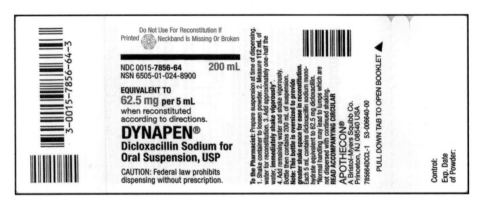

_____

55. Order: Urecholine 2.5 mg subcut stat.

    Available: 5 mg per mL

_____

56. Order: Glyburide 7.5 mg p.o. daily with breakfast.

    Available:

_____

57. Order: Biaxin 0.5 g p.o. q12h for 10 days.

    Available:

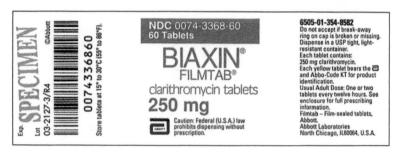

58. Order: Aricept 5 mg p.o. every day at bedtime.

    Available:

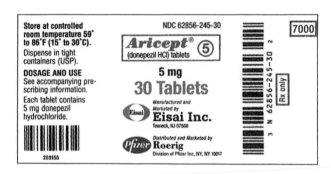

59. Order: Lasix 8 mg IM stat.

    Available: Lasix labeled 20 mg per 2 mL _____

60. Order: Toprol-XL 0.2 g p.o. every day.

    Available:

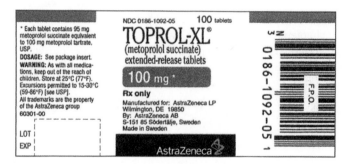

Answers on p. 621

 **For additional practice problems, refer to the Methods of Calculating Dosages section of Drug Calculations Companion, Version 4, on Evolve.**

# Dosage Calculation Using the Dimensional Analysis Method

## Objectives

*After reviewing this chapter, you should be able to:*
1. Define dimensional analysis
2. Implement unit cancellation in dimensional analysis
3. Perform conversions using dimensional analysis
4. Use dimensional analysis to calculate dosages

*Dimensional analysis* is the use of a simple technique with a fancy name for the process of manipulating units. By manipulating units you are able to eliminate or cancel unwanted units. It is considered to be a common-sense approach that eliminates the need to memorize a formula. Once the concepts related to dimensional analysis are mastered it can be used to calculate dosages.

Dimensional analysis is also referred to as the *factor-label method* or the *unit factor method*. Dimensional analysis can be viewed as a problem-solving method. The advantage of dimensional analysis is that because only one equation is needed, it eliminates memorization of formulas. Dimensional analysis can be used for all calculations you may encounter once you become comfortable with the process. This chapter will discuss dimensional analysis and provide examples of how it might be used in calculating dosages. Although some may find the formalism of the term *dimensional analysis* intimidating at first, you will find it is quite simple once you have worked a few problems. This method as stated can be used for all calculations. Dimensional analysis will be demonstrated as we proceed through the chapters. *Note:* Remember, as stated in the discussion of calculation methods, that it is important that you understand that you as the learner must choose a method of calculation you are comfortable with and use it consistently.

## UNDERSTANDING THE BASICS OF DIMENSIONAL ANALYSIS

To introduce the basics relating to dimensional analysis, let's begin by looking at how the process works in making conversions before we look at its use in calculating dosages. As you recall from previous chapters, you learned what were referred to as *equivalents* or *conversion factors:* for example, 1 g = 1,000 mg, 1 grain = 60 mg. When we begin using this process for dosage calculations, you will quickly see how dimensional analysis allows multiple factors to be entered in one equation. This method is particularly useful when you have a medication ordered in one unit and it is available in another unit. Although multiple factors can be placed in a dimensional analysis equation, you can decide to do the conversion before you set up the equation using one of the methods learned in earlier chapters, or you can use dimensional analysis to perform the conversion before calculating the dosage.

## Performing Conversions Using Dimensional Analysis

The equivalents or conversion factors you learned can be written in a fraction format, which is important to understand in using dimensional analysis. Let's look at the equivalent 1 kg = 1,000 g.

This can be written as:

$$\frac{1 \text{ kg}}{1,000 \text{ g}} \quad or \quad \frac{1,000 \text{ g}}{1 \text{ kg}}$$

**NOTE**

You have not changed the value of the unit: you have simply rewritten the equivalency or conversion factor in a fraction format.

Now let's look at the basics in using dimensional analysis for converting units of measure. It is necessary to state the equivalent (conversion factor) in fraction format, maintaining the desired unit in the numerator.

An equivalent (conversion factor) will give you two fractions:

**Example:** $\quad 2.2 \text{ lb} = 1 \text{ kg} = \dfrac{2.2 \text{ lb}}{1 \text{ kg}} \quad or \quad \dfrac{1 \text{ kg}}{2.2 \text{ lb}}$

**NOTE**

How the fraction is written depends on the unit you want to cancel or eliminate to get the unit desired.

$$1,000 \text{ mcg} = 1 \text{ mg} = \frac{1,000 \text{ mcg}}{1 \text{ mg}} \quad or \quad \frac{1 \text{ mg}}{1,000 \text{ mcg}}$$

## To Make Conversions Using Dimensional Analysis

1. Identify the desired unit.
2. Identify the equivalent needed.
3. Write the equivalent in fraction format, keeping the desired unit in the numerator of the fraction. This is written first in the equation.
4. Label all factors in the equation, and label what you desire *x* (unit desired).
5. Identify unwanted or undesired units, and cancel them. Reduce to lowest terms if possible.
6. If all the labels except the answer label are not eliminated, recheck the equation.
7. Perform the mathematical process indicated.

## Critical Thinking

Stating the equivalent incorrectly will not allow you to eliminate desired units. Knowing when the equation is set up correctly is an important part of the concept of dimensional analysis.

Let's look at examples to demonstrate the dimensional analysis process.

**Example 1:**  1.5 g = _____ mg
1. The desired unit is mg.
2. Equivalent: 1,000 mg = 1 g
3. Write the equivalent, keeping mg in the numerator to allow you to cancel the unwanted unit, g.
4. Write the equivalent first stated as a fraction, followed by a multiplication sign (×).
5. Perform the indicated mathematical operations.

Setup:

$$x \text{ mg} = \frac{1,000 \text{ mg}}{1 \text{ g}} \times 1.5 \text{ g}$$

$$or$$

$$x \text{ mg} = \frac{1,000 \text{ mg}}{1 \text{ g}} \times \frac{1.5 \text{ g}}{1}$$

$$1,000 \times 1.5 = 1,500 \text{ mg}$$

$$x = 1,500 \text{ mg}$$

The problem in Example 1 could be done by decimal movement. It is shown in this format to illustrate dimensional analysis.

**Example 2:**    110 lb = _____ kg
1. The desired unit is kg.
2. Equivalent: 2.2 lb = 1 kg
3. Proceed to set up the problem as outlined.

**RULE**

Placing a 1 under a value does not alter the value of the number. What you desire or are looking for is labeled *x*.

Setup:

$$x \text{ kg} = \frac{1 \text{ kg}}{2.2 \text{ lb}} \times 110 \text{ lb}$$

*or*

$$x \text{ kg} = \frac{1 \text{ kg}}{2.2 \text{ lb}} \times \frac{110 \text{ lb}}{1}$$

$$x = \frac{110}{2.2}$$

$$x = 50 \text{ kg}$$

**RULE**

All factors entered in the equation must always include the quantity and unit of measure. State all answers following the rules of the system. When there is more than one equivalent for a unit of measure, use the conversion factor used most often.

 **Practice Problems**

Set up the following problems using the dimensional analysis format; cancel the units. Do not solve.

1.  15 mg = gr _____

2.  gr 5 = _____ mg

3.  400 mcg = _____ mg

4.  2 tbs = _____ mL

5.  0.007 g = _____ mg

6.  0.5 L = _____ mL

7.  529 mg = _____ g

8.  1,600 mL = _____ L

9. 46.4 kg = _____ lb

10. 5 cm = _____ in

Answers on p. 622

---

## ■ Points to Remember

- Identify the desired unit, and label it *x*.
- State the equivalent (conversion factor) in fraction format with the desired unit in the numerator.
- Label all factors in the equation, including "*x*."
- State the equivalent first in the equation, followed by a multiplication sign (×).
- Remember the rules relating to conversions.
- Cancel the undesired units.

## DOSAGE CALCULATION USING DIMENSIONAL ANALYSIS

As stated previously, dimensional analysis can be used to calculate dosages with the use of a single equation. A single equation can also be used to calculate the dosage when the dosage desired is in units that differ from what is available. When using dimensional analysis to calculate dosages, it is important to extract the essential information needed from the problem.

In earlier chapters relating to calculating dosages, you learned how to read medication labels. Remember, dosages are always expressed in relation to the form or unit of measure (e.g., milliliters) that contains them.

**Examples:**    100 mg per tab, 500 mg per cap, 40 mg per 2 mL.

When dimensional analysis is used to calculate dosages, the above examples become crucial factors in the equation and are entered as a fraction with a numerator and denominator.

### Steps in Calculating Dosages Using Dimensional Analysis

1. Identify the unit of measure desired in the calculation. With solid forms the unit will be tab or cap. For parenteral and oral liquids the unit is milliliter.
2. On the left side of the equation, place the name or appropriate abbreviation for *x*, what you desire or are looking for (e.g., tab, cap, mL).
3. On the right side of the equation, place the available information from the problem in a fraction format. The abbreviation or unit matching the desired unit must be placed in the numerator.
4. Enter the additional factors from the problem, usually what is ordered. Set up the numerator so that it matches the unit in the previous denominator.
5. Cancel out the like units of measurement on the right side of the equation. The remaining unit should match the unit on the left side of the equation and be the unit desired. Reduce to lowest terms if possible.
6. Solve for the unknown *x*.

Let's look at an example using these steps.

**Example 1:**    Order: Lasix 40 mg p.o. daily

Available: Tablets labeled 20 mg

1. Place the unit of measure desired in the calculation on the left side of the equation, and label it $x$.

$$x \text{ tab} =$$

2. Place the information from the problem on the right side of the equation in a fraction format with the unit matching the desired unit in the numerator. (In this problem each tab contains 20 mg.) You must always think about what is a reasonable answer.

$$x \text{ tab} = \frac{1 \text{ tab}}{20 \text{ mg}}$$

3. Enter the additional factors from the problem, what is ordered, matching the numerator in the previous denominator (in the problem the order is 40 mg). Placing a 1 under it does not change the value.

$$
\begin{array}{ccc}
\text{Amount to} & \text{Available} & \text{Ordered} \\
\text{administer} & \text{dosage} & \text{dosage} \\
\downarrow & \downarrow & \downarrow
\end{array}
$$

$$x \text{ tab} = \frac{1 \text{ tab}}{20 \text{ mg}} \times \frac{40 \text{ mg}}{1}$$

4. Cancel the like units of measurement on the right side of the equation. The remaining unit of measurement should be what is desired. Match the unit of measurement on the left side. Proceed with the mathematical process. Notice that after cancellation of units (mg) the desired unit of measure to be administered remains (e.g., tabs in this problem).

$$x \text{ tab} = \frac{1 \text{ tab}}{20 \text{ m\!\!\!/g}} \times \frac{40 \text{ m\!\!\!/g}}{1}$$

$$x = \frac{1 \times 40}{20}$$

$$x = \frac{40}{20}$$

$$x = 2 \text{ tabs}$$

Now let's look at an example with parenteral medications. You would follow the same steps illustrated in Example 1.

**Example 2:**    Order: Gentamicin 55 mg IM q8h

Available: Gentamicin 80 mg per 2 mL (round to the nearest tenth)

1. On the left side of the equation, place the unit desired in this problem (mL).

$$x \text{ mL} =$$

2. On the right side, place the available information from the problem in fraction format, placing the unit matching the unit desired in the numerator. Think what is reasonable to administer.

$$x \text{ mL} = \frac{2 \text{ mL}}{80 \text{ mg}}$$

3. Enter the additional factors from the problem, what is ordered matching the numerator in the previous denominator (in this problem the order is 55 mg).

$$x \text{ mL} = \underset{\underset{\text{dosage}}{\underset{\downarrow}{\text{Available}}}}{\frac{2 \text{ mL}}{80 \text{ mg}}} \times \underset{\underset{\text{dosage}}{\underset{\downarrow}{\text{Ordered}}}}{\frac{55 \text{ mg}}{1}}$$

with "Amount to administer" ↓ pointing to $x$ mL.

4. Cancel out the like units of measurement on the right side of the equation. The remaining unit of measurement should match the unit on the left side of the equation and be the unit desired.

$$x \text{ mL} = \frac{2 \text{ mL}}{80 \text{ mg}} \times \frac{55 \text{ mg}}{1}$$

$$x = \frac{2 \times 55}{80}$$

$$x = \frac{110}{80} = 1.37$$

$$x = 1.4 \text{ mL}$$

As previously mentioned, dimensional analysis can be used when a medication is ordered in one unit of measurement and available in another, thereby necessitating a conversion. However, the same steps are followed as previously shown.

- An additional fraction is entered into the equation as the second fraction. This fraction is the equivalent or the conversion factor needed. The numerator must match the unit of the previous denominator.
- The last fraction is the medication ordered. This is written so that the numerator of the fraction matches the unit in the denominator of the fraction immediately before.

Let's look at an example:

**Example 3:**  Order: Ampicillin 0.5 g IM q6h

Available: Ampicillin labeled 250 mg per mL

1. On the left side of the equation, place the unit of measure desired in the calculation and label it *x*.

$$x \text{ mL} =$$

2. Place the information from the problem on the right side of the equation in a fraction format, placing the unit matching the unit desired in the numerator. Think about what is a reasonable amount to administer.

$$x \text{ mL} = \frac{1 \text{ mL}}{250 \text{ mg}}$$

3. The order is for 0.5 g, and the medication is available in 250 mg; a conversion is therefore needed.
   From previous chapters we know 1 g = 1,000 mg; this fraction is placed next in the form of a fraction (the numerator of the fraction must match the denominator of the immediately previous fraction).

$$x \text{ mL} = \frac{1 \text{ mL}}{250 \text{ mg}} \times \frac{1,000 \text{ mg}}{1 \text{ g}}$$

4. Next place the amount of medication ordered in the equation. This will match the denominator of the fraction immediately before. In this problem it is 0.5 g.

$$x \text{ mL} = \underbrace{\frac{1 \text{ mL}}{250 \text{ mg}}}_{\substack{\text{Available} \\ \text{dosage} \\ \downarrow}} \times \underbrace{\frac{1,000 \text{ mg}}{1 \text{ g}}}_{\substack{\text{Conversion} \\ \text{factor} \\ \downarrow}} \times \underbrace{\frac{0.5 \text{ g}}{1}}_{\substack{\text{Dose} \\ \text{ordered} \\ \downarrow}}$$

5. Cancel out like units of measurement on the right side of the equation; the remaining unit of measurement should match the unit on the left side of equation and be the desired unit. Notice that mg and g cancel, leaving the desired unit, mL.

$$x \text{ mL} = \frac{1 \text{ mL}}{250 \text{ mg}} \times \frac{1,000 \text{ mg}}{1 \text{ g}} \times \frac{0.5 \text{ g}}{1}$$

$$x = \frac{1,000 \times 0.5}{250}$$

$$x = \frac{500}{250}$$

$$x = 2 \text{ mL}$$

> **CAUTION**
>
> Incorrect placement of units of measure into the equation will not allow cancellation of units and can result in an error in calculation. Dimensional analysis does not eliminate thinking about what a reasonable answer should be.

## ■ Points to Remember

When using dimensional analysis to calculate dosages:
- First determine units of the medication you want to administer: for example, tablets, capsules, mL, and so on. The unit desired is written **FIRST** to the left of the equation followed by an equals sign (=).
- The units in the numerator on the left of the equals sign are the same units placed in the numerator of the **first fraction** on the right side of the equation.
- If a conversion is necessary the conversion factor is also entered into the right side of the equation, as the second fraction.
- The ordered dosage is added at the end as the final fraction.
- Cancel the like units. When all the cancellations have been made, only the units desired remain (e.g., tab, caps, mL).
- Always determine the units and **THINK** about what a reasonable answer is, set up the equation, and cancel the units.
- All factors entered into the equation must include the quantity and unit of measure.
- Incorrect placement of units of measurement will not allow you to cancel units and can result in an incorrect answer.
- Thinking and reasoning are essential even with dimensional analysis.

**Practice Problems**

Set up the following problems using dimensional analysis. Do not solve.

11. A dose strength of 0.3 g has been ordered.

    Available: 0.4 g per 1.5 mL _____

12. A dose strength of gr $^1/_4$ is ordered.

    Available: 15 mg per mL _____

13. Order: Ampicillin 1 g p.o. stat.

    Available: Ampicillin capsules labeled 500 mg _____

14. Order: Augmentin 400 mg p.o. q8h.

    Available: Augmentin oral suspension 400 mg per 5 mL _____

15. Order: Zantac 150 mg I.V. daily.

    Available: Zantac 25 mg per mL _____

16. Order: Aldomet 0.5 g p.o. daily.

    Available:

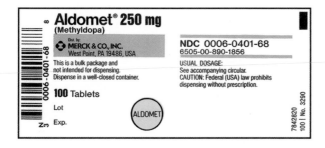

_____

17. Order: Digoxin 0.125 mg p.o. daily.

    Available: Scored tablets (can be broken in half)

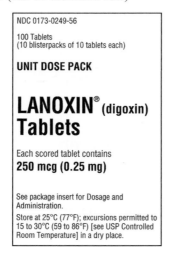

_____

18. Order: Dilantin 300 mg p.o. t.i.d.

    Available: Dilantin oral suspension labeled
    125 mg per 5 mL                                    _____

19. Order: Keflex 1 g p.o. q6h.

    Available: Keflex oral suspension labeled
    125 mg per 5 mL                                    _____

20. Order: Clindamycin 0.3 g IV q6h.

    Available:

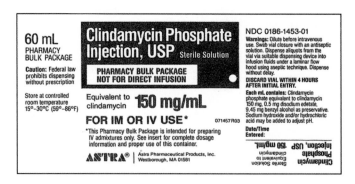

                                                        _____

Answers on p. 622

_____

✓ **CHAPTER REVIEW**

Calculate the following drug dosages using the dimensional analysis method. Use medication labels or information provided. Label answers correctly: tab, caps, mL. Answers expressed in milliliters should be expressed to the nearest tenth, except where indicated.

1. Order: Antivert 50 mg p.o. daily.

    Available:

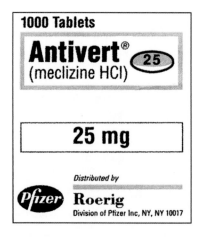

                                                        _____

2. Order: Potassium chloride 20 mEq in 1 L of D5W.

    Available: Potassium chloride
    30 mEq per 15 mL                    _____

3. Order: Morphine sulfate 20 mg IM stat.

    Available: Morphine sulfate 15 mg per mL    _____

4. Order: Kefzol 0.5 g IV q6h.

    Available: Kefzol labeled 225 mg per mL    _____

5. Order: Capoten 25 mg p.o. daily.

    Available:

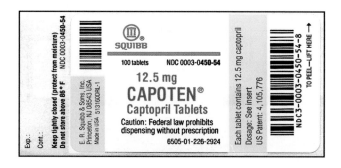

                                    _____

6. Order: Thiamine 80 mg IM stat.

    Available: Thiamine 100 mg per mL    _____

7. Order: Heparin 6,500 units subcut q12h.

    Available:
    (Express answer in hundredths.)

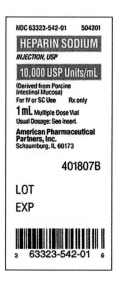

$$\frac{600 mg}{4 mL} \times \frac{300}{mg} \quad \frac{1200}{600} = 2$$

                                    _____

8. Order: Cleocin 300 mg IV q6h.

    Available: Cleocin 0.6 g per 4 mL    _____

9. Order: Trandate 300 mg p.o. b.i.d.

   Available: Trandate tablets labeled
   150 mg

   _____

10. Order: Solu-Medrol 175 mg IV daily.

    Available: Solu-Medrol labeled
    62.5 mg per mL

    _____

11. Order: Trental 0.4 g p.o. t.i.d.

    Available:

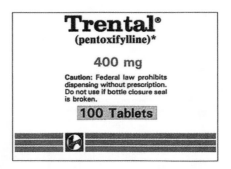

    _____

12. Order: Biaxin 0.5 g p.o. q12h for 7 days.

    Available:

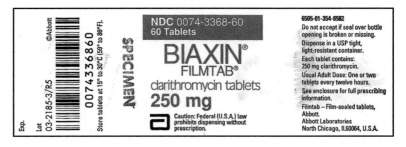

    _____

13. Order: Klonopin 0.5 mg p.o. b.i.d.

    Available:

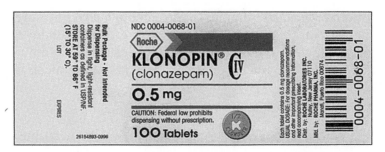

    _____

14. Order: Quinidine gluconate 200 mg IM q8h.

    Available:

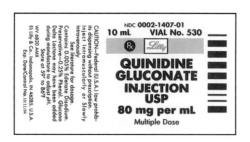

    _____

15. Order: Protamine sulfate 25 mg IV stat.

    Available:

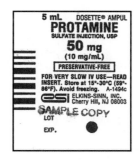

    _____

16. Order: Methotrexate 15 mg IM every week (on Monday).

    Available:

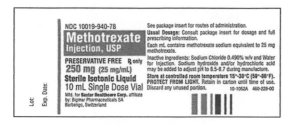

    _____

17. Order: Potassium chloride 15 mEq in 1,000 mL D5W.

    Available:

$\dfrac{2mEq}{1mL} \quad \dfrac{15mEq}{2}$

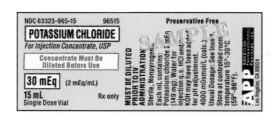

    _____

18.  Order: Benadryl 60 mg IM stat.

Available:

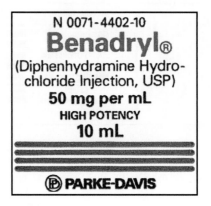

_____

19.  Order: Ceclor 0.4 g p.o. q8h.

Available: Ceclor labeled 375 mg per 5 mL    _____

20.  Order: Synthroid 0.075 mg po daily.

Available: Scored tablets (can be broken in half).

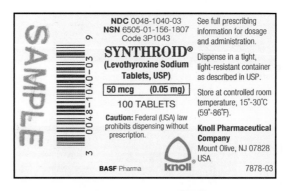

_____

For questions 21 through 35, set up the problem using dimensional analysis and make the conversion as indicated.

21.  3 qt =                                   _____ mL

22.  79 lb =                                  _____ kg
                                                (round to nearest tenth)

23.  5 mcg =                                  _____ mg

24.  2,400 mL =                               _____ L

25.  8 in =                                   _____ cm

26.  1.25 mcg =                               _____ mg

27. 240 mL = _____ oz

28. 1.75 mg = _____ mcg

29. 125 mL = _____ L

30. 8.5 L = _____ mL

31. 140$^1/_2$ lb = _____kg
    (round to nearest tenth)

32. 127.5 mL = _____ tbs

33. 25 oz = _____ mL

34. 36 cm = _____in

35. 50 mm = _____ cm

Answers on pp. 622-625

**For additional practice problems, refer to the Methods of Calculation Dosages section of Drug Calculating Companion, Version 4, on Evolve.**

# Oral and
# Parenteral Dosage
# Forms and Insulin

Oral medications are the easiest, most economical, and most frequently used medications, but sometimes parenteral (nongastrointestinal tract) dosage routes are necessary. Both oral and parenteral medications are available in liquid or powder form. Medications that are available in powdered form must be reconstituted and administered in liquid form. In addition to oral and parenteral dosage forms, this unit examines the varying types of insulin.

# CHAPTER
## 17
# Calculation of Oral Medications

## Objectives

*After reviewing this chapter, you should be able to:*
1. Identify the forms of oral medication
2. Identify the terms on the medication label to be used in calculation of dosages
3. Calculate dosages for oral and liquid medications using ratio and proportion, the formula method, or dimensional analysis
4. Apply principles learned concerning tablet and liquid preparations to obtain a rational answer

The easiest, most economical, and most commonly used method of medication administration is by mouth (p.o.). Medications for oral administration are available in solid forms such as tablets and capsules or as liquid preparations. To calculate dosages appropriately the nurse needs to understand the principles that apply to administration of medications by this route.

## FORMS OF SOLID MEDICATIONS

### Tablets

Tablets are preparations of powdered medications that have been molded into various sizes and shapes. Tablets come in a variety of dosages that can be expressed in metric or apothecary units—for example, milligrams and grains. There are different types of tablets and shapes (Figure 17-1, *A*).

*CAPLETS*   A caplet is a tablet that has an elongated shape like a capsule and is coated for ease of swallowing. Tylenol is available in caplet form.

*SCORED TABLETS*   Scored tablets are designed to administer a dosage that is less than what is available in a single tablet. In other words, scored tablets have indentations or markings that allow you to break the tablet into halves or quarters. Only scored tablets should be broken because there is no way to determine the dosage being administered when a nonscored tablet is broken. Breaking a tablet that is not scored could lead to the administration of an inaccurate dosage if the tablet is not divided equally. The purpose of the groove or indentation is to provide a guide for breaking a whole tablet into a fractional part (Figure 17-1, *B*). Figure 17-2 shows an example of a scored tablet.

**254**

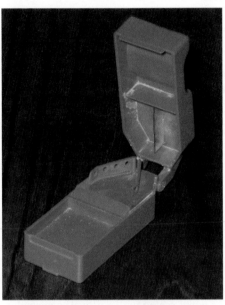

**Figure 17-1**  **A,** Various shapes of tablets. **B,** Tablets scored in halves and fourths. (From Kee JL, Marshall SM: *Clinical calculations: with applications to general and specialty areas,* ed. 6, St. Louis, 2009, Saunders.)

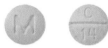

**Figure 17-2**  Clonazepam tablet scored. (From *Mosby's drug consult 2007,* St. Louis, 2007, Mosby.)

**Figure 17-3**  Pill/tablet cutter. (From Kee JL, Marshall SM: *Clinical calculations: with applications to general and specialty areas,* ed. 6, St. Louis, 2009, Saunders.)

**CAUTION**

Breaking an unscored tablet is risky and dangerous and can lead to the administration of an unintended dosage.

A pill or tablet cutter is readily available in most pharmacies that can be used to evenly cut tablets appropriately. Figure 17-3 shows a pill/tablet cutter. An appropriate medication reference should always be consulted before cutting a tablet. Many tablets come in a form that allows slow and steady release of the active drug. These forms cannot be cut, crushed, or chewed. Capsules and enteric-coated, timed-release, sustained-release, and controlled-release tablets cannot be cut. Nurses must use caution when instructing clients to cut tablets.

## Tips for Clinical Practice

If a tablet is not scored, it should not be divided. If the calculation of a medication dosage requires that a tablet be cut in half, divide the tablet along the scoring created by the manufacturer. If possible use a pill or tablet cutter to divide a tablet in half to help ensure acccuracy of a dose.

**Figure 17-4**   Layered tablet. (From Clayton BD, Stock YN, Harroun RD: *Basic pharmacology for nurses,* ed. 14, St. Louis, 2007, Mosby.)

*ENTERIC-COATED TABLETS*   Enteric-coated tablets have a special coating that protects them from the effects of gastric secretions and prevents them from dissolving in the stomach. They are dissolved and absorbed in the intestines.

The enteric coating also prevents the medication from becoming a source of irritation to the gastric mucosa, thereby preventing gastrointestinal upset. Examples include enteric-coated aspirin and iron tablets, such as ferrous gluconate. **Enteric-coated tablets should never be crushed, because crushing them destroys the special coating and defeats its purpose.** Always consult an appropriate medication reference or the pharmacist when in doubt about the safety of crushing a tablet or opening a capsule.

*SUBLINGUAL TABLETS*   Sublingual tablets are designed to be placed under the tongue, where they dissolve in saliva and the medication is absorbed. Sublingual tablets should never be swallowed because this will prevent them from achieving their desired effect. Nitroglycerin, which is used for the relief of acute chest pain, is usually administered sublingually.

*LAYERED TABLETS*   Some tablets contain different layers or have cores that separate different medications that may be incompatible with one another; thus incompatible ingredients may be separated and released at different times as the tablet passes through the gastrointestinal tract (Figure 17-4).

Medications in a layered form have become available in which one or more medications can be released immediately from the coating, whereas the same or other medications can be released on a sustained basis from the tablet core. An example of this is Ambien CR. Ambien CR is formulated in a two-layer tablet. The first layer of the tablet dissolves quickly to help in falling asleep, and the second layer dissolves slowly over the night to help the person stay asleep.

*FILM TAB*   A film tab is a tablet sealed with a film. The special coating helps to protect the stomach. Some medications that come as film tabs include Biaxin (clarithromycin) and E.E.S. 400 (erythromycin).

*TIMED-RELEASE AND EXTENDED-RELEASE TABLETS*   Look for abbreviations such as SA, LA, or XL. Medication from these types of tablets is not released immediately but released over a period of time at specific intervals. These types of preparations should not be crushed, chewed, or broken. These types of preparations should be swallowed whole. If a timed-release or extended-release tablet is crushed, chewed, or broken, all of the medication will be administered at one time and absorbed rapidly. Examples include Procardia, Calan, and theophylline.

**CAUTION**

Not all medications can be crushed. Medications such as timed-release or extended-release tablets and capsules have special coatings to prevent the medicaion from being absorbed too quickly. Always refer to a medication manual or some other reference book before crushing a medication to ensure that a medication can be safely crushed to avoid harm to the client.

## Capsules

A capsule is a form of medication that contains a powder, liquid, or oil enclosed in a hard or soft gelatin. Capsules come in a variety of colors, sizes, and dosages. Some capsules have special shapes and colorings to identify which company produced them. Capsules are also available as timed release, sustained release, and spansules and work over a period of time.

Capsules should always be administered whole to achieve the desired result (e.g., sustained release). Sustained-release and timed-release capsules cannot be divided or crushed (Figure 17-5). Always consult an appropriate reference or pharmacist when in doubt as to whether to open a capsule.

Examples of medications that come in capsule form are ampicillin, tetracycline, Colace, and Lanoxicaps. Lanoxicaps are an example of a capsule that has liquid medication contained in a gelatin capsule (Figure 17-6, *A*). On some labels, in addition to capsules, may be seen the term *kapseals* (e.g., kapseals is seen on a label for Dilantin extended capsules).

Although there are other forms of solid preparations for oral administration—such as lozenges and troches—tablets, capsules, and pulvules (proprietary capsules containing a dosage of a medication in powdered form) are the most common forms of solids requiring calculation encountered by the nurse. Figure 17-6 shows forms of solid oral medications, including capsules. Figures 17-6 through 17-8 show various types of capsules and an enteric-coated tablet.

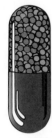

**Figure 17-5**   Timed-release capsule. (From Clayton BD, Stock YN, Harroun RD: *Basic pharmacology for nurses,* ed. 14, St. Louis, 2007, Mosby.)

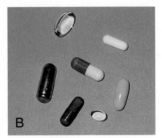

**Figure 17-6**   Various types of capsules. **A,** Lanoxicap. **B,** Different types of capsules. (**A** from *Mosby's drug consult 2003,* St. Louis, 2003, Mosby. **B** courtesy Amanda Politte, St. Louis.)

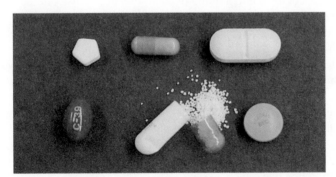

**Figure 17-7**   Forms of solid oral medications. *Top row,* Uniquely shaped tablet, capsule, scored tablet; *bottom row,* gelatin-coated liquid capsule, extended-release capsule, enteric-coated tablet. (From Potter PA, Perry AG: *Fundamentals of nursing,* ed. 7, St. Louis, 2009, Mosby.)

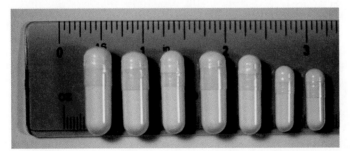

**Figure 17-8**   Various sizes of gelatin capsules. (Courtesy Oscar H Allison. From Clayton BD, Stock YN, Harroun RD: *Basic pharmacology for nurses,* ed. 14, St. Louis, 2007, Mosby.)

## CALCULATING DOSAGES INVOLVING TABLETS AND CAPSULES

When administering medications, you will have to calculate the number of tablets or capsules needed to administer the dosage ordered. To help determine if your calculated dosage is sensible, accurate, and safe, remember the following points:

### ■ Points to Remember

- Converting medication measures from one system to another and one unit to another to determine the dosage to be administered can result in discrepancies, depending on the conversion factor used.
- Example: Aspirin may indicate on the label 5 grains (325 mg). This is based on the equivalent 65 mg = gr 1. On the other hand, another label on aspirin may indicate 5 grains (300 mg). Here the equivalent 60 mg = gr 1 was used. Both of the equivalents are correct. **Remember, equivalents are not exact.** Use the common equivalents when making conversions—for example, 60 mg = gr 1.
- When the precise number of tablets or capsules is determined and you find that administering the amount calculated is unrealistic or impossible, always use the following rule to avoid an error in administration: *No more than 10% variation should exist between the dosage ordered and the dosage administered.* For example, you may determine that a client should receive 0.9 tablet or 0.9 capsule. Administration of such an amount accurately would be impossible. Following the stated rule, if you determined that 0.9 tablet or 0.9 capsule should be given, you could safely administer 1 tab or 1 cap. This variation should only occur when conversions are made between apothecary and metric measurements because approximate equivalents are used.
- Capsules are not scored and cannot be divided. They are administered in whole amounts only. If a client has difficulty swallowing a capsule, check to see if a liquid preparation of the same drug is available. Never crush or open a timed-release capsule or empty its contents into a liquid or food; this may cause release of all the medication at once. There are, however, some instances in which a soft gelatin capsule filled with liquid may be pierced with a small sterile needle and the medication squeezed out for sublingual use. For example, Procardia (nifedipine) has been used in this way for severe hypertension. This drug is not approved by the Food and Drug Administration (FDA) for use in this manner. When used in this manner, the action of the medication is erratic and short term. When administered in this manner, it can cause a hypotensive effect that is not easy to control. Precipitous drops in blood pressure can spell disaster for some clients. Over the years there have been reports of stroke and other complications resulting from lowering the blood pressure too much. It is important to note that administration of this medicine in this manner is not a common practice.
- Pulvules are proprietary capsules containing a dosage of a medication in powder form. For example, the popular antidepressant Prozac comes in pulvule form (proprietary capsules owned by a corporation under a trademark or patent).
- Tablets and capsules may be available in different strengths for administration, and you may have a choice when giving a dosage. For example, 75 mg of a medication may be ordered. When you check what is available, it may be in tablet or capsule form as 10, 25, or 50 mg. In deciding the best combination of tablets or capsules to give, the nurse should always choose the strength that would allow the least number of tablets or capsules to be administered without breaking a tablet, if possible, because breaking is found to result in variations in dosage. In the example given, the best combination for administering 75 mg is one 50 mg tablet or capsule and one 25 mg tablet or capsule.
- Only scored tablets are intended to be divided. It is safest and most accurate not to divide tablets, and give the fewest number of whole, undivided tablets possible.

- The maximum number of tablets or capsules given to a client to achieve a single dosage is usually three. Recheck your calculation if a single dose requires more. It is important to note that although the maximum number of tablets or capsules given to a client to administer a single dosage is usually three, for some medications the client may have to take more than three to achieve the desired dosage. This is true with some of the solid forms of HIV medications (e.g., tablets, capsules). Examples: Viracept 1,250 mg p.o. b.i.d. (available 250 mg per tab), ritonavir 400 mg p.o. q12h (available 100 mg per tab). Although many HIV medications come in liquid form, many clients prefer to take tablets or capsules. ***Remember:*** Except for special medications, any more than three capsules or tablets to achieve a single dosage is unusual and may indicate an error in interpretation of the order, transcription, or calculation. Think! Always question any order that exceeds this amount.
- When using ratio and proportion, the formula method, or dimensional analysis to calculate tablet and capsule problems, remember that each tablet or capsule contains a certain weight of the medication. The weight indicated on a label is per tablet or per capsule. This is particularly important when you are reading a medication label on a bottle or single unit-dose package.
- In calculating oral dosages you may encounter measures other than apothecary or metric measures. For example, electrolytes such as potassium will indicate the number of milliequivalents (mEq) per tablet. Units is another measure you may see for oral antibiotics or vitamins. For example, a vitamin E capsule will indicate 400 units per capsule. Measurements of units and milliequivalents are specific to the drug they are being used for. There is no conversion between these and apothecary or metric measures. (These are discussed in Chapter 18.)
- Always consult a medication reference or pharmacist when in doubt as to whether a capsule may be opened or pierced or whether a tablet can be crushed.

Remembering the points mentioned will be helpful before starting to calculate dosages. Any of the methods presented in Chapters 14, 15, and 16 can be used to determine the dosage to be administered.

To compute dosages accurately it is necessary to review a few reminders that were presented in previous chapters.

## Reminders

1. Read the problem carefully and
   a. Identify known factors
   b. Identify unknown factors
   c. Eliminate unnecessary information that is not relevant
2. Make sure that what is ordered and what is available are in the same system of measurement and units, or a conversion will be necessary. When a conversion is necessary, it is usual to convert what is ordered into what you have available or what is indicated on the medication label. You can, however, convert the measure in which the medication is available into the same units and system of measure as the dosage ordered. The choice is usually based on whichever is easier to calculate. Use any of the methods presented in Chapters 8 and 16 to make conversions consistent to avoid confusion. If necessary, go back and review these methods.
3. Consider what would be a reasonable answer based on what is ordered.
4. Set up the problem using ratio and proportion, the formula method, or dimensional analysis. Label each component in the setup, including *x*.
5. Label the final answer (tablet, capsule).
6. For administration purposes, for oral dosages that are given in fractional dosages (e.g., scored tablets), state answers to problems in fractions. Example: $\frac{1}{2}$ tab or $1\frac{1}{2}$ tabs, instead of 0.5 tabs or 1.5 tabs.

CAUTION

Question a dosage that seems unreasonable or requires administering a medication by a route other than what the form indicates. Regardless of the source of error, if you administer the wrong dosage or give a medication by a route other than that which is intended, you have committed a medication error and are legally responsible for the error.

Here are at some sample problems calculating the number of tablets or capsules to administer.

**Example 1:**  Order: Digoxin 0.375 mg p.o. daily

Available: Digoxin (scored tablets) labeled 0.25 mg

 Problem Setup

1. No conversion is necessary; the units are in the same system of measure.
   Order: 0.375 mg
   Available: 0.25 mg
2. Think critically: Tablets are scored; 0.375 mg is larger than 0.25 mg; therefore you will need more than 1 tab to administer the correct dosage.
3. Solve using ratio and proportion, the formula method, or dimensional analysis.

 Solution Using Ratio and Proportion

$$0.25 \text{ mg} : 1 \text{ tab} = 0.375 \text{ mg} : x \text{ tab}$$

(known)                 (unknown)

(what is available)    (what is ordered)

$$\frac{0.25x}{0.25} = \frac{0.375}{0.25}$$

$$x = \frac{0.375}{0.25}$$

Therefore $x = 1.5$ tabs or $1\frac{1}{2}$ tabs. (It is best to state it as $1\frac{1}{2}$ tabs for administration purposes.)

**NOTE**

You can administer $1\frac{1}{2}$ tabs because the tablets are scored. The ratio and proportion method could have been written in fraction format as well. (If necessary, review Chapter 4 on ratio and proportion.)

 Solution Using the Formula Method

$$\frac{(D) \ 0.375 \text{ mg}}{(H) \ 0.25 \text{ mg}} \times (Q) \ 1 \text{ tab} = x \text{ tab}$$

$$x = \frac{0.375}{0.25}$$

$$x = 1\frac{1}{2} \text{ tabs}$$

 Solution Using Dimensional Analysis

$$x \text{ tab} = \frac{1 \text{ tab}}{0.25 \text{ mg}} \times \frac{0.375 \text{ mg}}{1}$$

$$x = \frac{0.375}{0.25}$$

$$x = 1\frac{1}{2} \text{ tabs}$$

**Example 2:**   Order: Ampicillin 0.5 g p.o. q6h

Available: Ampicillin capsules labeled 250 mg per capsule

1. Order: 0.5 g
   Available: 250 mg capsules
2. After making the necessary conversion, think about what is a reasonable amount to administer.
3. Calculate the dosage to be administered using ratio and proportion, the formula method, or dimensional analysis.
4. Label your final answer (tablets, capsules).

 Problem Setup

1. Convert grams to milligrams. Equivalent: 1,000 mg = 1 g

$$1{,}000 \text{ mg}:1 \text{ g} = x \text{ mg}:0.5 \text{ g}$$

$$x = 1{,}000 \times 0.5$$

$$x = 500 \text{ mg}$$

Therefore 0.5 g is equal to 500 mg. Converting the grams to milligrams eliminated a decimal, which is often the source of calculation errors. Converting milligrams to grams would necessitate a decimal. Whenever possible, conversions that result in a decimal should be avoided to decrease the chance of error in calculating. Remember, a ratio and proportion could also be stated as a fraction. If necessary, review Chapter 4 on ratio and proportion. Because the measures are metric in this problem (grams, milligrams), the other method that can be used is to move the decimal the desired number of places (0.5 g = 0.500 = 500 mg).

2. After making the conversion, you are now ready to calculate the dosage to be given, using ratio and proportion, the formula method, or dimensional analysis. In this problem we will use the answer obtained from converting what was ordered to what is available (0.5 g = 500 mg). Remember that if dimensional analysis is used, you need only one equation; even if conversion is required, you can choose to do conversion first and then set the problem up in dimensional analysis.

 Solution Using Ratio and Proportion

$$250 \text{ mg}:1 \text{ cap} = 500 \text{ mg}:x \text{ cap}$$

$$\frac{250x}{250} = \frac{500}{250}$$

$$x = \frac{500}{250}$$

$$x = 2 \text{ caps}$$

 Solution Using the Formula Method

$$\frac{\text{(D) } 500 \text{ mg}}{\text{(H) } 250 \text{ mg}} \times \text{(Q) } 1 \text{ cap} = x \text{ cap}$$

$$x = \frac{500}{250}$$

$$x = 2 \text{ cap}$$

**NOTE**

A conversion is necessary. The ordered dosage and the available dosage are in the same system of measurement (metric), but the units are different (g and mg). Before calculating the dosage to be administered, you must have the ordered dosage and the available dosage in the same units.

**NOTE**

Two caps is a logical answer. Capsules are administered in whole amounts; they are not divisible. Using the value obtained from converting milligrams to grams in this problem would also net a final answer of 2 caps.

Solution Using Dimensional Analysis

$$x \text{ caps} = \frac{1 \text{ cap}}{250 \text{ mg}} \times \frac{1{,}000 \text{ mg}}{1 \text{ g}} \times \frac{0.5 \text{ g}}{1}$$

$$x = \frac{1{,}000 \times 0.5}{250}$$

$$x = \frac{500}{250}$$

$$x = 2 \text{ caps}$$

Set up if conversion done first, then set up in dimensional analysis to calculate dosage:

$$x \text{ mg} = \frac{1{,}000 \text{ mg}}{1 \text{ g}} \times 0.5 \text{ g}$$

$$x = \frac{1{,}000 \times 0.5}{1}$$

$$x = \frac{500}{1}$$

$$x = 500 \text{ mg}$$

Set up in dimensional analysis after conversion made:

$$x \text{ caps} = \frac{1 \text{ cap}}{250 \text{ mg}} \times \frac{500 \text{ mg}}{1}$$

$$x = \frac{500}{250}$$

$$x = 2 \text{ caps}$$

*Note:* It is easier to set up the problem by using one equation that will allow you to convert and calculate the dosage required.

**Example 3:**    Order: Nitroglycerin gr $^{1}/_{150}$ sublingual p.r.n. for chest pain

Available: Sublingual nitroglycerin tablets labeled 0.4 mg

 Problem Setup

1.  Conversion is required.
    Order: gr $^{1}/_{150}$
    Available: 0.4 mg
    Equivalent: 60 mg = gr 1
    Convert what is ordered to the same system and units as what is available (gr is apothecary, mg is metric).

$$60 \text{ mg} : \text{gr } 1 = x \text{ mg} : \text{gr } \frac{1}{150}$$

$$x = 60 \times \frac{1}{150}$$

$$x = \frac{60}{150}$$

$$x = 0.4 \text{ mg}$$

2.  Think critically—it is obvious after making the conversion that you will give 1 tab.
3.  Solve to obtain the desired dosage.

Solution Using Ratio and Proportion

$$0.4 \text{ mg} : 1 \text{ tab} = 0.4 \text{ mg} : x \text{ tab}$$

$$\frac{0.4x}{0.4} = \frac{0.4}{0.4}$$

$$x = \frac{0.4}{0.4}$$

$$x = 1 \text{ tab}$$

 Solution Using the Formula Method

$$\frac{(D)\ 0.4 \text{ mg}}{(H)\ 0.4 \text{ mg}} \times Q\ (1 \text{ tab}) = x \text{ tab}$$

$$x = \frac{0.4}{0.4}$$

$$x = 1 \text{ tab}$$

 Solution Using Dimensional Analysis

$$x \text{ tab} = \frac{1 \text{ tab}}{0.4 \text{ mg}} \times \frac{60 \text{ mg}}{\text{gr } 1} \times \frac{\text{gr } \frac{1}{150}}{1}$$

$$x = \frac{60 \times \frac{1}{150}}{0.4 \text{ mg}}$$

$$x = \frac{\frac{60}{150}}{0.4}$$

$$x = \frac{60}{150} \times \frac{1}{0.4} = \frac{60}{60}$$

$$x = \frac{60}{60}$$

$$x = 1 \text{ tab}$$

**Example 4:**   Order: Nembutal gr $1\frac{1}{2}$ p.o. at bedtime p.r.n.

Available: Nembutal capsules labeled 100 mg; what should the nurse administer?

 Problem Setup

1. Convert gr $1\frac{1}{2}$ to mg. Equivalent: 60 mg = gr 1

$$60 \text{ mg} : \text{gr } 1 = x \text{ mg} : \text{gr } 1\frac{1}{2}$$

$$60 \text{ mg} : \text{gr } 1 = x \text{ mg} : \text{gr } \frac{3}{2}$$

$$x = 60 \times \frac{3}{2} = \frac{180}{2}$$

$$x = 90 \text{ mg}$$

2. Solve for the dosage to be administered.

 ## Solution Using Ratio and Proportion

$$100 \text{ mg} : 1 \text{ cap} = 90 \text{ mg} : x \text{ capsule}$$

$$\frac{100x}{100} = \frac{90}{100}$$

$$x = \frac{90}{100}$$

$$x = 0.9 \text{ cap}$$

Administer 1 capsule.

## Solution Using the Formula Method

$$\frac{(D) \ 90 \text{ mg}}{(H) \ 100 \text{ mg}} \times Q \ (1 \text{ cap}) = x \text{ cap}$$

$$\frac{90}{100} \times 1 = x$$

$$x = 0.9 \text{ cap}$$

Administer 1 capsule.

## Solution Using Dimensional Analysis

$$x \text{ cap} = \frac{1 \text{ cap}}{100 \text{ mg}} \times \frac{60 \text{ mg}}{\text{gr } 1} \times \frac{\text{gr } 1\frac{1}{2}}{1}$$

$$x = \frac{60 \times 1\frac{1}{2}}{100} = \frac{60 \times \frac{3}{2}}{100} = \frac{90}{100}$$

$$x = \frac{90}{100}$$

$$x = 0.9 \text{ cap}$$

Administer 1 capsule.

 ## Critical Thinking

Capsules are not dividable, 90 mg is closest to 100 mg. It is safe to administer 1 cap; 1 cap falls within the 10% variation allowed between the dosage ordered and the dosage administered.

**Example 5:**   Order: Thorazine 100 mg p.o. t.i.d.

Available: Thorazine tablets labeled 25 mg and 50 mg

 Problem Setup

1. No conversion is necessary.
2. Thinking critically: 100 mg is larger than 25 or 50 mg. Therefore more than 1 tab is needed to administer the dosage. The client should always be given the strength of tablets or capsules that would require the least number to be taken.
3. In this problem, selection of the 50-mg tablets would require the client to receive 2 tabs, whereas using 25 mg tablets would require 4 tabs to be administered.

 Solution Using Ratio and Proportion

$$50 \text{ mg} : 1 \text{ tab} = 100 \text{ mg} : x \text{ tab}$$

$$\frac{50x}{50} = \frac{100}{50}$$

$$x = 2 \text{ tabs (50 mg each)}$$

> **NOTE**
>
> In Example 5, not only is the number of tablets specified, but also the strength of tablets chosen is specified.

 Solution Using the Formula Method

$$\frac{(D)\ 100 \text{ mg}}{(H)\ 50 \text{ mg}} \times Q\ (1 \text{ tab}) = x \text{ tab}$$

$$x = \frac{100}{50}$$

$$x = 2 \text{ tabs (50 mg each)}$$

 Solution Using Dimensional Analysis

$$x \text{ tab} = \frac{1 \text{ tab}}{50 \text{ mg}} \times \frac{100 \text{ mg}}{1}$$

$$x = \frac{100}{50}$$

$$x = 2 \text{ tabs (50 mg each)}$$

## Variation of Tablet and Capsule Problems

You will at times find it necessary to decide how many tablets or capsules are needed. This requires knowing the dosage and frequency. Numerous scenarios could arise, but for the purpose of illustration, we will use one: A client is going out of town on vacation and needs to know whether it is necessary to refill the prescription before leaving.

**Example 1:**   A client has an order for Valium 10 mg p.o. q.i.d. and has 5 mg tablets. The client is leaving town for 7 days and asks how many tablets to bring.

**Solution:**   To obtain a dosage of 10 mg, the client requires two 5-mg tablets each time. Therefore eight 5-mg tablets are necessary to administer the dosage q.i.d. (four times a day).
Number of tablets needed per day (8) ×
Number of days needed for (7)
= Total number of tablets needed

$$8 \times 7 = 56$$

**Answer:**   The total number of tablets needed for 7 days would be 56 tablets.

### Determining the Dosage to Be Given Each Time

**Example 2:**   A client is to receive 1 gram of a drug p.o. daily. The drug should be given in four equally divided doses.

How many milligrams should the client receive each time the medication is administered?

**Solution:**   $\dfrac{\text{Total daily allowance}}{\text{Number of doses per day}} = \text{Dosage to be administered}$

**Answer:**   $\dfrac{1 \text{ g } (1,000 \text{ mg})}{4} = 250$ mg each time the medication is administered.

## ■ Points to Remember

- The maximum number of tablets and capsules to administer to achieve a single desired dosage is usually three. Question any order for more than this before administering.
- Before calculating a dosage, make sure that the dosage ordered and what is available are in the same system and units of measurement. When a conversion is required, it is usually best to convert the dosage ordered to what is available.
- No more than a 10% variation should exist between the dosage ordered and the dosage administered for adults. Remember this should only occur when you are converting between apothecary and metric systems because of using approximate equivalents.
- Regardless of the method used to calculate a dosage, it is important to develop the ability to think critically about what is a reasonable amount. Think and question any dosage that seems unreasonable.
- State dosages as you are actually going to administer them. Example: 0.5 tab = ½ tab.

## Practice Problems

Calculate the correct number of tablets or capsules to be administered in the following problems using the labels or information provided. Use any of the methods presented to calculate the dosage. Remember to label your answers correctly: tabs, caps.

1. Order: Synthroid 0.025 mg p.o. every day.

   Available: Scored tablets.

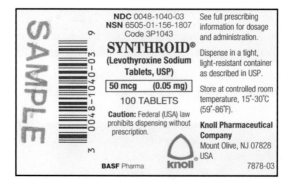

2. Order: Strattera 50 mg p.o. daily.

   Available:

   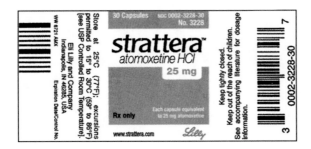

   _____

3. Order: Relafen 1 g p.o. daily.

   Available:

   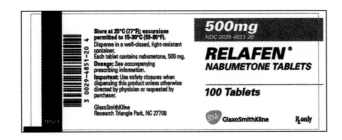

   _____

4. Order: Coumadin 7.5 mg p.o. at bedtime.

   Available: Scored tablets.

   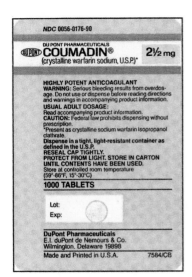 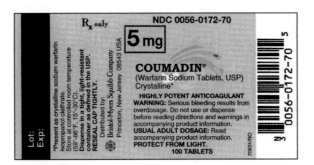

   What is the appropriate strength tablet to use? _____

5. Order: Lanoxin 0.125 mg p.o. daily.

   Available: Scored tablets.

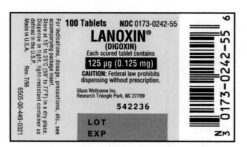 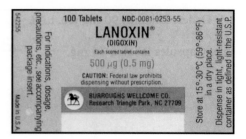

   a. What is the appropriate strength tablet to use?    _____

   b. What will you administer?    _____

6. Order: Ampicillin 1 g p.o. q6h.

   Available: Ampicillin capsules labeled 500 mg and 250 mg

   a. Which strength capsule is appropriate
      to use?    _____

   b. How many capsules are needed for one
      dosage?    _____

   c. What is the total number of capsules needed
      if the medication is ordered for 7 days?    _____

7. Order: Reglan 10 mg p.o. t.i.d. ½ hr a.c.

   Available: Reglan tablets labeled 5 mg    _____

8. Order: Baclofen 15 mg p.o. t.i.d. for 3 days.

   Available: Scored tablets.

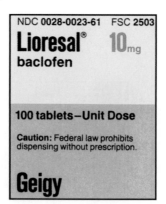

   a. How many tablets are needed for one
      dosage?    _____

   b. What is the total number of milligrams
      the client will receive in 3 days?    _____

9. Order: Synthroid 0.075 mg p.o. every day.

   Available: Synthroid scored tablets
   labeled 50 mcg                                    _____

10. Order: Calcium carbonate 1.3 g p.o. daily.

    Available: Calcium carbonate tablets
    labeled 650 mg                                   _____

11. Order: Dilantin 90 mg p.o. t.i.d.

    Available: Dilantin capsules labeled 30 mg       _____

12. Order: Tegretol 200 mg p.o. t.i.d.

    Available:

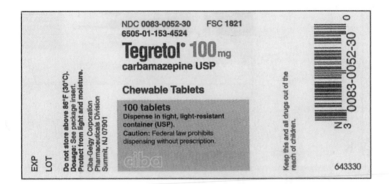

    How many tablets will you administer for
    each dosage?                                     _____

13. Order: Dicloxacillin 1 g p.o. as an initial dose and 0.5 g p.o. q6h thereafter.

    Available:

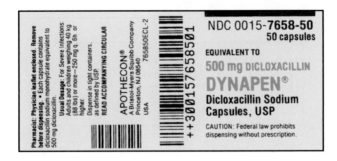

    a. How many capsules will you need for the
       initial dosage?                               _____

    b. How many capsules are needed for each
       subsequent dosage?                            _____

14. Order: Aldomet 250 mg p.o. b.i.d.

   Available:

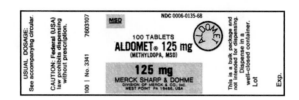

   How many tablets will you administer for
   each dosage?                                              _____

15. Order: Phenobarbital gr $1\frac{1}{2}$ p.o. at bedtime.

   Available: Phenobarbital 15 mg tabs and
   30 mg tabs.

   a. Which strength tablet is best to administer?           _____

   b. How many tablets of which strength will
      you prepare to administer?                             _____

16. Order: Decadron 3 mg p.o. b.i.d. for 2 days.

   Available:

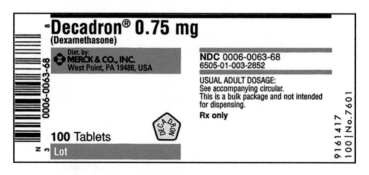

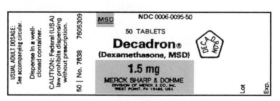

   a. Which is the best strength to administer?              _____

   b. How many tablets of which strength will
      you administer?                                        _____

17. Order: Thorazine 100 mg p.o. t.i.d.

    Available:

    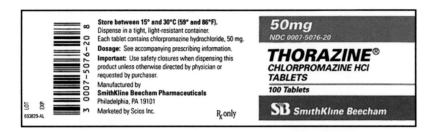

    How many tablets are needed for 3 days?      _____

18. Order: Verapamil 120 mg p.o. t.i.d. Hold for systolic blood pressure less than 100, heart rate less than 55.

    Available: Verapamil scored tablets labeled 80 mg and 40 mg

    How many tablets of which strength will
    you administer?      _____

19. Order: OxyContin (controlled-release) 20 mg p.o. q12h for pain management.

    Available:

    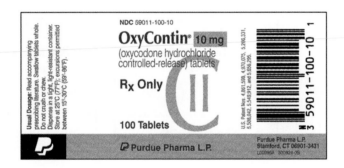

    _____

20. Order: Cogentin 1 mg p.o. t.i.d.

    Available:

    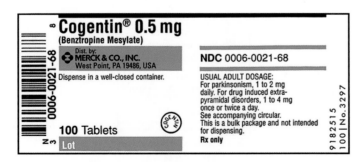

    _____

21. Order: Prazosin hydrochloride 3 mg p.o. b.i.d.

    Available: Prazosin hydrochloride capsules
    labeled 1 mg    _____

22. Order: Zyvox 0.6 g p.o. q12h for 10 days.

    Available:

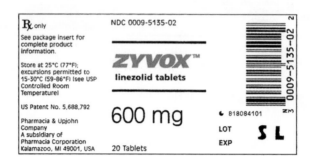

_____

23. Order: Dexamethasone 6 mg p.o. daily.

    Available: Scored tablets.

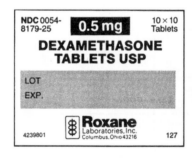 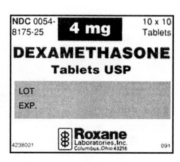 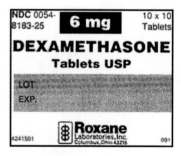

    How many tablets of which strength will
    you administer?    _____

24. Order: Pyridium 0.2 g p.o. q8h.

    Available:

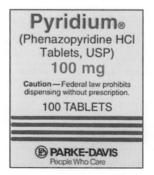

_____

25. Order: Torsemide 20 mg p.o. daily.

    Available:

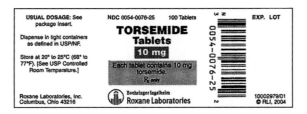

    _____

26. Order: Glyset 100 mg p.o. t.i.d. at the start of each meal.

    Available:

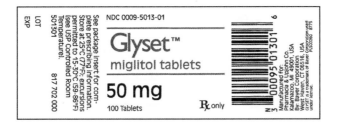

    _____

27. Order: Cimetidine (Tagamet) 400 mg p.o. b.i.d.

    Available:

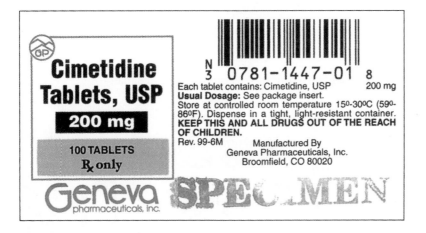

    How many tablets will you administer for
    each dosage?                                    _____

28. Order: Indocin SR 150 mg p.o. b.i.d.

    Available:

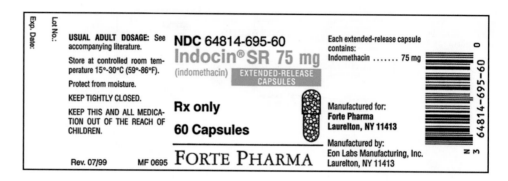

    How many capsules will you administer for
    each dosage?
    _____

29. Order: Sulfasalazine 1 g p.o. q6h.

    Available:

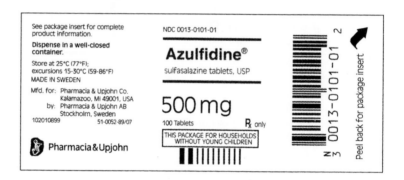

    How many tablets will you administer for
    each dosage?
    _____

30. Order: Cymbalta (delayed-release capsules) 60 mg p.o. daily.

    Available:

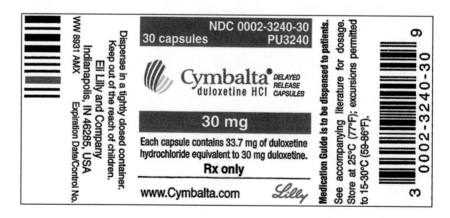

    How many capsules will you administer for
    each dosage?
    _____

31. Order: Synthroid 100 mcg p.o. daily.

    Available: Synthroid tablets labeled 75 mcg and 25 mcg

    How many tablets of which strength will you use to administer the dosage? _____

32. Order: Capoten 25 mg p.o. q8h.

    Available:

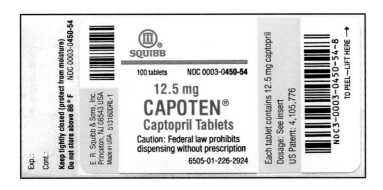

_____

33. Order: Clonazepam 0.25 mg p.o. b.i.d. and at bedtime.

    Available: Scored tablets.

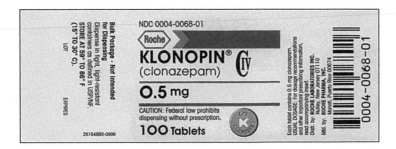

_____

34. Order: Augmentin 0.25 g p.o. q8h.

    Available:

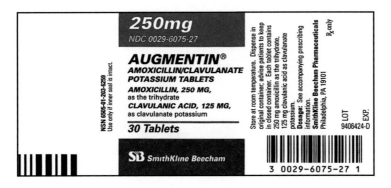

_____

35. Order: Synthroid 25 mcg p.o. every day.

    Available:

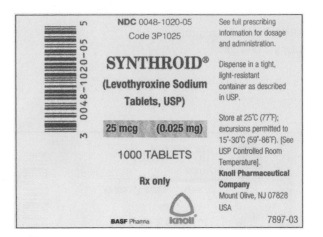

    _____

36. Order: Aspirin 650 mg p.o. q4h p.r.n. for pain.

    Available: Aspirin tablets labeled 325 mg     _____

37. Order: Dilantin (extended capsules) 0.2 g p.o. t.i.d.

    Available:

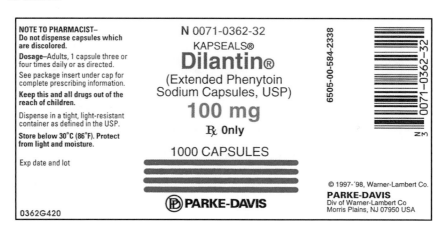

    _____

38. Order: Motrin 800 mg p.o. q6h p.r.n. for pain.

    Available:

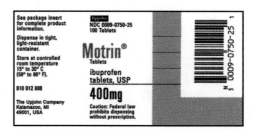

    _____

39. Order: Procardia XL 60 mg p.o. daily.

    Available: Procardia XL labeled 30 mg per tablet.   _____

40. Order: Minoxidil 0.03 g daily.

    Available:

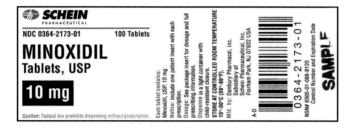

    _____

41. Order: Inderal LA 160 mg p.o. every day.

    Available: Inderal LA capsules labeled 80 mg  _____

Answers on pp. 625-629

## CALCULATING ORAL LIQUIDS

Medications are also available in liquid form for oral administration. Liquid medications are desirable to use for clients who have dysphagia (difficulty swallowing) or who are receiving medications through various types of tubes such as nasogastric (tube in nose to stomach), gastrostomy (tube placed directly into stomach), or jejunostomy (tube directly into intestines). Liquid medications are also desired for use in young children, infants, and elderly clients. When medications are ordered that cannot be crushed for administration, the availability of the medication in liquid form should be investigated. Medications in liquid form contain a specific amount or weight of a medication in a given amount of solution, which is indicated on the label. Liquid medications are prepared in different forms, as follows:

1. *Elixir*—Alcohol solution that is sweet and aromatic.
   Example: Phenobarbital elixir.
2. *Suspension*—One or more medications finely divided into a liquid such as water.
   Example: Penicillin suspension.
3. *Syrup*—Medication dissolved in concentrated solution of sugar and water.
   Example: Colace.

Liquid medications also come as tincture, emulsions, and extract preparations for oral use. Although oral liquids may be administered by means other than by mouth (e.g., nasogastric tube, gastrostomy), they should **never** be given by any other route, such as the intravenous (IV) route or by injection.

In solving problems that involve oral liquids, the methods presented in Chapters 14 to 16 can be used; you must calculate the volume or amount of liquid that contains the dosage of the medication. This information is usually indicated on the medication label and can be expressed per milliliter, ounce, etc.—for example, 25 mg per mL. The amount may also be expressed in terms of multiple milliliters. Examples: 80 mg per 2 mL, 125 mg per 5 mL.

When calculating liquid medications, the stock or what you have available is in liquid form; therefore the label on your answer will always be expressed in liquid measures, such as milliliters.

## MEASURING ORAL LIQUIDS

Liquid medications can be measured in several ways:

1. The standard measuring cup (plastic), which is calibrated in metric, apothecary, and household measures, can be used. When measuring liquid medications, pour them at eye level and read at the meniscus (a curvature made by the solution) while the cup is on a flat surface (Figure 17-9). Always pour liquid medications with the label facing you to avoid covering the label with your hand or obscuring label information if the medication drips down the side of the container.

2. Calibrated droppers are also used for measuring liquid medications (Figure 17-10).

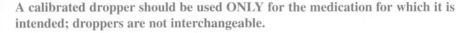

### Tips for Clinical Practice

A calibrated dropper should be used ONLY for the medication for which it is intended; droppers are not interchangeable.

If a dropper comes with a medication, it can only be used for that medication. Some medicine droppers are calibrated in milliliters or by actual dosage.

3. Syringes may also be used to measure medications. The medication is poured in a medication cup and drawn up in the syringe without the use of a needle. This is often done when the amount desired cannot be measured accurately in a cup. For example, 6.3 mL cannot be measured accurately in the standard medication cup; however, the medication may be drawn up in a syringe and then squirted into a cup or administered orally with the use of a syringe without the needle. Solutions can also be measured by using a specially calibrated *oral syringe* to ensure accurate and safe dosages (Figure 17-11). Oral syringes are not sterile, are often available in colors, and have an off-center (eccentric) tip. These features make it easy to distinguish them from hypodermic syringes. Oral syringes may also have markings such as teaspoon and tablespoon. Figure 17-12 shows how to fill a syringe from a medicine cup. Some oral liquid medications come in containers that allow the client to drink right out of the container, eliminating the need to transfer it to a medication cup.

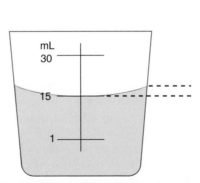

**Figure 17-9**    Reading meniscus. The meniscus is caused by the surface tension of the solution against the walls of the container. The surface tension causes the formation of a concave or hollowed curvature on the surface of the solution. Read the level at the lowest point of the concave curve. (From Clayton BD, Stock YN, Harroun RD: *Basic pharmacology for nurses,* ed. 14, St. Louis, 2007, Mosby.)

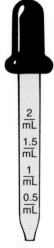

**Figure 17-10**    Medicine dropper. (Modified from Clayton BN, Stock YN, Harroun RD: *Basic pharmacology for nurses,* ed. 14, St. Louis, 2007 Mosby.)

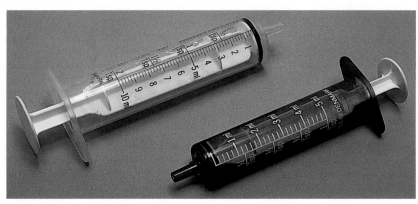

**Figure 17-11**   Oral syringes. (Courtesy Chuck Dresner. From Clayton BD, Stock YN, Harroun RD: *Basic pharmacology for nurses,* ed. 14, St. Louis, 2007, Mosby.)

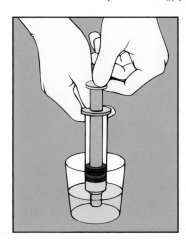

**Figure 17-12**   Filling a syringe directly from medicine cup. (Modified from Clayton BD, Stock YN, Harroun RD: *Basic pharmacology for nurses,* ed. 14, St. Louis, 2007, Mosby.)

Before we proceed to calculate liquid medications, let's review some helpful pointers.
1.  The label on the medication container must be read carefully to determine the dosage strength in the volume of solution, because it varies.

---

**CAUTION**

Do not confuse dosage strength with total volume. Read labels carefully. Confusing dosage strength with total volume can result in errors when performing calculations.

---

For example, the label on a medication may indicate a total volume of 100 mL, but the dosage strength may be 125 mg per 5 mL. It must be noted that dosage strength can be written on solutions in several ways to indicate the same thing. For example, 125 mg per 5 mL may be written as 125 mg/5 mL or 125 mg = 5 mL. Other examples of dosage strength are 20 mg per mL, 20 mg/mL, 200 mg/5 mL, and 200 mg per 5 mL.

---

**CAUTION**

Although dosage strengths may be written on solutions in several ways when dosages are written, for example, 40 mg per 2 mL or 40 mg/2 mL), ISMP (Institute for Safe Medication Practices) recommends that the "/" (slash mark) not be used to separate doses. The slash mark has been mistaken as the number 1. Use "per" rather than a slash mark to separate doses.

---

2.  Answers are labeled by using liquid measures. Example: mL.
3.  Calculations can be done by using the same methods (ratio and proportion, the formula method, or dimensional analysis) and the same steps as for solid forms of oral medications.

Now let's look at some sample problems that involve the calculation of oral liquids.

**Example 1:**    Order: Dilantin 200 mg p.o. t.i.d.

Available: Dilantin suspension labeled 125 mg per 5 mL

 ## Problem Setup

1. No conversion is required. Everything is in the same units of measure and the same system.
   Order: 200 mg
   Available: 125 mg per 5 mL
2. Think critically: What would be a logical answer? Looking at Example 1, you can assume the answer will be greater than 5 mL.
3. Set up the problem using ratio and proportion, the formula method, or dimensional analysis.
4. Label the final answer with the correct unit of measure. In this case the units will be milliliters. Remember: The answer has no meaning if written without the appropriate unit of measure.

 ## Solution Using Ratio and Proportion

$$125 \text{ mg} : 5 \text{ mL} = 200 \text{ mg} : x \text{ mL}$$

$$\text{(known)} \qquad \text{(unknown)}$$

$$125x = 200 \times 5$$

$$\frac{125x}{125} = \frac{1,000}{125}$$

$$x = \frac{1,000}{125}$$

$$x = 8 \text{ mL}$$

 ## Solution Using the Formula Method

$$\frac{\text{(D) } 200 \text{ mg}}{\text{(H) } 125 \text{ mg}} \times \text{(Q) } 5 \text{ mL} = x \text{ mL}$$

$$\frac{200}{125} \times 5 = x$$

$$\frac{1,000}{125} = x$$

$$x = 8 \text{ mL}$$

 ## Solution Using Dimensional Analysis

$$x \text{ mL} = \frac{5 \text{ mL}}{125 \text{ mg}} \times \frac{200 \text{ mg}}{1}$$

$$x = \frac{1,000}{125}$$

$$x = 8 \text{ mL}$$

**Example 2:**   Order: Lactulose 30 g p.o. b.i.d.

Available: Lactulose labeled 10 g per 15 mL

 Solution Using Ratio and Proportion

$$10 \text{ g} : 15 \text{ mL} = 30 \text{ g} : x \text{ mL}$$

$$\frac{10x}{10} = \frac{450}{10}$$

$$x = \frac{450}{10}$$

$$x = 45 \text{ mL}$$

 Solution Using the Formula Method

$$\frac{(D) \ 30 \text{ g}}{(H) \ 10 \text{ g}} \times (Q) \ 15 \text{ mL} = x \text{ mL}$$

$$\frac{30 \times 15}{10} = x$$

$$x = \frac{450}{10}$$

$$x = 45 \text{ mL}$$

 Solution Using Dimensional Analysis

$$x \text{ mL} = \frac{15 \text{ mL}}{10 \ \cancel{g}} \times \frac{30 \ \cancel{g}}{1}$$

$$x = \frac{450}{10}$$

$$x = 45 \text{ mL}$$

**Example 3:**   Order: Elixir of phenobarbital gr $1\frac{1}{2}$ p.o. daily

Available: Elixir of phenobarbital labeled 20 mg per 5 mL

Order: gr $1\frac{1}{2}$

Available: 20 mg per 5 mL

Equivalent: 60 mg = gr 1

$$60 \text{ mg} : \text{gr } 1 = x \text{ mg} : \text{gr } 1\frac{1}{2} \left( \frac{3}{2} \right)$$

$$60 \text{ mg} : \text{gr } 1 = x \text{ mg} : \text{gr } \frac{3}{2}$$

$$x = \frac{180}{2}$$

$$x = 90 \text{ mg}$$

> **NOTE**
>
> A conversion is necessary before calculating the dose. What the prescriber has ordered is different from what is available.

Solution Using Ratio and Proportion

$$20 \text{ mg}:5 \text{ mL} = 90 \text{ mg}:x \text{ mL}$$

$$\frac{20x}{20} = \frac{450}{20}$$

$$x = \frac{450}{20}$$

$$x = 22.5 \text{ mL}$$

**NOTE**

Some medication orders state the specific amount to be given and therefore require no calculation. Examples: milk of magnesia 1 ounce p.o. at bedtime; Robitussin 15 mL p.o. q4h p.r.n.; multivitamin 1 tab p.o. daily; Fer-In-Sol 0.2 mL p.o. daily.

 Solution Using the Formula Method

$$\frac{(D) \; 90 \text{ mg}}{(H) \; 20 \text{ mg}} \times (Q) \; 5 \text{ mL} = x \text{ mL}$$

$$\frac{90 \times 5}{20} = x$$

$$x = \frac{450}{20}$$

$$x = 22.5 \text{ mL}$$

Solution Using Dimensional Analysis

$$x \text{ mL} = \frac{5 \text{ mL}}{20 \text{ mg}} \times \frac{60 \text{ mg}}{\text{gr } 1} \times \frac{\text{gr } 1\frac{1}{2}}{1}$$

$$x = \frac{300 \times \frac{3}{2}}{20} = \frac{450}{20}$$

$$x = \frac{450}{20}$$

$$x = 22.5 \text{ mL}$$

## ■ Points to Remember

- Liquid medications can be calculated by using the same methods as those used for solid forms (tabs, caps).
- Read labels carefully on medication containers; identify the dosage strength contained in a certain amount of solution.
- Administration of accurate dosages of liquid medications may require the use of calibrated droppers or syringes. Oral syringes are designed for oral use; they are not sterile.
- The use of ratio and proportion, the formula method, or dimensional analysis is a means of validating an answer; however, it still requires thinking in terms of the dosage you will administer and applying principles learned to calculate dosages that are sensible and safe.
- Dosage strength on solutions can be written several ways. Do not confuse it with total volume (total amount in container). Use "per" to separate dosages when writing.
- For accurate measurement, oral solutions are poured at eye level and read at eye level while resting on a flat surface.
- Always pour away from the label to keep hands from covering it and spills from obscuring it.
- Calibrated droppers should be used only for the medication for which they are intended.

## Practice Problems

Calculate the following dosages for oral liquids in milliliters using the labels or information provided. Do not forget to label your answer. Round answers to the nearest tenth where indicated.

42. Order: Colace syrup 100 mg by jejunostomy tube t.i.d.

    Available: Colace syrup 50 mg per 15 mL          _____

43. Order: Biaxin 100 mg p.o. q12h.

    Available:

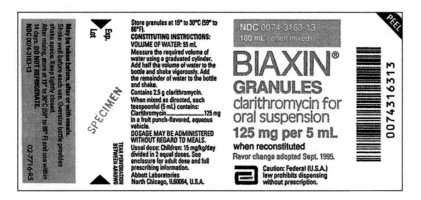

          _____

44. Order: Kaon-Cl (potassium chloride) 40 mEq p.o. daily.

    Available:

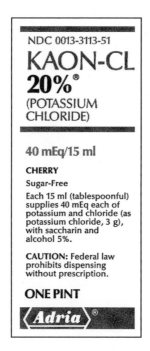

          _____

45. Order: Theophylline elixir 120 mg p.o. b.i.d.

    Available: Theophylline elixir 80 mg per 15 mL  _____

46. Order: Erythromycin oral suspension
    250 mg po q6h.

    Available:

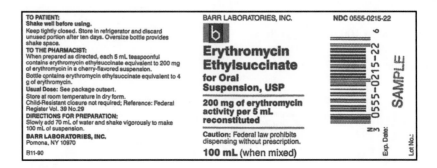

    _____

47. Order: Dilantin 100 mg p.o. t.i.d.

    Available: Dilantin suspension 125 mg per 5 mL  _____

48. Order: Digoxin 125 mcg p.o. every day.

    Available:

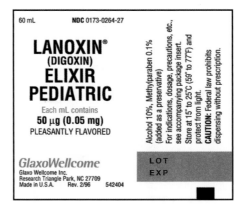

    _____

49. Order: Imodium (loperamide hydrochloride) 4 mg p.o. as initial dose and then 2 mg after each loose stool.

Available:

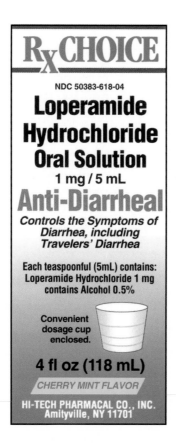

How many mL will you administer for the initial dose? _____

50. Order: Amoxicillin 0.5 g p.o. q6h.

Available:

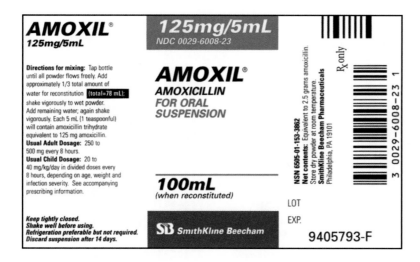

_____

51. Order: Phenobarbital 60 mg p.o. at bedtime.

    Available: Phenobarbital elixir 20 mg per 5 mL    _____

52. Order: Mellaril 150 mg p.o. b.i.d.

    Available:

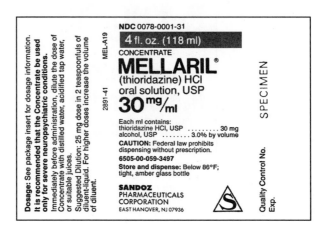

    _____

53. Order: Diphenhydramine HCl 25 mg p.o. b.i.d. p.r.n. for agitation.

    Available: Diphenhydramine hydrochloride
    elixir 12.5 mg per 5 mL    _____

54. Order: Lithium carbonate 600 mg p.o. at bedtime.

    Available: Lithium citrate syrup. Each 5 mL contains lithium carbonate 300 mg.
    Each unit-dose container contains 5 mL

    a. How many milliliters are needed to administer
       the required dosage?    _____

    b. How many containers of the medication will
       you need to administer the dosage?    _____

55. Order: Haldol 10 mg p.o. b.i.d.

    Available: Haldol concentrate labeled 2 mg per mL    _____

56. Order: Dicloxacillin sodium 0.5 g by gastrostomy tube q6h.

    Available:

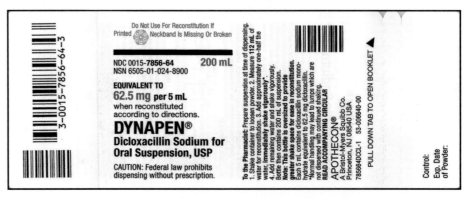

    _____

57. Order: V-Cillin K suspension 500,000 units p.o. q.i.d.

    Available: V-Cillin K oral solution 200,000 units
    per 5 mL                                                    _____

58. Order: Keflex 1 g by nasogastric tube q6h.

    Available: Keflex oral suspension 125 mg per 5 mL    _____

59. Order: Trilafon 24 mg p.o. b.i.d.

    Available: Trilafon concentrate labeled
    16 mg per 5 mL                                              _____

60. Order: Acetaminophen elixir 650 mg by nasogastric tube q4h p.r.n. for temperature
    greater than 101° F.

    Available:

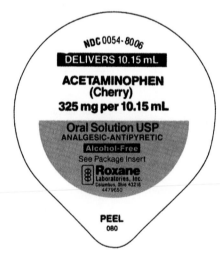

_____

61. Order: Tagamet 400 mg p.o. q6h.

    Available:

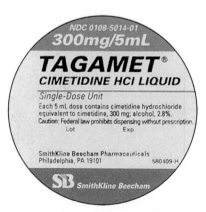

_____

62. Order: Epivir 150 mg p.o. b.i.d.

    Available:

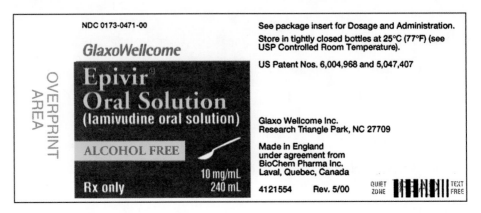

63. Order: Retrovir 0.3 g p.o. b.i.d.

    Available:

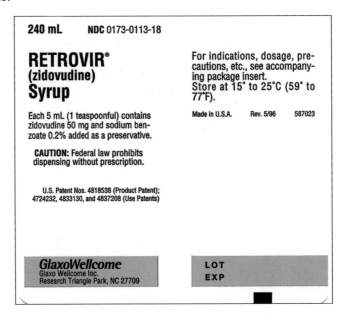

64. Order: Mycostatin suspension 200,000 units p.o. b.i.d.

    Available:

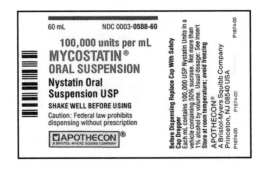

65. Order: Norvir 600 mg p.o. b.i.d.

    Available:

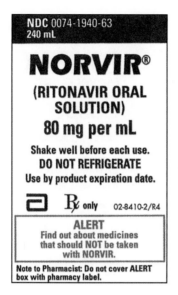

_____

66. Order: Augmentin 0.25 g p.o. q8h.

    Available:

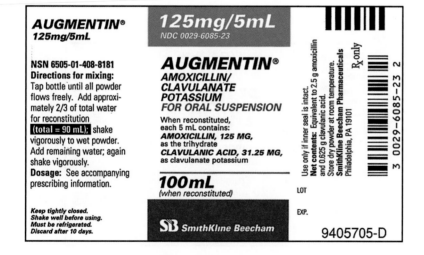

_____

67. Order: Zovirax 200 mg p.o. q4h for 5 days.

Available:

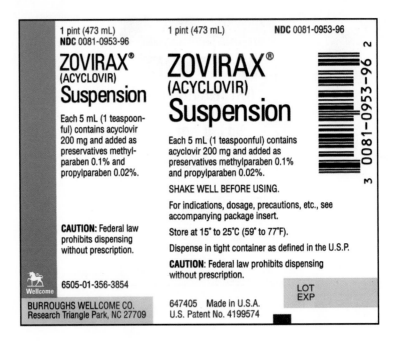

_____

68. Order: Prozac 30 mg p.o. every day in AM.

Available:

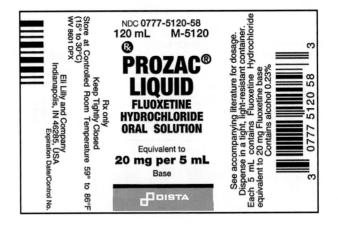

_____

69. Order: Zantac 150 mg b.i.d. by nasogastric tube.

    Available:

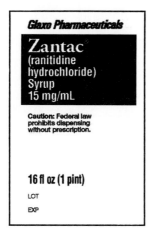

    _____

70. Order: OxyFast 30 mg p.o. q12h p.r.n. for pain.

    Available:

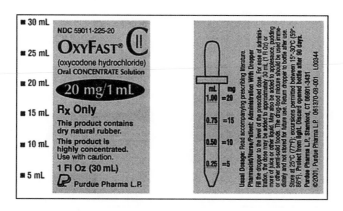

    _____

Answers on pp. 629-631

## Critical Thinking Questions

1. **Scenario:** Order: Digoxin 0.75 mg p.o. daily. In preparing to administer medications, you find 0.125 mg tabs (scored) in the medication drawer for the client.
   a. Based on the tablets available, how many would you have to administer? _____
   b. What action should you take? _____
   c. What is the rationale for your action? _____
2. **Scenario:** Order: Diflucan 150 mg p.o. daily. The pharmacy sends two 100-mg unscored tabs.
   a. What action should you take to administer the dosage ordered? _____
   b. What is the rationale for your action? _____

3. **Scenario:** Order: Percocet 2 tabs p.o. q4h p.r.n. for pain for a client who is allergic to aspirin. The nurse administers Percodan 2 tabs.

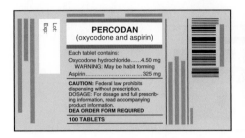

**PERCODAN**
(oxycodone and aspirin)

Each tablet contains:
Oxycodone hydrochloride......4.50 mg
 WARNING: May be habit forming
Aspirin.............................325 mg

**CAUTION:** Federal law prohibits dispensing without prescription.
DOSAGE: For dosage and full prescribing information, read accompanying product information.
**DEA ORDER FORM REQUIRED**
**100 TABLETS**

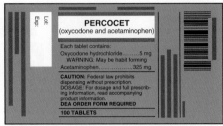

**PERCOCET**
(oxycodone and acetaminophen)

Each tablet contains:
Oxycodone hydrochloride.........5 mg
 WARNING: May be habit forming
Acetaminophen.................325 mg

**CAUTION:** Federal law prohibits dispensing without prescription.
DOSAGE: For dosage and full prescribing information, read accompanying product information.
**DEA ORDER FORM REQUIRED**
**100 TABLETS**

a. What client right was violated? _____

b. What contributed to the error? _____

c. What is the potential outcome of the error? _____

d. What preventive measures could have been taken to prevent the error? _____

Answers on p. 632

✓ **CHAPTER REVIEW**

Calculate the following dosages using the medication label or information provided. Express volume answers in milliliters; round answers to the nearest tenth as indicated. Remember to label answers: tab, caps, mL.

1. Order: Tylenol 975 mg p.o. q6h p.r.n. for earache.

 Available:

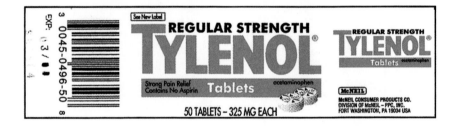

_____

2. Order: Zyvox 400 mg p.o. q12h.

 Available:

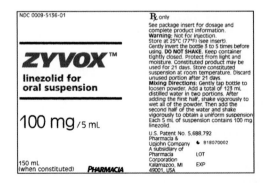

_____

3. Order: Lopressor 100 mg p.o. b.i.d. Hold for blood pressure less than 100/60.

   Available:

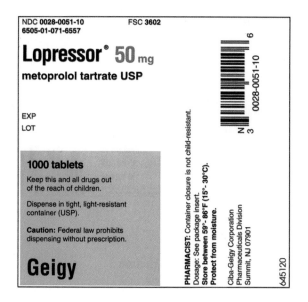

4. Order: Pravachol 30 mg p.o. at bedtime.

   Available:

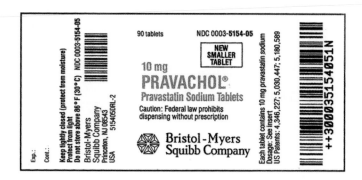

5. Order: Atacand 8 mg p.o. daily. Hold if systolic blood pressure less than 100.

   Available:

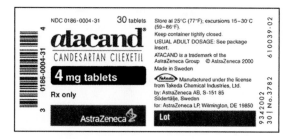

6. Order: Depakote 500 mg p.o. at bedtime.

   Available: Depakote syrup labeled 200 mg per 5 mL _____

7. Order: Levitra 5 mg p.o. 1 hr before sexual activity for a client with erectile dysfunction.

   Available:

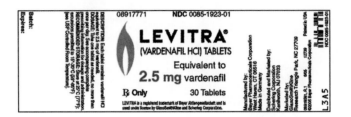

   _____

8. Order: Ativan 1 mg p.o. q4h p.r.n. for agitation.

   Available:

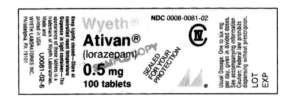

   _____

9. Order: Lopressor 25 mg per nasogastric tube b.i.d.

   Available: Scored Lopressor tablets labeled 50 mg _____

10. Order: Aldactone 100 mg p.o. daily.

    Available:

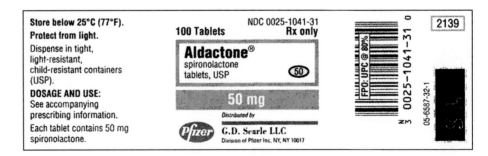

    _____

11.  Order: Digoxin 0.1 mg p.o. daily.

Available:

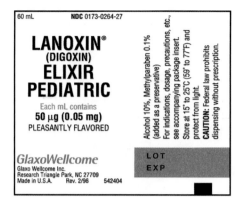

_____

12.  Order: Amoxicillin 0.375 g p.o. q6h.

Available:

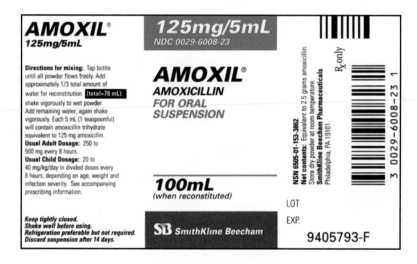

_____

13.  Order: Hydrochlorothiazide 12.5 mg p.o. daily. Hold for blood pressure less than 90/60.

Available (scored tablets):

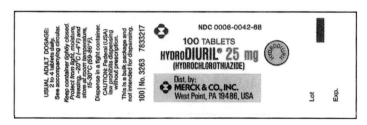

_____

14. Order: Tylenol 650 mg by nasogastric tube q4h p.r.n. for temp greater than 101.4° F.

Available:

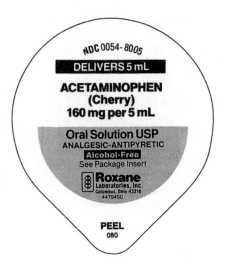

_____

15. Order: Lexapro 20 mg p.o. daily in the PM.

Available:

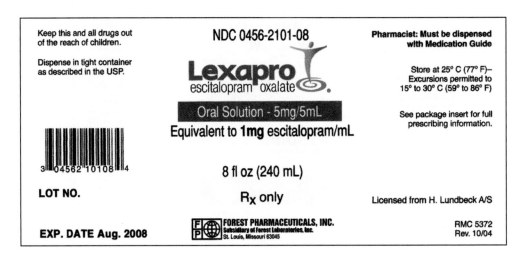

_____

16. Order: Elixophyllin Elixir 300 mg by nasogastric tube b.i.d.

Available: Elixophyllin liquid labeled 160 mg per 15 mL

_____

17. Order: Xanax 0.75 mg p.o. t.i.d.

Available: Xanax tabs labeled 0.25 mg

_____

18.  Order: Mevacor 20 mg p.o. daily.

Available:

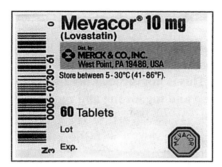

_____

19.  Order: Meclizine HCl (Antivert) 25 mg p.o. every day.

Available:

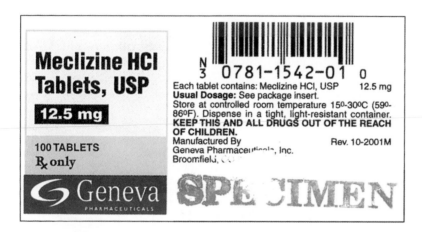

_____

20.  Order: Erythromycin suspension 0.25 g p.o. q.i.d.

Available:

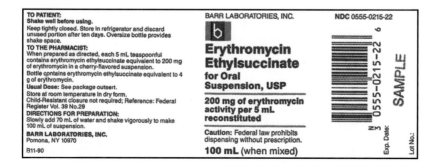

_____

21. Order: Clonidine 0.5 mg p.o. t.i.d. Hold for blood pressure less than 100/60.

   Available: Clonidine tablets labeled 0.1 mg, 0.2 mg, 0.3 mg

   Which would be the best combination to administer to the client? _____

22. Order: Nitrostat 0.3 mg SL stat.

   Available:

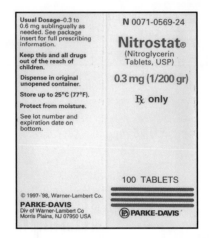

   _____

23. Order: Procanbid extended release 1 g p.o. q12h.

   Available:

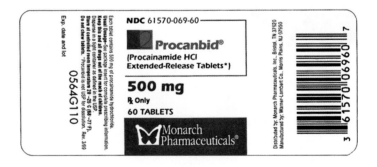

   _____

24. Order: Lactulose 20 g by gastrostomy tube b.i.d.

    Available:

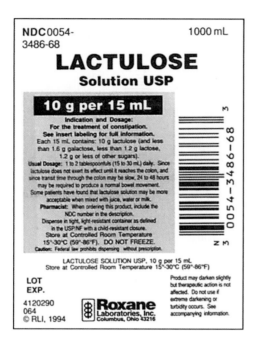

_____

25. Order: Kanamycin (Kantrex) 1 g p.o. q6h for 5 days.

    Available:

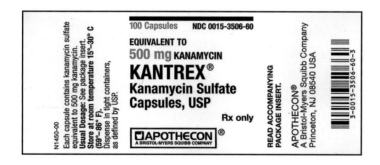

_____

26. Order: Ambien 10 mg p.o. at bedtime for 4 nights.

Available:

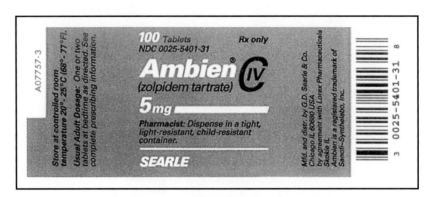

a. How many tabs will you administer for
each dosage? _____

b. How many tabs will be needed for the 4 nights? _____

27. Order: Lipitor 30 mg p.o. every day.

Available:

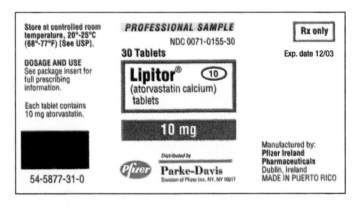

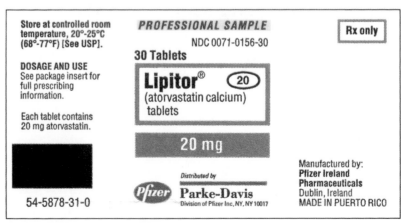

What will you administer to the client? _____

28. Order: Cimetidine 0.8 g p.o. t.i.d.

Available:

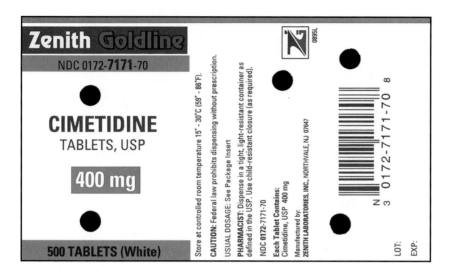

_____

29. Order: Lorabid 500 mg p.o. q12h.

Available:

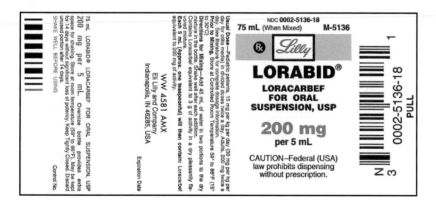

_____

30. Order: Nexium (delayed release) 40 mg p.o. every day for 4 weeks.

    Available:

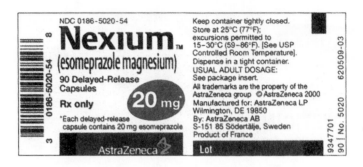

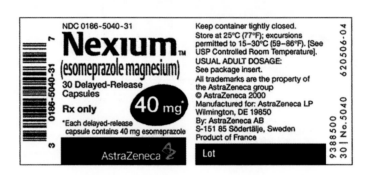

    What will you administer to the client?     _____

31. Order: Compazine 7.5 mg p.o. t.i.d.

    Available:

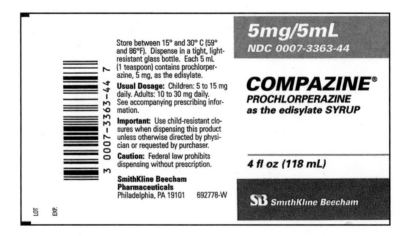

         _____

32. Order: Avandia 8 mg p.o. daily.

    Available:

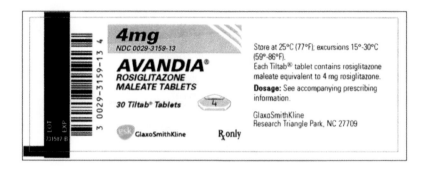

_____

33. Order: Allopurinol 0.25 g p.o. every day.

    Available: Scored tabs.

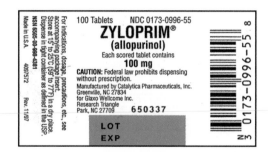

_____

34. Order: Geodon 120 mg p.o. b.i.d.

    Available:

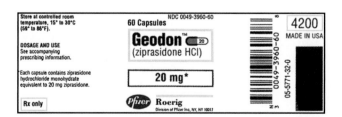

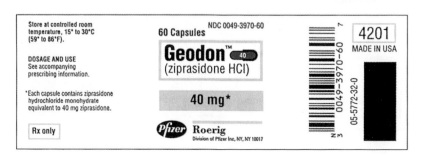

    What will you administer to the client?          _____

35.  Order: Lasix (furosemide) 100 mg by gastrostomy tube once a day.

Available:

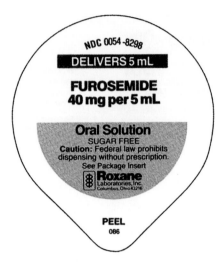

_____

36.  Order: Voltaren 0.1 g p.o. b.i.d.

Available:

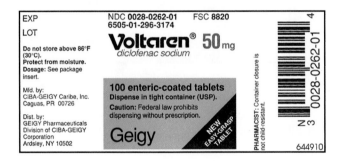

_____

37.  Order: Viagra 50 mg p.o. ½ hour before sexual activity for a client with erectile dysfunction.

Available:

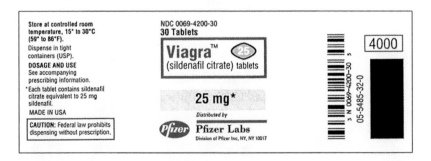

_____

38. Order: Tranxene 15 mg p.o. b.i.d.

    Available:

    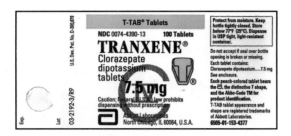

    _____

39. Order: Valproic acid (Depakene) 1 g p.o. every day.

    Available:

    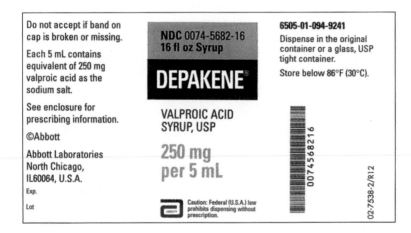

    _____

40. Order: Synthroid 175 mcg p.o. daily.

    Available:

    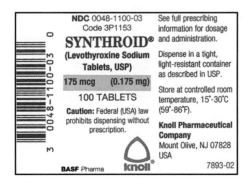

    _____

41.  Order: Zyprexa 10 mg p.o. b.i.d.

Available:

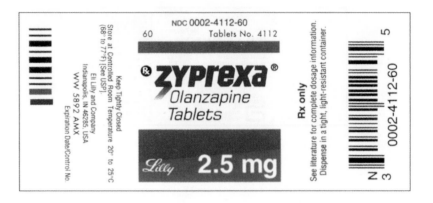

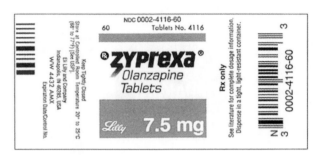

What will you administer to the client?    _____

42.  Order: Wellbutrin 150 mg p.o. b.i.d.

Available:

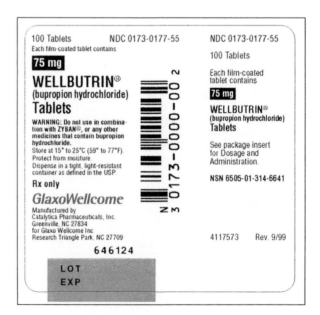

_____

43. Order: Ceftin 500 mg p.o. q12h.

    Available:

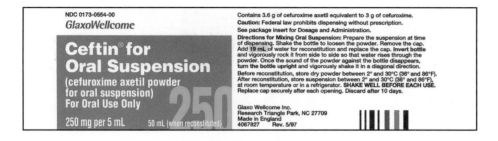

_____

44. Order: Paxil 40 mg p.o. every day in AM.

    Available:

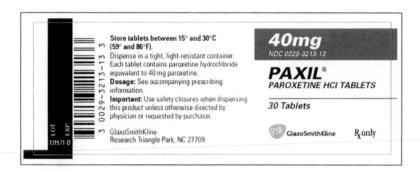

_____

45. Order: Cytotec 200 mcg p.o. q.i.d.

    Available:

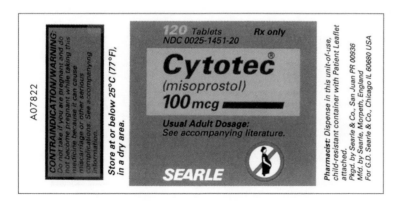

_____

46. Order: Claritin Syrup 4 mg p.o. every day.

    Available:

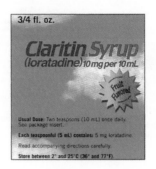

_____

47. Order: Benadryl 100 mg p.o. at bedtime.

    Available:

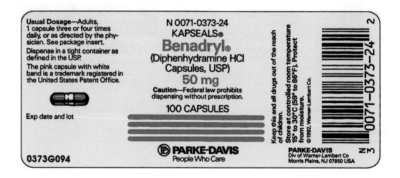

_____

48. Order: Zofran 8 mg p.o. ½ hour before chemotherapy.

    Available:

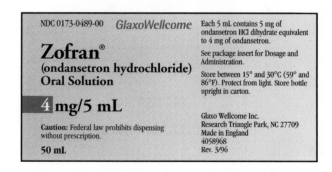

_____

49. Order: BenicarHCT 20 mg p.o. daily.

    Available:

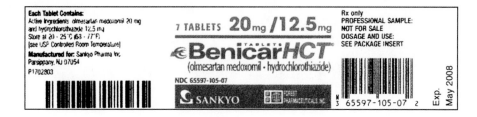

_____

50. Order: Ery-Tab 0.666 g p.o. q6h.

    Available:

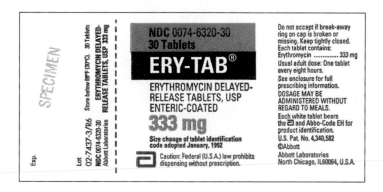

_____

Answers on p. 632

 **For additional practice problems, refer to the Basic Calculations section of Drug Calculations Companion, Version 4, on Evolve.**

# CHAPTER
# 18

# Parenteral Medications

## Objectives

*After reviewing this chapter, you should be able to:*
1. Identify the various types of syringes used for parenteral administration
2. Read and measure dosages on a syringe
3. Read medication labels on parenteral medications
4. Calculate dosages of parenteral medications already in solution
5. Identify appropriate syringes with which to administer dosages calculated

The term *parenteral* is used to indicate medications that are administered by any route other than through the digestive system. However, the term *parenteral* is commonly used to refer to the administration of medications by injection with the use of a needle and syringe into body tissue. In this text use of parenteral always means injection routes. Examples of common parenteral routes are intramuscular (IM), subcutaneous (subcut), intradermal (ID), and intravenous (IV). Medications administered by the parenteral route generally act more quickly than oral medications because they are absorbed more rapidly into the bloodstream. The parenteral route may be desired when rapid action of a drug is necessary, for a client who is unable to take a medication orally because of emesis (vomiting) or nonfunctioning gastrointestinal (GI) tract or for a client who is unconscious.

Medications for parenteral use are available as a sterile solution or liquid that can be absorbed and distributed without causing irritation to the tissues. Parenteral medications are also available in powder form that must be diluted with a liquid or solvent (reconstituted) before they can be used. Reconstitution of medications in powder form will be covered in Chapter 19. Medications for parenteral use come packaged in vials, ampules, and premeasured (prefilled) syringes and cartridges.

## PACKAGING OF PARENTERAL MEDICATIONS

Parenteral medications are packaged in various forms:
1. Ampule—An ampule is a sealed glass container designed to hold a single dose of medication. Ampules have a particular shape with a constricted neck. They are designed to snap open. The neck of the ampule may be scored or have a darkened line or ring around it to indicate where it should be broken to withdraw medication (Figure 18-1).

    When medication is withdrawn from an ampule, the neck is snapped off by grasping it with an alcohol wipe or sterile gauze and breaking it off. Aspiration of the medication into a syringe occurs easily and may be accomplished with a filter needle, if required by institutional policy. A filter needle prevents withdrawal of glass or rubber particulate (Elkin et al, 2007).

When the needle is inserted into an ampule, care must be taken to prevent the shaft and tip of the needle from touching the rim of the ampule. Medication is withdrawn into the syringe by gently pulling back on the plunger, which creates a negative pressure and allows the medication to be pulled into the syringe.

2. Vial—A vial is a plastic or glass container that has a rubber stopper (diaphragm) on the top. The rubber stopper is covered with a metal lid or plastic cover to maintain sterility until the vial is used for the first time (Figure 18-2). Some manufacturers do not guarantee a sterile top even though it is covered, and therefore it is necessary to wipe the top with alcohol even with first use. Vials are available in different sizes. Multidose vials contain more than one dosage of the medication. The label on the vial will specify the amount of medication in a certain amount of solution, for example, 60 mg per mL or 0.2 mg per 0.5 mL. Single-dose vials contain a single dosage of medication for injection. Many vials are single dose, because it is safer. Even if medication is in a single-dosage vial, it should still be measured and not just drawn up. The medication in a vial may be in liquid (solution) form, or it may contain a powder that must be reconstituted before administration.

Before medication is withdrawn from a vial, the top is wiped with alcohol and allowed to dry. Air equal to the amount of solution being withdrawn is injected into the air space between the solution and the rubber stopper, the vial is inverted, and the desired volume of medication is withdrawn.

In contrast to the ampule, the vial is a closed system, and air must be injected into it to allow for withdrawal of the medication. If air is not injected into the vial before the medication is withdrawn, a vacuum remains in the vial that makes the withdrawal of medication difficult. When large volumes of solution are to be withdrawn from a vial, a small volume of air is required to initiate the flow of medication. Injecting large volumes of air into the vial can create too much pressure in the vial and cause the top of the vial to be popped off, or the plunger of the syringe could be rapidly forced backward by the air pressure within the vial.

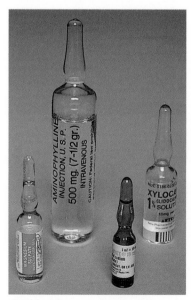

**Figure 18-1**    Medication in ampules. (From Elkin MK, Perry AG, Potter PA: *Nursing interventions and clinical skills,* ed. 4, St. Louis, 2007, Mosby.)

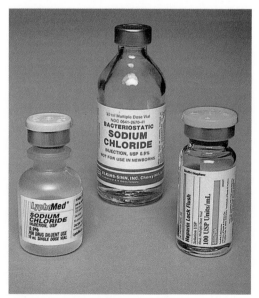

**Figure 18-2**    Medication in vials. (From Elkin MK, Perry AG, Potter PA: *Nursing interventions and clinical skills,* ed. 4, St. Louis, 2007, Mosby.)

## Tips for Clinical Practice

It is important to note that for both single-dose vials and ampules, there is a little extra medication present; it is most important to measure the amount of medication carefully.

3. Mix-o-vial—Some medications come in mix-o-vials (Figure 18-3), for example, Solu-Medrol and Solu-Cortef. The vial usually contains a single dosage of medication. The mix-o-vial has two compartments separated by a rubber stopper. The top compartment contains the sterile liquid (diluent), and the bottom compartment contains the powdered medication. When pressure is applied to the top of the vial, the rubber stopper that separates the medication and liquid is released. This allows the liquid and medication to be mixed, thereby dissolving the medication (Figure 18-4).

   A needle is inserted into the rubber stopper to withdraw the medication.

4. Cartridge—Some medications are packaged in a prefilled glass or plastic container. The cartridge is clearly marked, indicating the amount of medication in it. Certain cartridges require a special holder called a *Tubex* or *Carpuject* to release the medication from the cartridge. The cartridge contains a single dosage of medication.

   If the dosage to be administered is less than the amount contained in the unit, discard the unneeded portion if any, and then administer the medication (Figure 18-5).

5. Prepackaged syringe (premeasured)—The medication comes prepared for administration in a syringe with the needle attached or without a needle attached. A specific amount of medication is contained in the syringe. The amount desired is calculated, the excess disposed of, and the calculated dosage is administered. These syringes are for single use only. Valium and Lovenox are examples of medications that come in prepackaged syringes (see Figure 18-5, *B*).

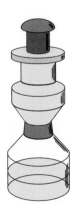

**Figure 18-3**   Mix-o-vial. (From Clayton BD, Stock YN, Harroun RD: *Basic pharmacology for nurses,* ed. 14, St. Louis, 2007, Mosby.)

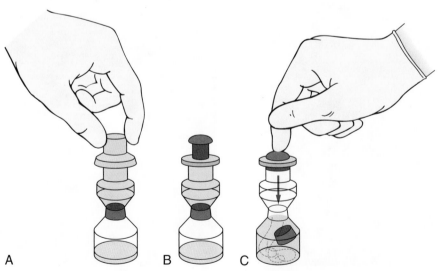

A          B          C

**Figure 18-4**   Mix-o-vial directions. **A,** Remove plastic lid protector. **B,** Powdered drug is in lower half; diluent is in upper half. **C,** Push firmly on the diaphragm-plunger. Downward pressure dislodges the divider between the two chambers. (Modified from Clayton BD, Stock YN, Harroun RD: *Basic pharmacology for nurses,* ed. 14, St. Louis, 2007, Mosby.)

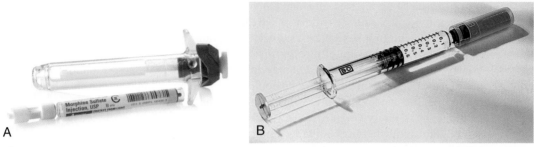

**Figure 18-5** **A,** Carpuject syringe holder and needleless, prefilled sterile cartridge. **B,** BD-Hypak prefilled syringe. (**A,** From Hospira, Inc., Lake Forest, IL. **B,** From Becton, Dickinson, and Company, Franklin Lakes, N.J.)

## SYRINGES

Various-sized syringes are available for use. They have different capacities and specific calibrations. Syringes are made of plastic and glass, but plastic syringes are more commonly used. They are disposable and designed for one-time use only. Syringes have three parts (Figure 18-6):

1. The barrel—The outer calibrated portion that holds the medication.
2. The plunger—The inner device that is moved backward to withdraw and measure the medication and is pushed to eject the medication from the syringe.
3. The tip—The end of the syringe that holds the needle. The tip can be plain (slip tip) or Luer-Lok (Figure 18-7).

Syringes are classified as being Luer-Lok or non–Luer-Lok (have a slip tip). They are disposable and designed for one-time use. Luer-Lok syringes require special needles, which are twisted onto the tip and lock themselves in place, which prevents inadvertent removal of the needle. Non–Luer-Lok syringes require needles that slip onto the tip (Potter and Perry, 2009). The needle fits onto the tip of the syringe. Needles come in various lengths and diameters. The nurse chooses the needle according to the client's size, the

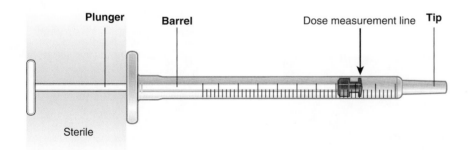

**Figure 18-6** Parts of a syringe. (From Harkreader H, Hogan MA: *Fundamentals of nursing: caring and clinical judgement,* ed. 3, St. Louis, 2007, Saunders.)

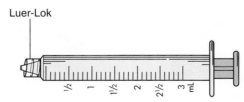

**Figure 18-7** 3-mL Luer-Lok syringe. (From Potter PA, Perry AG: *Fundamentals of nursing,* ed. 7, St. Louis, 2009, Mosby.)

type of tissue being injected into, and the viscosity of the medication to be injected. Some syringes also come with a needle attached that cannot be detached from the syringe.

It is important to note that needle-stick prevention has become increasingly important in preventing transmission of blood-borne infections from contaminated needles. Consequently, this has resulted in special prevention techniques (e.g., no recapping of a needle after use) and development of special equipment, such as syringes with a sheath or guard that covers the needle after it is withdrawn from the skin, thereby decreasing the chance of needle-stick injury (Figure 18-8). Another advance in safety needle technology is the safety glide syringe, which contains a protective needle guard that can be activated by a single finger to cover and seal the needle after injection (Figure 18-9). Needleless syringe systems have also been designed to prevent needle sticks during intravenous administration (Figure 18-10).

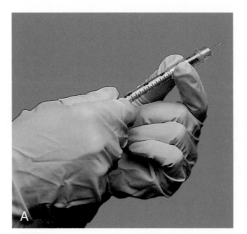
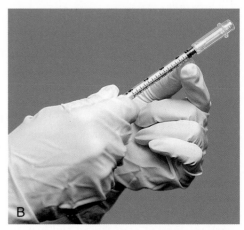

**Figure 18-8** Needle with plastic guard to prevent needle sticks. **A,** Position of guard before injection. **B,** After injection the guard locks in place, covering the needle. (From Elkin MK, Perry AG, Potter PA: *Nursing interventions and clinical skills,* ed. 4, St. Louis, 2007, Mosby.)

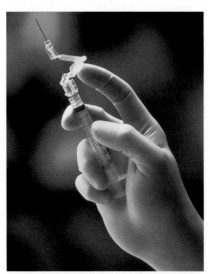

**Figure 18-9** BD SafetyGlide™ needle. (From Becton, Dickinson, and Company, Franklin Lakes, N.J.)

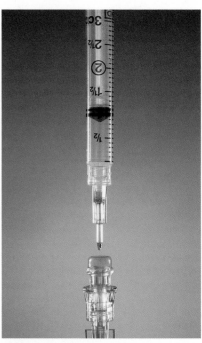

**Figure 18-10** Needleless syringe system. (From Becton, Dickinson, and Company, Franklin Lakes, N.J.)

## Types of Syringes

The three types of syringes are hypodermic, tuberculin, and insulin.

*HYPODERMIC SYRINGES*

Hypodermic syringes come in a variety of sizes from 0.5 to 60 mL and larger. Syringes are calibrated or marked in milliliters but hold varying capacities. Of the small-capacity syringes, the 3-mL syringe is used most often for the administration of medication that is more than 1 mL; however, hypodermic syringes are also available in larger sizes (10 mL 20 mL, 50 mL, and larger). Although many syringes are labeled in milliliters, a few syringes are still labeled with cubic centimeters (cc). **It is important to note that milliliter (mL) is correct. The milliliter is a measure of volume, the cubic centimeter is a three-dimensional measure of space and represents the space that a milliliter occupies. The terms, although sometimes used interchangeably, are not the same.** Many institutions are now purchasing syringes that indicate mL as opposed to cc. This text shows mL on syringes, not cc. Some of the small-capacity syringes (1, 2, 3 mL) may still indicate minims. The use of the minim scale is rare and discouraged because of its inaccuracy. Although a few syringes still have minim markings, more institutions are purchasing syringes that do not have minim markings on them to discourage their use (Figure 18-11).

It has been found that most errors in dosage measurement occur from misreading the minim scale.

**CAUTION**

It is critical that the scale on small hypodermics be read carefully and that the minim (m.) scale not be misread as the metric scale or milliliter (mL). This mistake could lead to a medication error.

For small hypodermics, decimal numbers are used to express dosages (e.g., 1.2 mL, 0.3 mL). Notice that small hypodermics up to 3-mL size also have fractions on them (see Figure 18-11). There are, however, some syringes that indicate 0.5 mL, 1.5 mL, etc., instead of fractions. The use of decimals on the syringes correlates with the use of decimals in the metric system; therefore a dosage should be stated in milliliters as a decimal.

Notice the side that indicates mL. There are 10 spaces between the largest markings. This indicates that the syringe is marked in tenths of a milliliter. Each of the lines is 0.1 mL. The longer lines indicate half (0.5) and full milliliter measures.

When looking at the syringe shown in Figure 18-12, notice the rubber ring. When you are measuring medication and reading the medication withdrawn, the forward edge of the

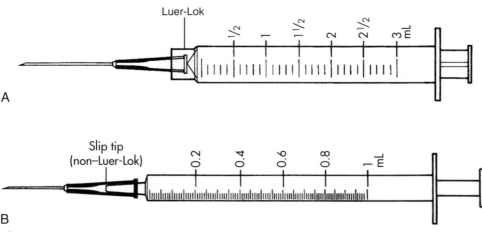

**Figure 18-11**   **A,** 3-mL Luer-Lok syringe and, **B,** 1-mL slip tip syringe.

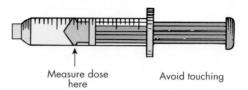

**Figure 18-12** Reading measured amount of medication in a syringe. (From Potter PA, Perry AG: *Fundamentals of nursing,* ed. 7, St. Louis, 2009, Mosby.)

plunger head indicates the amount of medication withdrawn. Do not become confused by the second, bottom ring or by the raised section (middle) of the suction tip. The point where the rubber plunger tip makes contact with the barrel is the spot that should be lined up with the amount desired.

Let's examine the syringes below to illustrate specific amounts in a syringe.

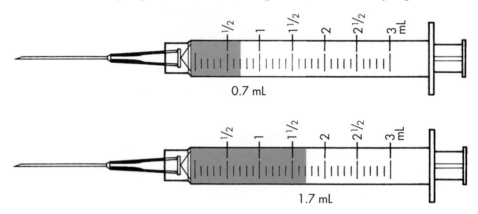

Because the small-capacity syringes are used most often to administer medications, it is very important to know how to read them to withdraw amounts accurately.

## ■ Points to Remember

- Small-capacity hypodermics are calibrated in milliliters; the 3-mL size syringe is used most often to administer dosages greater than 1 mL. Dosages administered with them must correlate to the calibration. Minims are no longer used.
- If minims are on a syringe, do not confuse the minim scale with the metric scale (mL); doing so can cause a serious medication error.
- Syringes are labeled with the abbreviation mL. More and more syringes are being manufactured with mL and no minim markings.
- The milliliter (mL) is the correct measure for volume. Although a few syringes may still indicate cubic centimeters (cc), technically this is incorrect.

 **Practice Problems**

Shade in the indicated amounts on the syringes in milliliters.
  1.  0.8 mL

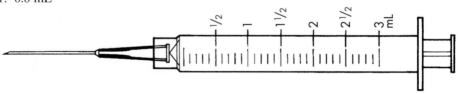

2. 1.2 mL

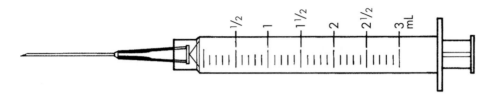

3. 1.5 mL

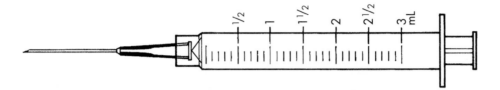

4. 2.4 mL

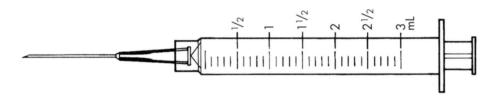

Indicate the number of milliliters shaded in on the following syringes.

5.

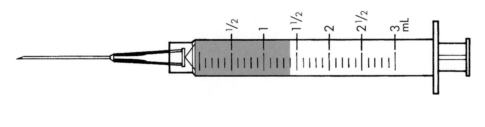

_____

6.

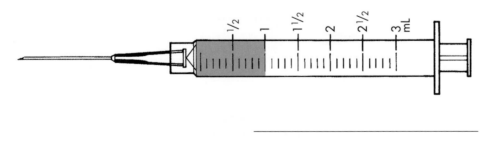

_____

7.

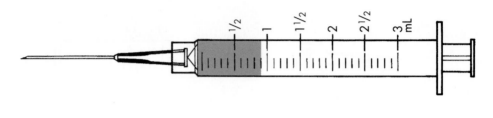

8.

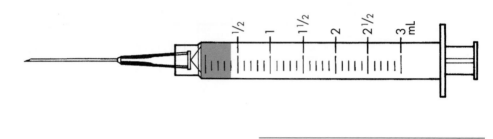

Answers on p. 633

The larger hypodermics (5, 6, 10, and 12 mL) are used when volumes larger than 3 mL are desired. These syringes are used to measure whole numbers of milliliters as opposed to smaller units such as a tenth of a milliliter. Syringes 5, 6, 10, and 12 mL in size are calibrated in increments of fifths of a milliliter (0.2 mL), with the whole numbers indicated by the long lines. Figure 18-13, *A,* shows 0.8 mL of medication measured in a 5-mL syringe, and Figure 18-13, *B,* shows 7.8 mL measured in a 10-mL syringe. Syringes that are 20 mL and larger are calibrated in whole milliliter increments and can have other measures, such as ounces, on them.

## Tips for Clinical Practice

The larger the syringe, the larger the calibration. Example: In 5-mL and 10-mL syringes, each shorter calibration measures two tenths of a milliliter (0.2 mL).

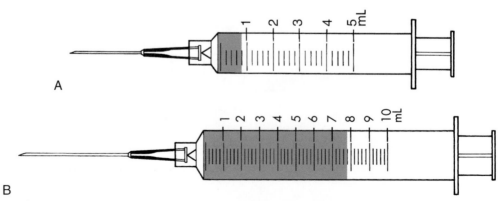

**Figure 18-13**   Large hypodermics. **A,** 5-mL syringe filled with 0.8 mL. **B,** 10-mL syringe filled with 7.8 mL.

## Practice Problems

Indicate the number of milliliters shaded in on the following syringes.

9.

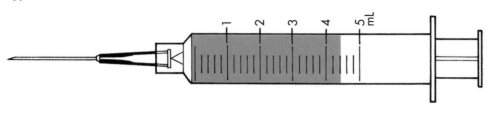

_____

10.

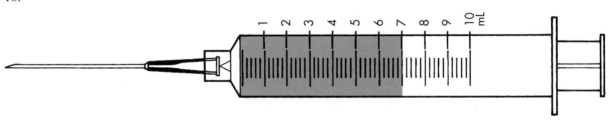

_____

11.

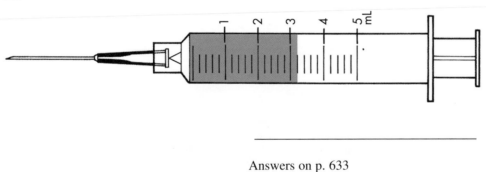

_____

Answers on p. 633

_____

*TUBERCULIN SYRINGE*   A tuberculin syringe is a narrow syringe that has a capacity of 0.5 mL or 1 mL. The 1-mL size is used most often. The volume of a tuberculin syringe can be measured on the milliliter scale. On the milliliter side of the syringe, the syringe is calibrated in hundredths (0.01 mL) and tenths (0.1 mL) of a milliliter. The markings on the syringe (lines) are closer together to indicate how small the calibrations are (Figure 18-14).

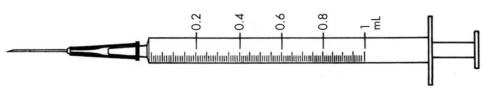

**Figure 18-14**   Tuberculin syringe. (From Potter PA, Perry AG: *Fundamentals of nursing,* ed. 7, St. Louis, 2009, Mosby.)

Tuberculin syringes are used to accurately measure medications given in very small volumes (e.g., heparin). This syringe is also often used in pediatrics and for diagnostic purposes (e.g., skin testing for tuberculosis). It is recommended that dosages less than 0.5 mL be measured with a tuberculin syringe to make certain that the correct dosage is administered to a client. Dosages such as 0.42 mL and 0.37 mL can be measured accurately with a tuberculin syringe. When a tuberculin syringe is used, it is important to read the markings carefully to avoid error.

*INSULIN SYRINGES*   Insulin syringes are designed for the administration of insulin only. Insulin dosages are measured in units. Insulin syringes are calibrated to match the dosage strength of the insulin being used. They are marked U-100 and are designed to be used with insulin that is marked U-100.

> **CAUTION**
>
> U-100 insulin should be measured only in a U-100 insulin syringe. It is important to note that for U-100 insulin, 100 units = 1 mL.

There are two types of insulin syringes: Lo-Dose and 1-mL size.

The *Lo-Dose syringe* is used to measure small dosages and is 0.5 mL or 0.3 mL in size. It may be used for clients receiving 50 units or less of U-100 insulin. It has a capacity of 50 units. The scale on the Lo-Dose syringe is easy to read. Each calibration (shorter lines) measures 1 unit, and each 5-unit increment is numbered (long lines) (Figure 18-15, *B*).

A 30-unit syringe, which is also a Lo-Dose syringe, is available for use with U-100 insulin only and is designed for small dosages of 30 units or less. Each increment on the

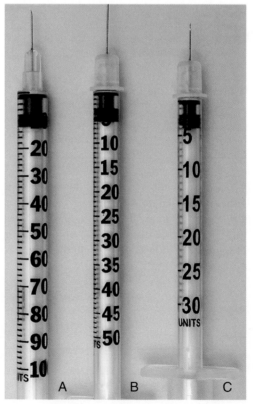

**Figure 18-15**   Insulin syringes. **A,** 1-mL size (100 units). **B,** Lo-Dose (50 units). **C,** Lo-Dose (30 units).

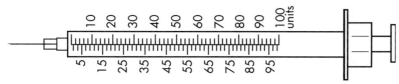

**Figure 18-16**   1-mL capacity insulin syringe (100 units) with dual scale odd and even calibrations.

syringe represents 1 unit (Figure 18-15, *C*). A 30-unit insulin syringe is commonly used in pediatrics to administer insulin.

The *1-mL size syringe* is designed to hold 100 units. There are currently two types on the market. One type of 1-mL (100-unit) capacity has each 10-unit increment numbered. This syringe is calibrated in 2-unit increments (see Figure 18-15, *A*). Odd-numbered units are therefore measured between the even calibrations. Measurement of dosages that are approximate (in between lines) should be avoided. The second type of 1-mL–capacity syringe has two scales on it. The odd numbers are on the left of the syringe, and the even numbers are on the right. The calibrations are in 1-unit increments. The best method for using this type of syringe is the following: Measure uneven dosages on the left, and measure even dosages using the scale on the right (see Figure 18-16). The calculation of insulin dosages and reading of the calibrations are discussed in more detail in Chapter 20.

## Tips for Clinical Practice

It is important to note that insulin syringes do not have detachable needles. The needle, hub, and barrel are inseparable.

## Critical Thinking

- Dosages must be measurable and appropriate for the syringe used.
- When reading syringes with both minim (m.) and milliliter (mL) calibration, remember that they are not the same measurement. It is critical to avoid making errors with m. and mL. Do not use the minim scale on any syringe.
- The insulin syringe and the tuberculin syringe are different. Confusion of the two can cause a medication error.
- Measure insulin in an insulin syringe only.
- If the dosage cannot be accurately measured, do not administer.

## Points to Remember

- When parenteral medications are prepared for administration, it is important to use the correct syringe for accurate administration of the dosage.
- Most medications are prepared and labeled with the dosage strength given per milliliter (mL). Remember that although you may see these terms used interchangeably and as equivalent measures (1 cc = 1 mL), technically they are not equivalents; milliliter should be used instead of cubic centimeter.
- Syringes are available with milliliters and without minims.
- Small-capacity hypodermic syringes are marked in tenths of a milliliter (0.1 mL). The 3-mL size is used most often to administer medication volumes greater than 1 mL. If minims are on a syringe, it is *important* not to confuse the minim scale with the metric scale (mL). The use of minims is discouraged.

*Continued*

- Hypodermic syringes—5, 6, 10, and 12 mL—are marked in increments of 0.2 mL and 1 mL.
- Hypodermic syringes—20 mL and larger—are marked in 1-mL increments and may have other markings, such as ounces.
- Tuberculin syringes or 1-mL syringes are small syringes marked in tenths and hundredths of a milliliter. They are used to administer small dosages and are recommended for use with a dosage less than 0.5 mL.
- Insulin syringes are marked U-100 for administration with U-100 insulin only. Insulin is measured in units and should be administered only with an insulin syringe.
- Dosages involving milliliters should be expressed as decimals even when the syringe is marked with fractions. The milliliter is a metric measure.

Before proceeding to discuss calculation of parenteral dosages, it is necessary to review some specifics in terms of reading labels. Reading the label and understanding what information is essential are important in determining the correct dosage to administer.

## READING PARENTERAL LABELS

The information contained on the parenteral label is similar to the information on an oral liquid label. It contains the total volume of the container and the dosage strength (amount of medication in solution) expressed in milliliters. It is important to read the label carefully to determine the dosage strength and volume. Example: 25 mg per mL. Let's examine some labels.

The diazepam label in Figure 18-17 tells us that the total size of the vial is 10 mL. The dosage strength is 5 mg per mL. The Corvert label shown in Figure 18-18 indicates that the total vial size is 10 mL and there are 0.1 mg per mL.

Some labels may contain two systems of measurement (e.g., apothecary and metric). The dosage strength on parenteral labels can be expressed in the metric or apothecary system or in a combination of the two systems. When apothecary measures are indicated on a label, the equivalent in metric measures is indicated as well.

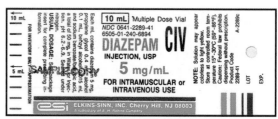

**Figure 18-17**    Diazepam label.

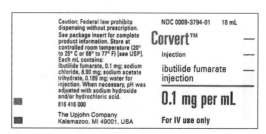

**Figure 18-18**    Corvert label.

**Practice Problems**

Use the labels provided to answer the questions.

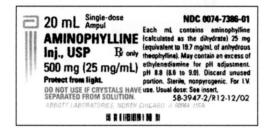

Using the aminophylline label above, answer the following questions:

12.  a.  What is the total volume of the ampule? _____

   b.  What is the dosage strength? _____

   c.  If 250 mg was ordered, how many
       milliliters would this be? _____

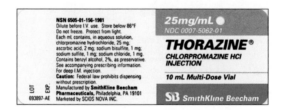

Using the Corvert label above, answer the following questions:

13.  a.  What is the total volume of the vial? _____

   b.  What is the dosage strength? _____

   c.  What is the route of administration? _____

Using the Thorazine label above, answer the following questions:

14.  a.  What is the total volume of the vial? _____

   b.  What is the dosage strength? _____

   c.  If 50 mg was ordered, how many
       milliliters would this be? _____

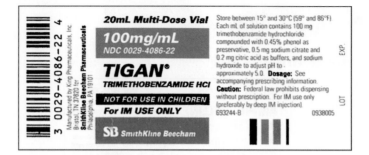

Using the Tigan label above, answer the following questions:

15. a. What is the total volume of the vial?          _____

    b. What is the dosage strength?          _____

    c. If 50 mg was ordered, how many
       milliliters would this be?          _____

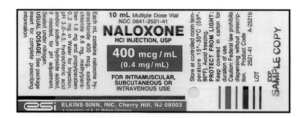

Using the naloxone label above, answer the following questions:

16. a. What is the total volume of the vial?          _____

    b. What is the dosage strength?          _____

    c. What is the route of administration?          _____

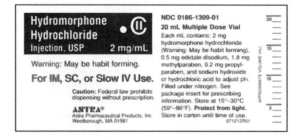

Using the hydromorphone label above, answer the following questions:

17. a. What is the total volume of the vial?          _____

    b. What is the dosage strength?          _____

    c. What is the controlled substance schedule?_____

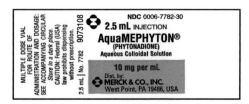

Using the AquaMEPHYTON label above, answer the following questions:

18.  a.  What is the total volume of the vial?  _____

b.  What is the dosage strength?  _____

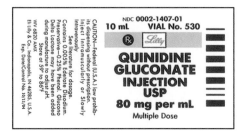

Using the quinidine gluconate label above, answer the following questions:

19.  a.  What is the total volume of the vial?  _____

b.  What is the dosage strength?  _____

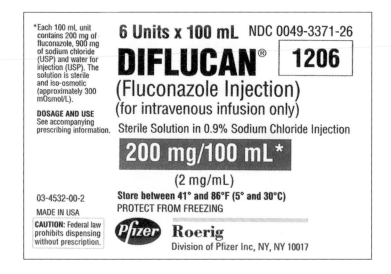

Using the Diflucan label above, answer the following questions:

20.  a.  What is the dosage strength?  _____

b.  What is the route of administration?  _____

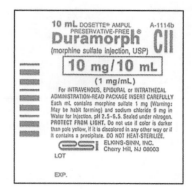

Using the Duramorph label above, answer the following questions:

21. a. What is the total volume of the ampule? _____

    b. What is the dosage strength? _____

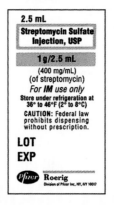

Using the streptomycin sulfate label above, answer the following questions:

22. a. What is the total volume? _____

    b. What is the dosage strength? _____

    c. What is the route of administration? _____

Answers on p. 633

Parenteral labels can express medications in percentage strengths, as well as units and milliequivalents.

## MEDICATIONS LABELED IN PERCENTAGE STRENGTHS

Medications that are labeled as percentage solutions give information such as the percentage of the solution and the total volume of the vial or ampule. Although percentage is used, metric measures are used as well. Example: In the figure below, which shows a label of lidocaine 1%, notice that there are 10 mg per mL. As discussed in Chapter 5, percentage solutions express the number of grams of the medication per 100 mL of solution. In the lidocaine label shown, lidocaine 1% contains 1 g of medication per 100 mL of solution, 1 g per 100 mL = 1,000 mg per 100 mL = 10 mg per mL.

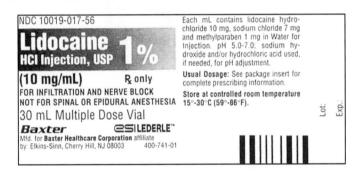

Often no calculation is necessary when medications expressed in percentage strength are given. The prescriber usually states the number of milliliters to prepare or may state it in the number of ampules or vials. Example: Calcium gluconate 10% may be ordered as "Administer one vial of 10% calcium gluconate or 10 mL of 10% calcium gluconate" (see label below).

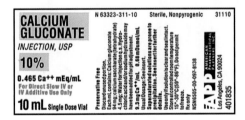

## SOLUTIONS EXPRESSED IN RATIO STRENGTH

A medication commonly expressed in terms of ratio strength is epinephrine. Medications expressed this way include metric measures as well and are often ordered by the number of milliliters. Example: Epinephrine may state 1:1,000 and indicate 1 mg per mL. Ratio solutions, as discussed in Chapter 4 on ratio and proportion, express the number of grams of the medication per total milliliters of solution. Epinephrine 1:1,000 contains 1 g medication per 1,000 mL solution, 1 g:1,000 mL = 1,000 mg:1,000 mL = 1 mg:1 mL. (See the label below.)

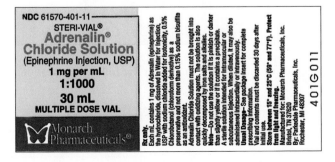

## PARENTERAL MEDICATIONS MEASURED IN UNITS

Some medications measured in units for parenteral administration are heparin, Pitocin, insulin, and penicillin. Notice that the labels indicate how many units per milliliters. Examples: Pitocin 10 units per mL, heparin 1,000 units per mL. Units express the amount of medication present in 1 mL of solution, and they are specific to the medication for which they are used. Units measure a medication in terms of its action (see heparin and insulin labels below).

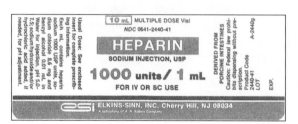
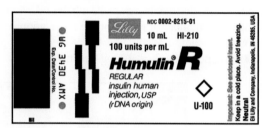

## PARENTERAL MEDICATIONS IN MILLIEQUIVALENTS

Potassium and sodium bicarbonate are medications that are expressed in milliequivalents. Like units, milliequivalents are specific measurements that have no conversion to another system and are specific to the medication used. Milliequivalents (mEq) are used to measure electrolytes (e.g., potassium) and the ionic activity of a medication. Milliequivalents are also defined as an expression of the number of grams of a medication contained in 1 mL of a normal solution. This definition is often used by a chemist or pharmacist. (See potassium label below.)

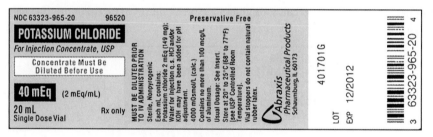

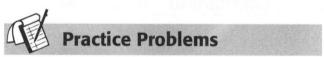
**Practice Problems**

Use the labels provided to answer the questions.

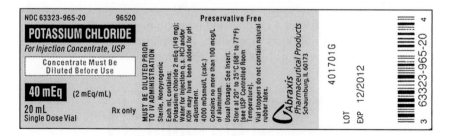

Use the potassium chloride label above to answer the following questions:

23. a. What is the total volume of the vial?  _____

    b. What is the dosage in milliequivalents per milliliter?  _____

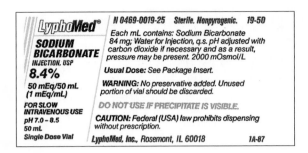

Use the sodium bicarbonate label above to answer the following questions:

24. a. What is the total volume of the vial? _____

    b. What is the dosage strength expressed
       in milliequivalents per milliliter? _____

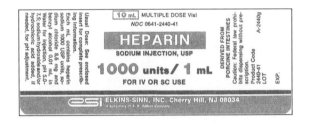

Use the heparin label above to answer the following questions:

25. a. What is the total volume of the vial? _____

    b. What is the dosage strength? _____

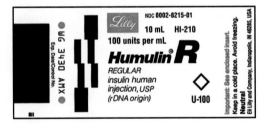

Use the insulin label above to answer the following questions:

26. a. What is the total volume of the vial? _____

    b. What is the dosage strength? _____

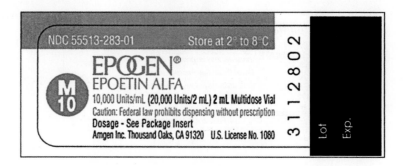

Use the Epogen label above to answer the following questions:

27. a.  What is the total volume of the vial?    _____

    b.  What is the dosage strength?    _____

Answers on p. 633

## Tips for Clinical Practice

It is important to read the labels on parenteral medications carefully. Labels on parenteral medications include a variety of units to express dosage strengths. To calculate dosages to administer it is important to know the strength of the medication in solution per milliliter. Confusing dosage strength with total volume can lead to a medication error.

## CALCULATING PARENTERAL DOSAGES

As previously stated, parenteral dosages can be calculated by using the same rules and methods used to compute oral dosages. Ratio and proportion, the formula method, and dimensional analysis have been presented in earlier chapters. The following guidelines will help you calculate a dosage that is logical, reasonable, and accurate.

### Guidelines for Calculating Parenteral Dosages

- To calculate parenteral dosages, convert if necessary, **THINK,** and calculate using one of the methods presented (ratio and proportion, the formula method, or dimensional analysis).

Calculate dosages and prepare injectable dosages using the following guidelines:
- The 3-mL syringe is calibrated in 0.1-mL increments. Round milliliters to the nearest tenth to measure in a 3-mL syringe; **never round to a whole unit.** If math calculation does not work out evenly to the tenths place, then carry division to the hundredths place (two decimal places) and round to the nearest tenth.
  **Example:**    1.75 mL = 1.8 mL
- The 1-mL (tuberculin syringe) is calibrated in 0.01-mL increments. If the math calculation does not work out evenly to the hundredths place, then the division is carried to the thousandths place and rounded to the hundredths place.
  **Example:**    0.876 mL = 0.88 mL. It is recommended that dosages less than 0.5 mL be measured with a 1-mL syringe.
- Large syringes (5-, 6-, 10-, and 12-mL) are calibrated in 0.2-mL increments. Dosages are also expressed to the nearest tenth.
- Dosages administered should be measured in milliliters, and the answer should be labeled accordingly.
- Insulin is measured and administered in units.

For injectable medications, there are guidelines as to the amount of medication that can be administered in a particular site.

> When the dosage for parenteral administration exceeds these guidelines, the dosage should be questioned, and the calculation should be double-checked.

- IM—According to Harkreader and Hogan (2007), the normal well-developed client can tolerate administration of 4 mL of medication into a well-developed muscle (e.g., the gluteus). A volume of 0.5 mL is recommended in the deltoid muscle, depending on client size. Children and older adults should not receive more than 1 or 2 mL. Wong and Hockenberry (2007) recommend giving no more than 1 mL to small children and older infants. Small infants should receive no more than 0.5 mL. (It should be noted that IM injections are less common today in the clinical setting than in the past.) Most IM injections do not exceed 2 or 3 mL.
- Subcutaneous—The volume that can be administered safely in an adult is 0.5 to 1 mL.

In administering medications by injection, the condition of the client, age of the client, site selected, and absorption and consistency of the medication must also be considered. For example, a dosage of 4 mL of a thick oily substance may be divided into two injections of 2 mL. Depending on his or her condition, a client may not be able to tolerate the maximum dosage volumes.

- Injectables that are added to an IV solution may have a volume greater than 5 mL.
- Always proceed with calculations in a logical and reasonable manner.

## Tips for Clinical Practice

It is critical to choose the correct size syringe to ensure accurate measurement.

## CALCULATING INJECTABLE MEDICATIONS ACCORDING TO THE SYRINGE

Now that you have an understanding of syringes and guidelines, let's begin calculating dosages.

Now, with the guidelines in mind, let's look at some sample problems. Regardless of what method you use to calculate, the following steps are used:
1. Check to make sure everything is in the same system and unit of measure.
2. Think critically about what the answer should logically be.
3. Consider the type of syringe being used. **The cardinal rule should always be that any dosage given must be able to be measured accurately in the syringe you are using.**
4. Use ratio and proportion, the formula method, or dimensional analysis to calculate the dosage. Let's look at some sample problems calculating parenteral dosages on the following pages.

**Example 1:**    Order: Gentamicin 75 mg IM q8h

Available: Gentamicin labeled 40 mg per mL

*Note:* No conversion is necessary here. Think—The dosage ordered is going to be more than 1 mL but less than 2 mL. Set up and solve.

### ➡ Solution Using Ratio and Proportion

$$40 \text{ mg} : 1 \text{ mL} = 75 \text{ mg} : x \text{ mL}$$

$$\frac{40x}{40} = \frac{75}{40}$$

$$x = 1.87 \text{ mL} = 1.9 \text{ mL}$$

**Answer:**    1.9 mL

The answer here is rounded to the nearest tenth of a milliliter. Remember that you are using a small hypodermic syringe marked in tenths of a milliliter.

### ➡ Solution Using the Formula Method

$$\frac{\text{(D) } 75 \text{ mg}}{\text{(H) } 40 \text{ mg}} \times \text{(Q) } 1 \text{ mL} = x \text{ mL}$$

$$x = \frac{75}{40}$$

$$x = 1.87 \text{ mL} = 1.9 \text{ mL}$$

**Answer:**    1.9 mL

### ➡ Solution Using Dimensional Analysis

$$x \text{ mL} = \frac{1 \text{ mL}}{40 \text{ mg}} \times \frac{75 \text{ mg}}{1}$$

$$x = \frac{75}{40}$$

$$x = 1.87 \text{ mL} = 1.9 \text{ mL}$$

**Answer:**    1.9 mL

Refer to the syringe below illustrating 1.9 mL shaded in on the syringe.

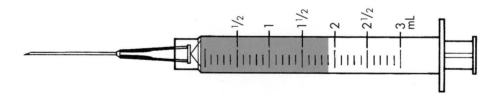

**Example 2:** Order: Kantrex 500 mg IM q12h

Available: Kanamycin (Kantrex) labeled 0.5 g per 2 mL

In this problem a conversion is necessary. Equivalent: 1,000 mg = 1 g. Convert what is ordered to what is available: 500 mg = 0.5 g. To get rid of the decimal point, convert what is available to what is ordered: 0.5 g = 500 mg. (Note setup in examples illustrating this.) Remember that either way will net the same final answer.

Think—The dosage you will need to give is greater than 1 mL, and it is being given intramuscularly. The dosage therefore should fall within the range that is safe for IM administration. The solution, after making conversion, is as follows:

 ## Solution Using Ratio and Proportion

$$0.5 \text{ g} : 2 \text{ mL} = 0.5 \text{ g} : x \text{ mL} \quad or \quad 500 \text{ mg} : 2 \text{ mL} = 500 \text{ mg} : x \text{ mL}$$

$$\frac{0.5x}{0.5} = \frac{1.0}{0.5} \qquad\qquad \frac{500x}{500} = \frac{1,000}{500}$$

$$x = \frac{1.0}{0.5} \qquad\qquad x = \frac{1,000}{500}$$

$$x = 2 \text{ mL} \qquad\qquad x = 2 \text{ mL}$$

**Answer:** 2 mL

 ## Solution Using the Formula Method

$$\frac{(D)\ 0.5 \text{ g}}{(H)\ 0.5 \text{ g}} \times (Q)\ 2 \text{ mL} = x \text{ mL} \quad or \quad \frac{(D)\ 500 \text{ mg}}{(H)\ 500 \text{ mg}} \times (Q)\ 2 \text{ mL} = x \text{ mL}$$

$$x = \frac{0.5 \times 2}{0.5} \qquad\qquad x = \frac{1,000}{500}$$

$$x = \frac{1}{0.5} \qquad\qquad x = 2 \text{ mL}$$

$$x = 2 \text{ mL}$$

 ## Solution Using Dimensional Analysis

$$x \text{ mL} = \frac{2 \text{ mL}}{0.5 \ \cancel{g}} \times \frac{1 \ \cancel{g}}{\underset{2}{\cancel{1,000} \ \text{mg}}} \times \frac{\overset{1}{\cancel{500}} \ \text{mg}}{1} \qquad \textit{(Note: Reduction was done here.)}$$

*Note:* Reduction was done here: $x = \dfrac{2}{1}$

$$x = 2 \text{ mL}$$

**Answer:** 2 mL

Refer to the syringe below illustrating 2 mL drawn up.

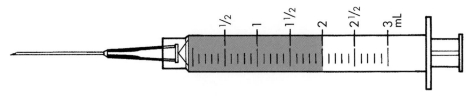

**Example 3:**   Order: Morphine sulfate gr ½ IM stat

Available: Morphine sulfate in a 20-mL vial, labeled 15 mg per mL

## Problem Setup

1. A conversion is necessary. Convert gr ½ to milligrams using the equivalent 60 mg = gr 1; gr ½ therefore is 30 mg.
2. Think—You will need more than 1 mL to administer the dosage.
3. Set up the problem, and calculate the dosage to be administered.

## Solution Using Ratio and Proportion

$$15 \text{ mg} : 1 \text{ mL} = 30 \text{ mg} : x \text{ mL}$$

$$\frac{\cancel{15}x}{\cancel{15}} = \frac{30}{15}$$

$$x = 2 \text{ mL}$$

**Answer:**   2 mL

## Solution Using the Formula Method

$$\frac{(D) \ 30 \text{ mg}}{(H) \ 15 \text{ mg}} \times (Q) \ 1 \text{ mL} = x \text{ mL}$$

$$x = \frac{30}{15}$$

$$x = 2 \text{ mL}$$

**Answer:**   2 mL

## Solution Using Dimensional Analysis

$$x \text{ mL} = \frac{1 \text{ mL}}{\underset{1}{\cancel{15} \text{ mg}}} \times \frac{\overset{4}{\cancel{60} \text{ mg}}}{\cancel{gr} \ 1} \times \frac{\cancel{gr} \ \dfrac{1}{2}}{1}$$

(*Note:* Reduction was done here.)

$$x = \frac{4 \times \dfrac{1}{2}}{1} = \frac{2}{1}$$

$$x = 2 \text{ mL}$$

**Answer:**   2 mL

Refer to Example 2 to visualize 2 mL in a syringe.

**Example 4:**   Order: Atropine sulfate gr $\frac{1}{100}$ IM stat

Available: Atropine sulfate in 20-mL vial labeled 0.4 mg per mL

 Problem Setup

1. A conversion is necessary. Convert gr $\frac{1}{100}$ to milligrams using the equivalent 60 mg = gr 1; gr $\frac{1}{100}$ is therefore 0.6 mg.
2. Think—You will need more than 1 mL to administer the required dosage.
3. Set up the problem, and calculate the dosage to be administered.

 Solution Using Ratio and Proportion

$$0.4 \text{ mg}:1 \text{ mL} = 0.6 \text{ mg}:x \text{ mL}$$

$$\frac{0.4x}{0.4} = \frac{0.6}{0.4}$$

$$x = \frac{0.6}{0.4}$$

$$x = 1.5 \text{ mL}$$

**Answer:**     1.5 mL

Note that some small hypodermics have fraction markings; however, milliliter is metric and should be stated by using a decimal.

 Solution Using the Formula Method

$$\frac{(D)\ 0.6 \text{ mg}}{(H)\ 0.4 \text{ mg}} \times (Q)\ 1 \text{ mL} = x \text{ mL}$$

$$x = \frac{0.6}{0.4}$$

$$x = 1.5 \text{ mL}$$

**Answer:**     1.5 mL

 Solution Using Dimensional Analysis

$$x \text{ mL} = \frac{1 \text{ mL}}{0.4 \text{ mg}} \times \frac{60 \text{ mg}}{\text{gr } 1} \times \frac{\text{gr } \frac{1}{100}}{1}$$

$$\left(\frac{4}{10}\right)$$

(*Note:* Reduction was done here.)

$$x = \frac{60 \times \frac{1}{10}}{4} = \frac{6}{4}$$

$$x = 1.5 \text{ mL}$$

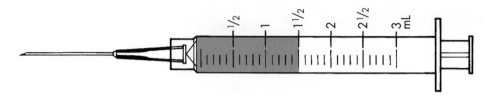

**Answer:** 1.5 mL

Refer to the illustration below showing 1.5 mL shaded in on the syringe.

## CALCULATING DOSAGES FOR MEDICATIONS IN UNITS

As previously mentioned, certain medications are measured in units. Some medications measured in units include vitamins, antibiotics, insulin, and heparin. The calculation of insulin will be discussed in Chapter 20. Insulin syringes are used for insulin only. In determining the dosage to administer when medications are measured in units, use the same steps as with other parenteral medications. Dosages of certain medications such as heparin are administered with a tuberculin syringe, as opposed to a hypodermic syringe (2, 2½, 3 mL). Because of its effects, heparin is never rounded off, but rather, exact dosages are given. Heparin will also be discussed in more detail in Chapter 23. Let's look at sample problems with units.

**Example 1:** Order: Heparin 750 units subcut daily

Available: Heparin 1,000 units per mL

Using a 1-mL (tuberculin) syringe, calculate the dosage to be administered.

 Problem Setup

1. No conversion is required. No conversion exists for units.
2. Think. The dosage to be given is less than 1 mL. This dosage can be accurately measured in a 1-mL tuberculin syringe. Heparin is administered in exact dosages.
3. Set up the problem, and calculate the dosage to be given.

**CAUTION**

Because of the action of heparin, an exact dosage is crucial; the dosage should not be rounded off.

Solution Using Ratio and Proportion

$$1,000 \text{ units} : 1 \text{ mL} = 750 \text{ units} : x \text{ mL}$$

$$\frac{1000x}{1000} = \frac{750}{1,000}$$

$$x = \frac{75}{1,000}$$

$$x = 0.75 \text{ mL}$$

**Answer:** 0.75 mL

Solution Using the Formula Method

$$\frac{\text{(D) 750 units}}{\text{(H) 1,000 units}} \times \text{(Q) 1 mL} = x \text{ mL}$$

$$x = \frac{750}{1,000}$$

$$x = 0.75 \text{ mL}$$

**Answer:**    0.75 mL

 Solution Using Dimensional Analysis

$$x \text{ mL} = \frac{1 \text{ mL}}{100\cancel{0} \text{ units}} \times \frac{75\cancel{0} \text{ units}}{1}$$    (Note cancellation of zeros to make numbers smaller.)

$$x = \frac{75}{100}$$

$$x = 0.75 \text{ mL}$$

**Answer:**    0.75 mL

Refer to the syringe illustrating 0.75 mL shaded in.

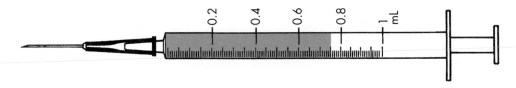

**Example 2:**    Order: Penicillin G procaine, 500,000 units IM b.i.d.

Available: Penicillin G procaine labeled 300,000 units per mL

 Problem Setup

1. No conversion is required.
2. Think—The dosage ordered is more than the available strength. Therefore more than 1 mL would be required to administer the dosage.
3. Set up the problem using ratio and proportion, the formula method, or dimensional analysis to calculate the dosage.

 Solution Using Ratio and Proportion

$$300,000 \text{ units} : 1 \text{ mL} = 500,000 \text{ units} : x \text{ mL}$$

$$300,000x = 500,000$$

$$x = \frac{500,000}{300,000}$$

$$x = 1.66 \text{ mL} = 1.7 \text{ mL}$$

**NOTE**

The division here is carried two decimal places. This answer is then rounded off to 1.7 mL. Remember that the hypodermic syringe (2, 2½, 3 mL) is marked in tenths of a milliliter.

**Answer:**    1.7 mL

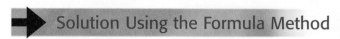

## Solution Using the Formula Method

$$\frac{(D)\ 500{,}000\ units}{(H)\ 300{,}000\ units} \times (Q)\ 1\ mL = x\ mL$$

$$x = \frac{500{,}000}{300{,}000}$$

$$x = 1.66\ mL = 1.7\ mL$$

**Answer:**    1.7 mL

## Solution Using Dimensional Analysis

$$x\ mL = \frac{1\ mL}{300{,}000\ units} \times \frac{500{,}000\ units}{1}$$

$$x = \frac{500{,}000}{300{,}000}$$

$$x = 1.66\ mL = 1.7\ mL$$

**Answer:**    1.7 mL

Refer to the syringe illustrating 1.7 mL shaded in.

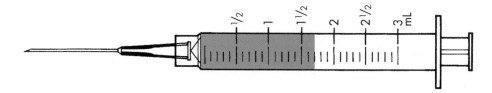

**CAUTION**

Read orders carefully when they are expressed in units. Units should *not* be abbreviated in orders. To avoid confusion, The Joint Commission (TJC) has placed the abbreviations for units (U) on the "do not use" list. This abbreviation is also on ISMP's (Institute for Safe Medication Practices) Error Prone Abbreviations, Symbols, and Dose Designations. Prescribers are required to write out the word *units* to help prevent misinterpretation of an order—for example, "50 ()" as "500 units." (Notice that the U is almost closed; it could be mistaken for a zero and misinterpreted as 500 units.) This error could be fatal.

## MIXING MEDICATIONS IN THE SAME SYRINGE

Two medications may be mixed in one syringe if they are compatible with each other and the total amount does not exceed the amount that can be safely administered in a site. Always consult a reliable reference in regard to compatibility of medications before mixing medications.

When mixing two medications for administration in one syringe, calculate the dosage to be administered in milliliters to the nearest tenth for each of the medications ordered. Then add the results to find the total volume to be combined and administered.

**Example:**   Order: Demerol 65 mg IM and Vistaril 25 mg IM q4h p.r.n. for pain

Available: Demerol 75 mg per mL and Vistaril 50 mg per mL

Solution: Demerol dosage 0.86 = 0.9 mL

Visatril dosage 0.5 mL

0.9 mL Demerol + 0.5 mL Vistaril = 1.4 mL (total volume)

Dosage shaded in one syringe:

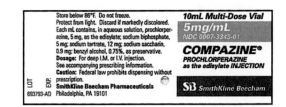

## Practice Problems

Calculate the dosages for the problems below, and indicate the number of milliliters you will administer. Shade in the dosage on the syringe provided. Use medication labels or information provided to calculate the volume necessary to administer the dosage ordered. Express your answers in milliliters to the nearest tenth except where indicated.

28. Order: Compazine 10 mg IM q4h p.r.n.

Available:

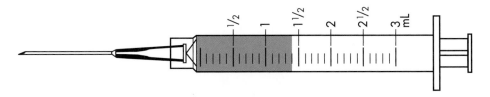

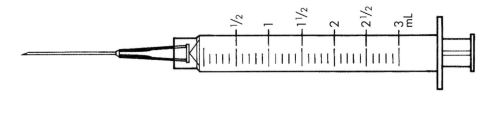

_____

29. Order: AquaMEPHYTON 5 mg subcut every day for 3 days.

    Available:

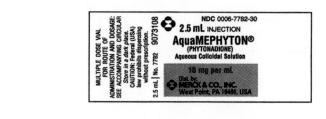

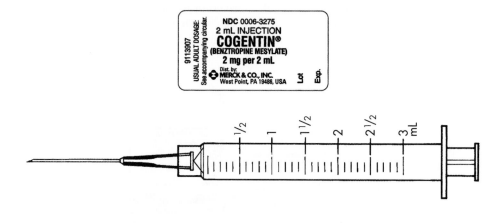

_____

30. Order: Cogentin 1 mg IM stat.

    Available:

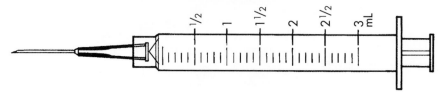

_____

31. Order: Valium (diazepam) 8 mg IM q4h p.r.n. for agitation.

    Available:

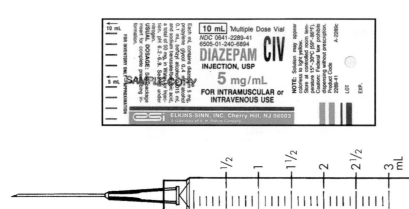

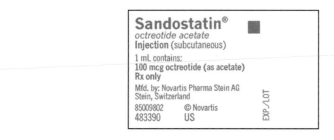

_____

32. Order: Sandostatin 0.05 mg subcut daily.

    Available:

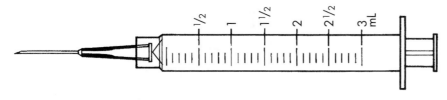

_____

33. Order: Demerol 50 mg IM and Vistaril 25 mg IM q4h p.r.n. for pain.

    Available: Demerol labeled 75 mg per mL
    Vistaril labeled 50 mg per mL

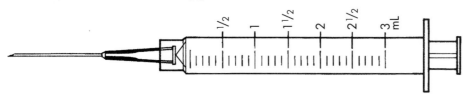

_____

34. Order: Reglan 5 mg IM b.i.d. ½ hour a.c.

Available:

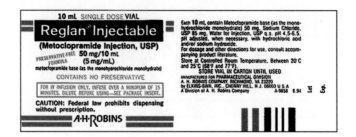

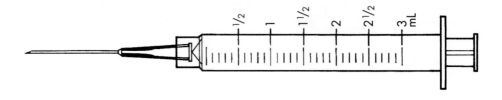

_____

35. Order: Heparin 5,000 units subcut b.i.d.

Available:

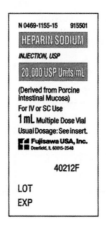

Express your answer in hundredths.    _____

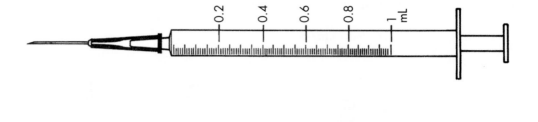

_____

36. Order: Morphine sulfate gr $\frac{1}{4}$ IM q4h p.r.n. for pain.

   Available:

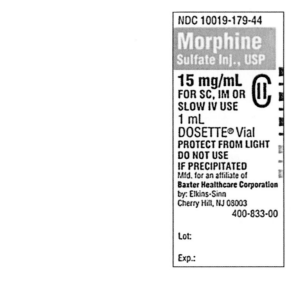

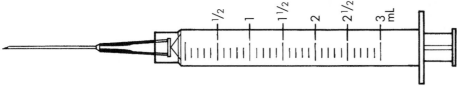

37. Order: Lasix (furosemide) 20 mg IM stat.

   Available:

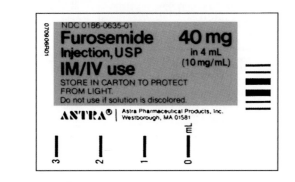

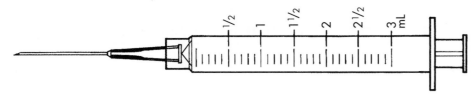

Answers on pp. 633-635

**Critical Thinking Question**

**Scenario:** Prescriber ordered the following:

Hydroxyzine 50 mg IM q4h p.r.n. for anxiety.

Available: Hydroxyzine 25 mg per mL.

The nurse, in error, administered hydralazine 50 mg IM from a vial labeled 20 mg per mL and administered 2.5 mL.

a. What client right was violated? _____

b. What contributed to the error made? _____

c. What is the potential outcome from the error? _____

d. What measures could have been taken to prevent the error? _____

Answers on p. 635

 **CHAPTER REVIEW**

Calculate the dosages for the problems that follow and indicate the number of milliliters you will administer. Shade in the dosage on the syringe provided. Use medication labels or information provided to calculate the volume necessary to administer the dosage ordered. Express your answers to the nearest tenth except where indicated.

1. Order: Clindamycin 0.3 g IM q6h.

   Available:

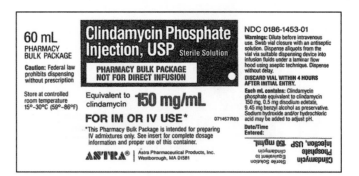

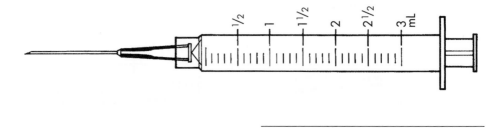

2. Order: Atropine 0.2 mg IM stat.

   Available:

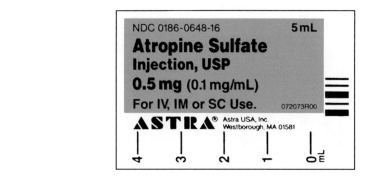

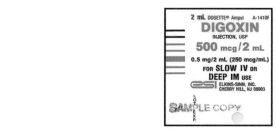

3. Order: Kefzol 0.5 g IM q6h.

   Available: Kefzol after reconstitution labeled 225 mg per mL

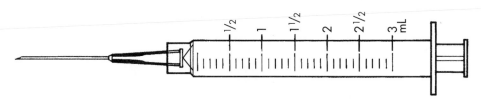

4. Order: Digoxin 100 mcg IM daily.

   Available:

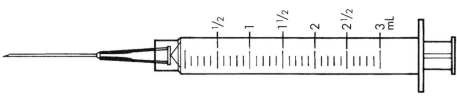

5. Order: Dilaudid HP 4 mg subcut q4h p.r.n. for pain.

   Available:

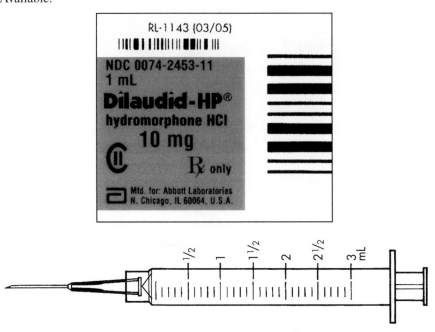

6. Order: Bicillin C-R (900/300) 1,200,000 units IM stat.

   Available:

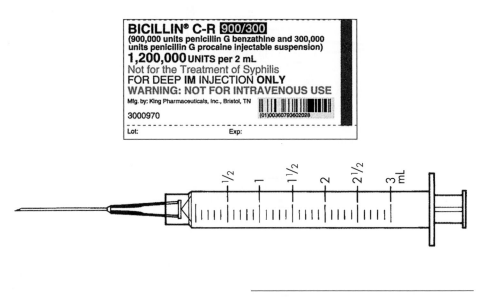

7. Order: Solu-Medrol 100 mg IM q8h for 2 doses.

   Available:

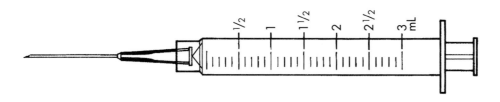

---

8. Order: Methergine 0.4 mg IM q4h for 3 doses.

   Available: Methergine labeled 0.2 mg per mL

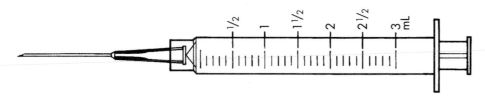

---

9. Order: Heparin 8,000 units subcut q12h.

   Available:

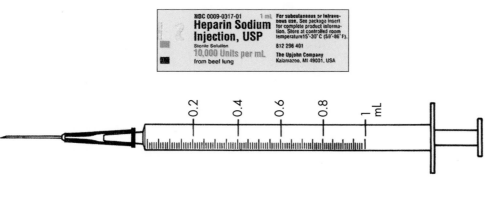

---

10. Order: Dilantin 200 mg IV stat.

    Available:

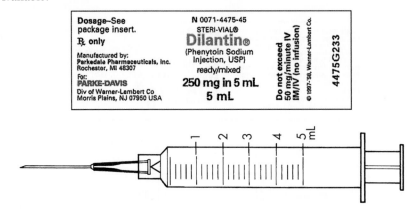

_____

11. Order: Vitamin K (AquaMEPHYTON) 10 mg IM daily for 3 days.

    Available:

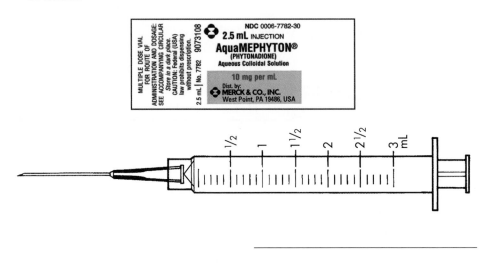

_____

12. Order: Codeine gr ¼ IM q4h p.r.n. for pain.

    Available:

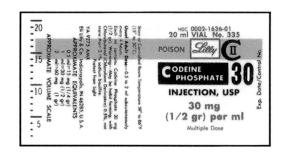

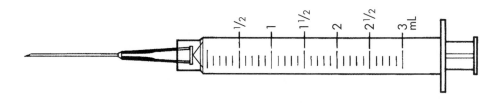

13. Order: Phenergan (promethazine HCl) 25 mg IM q4h p.r.n. for nausea.

    Available:

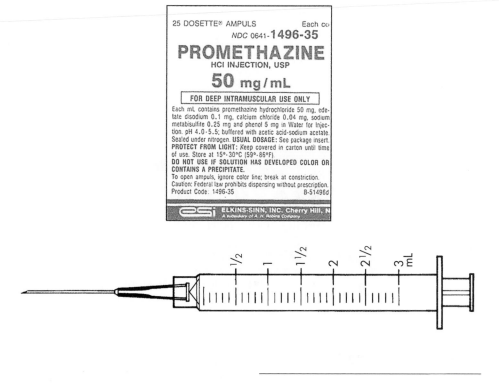

14.  Order: Stadol 1.5 mg IM q4h p.r.n. for pain.

Available: Stadol labeled 2 mg per mL

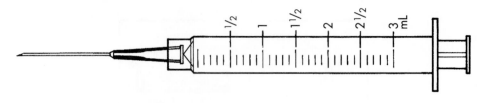

15.  Order: Tobramycin 50 mg IM q8h.

Available:

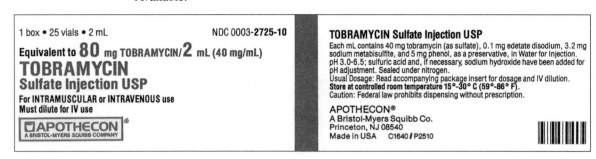

1 box • 25 vials • 2 mL                    NDC 0003-**2725-10**

Equivalent to **80** mg TOBRAMYCIN/**2** mL (40 mg/mL)
**TOBRAMYCIN**
**Sulfate Injection USP**
For INTRAMUSCULAR or INTRAVENOUS use
Must dilute for IV use
**APOTHECON**®
A BRISTOL-MYERS SQUIBB COMPANY

**TOBRAMYCIN Sulfate Injection USP**
Each mL contains 40 mg tobramycin (as sulfate), 0.1 mg edetate disodium, 3.2 mg sodium metabisulfite, and 5 mg phenol, as a preservative, in Water for Injection. pH 3.0-6.5; sulfuric acid and, if necessary, sodium hydroxide have been added for pH adjustment. Sealed under nitrogen.
Usual Dosage: Read accompanying package insert for dosage and IV dilution.
**Store at controlled room temperature 15°-30° C (59°-86° F).**
Caution: Federal law prohibits dispensing without prescription.
**APOTHECON**®
A Bristol-Myers Squibb Co.
Princeton, NJ 08540
Made in USA    C1640 / P2510

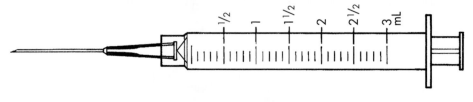

16.  Order: Romazicon 0.2 mg IV stat.

Available:

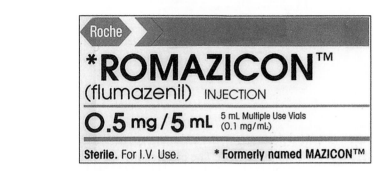

Roche ▸
**\*ROMAZICON**™
(flumazenil) INJECTION
**0.5** mg / **5** mL    5 mL Multiple Use Vials
(0.1 mg/mL)
Sterile. For I.V. Use.    \* Formerly named MAZICON™

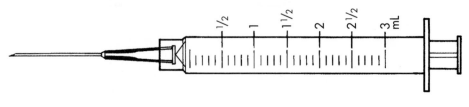

17. Order: Haldol 3 mg IM q6h p.r.n. for agitation.

    Available:

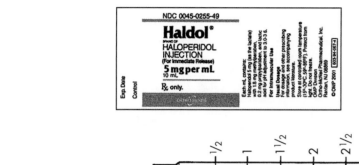

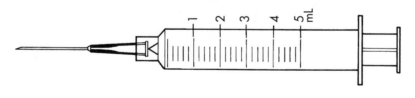

18. Order: Solu-Cortef 400 mg IV every day for a severe inflammation.

    Available:

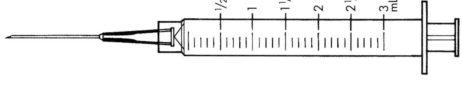

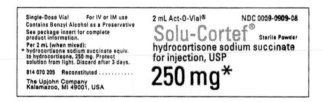

19. Order: Naloxone 0.2 mg IM stat.

    Available:

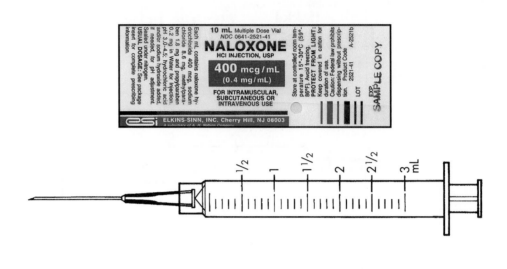

20. Order: Robinul 200 mcg IM on call to the O.R.

    Available:

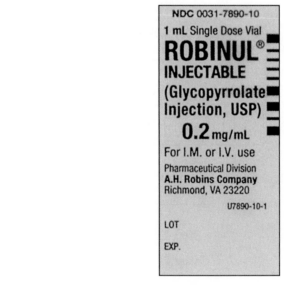

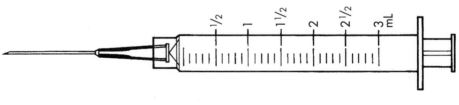

21. Order: Heparin 2,500 units subcut daily (express answer in hundredths).

   Available:

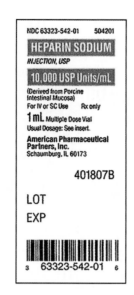

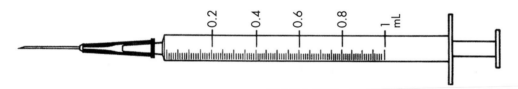

_____

22. Order: Vistaril 35 mg IM stat.

   Available:

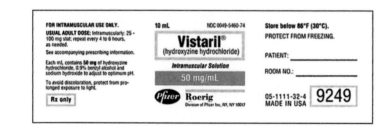

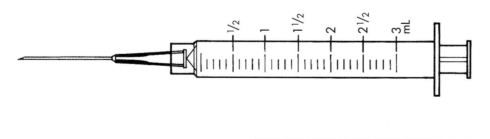

_____

23.  Order: Meperidine 60 mg IM q4h p.r.n. for pain.

Available:

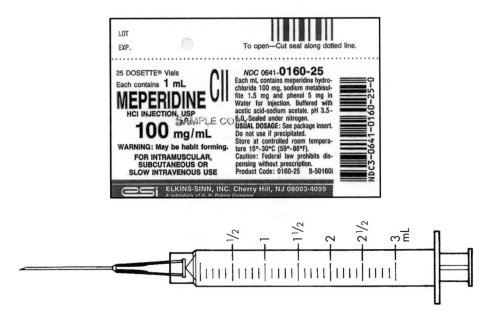

24.  Order: Bicillin 400,000 units IM q4h.

Available:

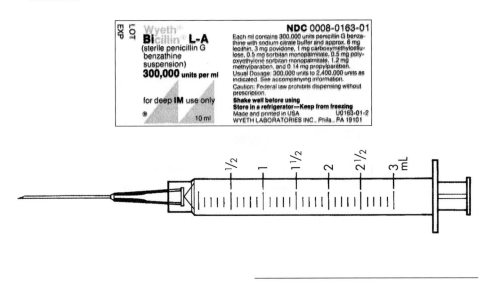

25.  Order: Lanoxin 0.4 mg IM stat.

Available:

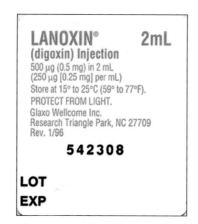

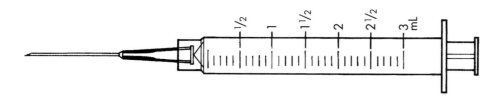

26.  Order: Amikin 100 mg IM q8h.

Available:

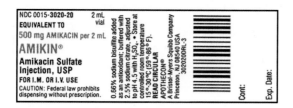

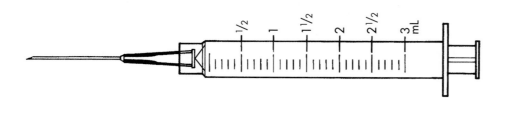

27. Order: Lincocin 500 mg IV q8h.

    Available:

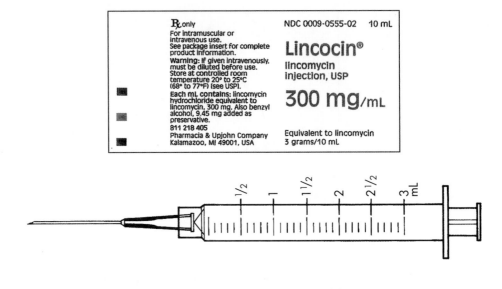

28. Order: Ativan 2 mg IM b.i.d. p.r.n. for agitation.

    Available:

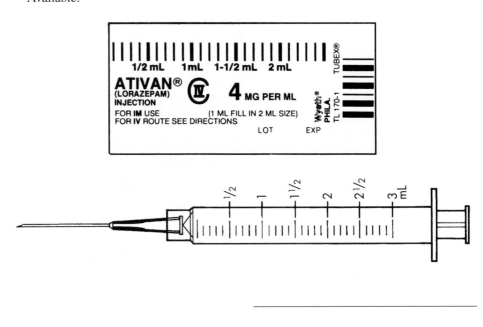

29.  Order: Thorazine 75 mg IM q4h p.r.n.

Available:

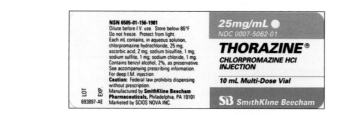

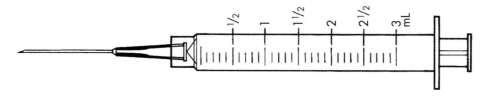

30.  Order: Nembutal sodium 120 mg IM at bedtime p.r.n.

Available:

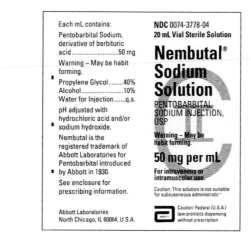

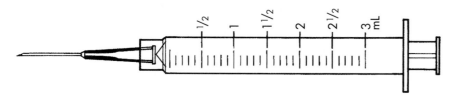

31. Order: Epogen 3,000 units subcut three times per week Monday, Wednesday, and Friday.

    Available: Epogen labeled 2,000 units per mL

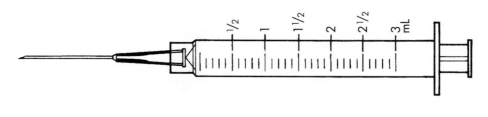

32. Order: Zantac 50 mg IM q8h.

    Available:

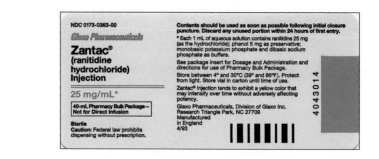

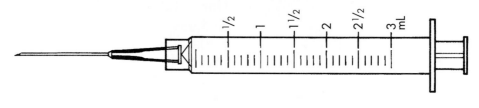

33. Order: Lovenox 30 mg subcut q12h.

    Available:

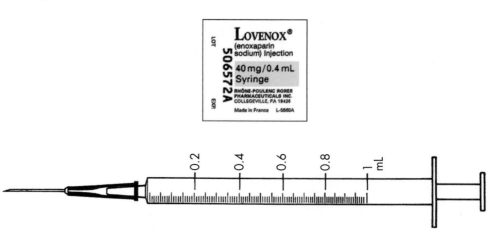

34. Order: Cimetidine 0.3 g IV t.i.d.

    Available:

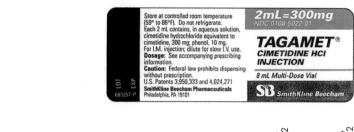

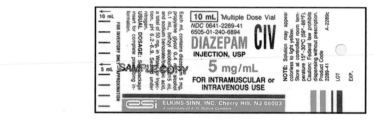

35. Order: Valium (diazepam) 7.5 mg IM stat.

    Available:

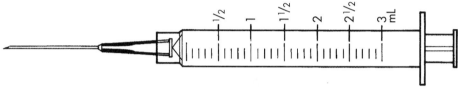

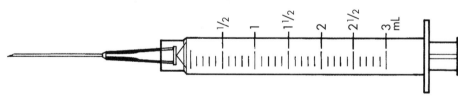

36. Order: Ketorolac 24 mg IV q6h p.r.n. for pain.

Available:

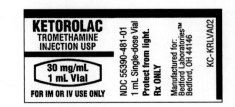

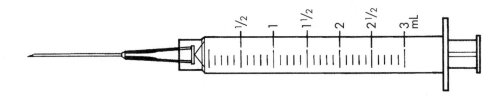

_____

37. Order: Luminal (phenobarbital sodium) 100 mg IM at bedtime.

Available:

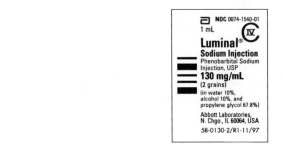

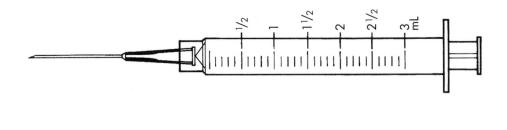

_____

38. Order: Celestone, Soluspan (betamethasone) 12 mg IM q24h for 2 doses.

Available:

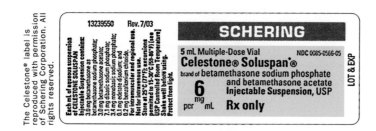

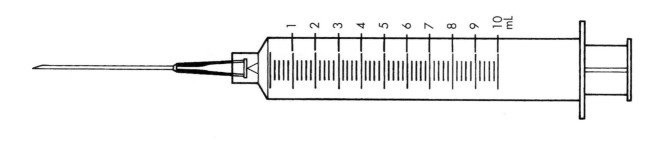

_____

39. Order: Aminophylline 0.25 g IV q6h.

Available:

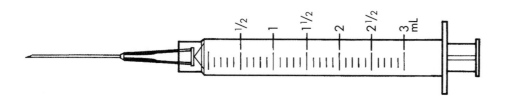

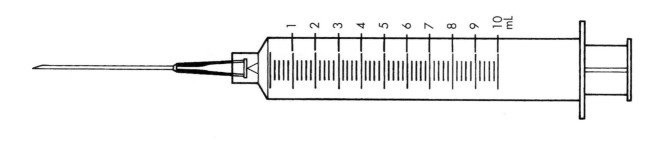

_____

40. Order: Pronestyl 0.5 g IV stat.

    Available:

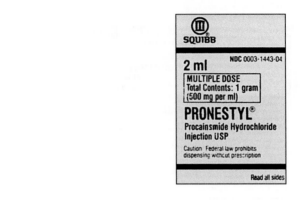

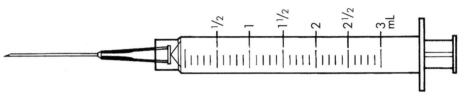

41. Order: Tigan 150 mg IM stat.

    Available:

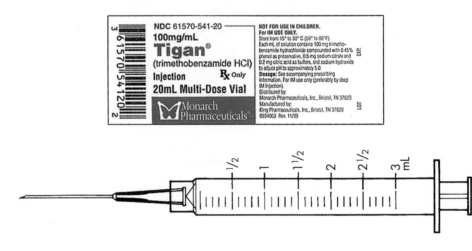

42. Order: Demerol (meperidine) 65 mg IM and Phenergan (promethazine) 25 mg IM q4h p.r.n. for pain.

    Available:

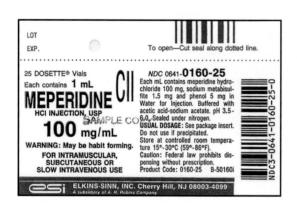

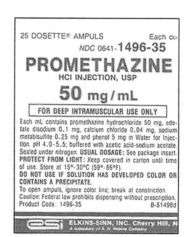

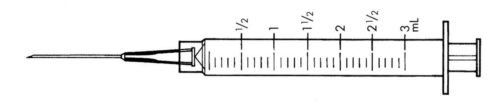

43. Order: Decadron (dexamethasone) 9 mg IV daily for 4 days.

    Available:

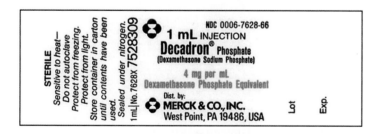

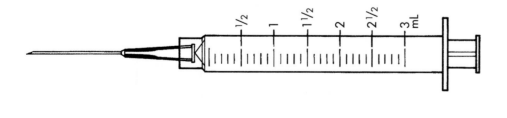

44. Order: Sublimaze (fentanyl) 60 mcg IM 30 minutes before surgery.

Available:

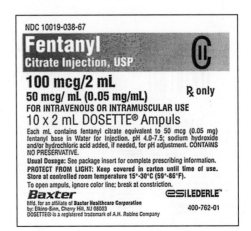

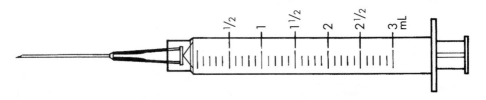

45. Order: Nubain 10 mg IV stat.

Available:

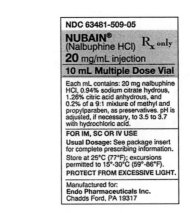

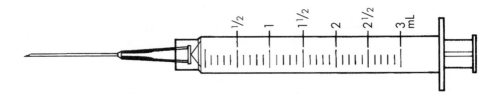

46. Order: Morphine 4 mg IV stat.

   Available:

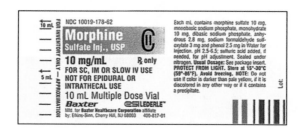

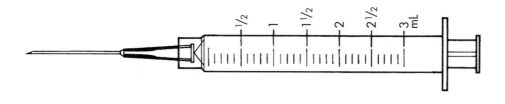

47. Order: Neupogen 175 mcg subcut every day for 2 weeks.

   Available:

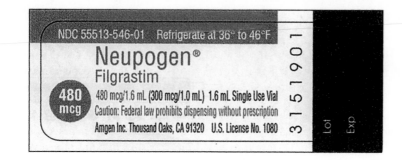

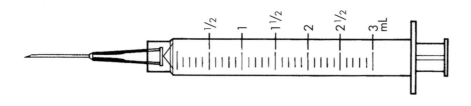

Answers on pp. 635-642

For additional practice problems, refer to the Basic Calculations
section of Drug Calculations Companion, Version 4, on Evolve.

# CHAPTER 19

# Reconstitution of Solutions

## Objectives

*After reviewing this chapter, you should be able to:*
1. Prepare a solution from a powdered medication according to directions on the vial or other resources
2. Identify essential information to be placed on the vial of a medication after it is reconstituted
3. Determine the best concentration strength for medications ordered when there are several directions for mixing
4. Identify the varying directions for reconstitution and select the correct directions to prepare the dosage ordered
5. Calculate dosages from reconstituted medications
6. Determine the rate in milliliters per hour for enteral feedings
7. Calculate the amount of solute and solvent needed to prepare a desired strength for enteral feedings

Some medications are unstable when stored in liquid form for long periods of time and therefore are packaged in powdered form. When medications come in powdered form, they must be diluted with a liquid referred to as a *diluent* or *solvent* before they can be administered to a client. Once a liquid is added to a powdered medication, the solution may be used for only 1 to 14 days, depending on the type of medication. The process of adding a solvent or diluent to a medication in powdered form to dissolve it and form a solution is referred to as *reconstitution*. Reconstitution is necessary for medications that come in powdered form before they can be measured and administered. If you think about it, this process is something you do in everyday situations. For example, when you make iced tea (powdered form), in essence you are reconstituting it. The iced tea, for example, is the powder, and the water you add to it is considered the diluent, or solvent.

As a safety precaution in some institutions, the pharmacy reconstitutes most medications. However, the nurse must understand the process of reconstitution because some medications may have to be reconstituted just before administration. Medications requiring reconstitution can be for oral or parenteral use; these are not always injectable medications. With emphasis being placed on home care, nurses and other health care providers may have to dilute things such as oral medications, irrigating solutions, and nutritional feedings. Sterile solutions are always used to reconstitute medications for injectable use. Special diluents, when required for reconstitution, are usually packaged with the powdered medication; but oral medications can often be, but are not always, reconstituted with tap water. Thus the nurse **must** know how the reconstitution process works. Understanding the terminology relating to reconstitution enables the nurse to understand the process:

- *Solute*—a powdered medication or liquid concentrate to be dissolved or diluted.

- *Solvent (diluent)*—a liquid that is added to the powder or liquid concentrate. The nurse must identify the solvent (diluent) to use. The type of solvent (diluent) varies according to the medication. The package insert or the medication label will indicate the solvent (diluent) to be used and the amount. If the information is not indicated on the label or the package insert is unavailable consult the pharmacy or a medication reference such as the *Physician's Desk Reference (PDR),* a medication reference, or the hospital formulary.
- *Solution*—the liquid that results when the solvent (diluent) dissolves the solute (powdered medication or liquid concentrate).

## BASIC PRINCIPLES FOR RECONSTITUTION

The first step in reconstitution is to find the directions and carefully read the information on the vial or the package insert. Medications labeled and packaged with reconstitution directions may indicate "oral, IM, or IV use only" or may say "can be used for any route." Carefully check the route of administration of the medication and the reconstitution directions. Examples of the several directions for reconstitution are shown in this chapter.

**CAUTION**

> Before reconstituting a medication, read and follow the directions on the label or package insert. This includes checking the expiration date on the medication and diluent. Never assume the type or amount of diluent to be used. Consult the appropriate resources if the information is not available.

1. The drug manufacturer provides directions for reconstitution, including information regarding the number of milliliters of diluent or solvent that should be added, as well as the type of solution that should be used to reconstitute the medication. The concentration (or strength) of the medication after it has been reconstituted according to the directions is also indicated on some medications. The directions for reconstitution must be read carefully and followed.
2. The diluent (solvent, liquid) commonly used for reconstitution is sterile water or sterile normal saline solution, prepared for injection. Other solutions that may be used are 5% dextrose and water and bacteriostatic water. Some powdered medications for oral use may be reconstituted with tap water. The manufacturer's directions will tell you which solution to use. If the medication requires a special solution for reconstitution, it is usually supplied by the drug manufacturer and packaged with the medication (e.g., Librium).
3. Once you have located the reconstitution directions on the label, you need to identify the following information:
   a. The type of diluent to use for reconstitution.
   b. The amount of diluent to add. This is essential because directions relating to the amount can vary according to the route of administration. There may be different dilution instructions for intravenous (IV) versus intramuscular (IM) administration.
   c. The length of time the medication is good once it is reconstituted. The length of time a medication can be stored once reconstituted can vary depending on how it is stored. When medications are reconstituted the solution must be used in a timely fashion. The potency (stability) of the medication may be several hours to several days or a week. Check the medication label, package insert, or appropriate resources for how long a medication may be used after reconstitution.
   d. Directions for storing the medication after mixing. Medications must be stored appropriately once reconstituted per manufacturer's instructions to ensure optimal potency of the medication. Medications can become unstable when stored incorrectly and for long periods. Example: A label may state a medication maintains its potency 96 hours at room temperature or 7 days when refrigerated.
   e. The strength or concentration of the medication after it has been reconstituted.
   Refer to Figure 19-1 showing the oxacillin sodium reconstitution procedure. Note that directions on the label say to add 2.7 mL sterile water for injection and that each 1.5 mL contains 250 mg. The available dosage after reconstitution is 250 mg of oxacillin per 1.5 mL solution (500 mg per 3 mL).

4. If there are no directions for reconstitution on the label or on a package insert, or if any of the information (listed in number 3) is missing, consult appropriate resources such as the *Physician's Desk Reference (PDR)*, a pharmacology text, the hospital drug formulary or the pharmacy.

5. Injectable medications for reconstitution can come in a single-dose vial or a multiple-dose vial. When medications are in single-dose vials, there is only enough medication for **one** dose and the contents are administered after reconstitution. In the case where the nurse reconstitutes a multiple-dose vial, there is enough medication for more than one dose. Therefore, when a multiple-dose vial is reconstituted, it is important to clearly label the vial after reconstitution with the following information:

   a. The date and time prepared, dosage strength prepared, the expiration date for the medication once reconstituted, and the time. *Note:* If all of the solution that is mixed is used, this information is not necessary. Information regarding the date and time of preparation and date and time of expiration is crucial when all of the medication is not used.

   b. Storage directions such as "Refrigerate."

   c. Your initials.

   If the medication label does not have room to clearly write the required information, add a label to the vial and indicate important information. Make certain the label is applied so that it does not obscure the medication name and dosage.

## Tips for Clinical Practice

When reconstituting a multiple-dose medication vial, label it with the required information and store it appropriately. If the vial is not labeled with a date and time, the medication must be discarded.

6. When reconstituting medications that are in multiple-dose vials or have several directions for preparation, **information regarding the dosage strength or final concentration (what the medication's strength or concentration is after you mixed it) must be on the label; for example, 500 mg per mL. This is important because others using the medication after you need this information to determine the dosage.**

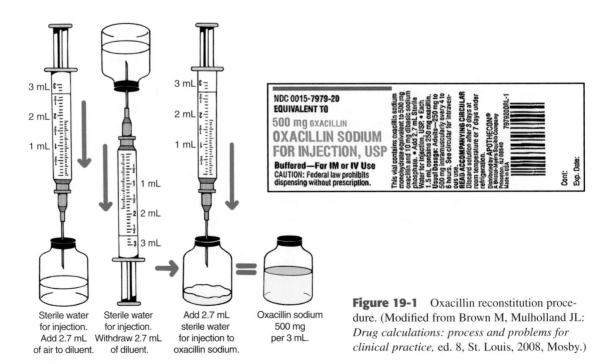

Sterile water for injection. Add 2.7 mL of air to diluent.

Sterile water for injection. Withdraw 2.7 mL of diluent.

Add 2.7 mL sterile water for injection to oxacillin sodium.

Oxacillin sodium 500 mg per 3 mL.

NDC 0015-7979-20
EQUIVALENT TO
**500 mg** OXACILLIN
**OXACILLIN SODIUM FOR INJECTION, USP**
Buffered—For IM or IV Use
CAUTION: Federal law prohibits dispensing without prescription.

**Figure 19-1** Oxacillin reconstitution procedure. (Modified from Brown M, Mulholland JL: *Drug calculations: process and problems for clinical practice,* ed. 8, St. Louis, 2008, Mosby.)

7. After the diluent is added to a powder, some medications completely dissolve and there is no additional volume added. Often, however, the powdered medication adds volume to the solution. The powdered medication takes up space as it dissolves and results in an increase in the amount of total (fluid) volume once it has dissolved. This is sometimes referred to as the *displacement factor,* or just *displacement.* The reconstituted material represents the diluent and powder. For example, directions for 1 g of powdered medication may state to add 2.5 mL sterile water for injection to provide an approximate volume of 3 mL (330 mg per mL). When the 2.5 mL of diluent is added, the 1 g of powdered medication displaces an additional 0.5 mL, for a total volume of 3 mL. The available dosage after reconstitution is 330 mg per milliliter of solution.

**CAUTION**

Always determine both the type and amount of diluent to be used for reconstituting medications. Read and follow the label or package insert directions carefully to ensure that your client receives the intended dosage. Consult a pharmacist or other appropriate resources if there are any questions. Never assume!

## Tips for Clinical Practice

If the powder displaces the liquid as it dissolves and increases the volume as illustrated in the example, the resulting volume and concentration must be considered when the correct dosage of medication is calculated. Whether a medication causes an increase in volume when it is reconstituted will be indicated on the medication label or the package insert.

The two types of reconstituted parenteral solutions are single strength and multiple strength. A single-strength solution has the directions for reconstitution printed on the label, as shown on the 500-mg oxacillin label in Figure 19-1. A multiple-strength solution usually has several directions for reconstitution and requires the nurse be even more attentive to the directions to select the best concentration to administer the required dosage.

**CAUTION**

Always consult the label, package insert, or other sources regarding directions for reconstituting medications in powdered form to ensure accurate reconstitution for administration.

Let's do some practice problems answering questions relating to single-strength solutions.

 **Practice Problems**

Using the label for ampicillin, answer the following questions.

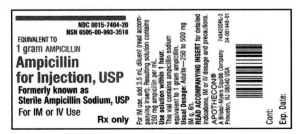

1. What is the total dosage strength of ampicillin in this vial?   _____

2. How much diluent is added to the vial to prepare the medication for IM use? _____

3. What diluent is recommended for reconstitution? _____

4. What is the final concentration of the prepared solution for IM administration? _____

5. How long will the reconstituted material retain its potency? _____

6. 500 mg IM q6h is ordered. How many milliliters will you give? Shade the dosage in on the syringe provided. _____

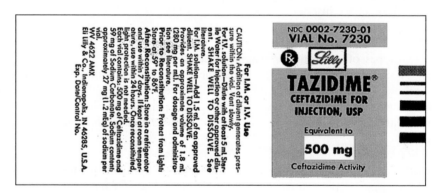

Using the label for Tazidime, answer the following questions.

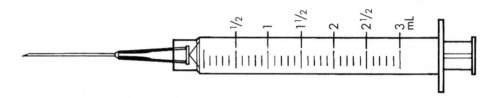

7. What is the total dosage strength of Tazidime in the vial? _____

8. How much diluent is added to the vial to prepare the medication for IM use? _____

9. What diluent is recommended for reconstitution for IM administration? _____

10. What is the final concentration of the solution prepared for IM administration? _____

11. How long does the medication retain its potency at room temperature? _____

12. How long does the medication retain its potency if it is refrigerated?   _____

13. 400 mg IM q8h is ordered. How many milliliters will you give? Shade the dosage in on the syringe provided.   _____

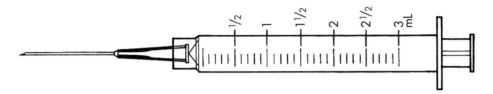

Using the label for Ticar, answer the following questions.

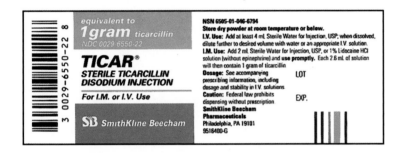

14. What is the total dosage strength of Ticar in the vial?   _____

15. What diluent is recommended to prepare an IV dosage?   _____

16. How many milliliters of diluent are needed to prepare an IM dosage?   _____

17. What is the final concentration of the solution prepared for IM administration?   _____

18. Ticar 500 mg IM q8h is ordered. How many milliliters will you give? Shade the dosage in on the syringe provided.   _____

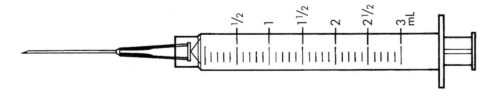

Using the label for Rocephin, answer the following questions.

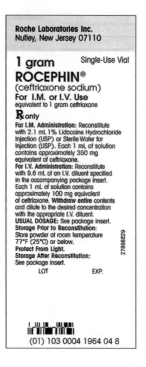

Roche Laboratories Inc.
Nutley, New Jersey 07110

**1 gram**    Single-Use Vial
**ROCEPHIN®**
(ceftriaxone sodium)
**For I.M. or I.V. Use**
equivalent to 1 gram ceftriaxone

**R** only

**For I.M. Administration:** Reconstitute with 2.1 mL 1% Lidocaine Hydrochloride Injection (USP) or Sterile Water for Injection (USP). Each 1 mL of solution contains approximately 350 mg equivalent of ceftriaxone.
**For I.V. Administration:** Reconstitute with 9.6 mL of an I.V. diluent specified in the accompanying package insert. Each 1 mL of solution contains approximately 100 mg equivalent of ceftriaxone. **Withdraw entire** contents and dilute to the desired concentration with the appropriate I.V. diluent.
**USUAL DOSAGE:** See package insert.
**Storage Prior to Reconstitution:** Store powder at room temperature 77°F (25°C) or below.
**Protect From Light.**
**Storage After Reconstitution:** See package insert.

LOT          EXP.

27868829

(01) 103 0004 1964 04 8

19. What is the total dosage strength of Rocephin in this vial? _____

20. For what routes of administration is the medication indicated? _____

21. How much diluent must be added to the vial to prepare the medication for IV use? _____

22. What kind of diluent is recommended for IV reconstitution? _____

23. What is the final concentration of the prepared solution for IV use? _____

24. How much diluent must be added to the vial to prepare the medication for IM use? _____

25. What kind of diluent is recommended for IM reconstitution? _____

26. 1 g IV q12h is ordered. How many milliliters will you give? Shade the dosage in on the syringe provided. _____

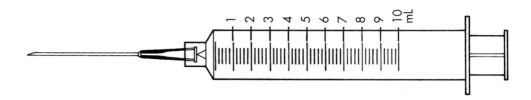

Using the label for Augmentin, answer the following questions.

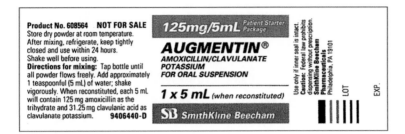

27. How much diluent must be added to prepare the solution?  _____

28. What type of solution is used for the diluent?  _____

29. What is the final concentration of the prepared solution?  _____

30. How should the medication be stored after it is reconstituted?  _____

Using the label for Zovirax and a portion of the package insert, answer the following questions.

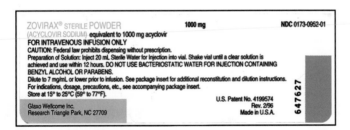

31. What is the total dosage strength of Zovirax in this vial?  _____

32. How much diluent must be added to prepare the solution?  _____

33. What diluent is recommended for reconstitution?  _____

34. What is the final concentration of the prepared solution?  _____

35. What is the route of administration?  _____

Using the label for erythromycin, answer the following questions.

**TO PATIENT:**
**Shake well before using.**
Keep tightly closed. Store in refrigerator
and discard unused portion after ten days.
Oversize bottle provides shake space.
**TO THE PHARMACIST:**
When prepared as directed, each 5 mL
teaspoonful contains erythromycin
ethylsuccinate equivalent to 200 mg of
erythromycin in a cherry-flavored
suspension.
Bottle contains erythromycin ethylsuccinate
equivalent to 8 g of erythromycin.
**Usual Dose:** See package outsert.
Store at room temperature in dry form.
Child-Resistant closure not required;
Reference: Federal Register Vol.39 No.29.
**DIRECTIONS FOR PREPARATION:** Slowly
add 140 mL of water and shake vigorously to
make 200 mL of suspension.
**BARR LABORATORIES, INC.**
Pomona, NY 10970
R11-90

BARR LABORATORIES, INC.

NDC 0555-0215-23
NSN 6505-00-080-0653

**Erythromycin
Ethylsuccinate**
**for Oral
Suspension, USP**

**200 mg of erythromycin
activity per 5 mL
reconstituted**

**Caution:** Federal law prohibits
dispensing without prescription.

**200 mL** (when mixed)

0555-0215-23

SAMPLE

Exp. Date:

Lot No.:

36. How much diluent must be added to
prepare the solution?

37. What is the volume of the solution after it
is mixed?

38. What is the final concentration of the
prepared solution?

39. For how long is the reconstituted solution
good?

Using the label for Zithromax, answer the following questions.

Store at or below 86°F (30°C).
**DOSAGE AND USE**
See accompanying prescribing information.
Constitute to 100 mg/mL* with
4.8 mL of Sterile Water For Injection.
**Must be further diluted before use.**
For appropriate diluents and storage
recommendations, refer to prescribing information.
*Each mL contains azithromycin dihydrate
equivalent to 100 mg of azithromycin,
76.9 mg of citric acid, and sodium hydroxide
for pH adjustment.
05-5191-32-0

**CAUTION:** Federal law prohibits
dispensing without prescription.

NDC 0069-3150-83

**Zithromax®**
(azithromycin for injection)

*For IV infusion only*
**STERILE**
equivalent to

**500 mg**

of azithromycin
*Distributed by*
*Pfizer* **Pfizer Labs**
Division of Pfizer Inc, NY, NY 10017

Lot No.

Exp. Date

40. What is the total dosage strength of
Zithromax in this vial?

41. How much diluent must be added to
prepare the solution?

42. What diluent is recommended for
reconstitution?

43. What is the final concentration of the
prepared solution?

44. What is the route of administration?

Using the label for cefazolin, answer the following questions.

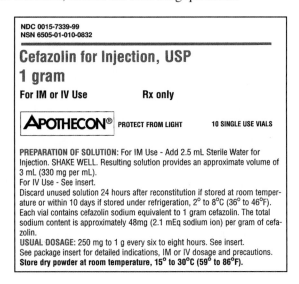

45. What is the total dosage strength of cefazolin in this vial?

_____

46. How many milliliters of diluent are needed to prepare an IM dosage?

_____

47. What diluent is recommended for reconstitution?

_____

48. What is the final concentration of the prepared solution?

_____

49. How long does the medication maintain its potency at room temperature?

_____

Using the label for fluconazole, answer the following questions.

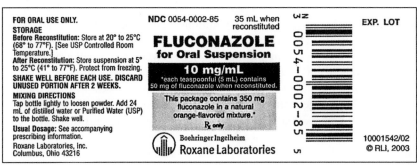

50. How much diluent must be added to prepare the solution?

_____

51. What diluent is recommended for reconstitution?

_____

52. What is the final concentration of the prepared solution?

_____

53. How should the medication be stored after it is reconstituted?

_____

Answers on pp. 642-643

## Calculation of Medications When the Final Concentration (Dosage Strength) Is Not Stated

Sometimes a medication comes with directions for only one way to reconstitute it, and the label does not indicate the final dosage strength after it is mixed, such as "becomes 250 mg per mL." Example: A particular medication is available in 1 g in powder. Directions tell you that adding 2.5 mL of sterile water yields 3 mL of solution. When you add 2.5 mL of sterile water to the powder, the volume expands to 3 mL. The concentration is not changing; you will get 3 mL of solution; however, it will be equal to 1 g.

The problem is therefore calculated by using 1 g = 3 mL.

# RECONSTITUTING MEDICATIONS WITH MORE THAN ONE DIRECTION FOR MIXING (MULTIPLE STRENGTH)

Remember the directions for reconstitution can be on the label or a package insert. At times the vial will contain minimal information. It may only include the dosage strength and state "see package insert for directions for reconstitution or storage."

Some medications in addition to giving the route of administration may come with several directions for preparing different solution strengths. In this case the nurse must choose the concentration or dosage strength appropriate for the dosage ordered. A common medication that has a choice of dosage strengths is penicillin. When a medication comes with several directions for preparation or offers a choice of dosage strengths, you must choose the strength most appropriate for the dosage ordered. The following guidelines may be used.

## Guidelines for Choosing Appropriate Concentrations

1. Consider the route of administration.
   a. IM—You are concerned that the amount does not exceed the maximum allowed for IM administration. However, you do not want to choose a concentration that will result in irritation when injected into a muscle. When a choice of strengths can be made, do not choose an amount that would exceed the amount allowed for IM administration or one that is very concentrated.
   b. IV—Keep in mind that this medication is usually further diluted because once reconstituted, the medication is then placed in additional fluid of 50 to 100 mL or more, depending on the medication being administered. Example: Erythromycin requires that the reconstituted solution be placed in 250 mL of fluid before administration to a client. In pediatrics a medication may be given in a smaller volume of fluid, depending on the child's age, the child's size, and the medication.
2. Choose the concentration or dosage strength that comes closest to what the prescriber has ordered. The dosage strengths are given for the amount of diluent used. Example: If the prescriber orders 300,000 units of a particular medication IM, and the choices of strength are 200,000 units per mL, 250,000 units per mL, and 500,000 units per mL, the strength closest to 300,000 units per mL is 250,000 units per mL. It allows you to administer a dosage within the range allowed for IM administration, and it is not the most concentrated.

> **CAUTION**
>
> When multiple directions are given for reconstituting medications, the smaller the amount of diluent used to reconstitute the medication, the more concentrated the resulting solution will be. Consider the route of administration when reconstituting medications. Always check the route and the directions related to reconstitution.

3. The word *respectively* may sometimes be used on a medication label for directions on reconstitution. For example, reconstitute with 23 mL, 18 mL, 8 mL of diluent to provide concentrations of 200,000 units per mL, 250,000 units per mL, 500,000 units per

mL, respectively. The word *respectively* means in the order given. In terms of the directions for reconstitution, this means that if you add 23 mL diluent, it will provide 200,000 units per mL, 18 mL diluent will provide 250,000 units per mL, etc. In other words, the amounts of diluent correspond to the order in which the concentrations are written. Remember: **When you are mixing a medication that is a multiple-strength solution, the dosage strength that you prepare must be written on the vial.**

Let's look at a sample label that shows a multiple-strength solution.

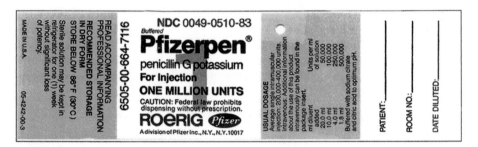

Notice that the penicillin label states one million units. This means a total of 1,000,000 units of penicillin is in the vial. The directions for reconstitution and the dosage strengths that can be obtained are listed on the right side of the label. If the dosage ordered for the client was, for example, 250,000 units q6h, the most appropriate strength to mix would be 250,000 units per mL. If you look next to the dosage strength in the directions, you will notice that 4 mL of diluent must be added to obtain a concentration of 250,000 units per mL. Because this is a multiple-strength solution, the dosage strength you choose must be indicated on the vial after you reconstitute it. Since the type of diluent is not indicated on the label, other resources, such as those recommended previously, must be consulted.

**CAUTION**

If a multiple-strength solution is prepared and not used in its entirety, the dosage strength (final concentration) you mixed must be indicated on the label to verify the dosage strength of the reconstituted solution. Proper labeling is a crucial detail.

 **Practice Problems**

Using the label for penicillin G potassium, answer the following questions.

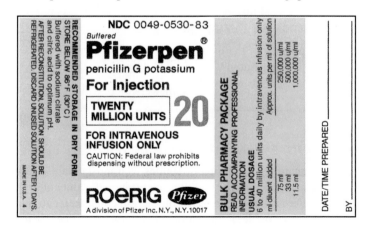

54. What is the total number of units of penicillin contained in the vial?
    (Write out in numbers.)                        _____

55. If you add 33 mL of diluent to the vial, what dosage strength will you print on the label? _____

56. If 2,000,000 units IV is ordered, which dosage strength would be appropriate to use? _____

57. How many milliliters will you administer? _____

58. How long will the medication maintain its potency if refrigerated? _____

Using the label for penicillin G potassium, answer the following questions.

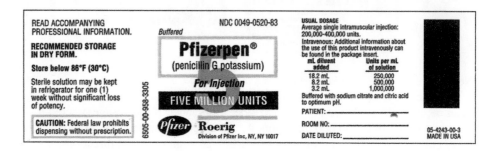

59. What is the total number of units of penicillin contained in the vial? (Write out in numbers.) _____

60. If 700,000 units IM is ordered, which dosage strength would be appropriate to use? _____

61. How many milliliters will you administer? _____

62. Where will you store any unused medication? _____

63. How long will the medication maintain its potency? _____

64. What concentration strength would be obtained if you added 18.2 mL of diluent? (Write out in numbers.) _____

65. How long can the potency of the medication be maintained if it is refrigerated? _____

Answers on p. 643

## RECONSTITUTION FROM PACKAGE INSERT DIRECTIONS

If the label does not contain reconstitution directions, you must obtain directions from the information insert that accompanies the vial. Pay attention to the amount in the vial and the route; there may be different directions based on these factors. Refer to the Tazicef label and insert that follow. For example, note that the directions for Tazicef IV infusion are different for reconstitution for a 1 gram vial and a 2 gram vial. Also, note that the Tazicef label has different directions for IM injection and IV infusion. Always carefully check the route ordered, and follow the directions corresponding to the route.

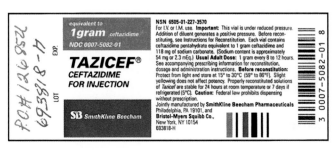

The reconstitution table:

**RECONSTITUTION**

**Single Dose Vials:**
For I.M. injection, I.V. direct (bolus) injection, or I.V. infusion, reconstitute with Sterile Water for injection according to the following table. The vacuum may assist entry of the diluent. SHAKE WELL.

**Table 5**

| Vial Size | Diluent to Be Added | Approx. Avail. Volume | Approx. Avg. Concentration |
|---|---|---|---|
| **Intramuscular or Intravenous Direct (bolus) Injection** | | | |
| 1 gram | 3.0 ml. | 3.6 ml. | 280 mg./ml. |
| **Intravenous Infusion** | | | |
| 1 gram | 10 ml. | 10.6 ml. | 95 mg./ml. |
| 2 gram | 10 ml. | 11.2 ml. | 180 mg./ml. |

Withdraw the total volume of solution into the syringe (the pressure in the vial may aid withdrawal). The withdrawn solution may contain some bubbles of carbon dioxide.

**NOTE: As with the administration of all parenteral products, accumulated gases should be expressed from the syringe immediately before injection of 'Tazicef'.**

These solutions of 'Tazicef' are stable for 18 hours at room temperature or seven days if refrigerated (5∞C.). Slight yellowing does not affect potency.

For I.V. infusion, dilute reconstituted solution in 50 to 100 ml. of one of the parenteral fluids listed under COMPATIBILITY AND STABILITY.

Label content:

NSN 6505-01-227-3570
For I.V. or I.M. use. **Important:** This vial is under reduced pressure. Addition of diluent generates a positive pressure. Before reconstituting, see Instructions for Reconstitution. Each vial contains ceftazidime pentahydrate equivalent to 1 gram ceftazidime and 118 mg of sodium carbonate. (Sodium content is approximately 54 mg or 2.3 mEq.) **Usual Adult Dose:** 1 gram every 8 to 12 hours. See accompanying prescribing information for reconstitution, dosage and administration instructions. **Before reconstitution:** Protect from light and store at 15° to 30°C (59° to 86°F). Slight yellowing does not affect potency. Properly reconstituted solutions of *Tazicef* are stable for 24 hours at room temperature or 7 days if refrigerated (5°C). **Caution:** Federal law prohibits dispensing without prescription.
Jointly manufactured by **SmithKline Beecham Pharmaceuticals**, Philadelphia, PA 19101, and **Bristol-Myers Squibb Co.,** New York, NY 10154
693818-H

equivalent to
**1 gram** ceftazidime
NDC 0007-5082-01
**TAZICEF®**
CEFTAZIDIME
FOR INJECTION
**SB** SmithKline Beecham

3 0007-5082-01 8

66. What is the dosage strength of the total vial? _____

67. How much diluent must be added to this vial for reconstitution for IM administration? _____

68. What kind of diluent must be used? _____

69. What is the concentration per milliliter for the IM solution? _____

70. How much diluent must be added to the vial for IV infusion? _____

71. What is the concentration per milliliter for the IV solution? _____

Answers on p. 643

Before we proceed to calculate dosages, let's review the steps to use with medications that have been reconstituted.

1. Ratio and proportion, the formula method, or dimensional analysis may be used to calculate the dosage. What is available becomes the dosage strength you obtain after mixing the medication according to the directions.
2. Powdered medications may increase in volume after a liquid is added (diluent + powder). The volume to which the medication expands must be considered when calculations are made.
3. When the final concentration is not stated, the total weight of the medication in powdered form is used, and the number of milliliters produced after the solvent or liquid has been added.
4. As with all calculation problems, check to make sure that the ordered and the available medications are in the same system of measurement and the same units.
5. Do not forget to label your answer.

## CALCULATION OF DOSAGES

To calculate the dosage to administer after reconstituting a medication, ratio and proportion, the formula method, or dimensional analysis may be used, as with other forms of medication. However, the H (have or what is available) is the dosage strength you obtain after you mix the medication according to the directions. If you are using ratio and proportion, therefore, the known ratio is also the dosage strength obtained after you mix the medication.

In $\dfrac{D}{H} \times Q = x$, Q is the volume of solution that contains the dosage strength.

In dimensional analysis, the first fraction written is the solution (volume) that contains the dosage strength.

**Example 1:**   To illustrate, let's calculate the dosage you would administer if you mixed penicillin and made a solution containing 1,000,000 units per mL. Order: 2,000,000 units IM q6h.

 ## Solution Using Ratio and Proportion

$$1,000,000 \text{ units} : 1 \text{ mL} = 2,000,000 \text{ units} : x \text{ mL}$$
$$\text{(known)} \qquad\qquad\qquad \text{(unknown)}$$

$$\frac{1,000,000\,x}{1,000,000} = \frac{2,000,000}{1,000,000}$$

(Note cancellation of zeros to make numbers smaller.)

$$x = \frac{2}{1}$$

$$x = 2 \text{ mL}$$

**Answer:**    2 mL

 ## Solution Using the Formula Method

$$\frac{D}{H} \times Q = x$$

$$\frac{2,000,000 \text{ units}}{1,000,000 \text{ units}} \times 1 \text{ mL} = x \text{ mL}$$

$$x = \frac{2,000,000}{1,000,000}$$

$$x = 2 \text{ mL}$$

**Answer:**    2 mL

 ## Solution Using Dimensional Analysis

$$x \text{ mL} = \frac{1 \text{ mL}}{1,000,000 \text{ units}} \times \frac{2,000,000 \text{ units}}{1}$$

$$x = \frac{2,000,000}{1,000,000}$$

$$x = \frac{2}{1}$$

$$x = 2 \text{ mL}$$

**Answer:**    2 mL

**Example 2:**   Order: 0.5 g of an antibiotic IM q4h

Available: 1 g of the medication in powdered form; the label reads: Add 1.7 mL of sterile water; each mL will then contain 500 mg

 Problem Setup

1. A conversion is necessary. Equivalent: 1,000 mg = 1 g. Convert what is ordered into the available units. This will eliminate a decimal point. Therefore 0.5 g = 500 mg.
2. Think: What would a logical answer be?

 Solution Using Ratio and Proportion

$$500 \text{ mg} : 1 \text{ mL} = 500 \text{ mg} : x \text{ mL}$$
$$\text{(known)} \qquad \text{(unknown)}$$

$$\frac{500x}{500} = \frac{500}{500}$$

$$x = \frac{500}{500}$$

$$x = 1 \text{ mL}$$

**Answer:**   1 mL

 Solution Using the Formula Method

$$\frac{D}{H} \times Q = x$$

$$\frac{500 \text{ mg}}{500 \text{ mg}} \times 1 \text{ mL} = x \text{ mL}$$

$$x = \frac{500}{500}$$

$$x = 1 \text{ mL}$$

**Answer:**   1 mL

 Solution Using Dimensional Analysis

$$x \text{ mL} = \frac{1 \text{ mL}}{500 \text{ mg}} \times \frac{1,000 \text{ mg}}{1 \text{ g}} \times \frac{0.5 \text{ g}}{1}$$

$$x = \frac{1,000 \times 0.5}{500}$$

$$x = \frac{500}{500}$$

$$x = 1 \text{ mL}$$

**Answer:**   1 mL

### ■ Points to Remember

- If the medication is not used in its entirety after it is mixed, any remaining must have the following information clearly written on the label:
  a. Initials of the preparer
  b. Dosage strength (if multichoice/multiple strengths)
  c. Date and time of preparation and date and time of expiration
- Read all directions carefully; if there are no instructions on the vial, then the package insert, pharmacy, or other reliable resources may be used to find the information needed for reconstitution.
- When directions on the label are for IM and IV reconstitution, read the label carefully for the solution you are preparing.
- The type and amount of diluent to be used for reconstitution must be followed exactly.
- Read directions relating to storage (room temperature, refrigeration) and the time period for maintaining potency.
- When dilution of powdered medication results in an increase in volume, this must be considered in calculating the dosage.
- Read instructions carefully. There may be different directions for mixing according to the amount in the vial and the route. Always check the route ordered and follow the directions corresponding to the route. Interchanging the dilution instructions for IV and IM administration can have serious outcomes.

## RECONSTITUTION OF NONINJECTABLE SOLUTIONS

The principles of reconstitution can be applied to nutritional liquids. Enteral feeding solutions are formulated to be administered in full strength; however, the nurse may, on occasion, need to dilute the enteral solution before administering it. Before beginning calculations, let's discuss enteral feedings.

### Enteral Feeding

Enteral nutrition involves the provision of nutrients to the gastrointestinal tract. This nutrition is provided to clients who are unable to ingest food safely or have eating difficulties. Enteral nutrition may be provided with a nasogastric, jejunal, or gastric tube. It may consist of blended foods or tube feeding formulas. Tube feedings can be administered in several ways. Depending on the client's needs, they may be given as a bolus amount by means of gravity several times per day by using a large-volume syringe, as a continuous gravity drip over a period of $\frac{1}{2}$ to 1 hour several times per day by using a pouch to hang the feeding, or as a continuous drip per infusion pump. When clients are receiving a continuous feeding, the feeding is placed in a special pouch or container and attached to a feeding pump. A common feeding pump is the Kangaroo pump (Figure 19-2). When the feeding pump is used, the feeding is delivered at a rate expressed in milliliters per hour. For the purpose of this chapter, we will focus on administering a feeding by the continuous drip method with an enteral infusion pump.

When an order is written for feedings by continuous infusion, the nurse attaches the feeding to a special pump and administers it at the prescribed rate in milliliters per hour. A sample order is Jevity at 65 mL per hour by PEG (percutaneous endoscopic gastrostomy) or by NG (nasogastric) tube. The feeding order also includes a certain volume of water with feeding (100 to 250 mL). Some orders may be written as follows: Pulmo Care 400 mL q8h followed by 100 mL of water after each feed. When the prescriber does not indicate milliliters per hour, the nurse uses the same formula as with IV calculation to determine the rate. In pediatrics the order often specifies the formula and the rate. Example: Similac 24 at 20 mL per hr continuously by NG tube.

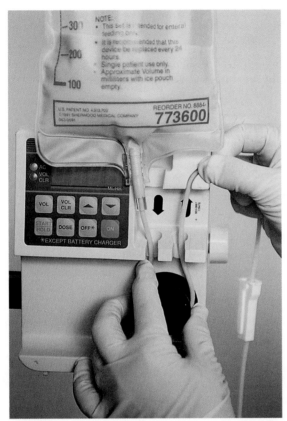

**Figure 19-2**    Kangaroo pump. (From Elkin MK, Perry AG, Potter PA: *Nursing interventions and clinical skills,* ed. 4, St. Louis, 2007, Mosby.)

**Example 1:**    Order: Pulmocare 400 mL q8h followed by 100 mL of water after each feed. Determine the rate in milliliters per hour.

$$\frac{400 \text{ mL}}{8 \text{ hr}} = 50 \text{ mL/hr}$$

The pump would be set at 50 mL/hr.

**Example 2:**    Order: Nepro 1,200 mL over 16 hours. Determine the rate in milliliters per hour.

$$\frac{1,200 \text{ mL}}{16 \text{ hr}} = 75 \text{ mL/hr}$$

The pump would be set to deliver 75 mL/hr.

> **NOTE**
>
> The amount of water given with a tube feeding and how it is administered vary from one institution to the next. Check the institution's policy relating to administering enteral feedings.

In addition to nutrients, medications may be given through a tube. Liquid medications are preferred; however, some tablets may be crushed, dissolved in water, and administered.

Never assume. Not all medications are designed for administration through a tube, so check with the pharmacist or other appropriate resources. A medication's effectiveness could depend on the location of the tube (e.g., stomach, jejunum).

**CAUTION**

Always verify that the medications to be administered are not sublingual, enteric-coated, or timed-release medications, because such medications are absorbed differently and the effects of the medication may be altered. Consult the pharmacist or medication guide before tablets are crushed and before capsules are opened and dissolved for tube feeding administration.

**Practice Problems**

Determine the rate in milliliters per hour for the following continuous feedings:
72. Ensure 480 mL by NG tube over 8 hr. Follow
    with 100 mL of water after each feeding. _____

73. Perative 1,600 mL over 24 hr by gastrostomy.
    Follow with 250 mL of water.         _____

Answers on p. 643

## Calculations of Solutions

Because of special circumstances in both adults and children, nutritional liquids may require dilution before they are used. Nutritional formulas may be diluted with sterile or tap water. **Always consult a reference regarding what should be used to reconstitute a nutritional formula.**

To prepare a prescribed solution of a certain strength from a solute, first let's review some basic terms.

---

Solute—a concentrated or solid substance to be dissolved or diluted
Solvent—a liquid substance that dissolves another substance
Solution—a solute plus a solvent

To prepare a solution of a specific strength, use the following steps:

1. Desired solution strength $\times$ $\dfrac{\text{Amount of}}{\text{desired solution}}$ = Solute (solution to be dissolved)

*Note:* The strength of the desired solution is written as a fraction; the amount of desired solution is expressed in milliliters or ounces, depending on the problem. This will give you the amount of solute you will need to add to the solvent to prepare the desired solution.

2. Amount of desired solution − Solute = $\dfrac{\text{Amount of liquid needed to}}{\text{dissolve substance (solvent)}}$

---

**Example 1:**   Order: $\frac{1}{3}$-strength Ensure 900 mL by NG tube over 8 hr

**Solution:**
$$\underset{\substack{\text{(desired} \\ \text{strength)}}}{\tfrac{1}{3}} \times \underset{\substack{\text{(amount of} \\ \text{solution)}}}{900 \text{ mL}} = \underset{\text{(solute)}}{x}$$

**Step 1:**
$$\frac{900}{3} = x$$
$$x = 300 \text{ mL}$$

You need 300 mL of the formula (solute).

**Step 2:**    $\underset{\substack{\text{(amount of} \\ \text{solution)}}}{900 \text{ mL}} - \underset{\text{(solute)}}{300 \text{ mL}} = \underset{\text{(amount needed to dissolve)}}{600 \text{ mL}}$

Therefore you would add 600 mL water to 300 mL of Ensure to make 900 mL of $\frac{1}{3}$-strength Ensure.

**Example 2:** ¾-strength Isomil 4 oz p.o. q4h for 24 hr

*Note:* 4 oz q4h = 6 feedings; 4 oz × 6 = 24 oz

1 oz = 30 mL; therefore 24 oz = 720 mL

$$\frac{3}{4} \times 720 \text{ mL} = x \text{ mL}$$

$$\frac{2,160}{4} = x$$

$$x = 540 \text{ mL of the formula (solute)}$$

720 mL     − 540 mL = 180 mL
(amount of    (solute)    (amount needed
solution)                 to dissolve)

Therefore you would add 180 mL water to 540 mL of Isomil to make 720 mL of ¾-strength Isomil for a 24-hour period.

 ## Practice Problems

Prepare the following strength solutions:.

74. ⅔-strength Sustacal 300 mL p.o. q.i.d.

75. ¾-strength Ensure 16 oz by nasogastric (NG) tube over 8 hr

76. ½-strength Ensure 20 oz by gastrostomy tube (GT) over 5 hr

Answers on p. 643

## Tips for Clinical Practice

Think and calculate with accuracy. Errors can be made in determining the dilution for an enteral solution if you incorrectly calculate the amount of solute and solvent for a required solution strength.

## Points to Remember

- Enteral feedings (continuous) are placed on an infusion pump and administered at a rate expressed in milliliters per hour. The prescriber usually orders the feeding rate in milliliters per hour. If not, the nurse must calculate the rate at which to deliver the feeding.
- To prepare a solution of a specific strength, write the desired solution strength as a fraction and multiply it by the amount of desired solution. This will give you the amount of solute needed.
- The amount of desired solution − solute = amount of liquid needed to dissolve the substance (solvent).
- Think and calculate with accuracy to avoid making errors in determining the dilution for a required solution strength.

**Critical Thinking Question**

1. **Scenario:** Order: Tazicef 250 mg IM q8h.
   The nurse had the package insert below and a 1-g vial.

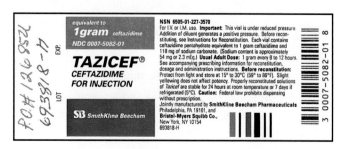

### RECONSTITUTION

**Single Dose Vials:**
For I.M. injection, I.V. direct (bolus) injection, or I.V. infusion, reconstitute with Sterile Water for injection according to the following table. The vacuum may assist entry of the diluent. SHAKE WELL.

**Table 5**

| Vial Size | Diluent to Be Added | Approx. Avail. Volume | Approx. Avg. Concentration |
|---|---|---|---|
| **Intramuscular or Intravenous Direct (bolus) Injection** | | | |
| 1 gram | 3.0 ml. | 3.6 ml. | 280 mg./ml. |
| **Intravenous Infusion** | | | |
| 1 gram | 10 ml. | 10.6 ml. | 95 mg./ml. |
| 2 gram | 10 ml. | 11.2 ml. | 180 mg./ml. |

Withdraw the total volume of solution into the syringe (the pressure in the vial may aid withdrawal). The withdrawn solution may contain some bubbles of carbon dioxide.

**NOTE: As with the administration of all parenteral products, accumulated gases should be expressed from the syringe immediately before injection of 'Tazicef'.**

These solutions of 'Tazicef' are stable for 18 hours at room temperature or seven days if refrigerated (5∞C.). Slight yellowing does not affect potency.

For I.V. infusion, dilute reconstituted solution in 50 to 100 ml. of one of the parenteral fluids listed under COMPATIBILITY AND STABILITY.

The medication was reconstituted with 10.6 mL of diluent.

Order: Tazicef 250 mg IM q8h.

Administered: Tazicef 2.6 mL.

a. What error occurred here?  _____

b. What concentration should have been made?  _____

c. What concentration did the nurse make and for which route?  _____

d. What is the potential outcome of the error?  _____

e. What measures could have been taken to prevent the error?  _____

Answers on p. 644

# ✓ CHAPTER REVIEW

Use the labels where provided to obtain the necessary information; shade the dosage on syringes where provided. Round the answers to the nearest tenth where indicated.

1. Order: Kefzol 250 mg IM q4h.

    Available:

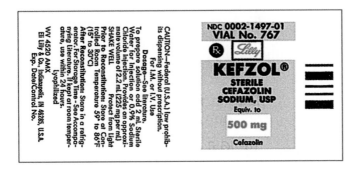

    a. How much diluent must be added to
       the vial for IM administration?            _____

    b. What is the final concentration of the
       solution prepared for IM administration? _____

    c. How many milliliters will you administer
       to provide the ordered dosage?            _____

    d. Shade the dosage calculated on the
       syringe provided.

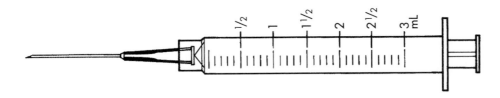

2. Order: Ampicillin 1 g IV q6h.

   Available: 1-g vial. Directions for IV administration state:
   Reconstitute with 10 mL of diluent.

   a.  How many milliliters will you administer? _____

   b.  Shade the dosage calculated on the syringe provided.

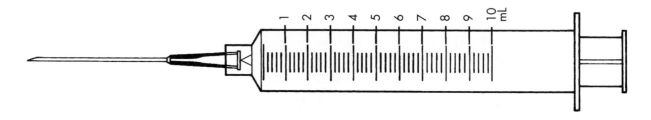

3. Order: Oxacillin 300 mg IM q6h.

   Available:

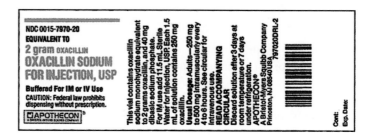

   a.  How much diluent must be added to
       the vial for IM administration?       _____

   b.  What is the final concentration of the
       solution prepared for IM administration? _____

   c.  How many milliliters will you administer? _____

   d.  Shade the dosage calculated on the syringe provided.

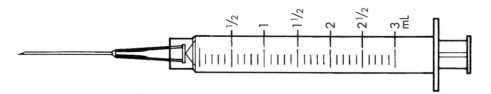

4. Order: Mezlocillin 1.5 g IV q6h.
   Label states: For IV use reconstitute with 30 mL sterile water for injection.
   Each 30 mL of reconstituted solution will contain 3 g mezlocillin.

   How many milliliters will you administer? _____

5. Order: Omnicef 300 mg p.o. q12h.

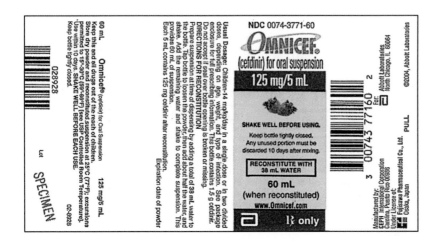

a. How much diluent must be added to prepare the solution? _____

b. What diluent is recommended for reconstitution? _____

c. What is the dosage strength of the reconstituted solution? _____

d. How many milliliters will you administer? _____

e. How long will the medication maintain its potency? _____

6. Order: Penicillin G potassium 600,000 units IV q4h.

Available:

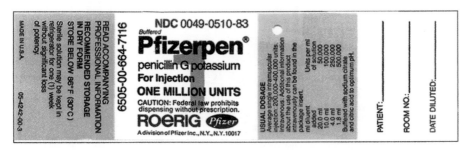

a. Which dosage strength would be best to choose? _____

b. How many milliliters of diluent would be
   needed to make the dosage strength? _____

c. How many milliliters will you administer? _____

d. Shade the dosage calculated on the syringe provided.

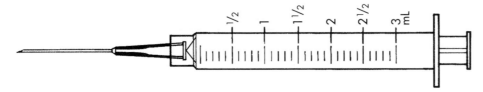

7. Order: Solu-Cortef 200 mg IV q6h for 1 week.

Available:

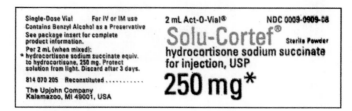

a. What is the concentration of the reconstituted material?

_____

b. How many milliliters will you administer?

_____

c. Shade the dosage calculated on the syringe provided.

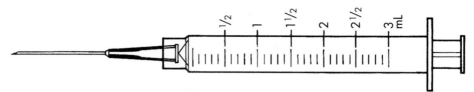

8. Order: methylprednisolone sodium succinate 175 mg IV q6h.

Available:

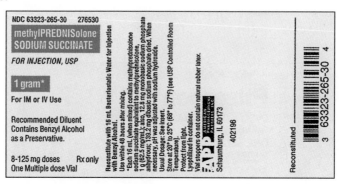

a. What is the total dosage strength of methylprednisolone sodium succinate in this vial?

_____

b. What diluent is recommended for reconstitution?

_____

c. How many milliliters will you administer?

_____

d. Shade the dosage calculated on the syringe provided.

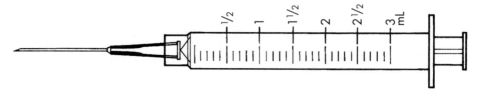

9. Order: Amoxicillin 500 mg p.o. q6h.

   Available:

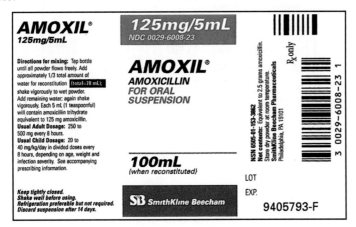

   a. How many milliliters of diluent must
      be added?    _____

   b. What is the dosage strength after
      reconstitution?    _____

   c. How many milliliters are needed to
      administer the required dosage?    _____

10. Order: Cefotan 1.2 g IM q12h.

    Available: Read the medication label and portion of the package insert.

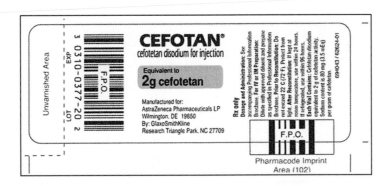

| Vial Size | Amount of Diluent Added (mL) | Approximate Withdrawable Vol (mL) | Approximate Average Concentration (mg/mL) |
|---|---|---|---|
| 1 gram | 2 | 2.5 | 400 |
| 2 gram | 3 | 4 | 500 |

   a. How many milliliters will you administer?  _____

   b. Shade the dosage calculated on the syringe provided.

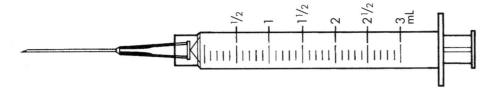

11. Order: Nafcillin 0.5 g IM q6h.

Available:

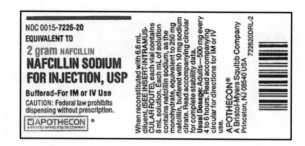

a. What is the dosage strength of the reconstituted nafcillin? _____

b. How many milliliters will you administer? _____

c. Shade the dosage calculated on the syringe provided.

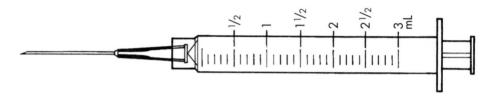

12. Order: Biaxin 350 mg p.o. q12h for 10 days.

Available:

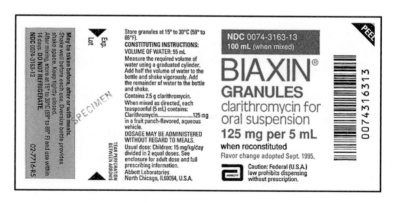

a. How many milliliters of diluent must be added? _____

b. What is the dosage strength after reconstituion? _____

c. How many milliliters will you administer? _____

13. Order: Ifex 2.4 g IV every day for 5 days.

    Available:

    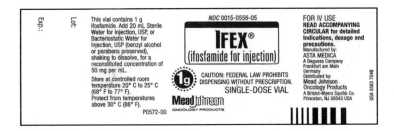

    a. What is the volume of diluent used
       for reconstitution?                     _____

    b. What is the dosage strength of the
       reconstituted Ifex?                     _____

    c. How many milliliters will you
       add to the IV?                          _____

14. Order: Penicillin G potassium 400,000 units IM q4h.

    Available:

    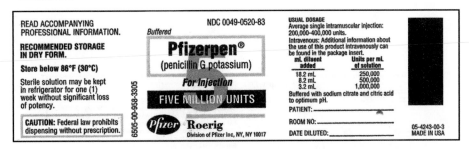

    a. How many milliliters will you
       administer?                             _____

    b. Shade the dosage calculated on the syringe provided.

    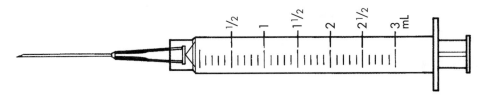

15. Order: Ceftazidime 250 mg IM q12h.

    Available:

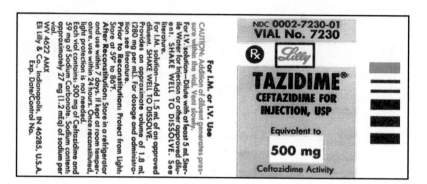

    a. How many milliliters will you administer?

    _____

    b. Shade the dosage calculated on the syringe provided.

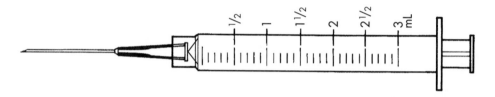

16. Order: Ticar 0.5 g IM q6h.

    Available:

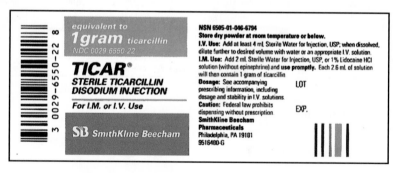

    a. How many milliliters will you administer?

    _____

    b. Shade the dosage calculated on the syringe provided.

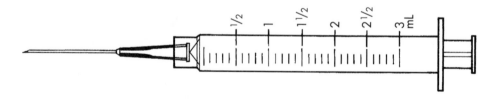

17. Order: Tazicef 0.4 g IV q8h.

    Directions for IV state: Add 10 mL of sterile water for injection. Each mL of solution contains 95 mg per mL.

    a. How many milliliters will you
       administer?                          _____

    b. Shade the dosage calculated on the syringe provided.

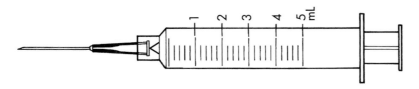

18. Order: Vancomycin 0.5 g IV q12h.

    Use the directions from the insert below.

    Available:

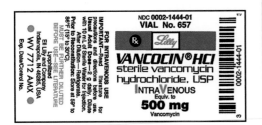

**PREPARATION AND STABILITY**
At the time of use, reconstitute by adding either 10 mL of Sterile Water for Injection to the 500-mg vial or 20 mL of Sterile Water for Injection to the 1-g vial of dry, sterile vancomycin powder. Vials reconstituted in this manner will give a solution of 50 mg/mL. FURTHER DILUTION IS REQUIRED.
After reconstitution, the vials may be stored in a refrigerator for 14 days without significant loss of potency. Reconstituted solutions containing 500 mg of vancomycin must be diluted with at least 100 mL of diluent. Reconstituted solutions containing 1 g of vancomycin must be diluted with at least 200 mL of diluent. The desired dose, diluted in this manner, should be administered by intermittent intravenous infusion over a period of at least 60 minutes.

    a. How many milliliters of diluent
       must be added to the vial?           _____

    b. What is the final concentration of
       the prepared solution?               _____

    c. How many milliliters will you
       administer?                          _____

    d. Shade the dosage calculated on the syringe provided.

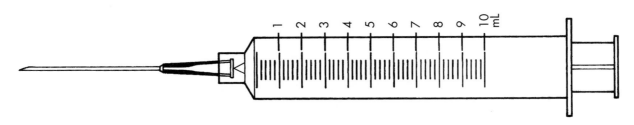

19. Order: Levothyroxine sodium 0.05 mg IV daily.

Available:

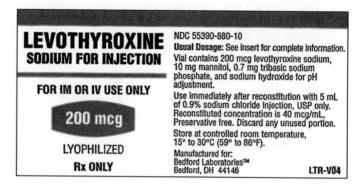

a. How many milliliters will you administer? _____

b. Shade the dosage calculated on the syringe provided.

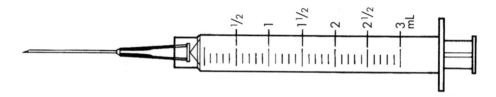

20. Order: Zovirax 0.25 g IV q8h for 5 days.

Use the directions from the insert below.

Available:

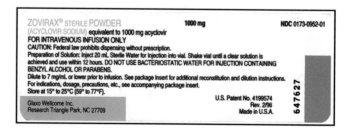

a. How many milliliters will you administer? _____

b. Shade the dosage calculated on the syringe provided.

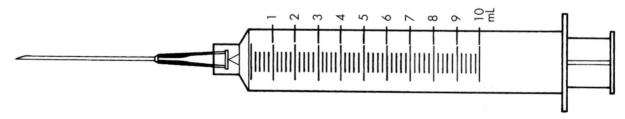

21. Order: Vantin 200 mg p.o. q12h.

    Available:

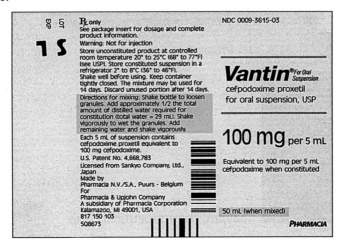

    How many milliliters will you
    administer using an oral syringe?   _____

22. Order: Timentin 2 g IV q12h.

    Available: Timentin 3.1 g. Directions state: Reconstitute with approximately 13 mL
    of sterile water for injection or sodium chloride for injection. The concentration will
    be approximately 200 mg per mL.

    a. How many milliliters will you
       administer?   _____

    b. Shade the dosage on the syringe provided.

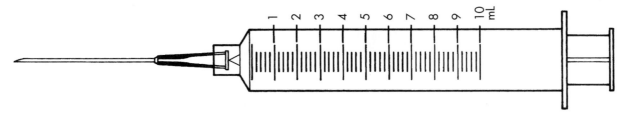

23. Order: Maxipime (cefepime hydrochloride) 2 g IV q12h.

    Available:

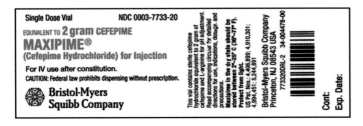

    When reconstituted, yields a concentration of 160 mg per mL.

    How many milliliters will you
    administer?   _____

24. Order: Nafcillin 300 mg IM q6h.

    Available:

    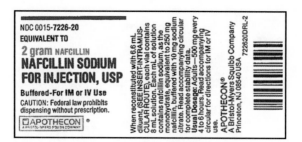

a. How many milliliters will you
   give?

_____

b. Shade the dosage on the syringe provided.

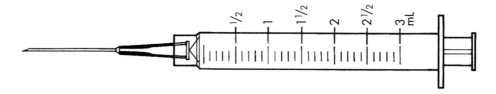

25. Order: Vancomycin 1 g IV q12h.

    Available:

    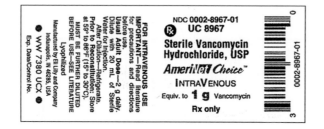

    **PREPARATION AND STABILITY**
    At the time of use, reconstitute by adding either 10 mL of
    Sterile Water for Injection to the 500-mg vial or 20 mL of
    Sterile Water for Injection to the 1-g vial of dry, sterile van-
    comycin powder. Vials reconstituted in this manner will give
    a solution of 50 mg/mL. FURTHER DILUTION IS RE-
    QUIRED.
    After reconstitution, the vials may be stored in a refrigerator
    for 14 days without significant loss of potency. Reconstituted
    solutions containing 500 mg of vancomycin must be diluted
    with at least 100 mL of diluent. Reconstituted solutions con-
    taining 1 g of vancomycin must be diluted with at least 200
    mL of diluent. The desired dose, diluted in this manner,
    should be administered by intermittent intravenous infusion
    over a period of at least 60 minutes.

a. How many milliliters of diluent
   must be added to the vial?

_____

b. How many milliliters will you
   administer?

_____

26. Order: Lorabid 375 mg p.o. q12h.

    Available:

    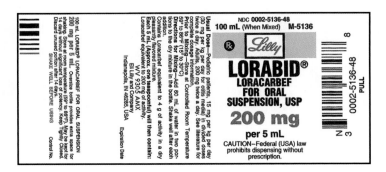

    a. How many milliliters of diluent are
       recommended for reconstitution?    _____

    b. How many milliliters will the bottle
       contain after reconstitution?    _____

    c. How many milliliters will you
       administer?    _____

27. Order: Zosyn 2.25 g q8h IV.

    Available:

    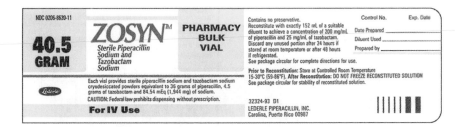

    a. How many milliliters of diluent are
       recommended for reconstitution?    _____

    b. What is the total strength of the vial?    _____

    c. How many milliliters will you
       administer?    _____

28. Order: Fortaz 1.5 g IV q8h for 5 days.

    Available:

    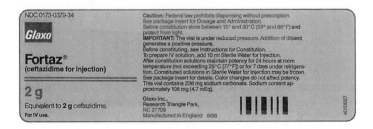

    How many milliliters will you
    administer?    _____

29. Order: Cefobid 1 g IM q12h for 5 days.

    Available:

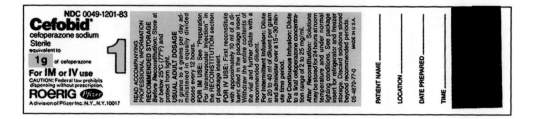

    Directions state: Add 1.4 mL of sterile water for injection. Each 2 mL yields 1 g.

    a. How many milliliters will you
       administer?          _____

    b. Shade the dosage on the syringe provided.

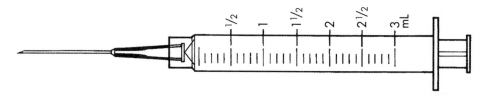

30. Order: Unasyn 1.5 g IV q6h.

    Available:

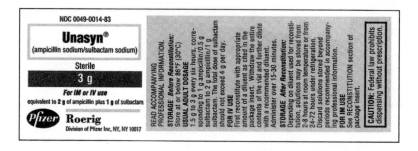

    Package insert states: Add 6.4 mL diluent to get 8 mL of solution.

    How many milliliters will you
    administer?          _____

31. Order: Pepcid 20 mg p.o. b.i.d.

    Available:

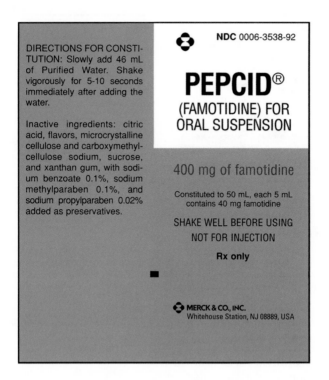

How many milliliters will you
administer using an oral syringe?  _____

32. Order: Nebcin 250 mg IV q8h.

    Available:

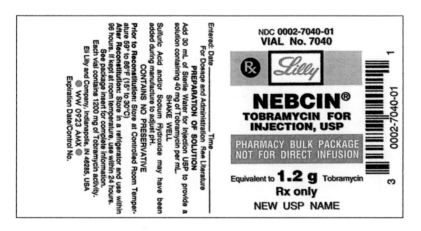

a. How many milliliters of diluent
   must be added to the vial?  _____

b. What is the final concentration of
   the solution per milliliter?  _____

c. How many milliliters will you
   administer?  _____

33. Order: Amphotericin B 45.5 mg IV every day.

    Available:

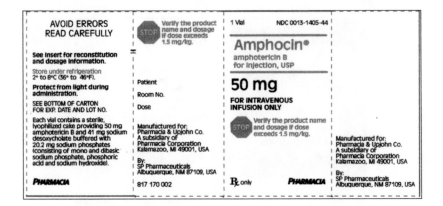

---

**PREPARATION OF SOLUTIONS**

Reconstitute as follows: An initial concentrate of 5 mg amphotericin B per mL is first prepared by rapidly expressing 10 mL 10 mL sterile water for injection, USP *without a bacteriostatic agent* directly into the lyephilized cake, using a sterile needle (minimum diameter: 20 gauge) and syringe. Shake the vial immediately until the colloidal solution is clear. The infusion solution, providing 0.1 mg amphotericin B per mL, is then obtained by further dilution (1:15) with 5% dextrose infection, USP.

---

Use the information from the partial package insert to answer the questions and calculate the number of milliliters you will administer.

a. How many milliliters of diluent must be added for the initial concentration?  _____

b. What is the recommended diluent?  _____

c. What is the final concentration of the prepared solution per milliliter?  _____

d. How many milliliters will you administer?  _____

34. Order: Cefadyl 850 mg IV q6h.

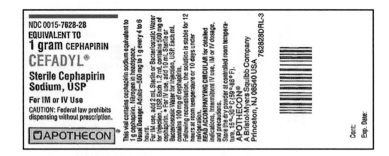

a. How many milliliters of diluent must be added to the vial for IV administration?  _____

b. What is the final concentration of the solution prepared for IV administration?  _____

c. How many milliliters will you administer?  _____

35. Order: Monocid 1 g IM 60 minutes before surgery.

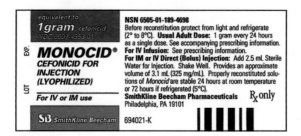

a. How many milliliters of diluent must be added to the vial for IM administration?

_____

b. What is the final concentration of the solution prepared for IM administration?

_____

c. How many milliliters will you administer?

_____

Prepare the following solutions from the nutritional formulas.

36. Order: $\frac{1}{4}$-strength Ensure 12 oz by nasogastric tube over 6 hr. _____

37. Order: $\frac{2}{3}$-strength Isomil 6 oz p.o. q4h for 24 hr. _____

38. A client has an order for Jevity 1,200 mL by continuous feeding through a gastrostomy tube over 16 hours, followed by 250 mL of free water. The feeding is placed on an infusion pump. Calculate the mL per hr to set the pump at. _____

39. Order: $\frac{1}{8}$-strength Ensure 4 oz by nasogastric tube q4h for 24h. _____

Answers on pp. 644-649

 **For additional practice problems, refer to the Basic Calculations section of Drug Calculations Companion, Version 4, on Evolve.**

# CHAPTER
# 20

# Insulin

## Objectives

*After reviewing this chapter, you should be able to:*
1. Identify important information on insulin labels
2. Read calibrations on 30-, 50-, and 100-unit syringes
3. Measure insulin in single dosages
4. Measure combined insulin dosages

Insulin, which is used in the treatment of diabetes mellitus, is a hormone secreted by the islets of Langerhans in the pancreas. It is a necessary hormone for glucose use by the body. Individuals who do not produce adequate insulin experience an increase in their blood sugar (glucose) level. These individuals may require the administration of insulin. Accuracy in insulin administration is extremely important because inaccurate dosages can lead to serious or life-threatening effects. Cohen (2007), in the book titled *Medication Errors,* identified some causes of errors that have occurred with insulin:

- Incorrect rates being programmed into infusion pumps
- Incorrect concentrations of insulin used to prepare a dose
- Use of tuberculin syringe to prepare a dose, which has resulted in tenfold overdoses
- Look-alike names and packaging
- Miscommunication of insulin orders
- "U" used as an abbreviation for units in orders, resulting in the "U" being misinterpreted as a zero (0) or a number

This is just a sample of the causes of errors with insulin and has serious implications for nurses.

**CAUTION**

Accuracy in insulin preparation and administration is crucial. Inaccurate dosages can lead to serious or life-threatening effects. Nurses must correctly interpret insulin orders and use the correct syringe to measure insulin for administration.

Insulin dosages are measured in units and administered with syringes that correspond to insulin U-100; U-100 insulin means 100 units per milliliter. The most common type of insulin is supplied in 10-mL vials and labeled U-100. Insulin is also available as U-500 (500 units per mL). U-500 is a more concentrated strength and is used for diabetic clients who have blood sugars that fluctuate to extremely high levels.

## TYPES OF INSULIN

Different types of insulin are available today. The choice of dosage and insulin preparation depends on the needs of the client. The source of insulin (animal or human), brand and generic names, the dosage strength or concentration, and storage information are indicated on the label. Currently, the only insulins distributed in the United States and other countries are synthetic "human" insulins or their analogs. Insulin from a human source is designated on the label as recombinant DNA (rDNA origin).

Humalog insulin (lispro), a fast-acting insulin analog also known as recombinant DNA insulin, became available in 1996. Lispro acts within 5 to 15 minutes. Lispro can be administered 5 minutes before meals, whereas regular insulin can be administered 30 to 60 minutes before meals. Lispro is intended for subcutaneous administration only. Errors have occurred from the timing of lispro as well as its similarity to regular insulin; both are clear. Other rapid-acting insulin analogs followed lispro, such as aspart (NovoLog) and glulisine (Apidra) in 2004. Like lispro and regular, these analogs are clear.

The long-acting insulin Lantus (insulin glargine) was first approved by the Food and Drug Administration (FDA) in 2000. It is an analog of human insulin. Lantus permits once-daily dosing. It may be administered at any time during the day for 24-hour coverage without a peak; however, it must be administered at the same time every day. It is clear in appearance and intended for subcutaneous use only and cannot be mixed with other insulins. Lantus comes in distinctive packaging. The vial is tall and narrow, and the name Lantus is written in purple letters. The latest long-acting insulin analog, detemir (Levemir), is also generally given once daily. Detemir does not last as long as Lantus so clients may need a nighttime dose of the medication.

The only insulin on the market today is recombinant DNA insulin because it causes fewer reactions than insulin from animal sources. It is essential that the nurse knows where to locate this information. When an insulin order is written, the label will specify the origin of the insulin. Also found on the label is the type of insulin. This is indicated by a letter that follows the trade name. (Figure 20-1 shows information that can be found on an insulin label.)

The letters that follow the trade name on insulin labels (e.g., Humulin R, Humulin N) identify the type of insulin by action and time (see Figure 20-1). Nurses must be familiar with the onset, peak, and duration of action, which vary depending on the type of insulin. There are three basic action types of insulins: rapid acting (regular, lispro [Humalog], aspart [NovoLog], glulisine [Apidra]); intermediate acting (NPH); and long acting (glargine [Lantus], detemir [Levemir]). The expiration date and concentration are also indicated on the label and are important to check. Notice the uppercase letters on all insulin labels, for example, N for NPH as in Figure 20-1. You will see R for regular insulin. Regular and NPH are the two types of insulin used most often.

Look at the Humulin insulin label in Figure 20-1. Notice that the label shows Humulin (trade name), followed by the letter N. N = NPH (intermediate acting). These letters are important identifiers for insulin.

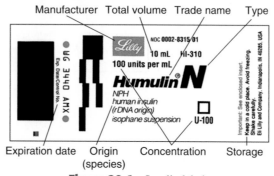

**Figure 20-1**   Insulin label.

**CAUTION**

Careful reading of insulin labels is essential to avoid a medication error that could be life-threatening. Always read the label and compare it with the medication order three times. Insulin dosages must be checked by two nurses. Reading the label carefully ensures selection of the correct action time and type of insulin.

### Types of U-100 Insulins

Nurses must be familiar with the three types of U-100 insulins. Below are samples of labels according to their action times.

*FAST ACTING (RAPID ACTING)*

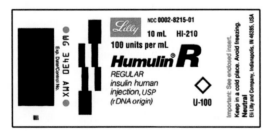
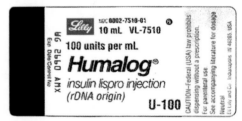

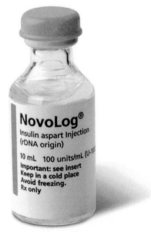

From Novo Nordisk, Inc., Princeton, NJ.

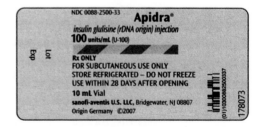

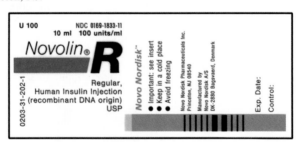

*INTERMEDIATE ACTING*

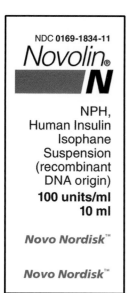

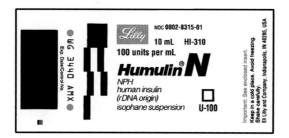

*LONG ACTING*

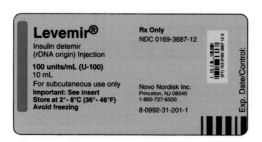

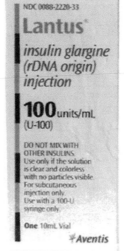

 **Practice Problems**

Using the labels below, identify the insulin trade name and action time (rapid acting, intermediate acting, or long acting).

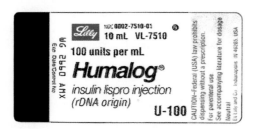

1. Trade name _____ Action time _____

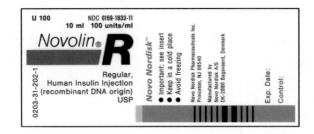

2. Trade name _____ Action time _____

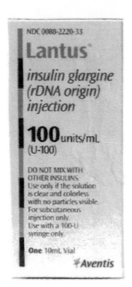

3. Trade name _____ Action time _____

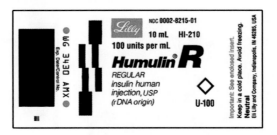

4. Trade name _____ Action time _____

Answers on p. 650

## APPEARANCE OF INSULIN

Regular insulin, Humalog (lispro), and Lantus (insulin glargine), Apidra (insulin glulisine), aspart (Novolog), and Levemir (insulin detemir) insulin are clear. All other insulin is cloudy. They include NPH and fixed combination insulins such as Humulin 70/30, 50/50, and Humalog 75/25.

## FIXED-COMBINATION INSULINS

Fixed-combination insulins are now available (Figure 20-2). These insulins have become popular for clients who must mix fast-acting and intermediate-acting insulins. The purpose of the fixed-combination insulins is to simulate the varying levels of insulin within the bod-

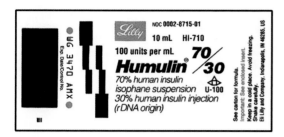

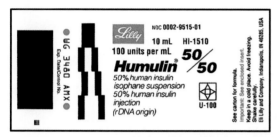

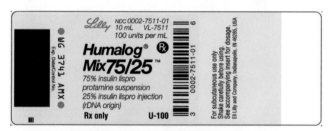

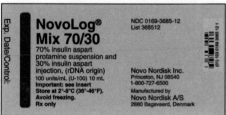

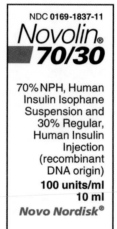

**Figure 20-2**   Fixed-combination insulins.

ies of diabetic persons. The availability of the premixed combination insulins has also decreased the need for clients to mix insulins. Examples of fixed-combination insulins are Humulin 70/30, Novolin 70/30, Humulin 50/50, and Humalog Mix 75/25. Humulin 70/30 is used most often.

To understand fixed-combination insulin orders, it is important for the nurse to understand that, for example, 70/30 concentration means there is 70% NPH insulin (isophane) and 30% regular insulin in each unit. Therefore if the order was 30 units of Humulin 70/30 insulin, the client would receive 21 units of NPH (70% or 0.7 × 30 units = 21 units) and 9 units of regular insulin (30% or 0.3 × 30 units = 9 units).

The 50/50 insulin concentration means there is 50% NPH insulin and 50% regular insulin in each unit. Therefore if the order was 20 units of 50/50 insulin, the client would receive 10 units of NPH (50% or 0.5 × 20 units = 10 units) and 10 units of regular insulin (50% or 0.5 × 20 units = 10 units). It is important to note that Humalog Mix 75/25 contains 75% lispro protamine insulin and 25% lispro "rapid insulin." Figure 20-2 shows labels of fixed-combination insulins.

**CAUTION**

Do not shake insulin. Mix by rolling gently between the palms of your hands.

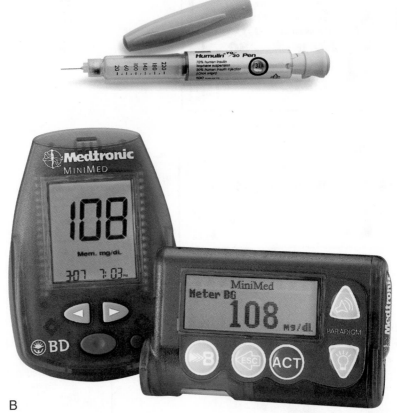

**Figure 20-3** **A,** Insulin pens. **B,** Paradigm® 515 insulin pump and Paradigm Link™ blood glucose monitor. (**A,** Copyright Eli Lilly and Company. All rights reserved. Used with permission. **B,** From Medtronic, Minneapolis, Minn.)

## INSULIN ADMINISTRATION

Insulin is available in 100 units per mL multidose vials and supplied in units that denote strength. The major route of administration for insulin is by subcutaneous injection; it is never administered intramuscularly. Regular insulin, aspart, and glulisine are approved insulins for intravenous administration. Dosage and frequency of insulin administration are highly individualized. It can also be administered with insulin pens that contain a cartridge filled with insulin or with a CSII pump (continuous subcutaneous [subcut] insulin infusion). The CSII pump is used to administer a programmed dose of a rapid-acting 100 units per mL–insulin at a set rate of units per hour. Figure 20-3 shows the various delivery systems used to administer insulin.

### Measuring Insulin in a U-100 Syringe

Insulin is always ordered in units, the medication is supplied in 100 units per mL, and the syringes are calibrated for 100 units per mL and marked U-100. Therefore no calculations are required to prepare insulin dosages subcutaneously. We will focus on the administration of insulin with the U-100 syringes, of which there are different types.

1. **Lo-Dose syringe**—It has a capacity of 50 units (0.5 mL). Each calibration on the syringe measures 1 unit. There is also a 30-unit (0.3 mL) syringe, which is used to accurately measure very small amounts of insulin. It is marked in units up to 30 units. Each calibration is 1 unit.

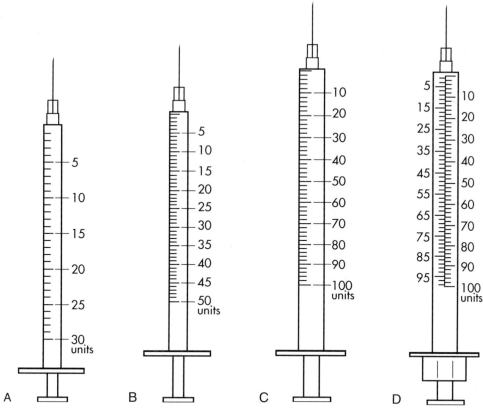

**Figure 20-4**   Types of insulin syringes. **A,** Lo-Dose insulin syringe (30 units). **B,** Lo-Dose insulin syringe (50 units). **C,** Single-scale syringe (100 units). **D,** Double-scale syringe (100 units).

2. **1-mL (100-unit) capacity syringe**—The 100-unit syringe comes with even and odd numbers on it. There are two types of 1-mL syringes in current use.
   a. The single-scale syringe is calibrated in 2-unit increments. Any dosage measured in an odd number of units is measured between the even calibrations. This would not be the desired syringe for clients with vision problems.
   b. The double-scale syringe has odd-numbered units on the left and even-numbered units on the right. To avoid confusion, the scale on the left should be used for odd numbers of units (e.g., 13 units) and the scale on the right, for even numbers of units (e.g., 26 units). When even numbers of units are measured, each calibration is then measured as 2 units.

**CAUTION**

Administer insulin in an insulin syringe used only for the administration of U-100 insulin. Do not use an insulin syringe to measure other medications that are measured in units. Syringes of 30 and 50 units measure a smaller volume of insulin but are intended for the measurement of U-100 insulin only. Use the smallest capacity insulin syringe available to ensure the accuracy of dosage preparation.

To review what the syringes look like, see Figure 20-4 for the four types of insulin syringes discussed.

## Lo-Dose Syringe

Let's look at some insulin dosages measured in the syringes to help you visualize the amounts in a syringe. Syringe *A* shows 30 units and syringe *B* shows 37 units in a Lo-Dose syringe.

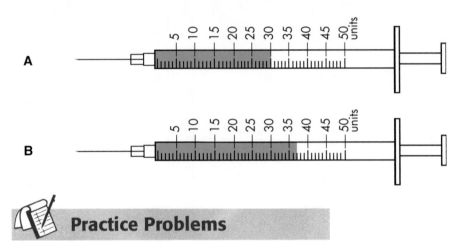

## Practice Problems

Using the syringes below, indicate the dosages shown by the arrows.

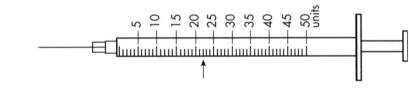

5. _____

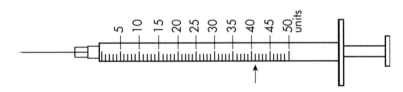

6. _____

Using the syringes below, shade in the dosages indicated.
7.  17 units

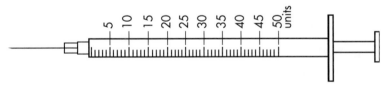

8.  47 units

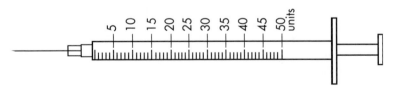

Answers on p. 650

## Single-Scale 1-mL Syringe

Now let's look at what dosages would look like on a single-scale 1-mL syringe. The syringes below show 25 units in syringe *A* and 55 units in syringe *B*. Notice that the dosages are drawn up between the even calibrations.

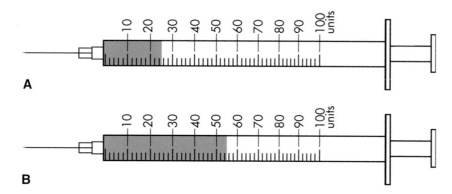

## Double-Scale 1-mL Syringe

Now let's look at the dosage indicated on a double-scale (100-unit) 1-mL syringe. Syringe *C* shows 37 units; notice that the scale on the left is used. Syringe *D* shows 54 units; notice that the scale on the right is used.

**CAUTION**

Look carefully at the increments when using a dual syringe.

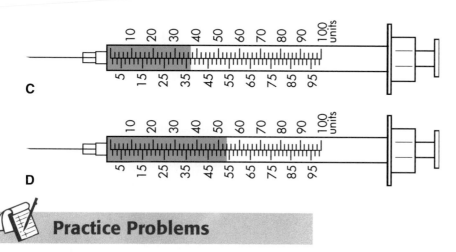

## Practice Problems

Indicate the following dosages shaded on the 100-unit (1-mL) syringes.

9. _____

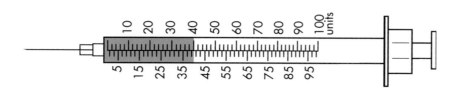

10. _____

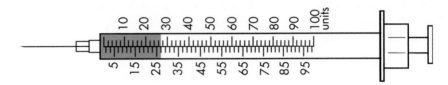

11. _____

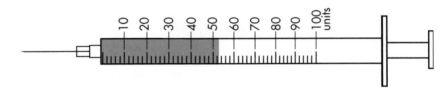

12. _____

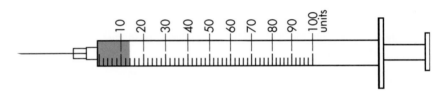

Shade the specified dosages on each of the U-100 syringes below.

13. 88 units

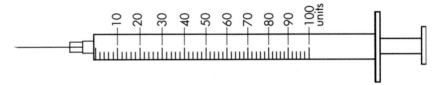

14. 44 units

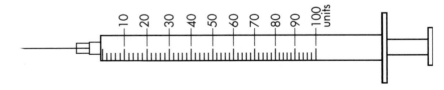

15. 30 units

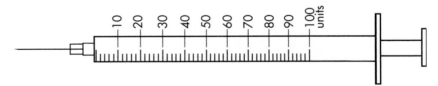

Answers on p. 650

## INSULIN ORDERS

Like any written medication order, an insulin order must be written clearly and contain certain information to prevent errors in administration. An error in administration can cause harmful effects to a client. Insulin orders should contain the following information:

    a. The brand name of insulin (which implies the origin) and the action time. Example: Humulin R indicates human origin. Regular indicates rapid action. Some orders may be written simply as Humulin Regular.

    b. The number of units to be administered. Example: 20 units, Humulin Regular.

    c. The route (subcut). Insulin is usually administered subcutaneously; however, regular insulin, aspart, and glulisine can be administered intravenously, as well.

    d. The time it should be given. Example: ½ hour before meals.

    e. The strength of the insulin to be administered. Example: U-100.

**Example of Insulin Order:** Regular Humulin insulin U-100 20 units subcut ½ hr $\overline{a}$ breakfast.

> **NOTE**
>
> Insulin is given subcutaneously unless IV is specified.

**CAUTION**

To avoid misinterpretation the abbreviation "U," which stands for units, should not be used when insulin orders are written. The word *units* should be written out. Errors have occurred as a result of the "U" being mistaken for a "0" in a hand-written order. Example: 6U subcut stat of Humulin Regular. The U is almost completely closed and could be misread as 60 units. The recommendation to write out the word *units* has also been issued by the Institute for Safe Medication Practices (ISMP) and should be included on each accredited organization's "do not use" list approved by The Joint Commission (TJC).

### Coverage Orders

Sometimes, in addition to standing insulin orders, clients may have orders for additional insulin to "cover" their increased blood sugar levels. (This is often referred to as a sliding scale.) The sliding scale indicates a certain dosage of insulin based on the client's blood glucose levels. The order may also state CBG (capillary blood glucose) to indicate checking blood glucose levels for the sliding scale. Regular insulin is used because of its immediate action and short duration. Lispro is also used. A coverage order specifies the dosage of insulin according to the blood sugar level and the frequency. The amount of insulin and the blood sugar level should be specific. The following is a sample coverage order (sliding scale).

### Tips for Clinical Practice

When orders are written for sliding scale, the abbreviation $\overline{ss}$ should not be used to mean sliding scale. In the apothecary system $\overline{ss}$ means 1/2, and ss could also be mistaken for the number 55. Write out sliding scale.

**Humulin Regular U-100 according to finger stick q8h.**

| | |
|---|---|
| 0-180 mg/dL | no coverage |
| 181-240 mg/dL | 2 units subcut |
| 241-300 mg/dL | 4 units subcut |
| 301-400 mg/dL | 6 units subcut |
| Greater than 400 mg/dL | 8 units subcut stat and notify doctor. |
| | Repeat finger stick in 2 hr. |

> **NOTE**
>
> This sliding scale is an example used for one patient. It is not a standard scale. Sliding scales are individualized for clients.

At some institutions there is a special record to document insulins given. A sample of an insulin therapy record is shown in Figure 20-5.

## ST. BARNABAS HOSPITAL
BRONX, NY 10457

INSULIN THERAPY RECORD

Addressograph or label (printed)
with client identification

DIAGNOSIS:
S/P I+D of Perineal Abscess

| ALLERGIC TO: NKDA | DATE 4/1/11 |
|---|---|

*USE ASTERISK (*) TO INDICATE DOSES NOT GIVEN-EXPLAIN IN NURSES NOTES.*

| ORDER DATE / EXP DATE | STANDING INSULIN ORDERS | DATE 2011 | 4/1 | 4/2 | 4/3 | 4/4 | 4/5 | 4/6 | 4/7 | 4/8 | 4/9 |
|---|---|---|---|---|---|---|---|---|---|---|---|
| RN. INIT. | MED-DOSE-FREQ-ROUTE | HOUR | INIT. | INIT. | INIT. | INIT. | INIT. | INIT. | INIT. | INIT. | INIT. |
| 4/1/11 DM | NPH 10 (ten) | 7³⁰A | DM | JN | DG | | | | | | |
| | units subcut q AM | site | RA | RT | LA | | | | | | |
| 5/1/11 | | | | | | | | | | | |
| RN. INIT. 4/1/11 DM | NPH 12 (twelve) | 4³⁰p | NN | NN | JJ | | | | | | |
| | units subcut q PM | site | LA | LT | RA | | | | | | |
| 5/1/11 | | | | | | | | | | | |
| RN. INIT. | | | | | | | | | | | |
| | | | | | | | | | | | |
| | | | | | | | | | | | |
| RN. INIT. | | | | | | | | | | | |
| | | | | | | | | | | | |
| | | | | | | | | | | | |

### SINGLE/STAT ORDERS

| ORDER DATE | NURSE INIT. | MED-DOSE-ROUTE | TO BE GIVEN DATE | TIME | NURSE INIT. | ORDER DATE | NURSE INIT. | MED-DOSE-ROUTE | TO BE GIVEN DATE | TIME | NURSE INIT. |
|---|---|---|---|---|---|---|---|---|---|---|---|
| | | | | | | | | | | | |
| | | | | | | | | | | | |
| | | | | | | | | | | | |
| | | | | | | | | | | | |
| | | | | | | | | | | | |

INJECTION CODES:   RT = RIGHT THIGH    RA = RIGHT ARM    ▲ RAB = UPPER RIGHT ABDOMEN    ▲ LAB = UPPER LEFT ABDOMEN
LT = LEFT THIGH    LA = LEFT ARM    ▼ RAB = LOWER RIGHT ABDOMEN    ▼ LAB = LOWER LEFT ABDOMEN

***Note**: At this institution, to reduce the potential for errors and eliminate misinterpretation of insulin orders, all handwritten orders for insulin *must* include the dose in both numerical and text form.

**Figure 20-5**    Insulin therapy record. (Used with permission from St. Barnabas Hospital, Bronx, New York.)

## INITIAL IDENTIFICATION

(NORMAL CBG RANGE 80 - 120 MG/DL)

| INITIAL | PRINT NAME, TITLE | INITIAL | PRINT NAME, TITLE | INITIAL | PRINT NAME, TITLE |
|---|---|---|---|---|---|
| 1 DM | Deborah C. Morris RN | 5 JJ | Jupiter Jones RN | 9 | |
| 2 NN | Nancy Nurse RN | 6 MS | Mary Smith RN | 10 | |
| 3 JN | Jane Nightingale RN | 7 | | 11 | |
| 4 DG | Deborah Gray RN | 8 | | 12 | |

## INSULIN COVERAGE

| INSULIN COVERAGE ORDERS | | |
|---|---|---|
| ORDER DATE / RN. INIT. 4/1/11 DM | ORDER DATE / RN. INIT. | ORDER DATE / RN. INIT. |
| CBG bid | | |
| BS 200-250 2 (two) units Reg. Insulin subcut | | |
| 251-300 4 (four) units Reg. Insulin subcut | | |
| 301-350 6 (six) units Reg. Insulin subcut | | |
| 351-400 8 (eight) units Reg. Insulin subcut | | |
| Call MD if less than 60 or greater than 400 | | |

| DATE | TEST TIME | URINE SUGAR | ACETONE | CBG RESULT | TIME GIVEN | INSULIN TYPE | DOSE | SITE | SIGNATURE/ TITLE | REMARKS (FBS RESULTS, TPN, ETC.) |
|---|---|---|---|---|---|---|---|---|---|---|
| 4/1/11 | 6A | | | 314 | 6A | Regular Insulin 6 units subcut LA | | | Mary Smith RN | |
| 4/1/11 | 4³⁰p | | | 243 | 4⁴⁰p | Regular Insulin 2 units subcut LT | | | Nancy Nurse RN | |

**Figure 20-5, cont'd** Insulin therapy record. *CBG,* Capillary blood glucose. (Used with permission from St. Barnabas Hospital, Bronx, New York.)

## PREPARING A SINGLE DOSAGE OF INSULIN IN AN INSULIN SYRINGE

Measuring insulin in an insulin syringe requires no calculation or conversion. An order must be written following the previously stated guidelines. Frequent errors have occurred with insulin dosages. To avoid insulin dosage errors remember the following:

> **RULE**
>
> Insulin dosages *must* be checked by two nurses. In the preparation of combination dosages (two insulins) two nurses must verify each step of the process.

**Example 1:** Order: Humulin R U-100 40 units subcut in AM ½ hr before breakfast

Available: Humulin R labeled U-100

To measure 40 units, withdraw U-100 insulin to the 40 mark on the U-100 syringe. A Lo-Dose syringe can also be used to draw up this dose, as shown below.

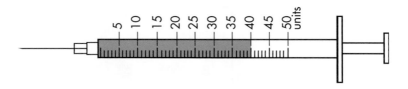

**Example 2:** Order: Humulin N U-100 70 units subcut daily at 7:30 AM

Available: Humulin N labeled U-100

There is no calculation or conversion required here. Draw up the required amount using a U-100 (1-mL) syringe.

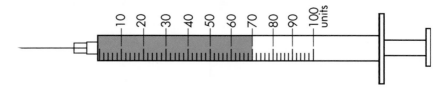

**Example 3:** Order: Humulin R U-100 5 units subcut stat

Available: Humulin R labeled U-100

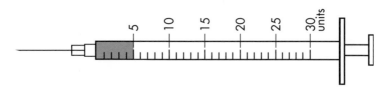

## MEASURING TWO TYPES OF INSULIN IN THE SAME SYRINGE

Sometimes individuals may require two different types of insulin for control of their blood sugar levels, for example, NPH and regular. To decrease the number of injections it is common to mix two insulins in a single syringe. To mix insulin in one syringe, remember:

> **RULE**
>
> Regular insulin is always drawn up in the insulin syringe first: clear then cloudy insulin.

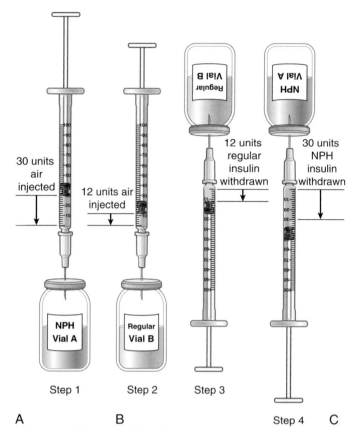

**Figure 20-6** Mixing insulins. Order: Humulin N (NPH) U-100 30 units subcut, Humulin R (Regular) U-100, 12 units subcut. **A,** Inject 30 units of air into Humulin N first; do not allow needle to touch insulin. **B,** Inject 12 units of air into Humulin R and withdraw 12 units; withdraw needle. **C,** Insert needle into vial of Humulin N and withdraw 30 units. Total 30 units Humulin N (NPH) + 12 units Humulin R (Regular) = 42 units. (Modified from Harkreader H, Hogan MA: *Fundamentals of nursing: caring and clinical judgement,* ed. 3, St. Louis, 2007, Saunders.)

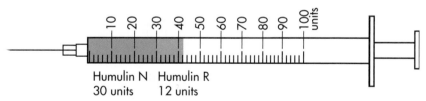

**Figure 20-7** Total of two insulins combined. Total = 42 units (30 units Humulin NPH + 12 units Humulin R).

Drawing regular insulin up first prevents contamination of the regular insulin with other insulin. This sequence is extremely important.

To prepare insulin in one syringe (mixing insulin), complete the following steps (Figures 20-6 and 20-7):

1. Cleanse tops of both vials with alcohol wipe.
2. Inject air equal to the amount being withdrawn into the vial of cloudy insulin first. When the air is injected, the tip of the needle should not touch the solution.
3. Remove the needle from the vial of cloudy insulin.
4. Using the same syringe, inject an amount of air into the regular insulin (clear) equal to the amount to be withdrawn, invert or turn the bottle up in the air, and draw up the desired amount.
5. Remove the syringe from the regular insulin, and check for air bubbles. If air bubbles are present, gently tap the syringe to remove them.
6. Next withdraw the desired dosage from the vial of cloudy insulin.
7. The total number of units in the syringe will be the sum of the two insulin orders.

**CAUTION**

Cloudy insulin should be rolled gently between the palms of the hands to mix it before it is drawn up. Do not shake insulin. Shaking creates bubbles in addition to breaking down the particles and causing clumping.

## Tips for Clinical Practice

Insulins mix instantly; they do not remain separated. Therefore insulin that has been overdrawn cannot be returned to the vial.

**Example 1:**    The order is to administer 18 units of regular U-100 subcut and 22 units subcut of NPH U-100.

The total amount of insulin is 40 units (18 units [regular] + 22 units [NPH] = 40 units).

To administer this dosage, a Lo-Dose syringe or a U-100 (1-mL) syringe can be used. However, because the dosage is 40 units, the Lo-Dose would be more desirable. (See syringes that follow, illustrating this dosage.)

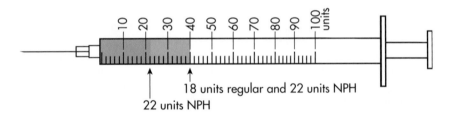

18 units regular and 22 units NPH

22 units NPH

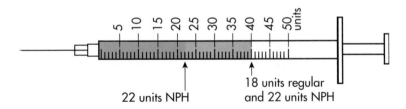

22 units NPH

18 units regular and 22 units NPH

## Tips for Clinical Practice

When mixing insulins, it is important to follow the steps outlined. Committing one of the following phrases to memory may help you remember the steps: (1) last injected is first drawn up; (2) run fast first (regular), then slow down (NPH); (3) clear to cloudy; or (4) it is alphabetical: <u>clear</u>, <u>cloudy</u>. Also remember when mixing insulins, only the same type should be mixed together, for example, Humulin and Humulin.

## ■ Points to Remember

- U-100 means 100 units per mL.
- Carefully read the prescriber's orders.
- To ensure accuracy, insulin should be given only with an insulin syringe. Insulin syringes should not be used to measure other medications measured in units.
- U-100 insulin is designed to be given with syringes marked U-100.
- Insulin dosages must be exact. Read the calibration on the insulin syringes carefully.
- Lo-Dose syringes are desirable for small dosages up to 50 units. The Lo-Dose 30-unit syringe may be used for dosages up to 30 units. Although Lo-Dose insulin syringes (30 units and 50 units) can hold a smaller volume, they are intended for U-100 insulin only.
- A U-100 (1-mL capacity) syringe is desirable when the dosage exceeds 50 units.
- Drawing up insulin correctly is critical to safe administration of insulin to clients.
- When insulins are mixed, regular insulin (clear) is always drawn up first, then cloudy.
- Do not shake insulin. Roll the insulin gently between the palms of the hands to mix.
- When insulins are mixed, the total volume is the sum of the two insulin amounts.
- Regular insulin, aspart, and glulisine are approved for IV administration.
- Lantus must not be mixed with any other insulin, and it must not be diluted.
- Read insulin labels to ensure that you have the correct type of insulin to avoid medication errors. Only mix the same types of insulin (e.g., Humulin R and Humulin N).
- Use the smallest-capacity syringe possible to ensure accuracy.
- Insulin orders should be written with units spelled out, not abbreviated U.
- Avoid insulin errors by always double-checking dosages with another nurse.

## ? Critical Thinking Questions

1. **Scenario:** Suppose the prescriber wrote the following insulin order:
   Humulin U-100 10 Ս subcut ā breakfast.
   The nurse assumed the order was for regular insulin 100 units and administered the insulin to the client.
   Later, it was discovered the insulin dose desired was NPH 10 units.
   a. What error occurred here? _____
   b. What client rights were violated? _____
   c. What is the potential outcome of the error? _____
   d. What measures could have been taken to prevent the error that occurred? _____

2. **Scenario:** A client is to receive Humulin R U-100 10 units subcut and Humulin N U-100 14 units subcut before breakfast. In drawing up the insulins in the same syringe, the nurse used the following technique:
   a. Injected 10 units of air into the regular vial.
   b. Injected 14 units of air into the NPH vial.
   c. Withdrew 14 units of NPH insulin, then the 10 units of regular insulin.
      (a) What is the error in the technique of drawing up the two insulins? _____
      (b) What is the potential outcome from the technique used? _____

Answers on p. 650.

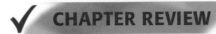

## CHAPTER REVIEW

Using the syringes below and the labels where provided, indicate the dosage you would prepare and shade the dosage on the syringe provided.

1. Order: Humulin R U-100 35 units subcut daily at 7:30 AM.

   Available:

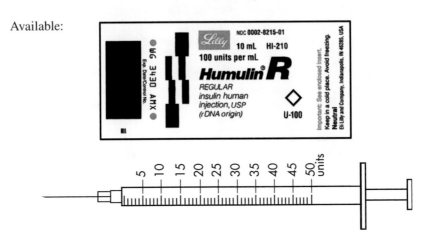

2. Order: Humulin N U-100 56 units subcut daily every AM ½ hour before breakfast.

   Available:

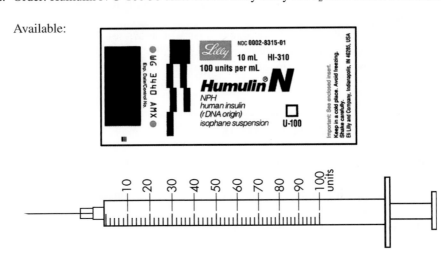

3. Order: Humulin R U-100 18 units subcut and Humulin N U-100 40 units subcut daily at 7:30 AM.

   Available:

   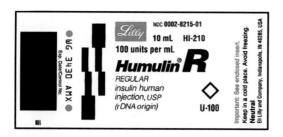

   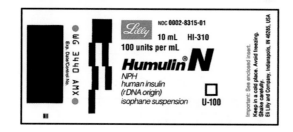

   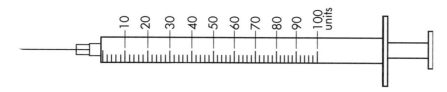

4. Order: Novolin R U-100 9 units subcut daily.

   Available:

   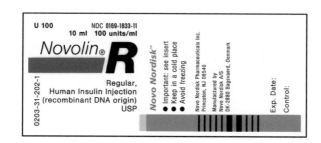

   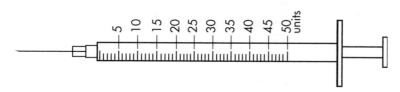

Indicate the number of units measured in the following syringes.

5. Units measured _____

   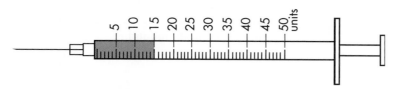

6. Units measured                              _____

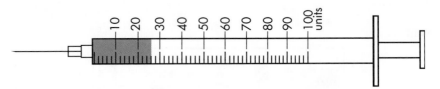

7. Units measured                              _____

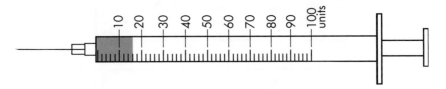

8. Units measured                              _____

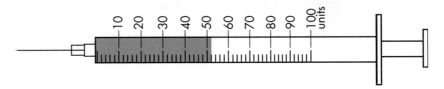

9. Units measured                              _____

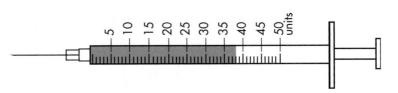

10. Units measured                             _____

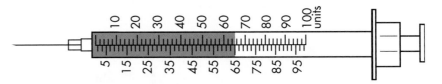

11. Units measured                             _____

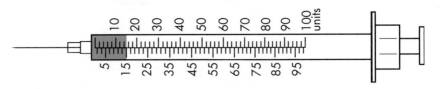

Calculate the dosage of insulin where necessary, and shade the dosage on the syringe provided. Labels have been provided for some problems.

12. Order: Humulin R U-100 10 units subcut at 7:30 AM.

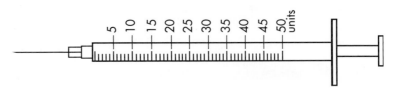

13. Order: Humulin R U-100 16 units subcut and Humulin N U-100 24 units subcut a.c. 7:30 AM.

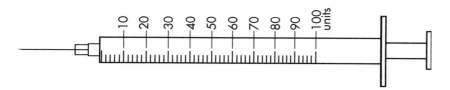

14. Order: Humulin R U-100 10 units subcut and Humulin N U-100 15 units subcut a.c. 7:30 AM.

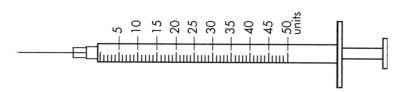

15. Order: Humulin R U-100 5 units subcut and Humulin N U-100 25 units subcut a.c. 7:30 AM.

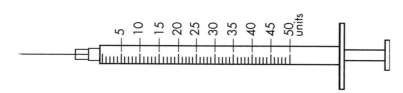

16. Order: Novolin R U-100 40 units subcut and Novolin N U-100 10 units subcut at 7:30 AM.

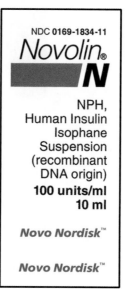

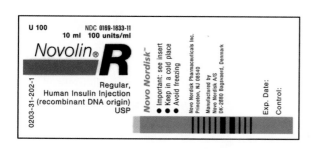

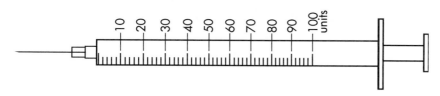

17. Order: Humulin N U-100 48 units subcut and Humulin R U-100 30 units subcut a.c. 7:30 AM.

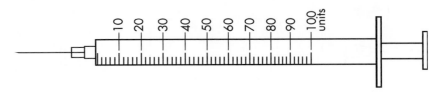

18. Order: Novolin R U-100 16 units subcut and Novolin N U-100 12 units subcut 7:30 AM.

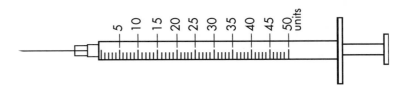

19. Order: Novolin R U-100 17 units subcut 5 PM.

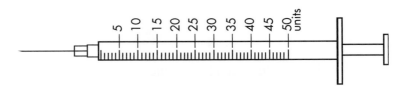

20. Order: Humalog U-100 15 units subcut daily at 7:30 AM.

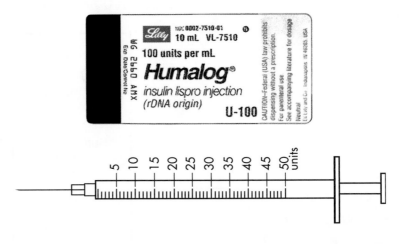

21. Order: Humulin R U-100 26 units subcut and Humulin N U-100 48 units subcut daily.

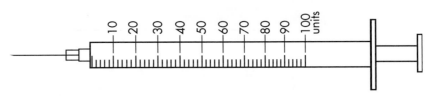

22. Order: Humulin 70/30 U-100 27 units subcut at 5 PM.

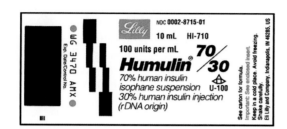

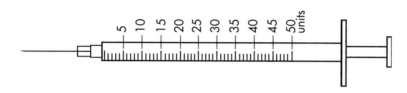

23. Order: Novolin R U-100 21 units subcut and Novolin N U-100 35 units subcut daily at 7:30 AM.

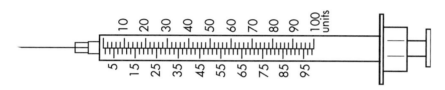

24. Order: Novolin Regular U-100 5 units subcut and Novolin N U-100 35 units subcut 7:30 AM.

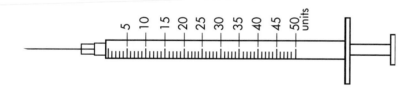

25. Order: NovoLog U-100 36 units subcut 7:30 AM before breakfast.

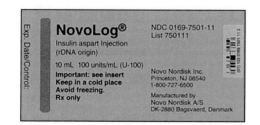

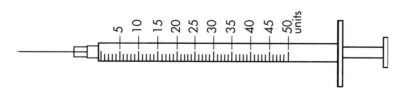

26. A client has a sliding scale for insulin dosages. The order is for Humulin Regular insulin U-100 q6h as follows:

| Finger stick | 0-180 mg/dL | no coverage |
|---|---|---|
| Blood sugar | 181-240 mg/dL | 2 units subcut |
| | 241-300 mg/dL | 4 units subcut |
| | 301-400 mg/dL | 6 units subcut |
| | Greater than 400 mg/dL | 8 units subcut and repeat finger stick in 2 hr |

At 11:30 AM the client's finger stick is 364 mg/dL. Shade the syringe to indicate the dosage that should be given.

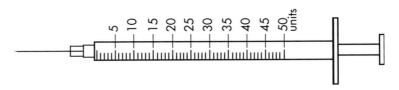

27. Order: Humulin N U-100 66 units subcut 10 PM.

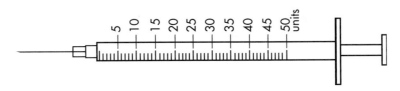

28. Order: Humulin R U-100 32 units subcut every morning at 7:30 AM.

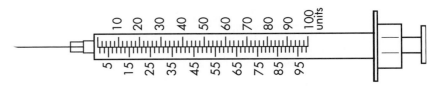

29. Order: Humulin N U-100 35 units subcut daily at 7:30 AM.

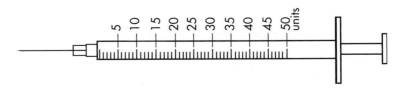

30. Order: Humulin R U-100 9 units subcut 5 PM.

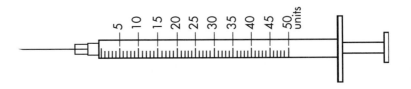

31. Order: Humulin N U-100 24 units subcut 10 PM.

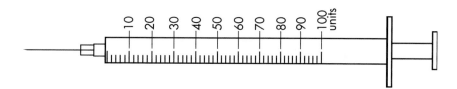

32. Order: Humulin R U-100 8 units subcut, and Humulin N U-100
    18 units subcut at 7:30 AM.

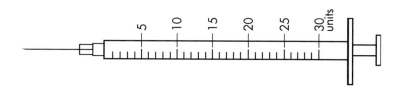

33. Order: Humulin N U-100 11 units subcut at bedtime.

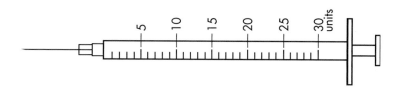

34. Order: Humulin 70/30 U-100 20 units subcut ½ hr before breakfast.

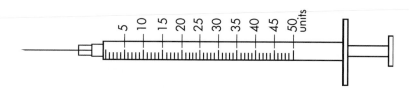

35. Order: Humulin R U-100 10 units subcut and Humulin N U-100 42 units subcut at
    4:30 PM.

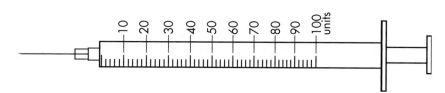

36. Order: Novolin R U-100 8 units subcut and Novolin N U-100 15 units subcut at
    7:30 AM.

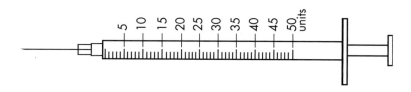

37. Order: Humalog Insulin U-100 35 units subcut at 7:30 AM.

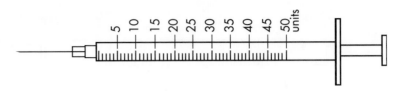

38. Order: Humulin R U-100 30 units subcut and Humulin N U-100 40 units subcut every day at 8:00 AM.

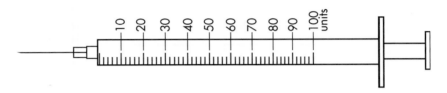

39. A client has a sliding scale for insulin dosages. The order is for Humulin R U-100 q6h as follows:

| Finger stick | 201-250 mg/dL | 4 units subcut |
|---|---|---|
| Blood sugar | 251-300 mg/dL | 6 units subcut |
| (mg/dL) | 301-350 mg/dL | 8 units subcut |
| | 351-400 mg/dL | 10 units subcut |
| | Greater than 400 mg/dL | call MD |

At 6:00 PM the client's blood sugar is 354 mg/dL. Shade the syringe to indicate the dosage that should be administered.

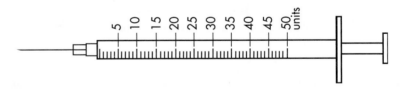

Answers on pp. 650-652

---

○ℓ **For additional practice problems, refer to the Advanced Calculations section of Drug Calculations Companion, Version 4, on Evolve.**

# UNIT Five

# Intravenous, Heparin, and Critical Care Calculations and Pediatric Dosage Calculations

The ability to accurately calculate flow rates for intravenous medications is essential to both heparin administration and critical care calculations.

# CHAPTER
# 21

# Intravenous Solutions and Equipment

## Objectives

*After reviewing this chapter, you should be able to:*
1. Identify common intravenous (IV) solutions and abbreviations
2. Calculate the amount of specific components in IV solutions
3. Define the following terms associated with IV therapy: peripheral line, central line, primary line, secondary line, saline/heparin locks, IV piggyback (IVPB), and IV push
4. Differentiate among various devices used to administer IV solutions (e.g., patient-controlled analgesia [PCA] pumps, syringe pumps, volumetric pumps)

The calculations associated with IV therapy will be discussed in the next chapter (Chapter 22). A general discussion of IV therapy will make it easier to understand the calculations that are performed involving IV therapy. Intravenous (IV) means the administration of fluids or medications through a vein. Medications, electrolyte solutions, and blood and blood products are frequently ordered and administered directly into the vein. The advantage of administering medications by this route is the immediate availability of the medication to the body and the rapidity of action. IV fluids are ordered for varied reasons. They may be ordered to restore or maintain fluid and electrolyte balance, to replace lost fluids, and to act as a medium for administering medications directly into the bloodstream. *Replacement fluids* are ordered for a client who has lost fluids because of things such as diarrhea, vomiting, or hemorrhage. *Maintenance fluids* help to sustain normal levels of fluids and electrolytes for clients at risk for depletion (e.g., a client NPO).

IV fluids and medications can be administered by continuous and intermittent infusion. *Continuous IV* infusions replace or maintain fluids and electrolytes. *Intermittent IV* infusions, for example, IV piggyback (IVPB) and IV push, are used to administer medications and supplemental fluids. Intermittent peripheral infusion devices known as saline or heparin locks are used to maintain venous access without the need of continuous infusion.

Nursing responsibility includes administration of IV fluids at the correct rate and monitoring the client during the therapy.

Calculations related to IV therapy may include calculating infusion rates in drops per minute (gtt/min) or milliliters per hour (mL/hr). The calculations necessary for the safe administration of IV fluids will be presented in Chapter 22.

If a client receives an IV infusion too rapidly and is not monitored closely, reactions can vary from mild to severe (death). Administration of IV fluids at a proper rate is a priority and an essential nursing responsibility.

The prescriber is responsible for writing the IV order, which **must** specify the following:
1. Name of the IV solution
2. Name of medication to be added, if any
3. Amount (volume) to be administered
4. Time period during which the IV is to infuse

For example, an IV order might read:

1,000 mL 5% D/W IV in 8 hours.

In this case the order is for an IV solution in which the name of the solution is 5% dextrose and water, the route of administration is IV, and the duration is 8 hours.

## IV FLUIDS

There are several types of IV fluids. The type of fluid used is individualized according to the client and the reason for its use. IV solutions come prepared in plastic bags or glass bottles ranging from 50 mL (bags only) to 1,000 mL. IV plastic bags are more commonly used. IV solutions are clearly labeled with the exact components and amount of solution. When IV solutions are written in orders and charts, abbreviations are used. Example: D5W means dextrose 5% in water. You may encounter various abbreviations; however, the percentage and initials, regardless of how they are written, have the same meaning: "D" is for dextrose, "W" is for water, "S" is for saline, and "NS" is for normal saline. Ringer lactate (lactated Ringer), a commonly used electrolyte solution, is abbreviated "RL" or "LR" and occasionally "RLS." Potassium chloride (KCl) is commonly added to IV solutions. Potassium chloride is measured in milliequivalents (mEq). The order is usually written to indicate the amount of milliequivalents per liter (1,000 mL) to be added to the IV fluid. Example: 0.9 % NS 1,000 mL IV with 20 mEq KCl per L q8h; this is interpreted as "infuse 1,000 mL 0.9 % normal saline IV solution with 20 milliequivalents potassium chloride added per liter every 8 hours." Saline (sodium chloride or NaCl) is also found in IV fluids. Refer to Box 21-1, and learn the common abbreviations for IV solutions. Figures 21-1 to 21-5 show various IV solutions.

Pay close attention to IV abbreviations. The letters indicate the solution compounds, whereas the numbers indicate the solution strength.

### BOX 21-1 Abbreviations for Common IV Solutions

| | |
|---|---|
| NS | Sodium chloride 0.9% |
| ½ NS | Sodium chloride 0.45% |
| D5W or 5% D/W | Dextrose 5% in water |
| D5RL | Dextrose 5% and lactated Ringer (Ringer lactate) |
| RL or RLS | Lactated Ringer solution (electrolytes) |
| D5NS | Dextrose 5% in sodium chloride |
| D5 and ½ NS (0.45%) | Dextrose 5% in 0.45% sodium chloride |

From Brown M, Mulholland J: *Drug calculations: process and problems for clinical practice,* ed. 8, St. Louis, 2008, Mosby.
IV bags are labeled as sodium chloride, although frequently referred to as normal saline (NS).

Normal saline solutions are often written with 0.9 or the percent sign included (e.g., D5 0.9% NS). NS is the abbreviation used for normal saline. Normal saline is also referred to as sodium chloride (NaCl). Saline is available in different percentages. Normal saline is the common term used for 0.9% sodium chloride. Another common saline IV concentration is 0.45% NaCl, often written as "¹/₂ NS" (0.45% is half of 0.9%).

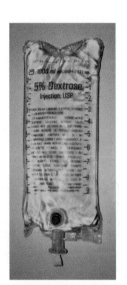
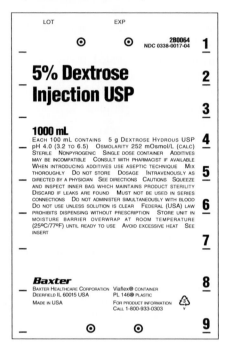

**Figure 21-1** 5% Dextrose. (From Brown M, Mulholland JL: *Drug calculations: process and problems for clinical practice,* ed. 8, St. Louis, 2008, Mosby.)

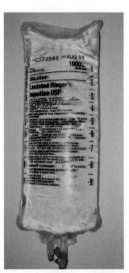
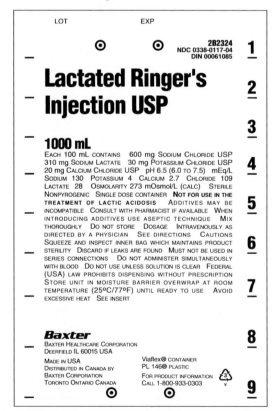

**Figure 21-2** Lactated Ringer solution. (From Brown M, Mulholland JL: *Drug calculations: process and problems for clinical practice,* ed. 8, St. Louis, 2008, Mosby.)

Other saline solution strengths include 0.33% NaCl, also abbreviated as "1/3 NS," and 0.225% NaCl, also abbreviated as "1/4 NS." Some orders for IV fluids may therefore be written as D5 $\frac{1}{2}$ NS, D5 $\frac{1}{4}$ NS. *Note:* IV fluids can contain saline only (see Figure 21-4) or saline mixed with dextrose, which would be indicated with the percentage of dextrose (e.g., D5 0.9% sodium chloride). Figures 21-3 and 21-5 show saline solution (NaCl) mixed with dextrose.

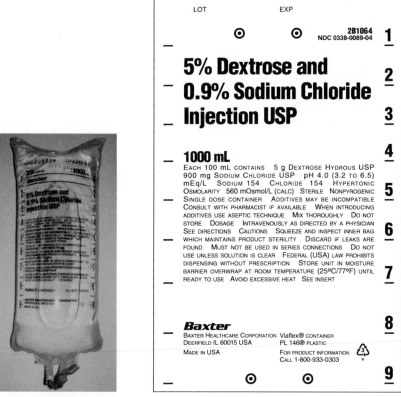

**Figure 21-3** 5% Dextrose in 0.9% sodium chloride. (From Brown M, Mulholland JL: *Drug calculations: process and problems for clinical practice,* ed. 8, St. Louis, 2008, Mosby.)

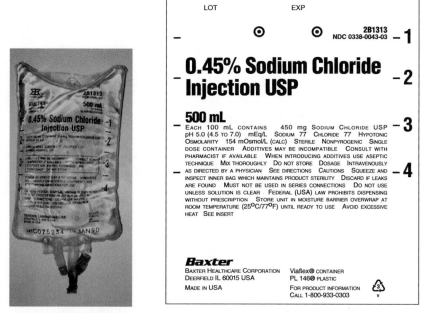

**Figure 21-4** 0.45% Sodium chloride. (From Brown M, Mulholland JL: *Drug calculations: process and problems for clinical practice,* ed. 8, St. Louis, 2008, Mosby.)

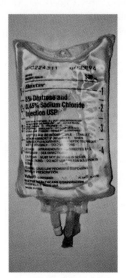
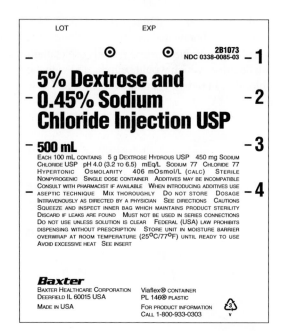

**Figure 21-5** 5% Dextrose in 0.45% sodium chloride. (From Brown M, Mulholland JL: *Drug calculations: process and problems for clinical practice,* ed. 8, St. Louis, 2008, Mosby.)

## Charting of IV Solution

IV fluids are charted on the intake and output (I&O) sheet; in some institutions they are also charted on the medication administration record (MAR). Figure 21-6 is a sample I&O charting record.

Juice glass – 180 mL    Small water cup – 120 mL
Water glass – 210 mL    Jello cup – 150 mL
Coffee cup – 240 mL     Ice cream – 120 mL
Soup bowl – 180 mL      Creamer – 30 mL

**Date:** 8/17/11

| Client information |
|---|
|  |

| INTAKE | | | | | OUTPUT | | | |
|---|---|---|---|---|---|---|---|---|
| Time | Type | Amt | Time | IV/ Blood type | Amount absorbed | Time | Urine | Stool | Other |
|  |  |  | 7A | 1,000 mL D5W | 800 mL | 9A | 400 mL |  |  |
|  |  |  | 12P | IVPB | 100 mL | 1P | 500 mL |  |  |
|  |  |  |  |  |  |  |  |  |  |
|  |  |  |  |  |  |  |  |  |  |
|  |  |  |  |  |  |  |  |  |  |
|  |  |  |  |  |  |  |  |  |  |
|  |  |  |  |  |  |  |  |  |  |
|  |  |  |  |  |  |  |  |  |  |
| 8 hr total |  |  |  |  | 900 mL |  | 900 mL |  |  |

**Figure 21-6** Sample of charting IV fluids on I&O record.

## Calculating Percentage of Solute in IV Fluids

The amount of each ingredient in an IV fluid can be calculated; however, it is not necessary because the label on the IV solution indicates the amount of each ingredient. Calculation of the percentage of solutions was presented in Chapter 5, which deals with percentages.

As you may recall, it is possible to determine the percentage of substances such as dextrose in IV solutions. It is important to remember that **solution strength expressed as a percentage means grams of solute per 100 mL of fluid.** Therefore 5% dextrose solution will have 5 g of dextrose in each 100 mL. In addition to the amount of dextrose in the solution, amounts of other components, such as sodium chloride, can be determined. To calculate the amount of a specific component in an IV solution, a ratio and proportion or dimensional analysis can be used.

**Example 1:**   Calculate the amount of dextrose in 500 mL D5W. Remember % = g per 100 mL; therefore 5% dextrose = 5 g dextrose per 100 mL.

 Solution Using Ratio and Proportion

$$5 \text{ g}:100 \text{ mL} = x \text{ g}:500 \text{ mL}$$

$$\frac{100x}{100} = \frac{2{,}500}{100}$$

$$x = 25 \text{ g}$$

500 mL D5W contains 25 g of dextrose

Remember that ratios and proportions can be stated in various ways. This ratio and proportion could also be stated as follows:

$$\frac{5 \text{ g}}{100 \text{ mL}} = \frac{x \text{ g}}{500 \text{ mL}}$$

 Solution Using Dimensional Analysis

5% dextrose = 5 g dextrose per 100 mL. Enter it as the starting fraction, and determine the number of grams in the solution.

$$x \text{ g} = \frac{5 \text{ g}}{\underset{1}{\cancel{100 \text{ mL}}}} \times \frac{\overset{5}{\cancel{500 \text{ mL}}}}{1}$$

$$x = 25 \text{ g dextrose}$$

500 mL D5W contains 25 g dextrose

**Example 2:**   Calculate the amount of sodium chloride (NaCl) in 1,000 mL NS.

$$0.9\% = 0.9 \text{ g NaCl per 100 mL}$$

 Solution Using Ratio and Proportion

$$0.9 \text{ g}:100 \text{ mL} = x \text{ g}:1{,}000 \text{ mL} \quad or \quad \frac{0.9 \text{ g}}{100 \text{ mL}} = \frac{x \text{ g}}{1{,}000 \text{ mL}}$$

$$\frac{100x}{100} = \frac{900}{100}$$

$$x = 9 \text{ g NaCl}$$

1,000 mL of NS contains 9 g of sodium chloride

Solution Using Dimensional Analysis

0.9% = 0.9 g NaCl per 100 mL. Use the grams of solute per 100 mL of fluid as the starting fraction.

$$x\,g = \frac{0.9\,g}{\overset{1}{\cancel{100\,mL}}} \times \frac{\overset{10}{\cancel{1,000}}\,mL}{1}$$

$$x = 9\,g\,NaCl$$

1,000 mL of NS contains 9 g of NaCl

**Example 3:** Calculate the amount of dextrose and sodium chloride in 1,000 mL of 5% dextrose and 0.45% normal saline (D5 and ½ NS).

 Solution Using Ratio and Proportion

D5 = dextrose 5% = 5 g dextrose per 100 mL

0.45% NS = 0.45 g NaCl per 100 mL

Dextrose: 5 g : 100 mL = $x$ g : 1,000 mL   *or*   $\dfrac{5\,g}{100\,mL} = \dfrac{x\,g}{1,000\,mL}$

$$\frac{100x}{100} = \frac{5,000}{100}$$

$$x = 50\,g\,dextrose$$

NaCl: 0.45 g : 100 mL = $x$ g : 1,000 mL

$$\frac{100x}{100} = \frac{450}{100}$$

$$x = 4.5\,g\,NaCl$$

1,000 mL D5 0.45% NS contains 50 g of dextrose and 4.5 g of NaCl

 Solution Using Dimensional Analysis

5% dextrose = 5 g dextrose per 100 mL

0.45% NS = 0.45 g NaCl per 100 mL

Dextrose: $x\,g = \dfrac{5\,g}{\overset{1}{\cancel{100\,mL}}} \times \dfrac{\overset{10}{\cancel{1,000}}\,mL}{1}$

$$x = 50\,g\,dextrose$$

NaCl: $x\,g = \dfrac{0.45\,g}{\overset{1}{\cancel{100\,mL}}} \times \dfrac{\overset{10}{\cancel{1,000}}\,mL}{1}$

$$x = 4.5\,g\,NaCl$$

1,000 mL D5 0.45% NS contains 50 g of dextrose and 4.5 g of NaCl

**Example 4:** Calculate the amount of dextrose and sodium chloride in 1,000 mL of D5 NS.

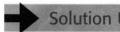 Solution Using Ratio and Proportion

D5 = dextrose 5% = 5 g dextrose per 100 mL

NS = 0.9 g NaCl per 100 mL

Dextrose: 5 g : 100 mL = $x$ g : 1,000 mL   *or*   $\dfrac{5 \text{ g}}{100 \text{ mL}} = \dfrac{x \text{ g}}{1,000 \text{ mL}}$

$$\frac{100x}{100} = \frac{5,000}{100}$$

$$x = 50 \text{ g dextrose}$$

NaCl: 0.9 g : 100 mL = $x$ g : 1,000 mL   *or*   $\dfrac{0.9 \text{ g}}{100 \text{ mL}} = \dfrac{x \text{ g}}{1,000 \text{ mL}}$

$$\frac{100x}{100} = \frac{900}{100}$$

$$x = 9 \text{ g NaCl}$$

1,000 mL D5NS contains 50 g of dextrose and 9 g of NaCl

 Solution Using Dimensional Analysis

D5 = dextrose 5% = 5 g dextrose per 100 mL

NS = 0.9 g NaCl per 100 mL

Dextrose: $x$ g = $\dfrac{5 \text{ g}}{\cancel{100}^{1} \text{ mL}} \times \dfrac{\cancel{1,000}^{10} \text{ mL}}{1}$

$$x = 50 \text{ g dextrose}$$

NaCl: $x$ g = $\dfrac{0.9 \text{ g}}{\cancel{100}^{1} \text{ mL}} \times \dfrac{\cancel{1,000}^{10} \text{ mL}}{1}$

$$x = 9 \text{ g NaCl}$$

1,000 mL D5NS contains 50 g of dextrose and 9 g of NaCl

## Parenteral Nutrition

Parenteral nutrition is a form of nutritional support in which the nutrients are provided by the IV route. Parenteral nutrition solutions consist of glucose, amino acids, minerals, vitamins, and/or fat emulsions. The nutrients are infused by a peripheral or central line. Solutions less than 10% dextrose may be given through a peripheral vein; parenteral nutrition with greater than 10% dextrose requires administration by a central venous catheter. A central venous catheter is placed into a high-flow central vein, such as the superior vena cava, by the health care provider. Lipid emulsions are also given when the client is receiving parenteral nutrition. They provide supplemental kilocalories and prevent fatty acid deficiencies. These emulsions can be administered through a separate peripheral line, through a central line by a Y connector tubing, or as mixtures with the parenteral nutrition solution.

Clients who are unable to digest or absorb enteral nutrition are candidates for parenteral nutrition. Parenteral nutrition is referred to as TPN (total parenteral nutrition) and hyperalimentation. The same principles relating to IV therapy are applicable to parenteral nutrition, but more emphasis is placed on care for the site to prevent infection. Further discussion of parenteral nutrition can be found in nursing reference books. Flow rate and

**NOTE**

Always adhere to the protocol for administering IV medications.

calculation of infusion times, which will be discussed in this chapter, are also applicable to parenteral nutrition solutions.

*IV medication protocols* are valuable references, often posted in the medication room of an institution. They provide nurses with specifics about usual medication dosage, dilution for IV administration, compatibility, and specific observations of a client that need to be made during medication administration.

## Administration of Blood and Blood Products

Blood and blood products are also administered intravenously. When blood is administered, specific protocols must be followed. These can be found in nursing reference books. Flow rates and calculation of infusion times are also applicable to blood and blood products. When blood is administered, a standard blood set or Y-type blood set is commonly used. The Y refers to two spikes above the drip chamber of the IV tubing. One spike is attached to the blood container, and the other is attached to a container of normal saline (NaCl) solution. Normal saline (NaCl) is used to flush the IV tubing at the start of the transfusion and at the end. Blood may be administered by gravity or electronic pump (Figure 21-7). Tubing for blood administration has an in-line filter.

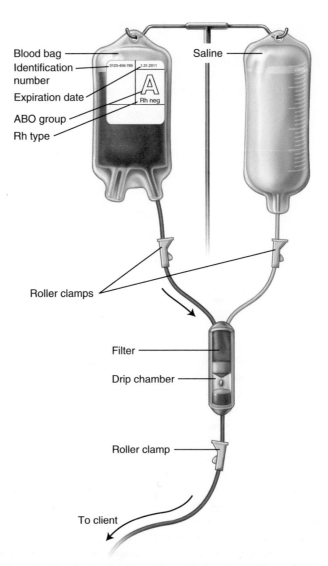

**Figure 21-7** Setup for blood administration. (From Harkreader H, Hogan MA: *Fundamentals of nursing: caring and clinical judgment,* ed. 3, St. Louis, 2007, Saunders.)

## ADMINISTRATION OF IV FLUIDS

IV fluids are administered by an IV infusion set, which includes a sealed bag containing the fluids. A drip chamber is connected to the IV bottle or bag. The flow rate is adjusted to drops per minute (gtt/min) by use of a roller clamp. Some IV tubings have a sliding clamp attached, which can be used to temporarily stop the IV infusion. Injection ports are located on the IV tubing and on most IV solution bags. Injection ports allow for injection of medications directly into the bag of solution or line. The injection ports also allow for attachment of secondary IV lines that contain fluids or medications to the primary line. Figure 21-8 shows a primary line infusion set. IV fluids infuse by gravity flow. This means that for the IV solution to infuse, it must be hung above the level of the client's heart, which will allow for adequate pressure to be exerted for the IV to infuse. The height of the IV bag therefore has a relationship to the rate of flow. The higher the IV bag is hung, the greater the pressure; therefore the IV will infuse at a more rapid rate.

### IV Sites

IV fluids may be administered through a peripheral line or a central line. IV lines are referred to as either *peripheral* or *central* lines, terms used in relation to the primary line. The infusion site of a **peripheral line** is a vein in the arm, hand, or scalp in an infant; or if other sites are not accessible and on rare occasions, a vein in the leg. For a **central line,** a special catheter is used to access a large vein such as the subclavian or jugular vein. The special catheter is threaded through a large vein into the right atrium. Examples of central catheters include triple-lumen, Hickman, Broviac, and Groshong catheters. When a peripheral vein is used to access a central vein, you may see the term *peripherally inserted central catheter* or *PICC* line. A PICC line is inserted into the antecubital vein in the arm and is advanced into the superior vena cava.

### Primary and Secondary Lines

Medications may be added to a primary line either before the IV is started or after it has been infusing. Examples of medications added include electrolytes, such as potassium chloride, and vitamins, such as multivitamins (MVI). These medications are usually diluted in a large volume of fluid (1,000 mL), particularly potassium chloride, because of the side effects and untoward reactions that can occur. In some institutions IV solutions containing potassium chloride are stocked by the pharmacy and obtained on request by the unit, eliminating the need to add it to an IV bag. **Secondary lines** attach to the primary line at an injection port. The main purpose of secondary lines is to infuse medications on an intermittent basis (e.g., antibiotics every 6 hr). They can also be used to infuse other IV fluids, as long as they are compatible with the fluid on the primary line. A secondary line is referred to as an IV piggyback (IVPB). Notice that the IVPB is hanging higher than the primary line (Figure 21-9*A*).

The IVPB is hanging higher than the primary line so that it gives it greater pressure than the primary, thereby allowing it to infuse first. Most secondary administration sets come with an extender that allows the nurse to lower the primary bag. Notice that the secondary bags are smaller than the primary. Amounts of 50 to 100 mL are seen most often. The amount of solution used for the IVPB is determined by the medication being added. Some medications may have to be mixed in 250 mL of fluid for administration. IVPB medications can come premixed by the manufacturer or pharmacist, depending on the institution, or the nurse may have to prepare them. The rate for an IVPB to infuse should be checked. The manufacturer's insert provides recommended times for infusion if not stated in the prescriber's order.

### Systems for Administering Medications by Intravenous Piggyback

*TANDEM PIGGYBACK SETUP*   The tandem piggyback setup is a small IV bag connected to the port of a primary infusion line or to an intermittent venous access. Unlike the piggyback setup, however, the small IV bag that is to infuse is placed at the same height as the primary infusion bag or bottle. In this  setup the tandem and primary IV solution infuse simultaneously (see Figure 21-9, *B*). The nurse must monitor the tandem system closely and clamp the tandem setup immediately once the medication has infused to prevent the IV solution from the primary line from backing up into the tandem line.

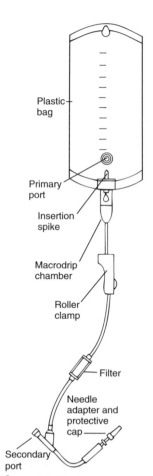

**Figure 21-8**    Intravenous infusion set. (From Clayton BD, Stock YN, Harroun RD: *Basic pharmacology for nurses,* ed. 14, St. Louis, 2007, Mosby.)

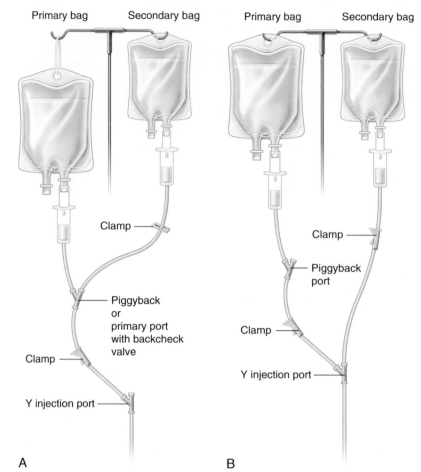

**Figure 21-9**    Intermittent IV medication administration can be accomplished with the use of IV piggyback. **A,** Piggyback. **B,** Tandem. (From Harkreader H, Hogan MA: *Fundamentals of nursing: caring and clinical judgment,* ed. 3, St. Louis, 2007, Saunders.)

Another type of secondary medication setup used in some institutions is called the **ADD-Vantage system.** This system requires a special type of IV bag that has a port for inserting the medication (usually in powder form and mixed with the IV solution as a diluent). The contents of the vial are therefore mixed into the total solution and then infused (Figure 21-10).

The Baxter Mini-Bag Plus is also used to administer piggyback medication. The mini-bag, which is dispensed by the pharmacy, has a vial of unreconstituted medication attached to a special port. You break an internal seal and mix the medication and diluent just before administration. The medication vial remains attached to the mini-bag (Figure 21-11).

**Volume control devices** are used for accurate measurement of small-volume medications and fluids. Most volume control devices have a capacity of 100 to 150 mL and can be used with secondary or primary lines. They are also used intermittently for medication purposes. They have a port that allows medication to be injected and a certain amount of IV fluid to be added as a diluent (Figure 21-12). Volume control devices are referred to by their trade names (Volutrol, Soluset, or Buretrol) depending on the institution. They are used mostly in pediatrics and critical care settings. These devices allow for precise control of the infusion and the medication.

**CAUTION**

When an infusion time is not stated for IVPB, check appropriate resources, such as a medication book or the hospital pharmacy. The nurse is responsible for any error that occurs in reference to IV administration, including incorrect rate of administration.

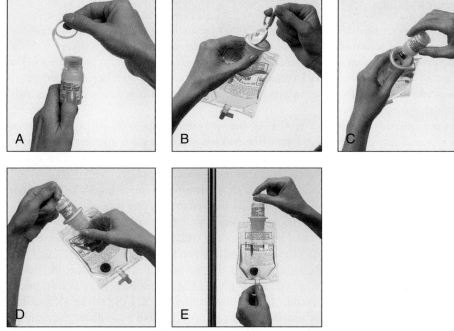

**Figure 21-10** Assembling and administering medication with the ADD-Vantage® system.
**A,** Swing the pull ring over the top of the vial, and pull down far enough to start the opening. Then pull straight up to remove the cap. Avoid touching the rubber stopper and vial threads. **B,** Hold diluent container, and gently grasp the tab on the pull ring. Pull up to break the tie membrane. Pull back to remove the cover. Avoid touching the inside of the vial port. **C,** Screw the vial into the vial port until it will go no farther. Recheck the vial to ensure that it is tight. Label appropriately. **D,** Mix container contents thoroughly to ensure complete dissolution. Look through bottom of vial to verify complete mixing. Check for leaks by squeezing container firmly. If leaks are found, discard unit. **E,** When ready to administer, remove the white administration port cover and pierce the container with the piercing pin. (From Hospira, Inc, Lake Forest, Ill.)

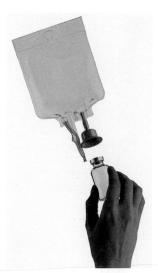

**Figure 21-11** Mini-Bag Plus. (From Baxter Healthcare Corporation, Deerfield, Ill.)

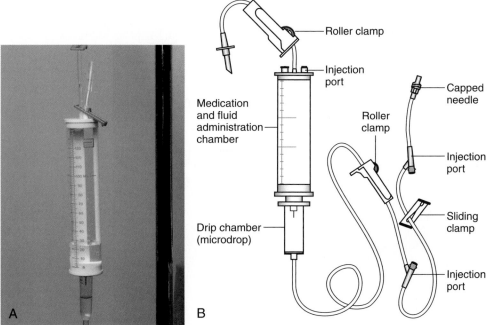

Roller clamp

Injection port

Medication and fluid administration chamber

Drip chamber (microdrop)

Roller clamp

Capped needle

Injection port

Sliding clamp

Injection port

**Figure 21-12** **A,** Volume-controlled device. **B,** Parts of a volume control set. (**A** from Potter PA, Perry AG: *Fundamentals of nursing,* ed. 7, St. Louis, 2009, Mosby.)

## Saline and Heparin IV Locks

Intermittent venous access devices (Figure 21-13) are used for the purpose of administering IV medication intermittently or for access to a vein in an emergency situation. Intermittent venous access devices are referred to as *medlocks, saline locks,* or *heplocks.* The line is usually kept free from blockage or clotting by irrigating it with heparin (anticoagulant) or sterile saline solution. The solution used and the amount of solution vary from institution to institution.

Various institutions have purchased a needleless system (Figure 21-14) for administration of medications through the primary line and for access devices such as saline locks. The needleless system does not require attachment of a needle by the nurse. The system allows for administration by IV push, bolus, or piggyback.

When medications are administered through intermittent venous access devices (also called *access devices*), they must be periodically flushed to maintain patency. Due to bolusing of clients when heparin is used, heparin (a potent anticoagulant despite its use in dilute forms) is now used only on the initial insertion of the catheter. For subsequent flushings of the port, normal saline solution is used (1 to 3 mL, depending on institution policy).

When medications are administered through an intermittent access device, the device must be flushed before and after medication is given. The letters used in most institutions to remember the technique for medication administration are S, I, S (saline, IV medications, saline). Some institutions use the acronym SAS (saline, administer medication, saline). With early discharge and an increased number of home care clients discharged with access devices in place, it is imperative that clients be taught about the care of the intermittent access device.

**CAUTION**

Always refer to the policy at your institution or health care agency regarding the frequency, volume, and concentration of saline or heparin to be used to maintain the IV lock.

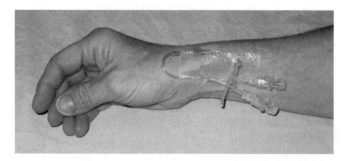

**Figure 21-13**    Intermittent lock covered with a rubber diaphragm. (From Potter PA, Perry AG: *Fundamentals of nursing,* ed. 7, St. Louis, 2009, Mosby.)

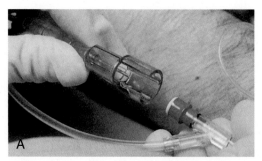
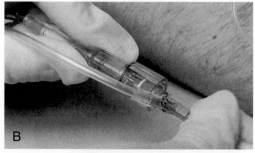

**Figure 21-14**    **A,** Needleless infusion system. **B,** Connection into an injection port. (From Elkin MK, Perry AG, Potter PA: *Nursing interventions and clinical skills,* ed. 4, St. Louis, 2007, Mosby.)

Medications can be administered through a port used for direct injection of medication by syringe or directly into the vein by venipuncture. This is referred to as IV **push** or **bolus.** IV *push* indicates that a syringe is attached to the lock and the medication is pushed in. IV *bolus* indicates that a volume of IV fluid is infused over a specific period of time through an IV administration set attached to the lock. There are guidelines, however, relating to the acceptable rate for IV push administration. **Check appropriate references for the rate (per minute) for IV push medication administration.** Also check the institution's policy and a pharmacology reference regarding administration by IV push or bolus.

### Electronic Infusion Devices

Several electronic infusion devices are on the market today (Figure 21-15). Special tubing is supplied by the manufacturers of these electronic devices. Each device can be set for a specific flow rate and generally emits an alarm if the rate is interrupted. The use of electronic infusion devices is based on the need to strictly regulate the IV. Electronic infusion devices are essential in pediatrics and the critical care setting, where they provide for infusion of small amounts of fluids or medications with precision.

*ELECTRONIC VOLUMETRIC PUMPS* Electronic volumetric pumps infuse fluids into the vein under pressure and against resistance and do not depend on gravity. The pumps are programmed to deliver a set amount of fluid per hour (see Figure 21-15). There is a

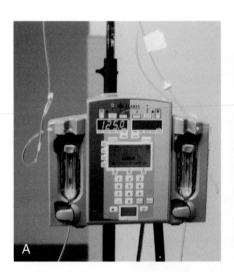
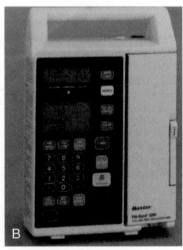
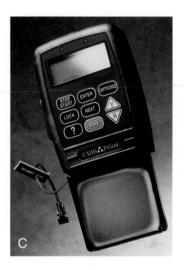
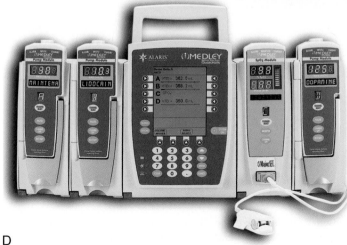

**Figure 21-15** **A,** Dual-channel infusion pump. **B,** Single-channel infusion pump. **C,** CADD-Prizm® VIP ambulatory battery-operated infusion device used for IV parenteral nutrition. **D,** Alaris® System. (**A** from Kee JL, Marshall SM: *Clinical calculations: With applications to general and specialty areas,* ed. 6, St. Louis, 2009, Saunders. **B** from Baxter Healthcare Corporation, Deerfield, Ill. **C** from Smiths Medical MD, Inc., St. Paul, Minn. **D** from Cardinal Health, San Diego, Calif.)

wide range of electronic pumps. Because these pumps deliver milliliters per hour (mL/hr), any milliliter calculation that results in a decimal fraction must be rounded to a whole milliliter. There has been the advent of more sophisticated pumps that allow infusions to be set by pump rate and the medication dosage to be administered. Some pumps allow decimal increments per milliliter. These pumps may be seen in some intensive care units and are also used to administer chemotherapeutic agents.

*SYRINGE PUMPS*    Syringe pumps are electronic devices that deliver medications or fluids by use of a syringe. The medication is measured in a syringe and attached to the special pump, and the medication is infused at the rate set (Figure 21-16). These pumps are useful in pediatrics and intensive care units, as well as in labor and delivery areas.

*PATIENT-CONTROLLED ANALGESIA DEVICES*    Patient-controlled analgesia is a form of pain management that allows the client to self-administer IV analgesics. This is accomplished by using a computerized infuser pump attached to the IV line (Figure 21-17, *B*). The patient-controlled analgesia (PCA) pump is programmed to allow dosages of narcotics only within specific limits to be delivered to prevent overdosage. The dosage and frequency of

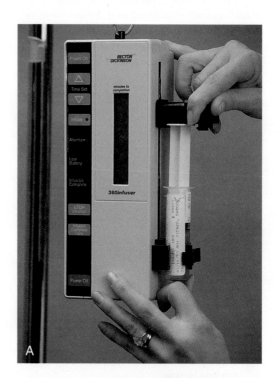

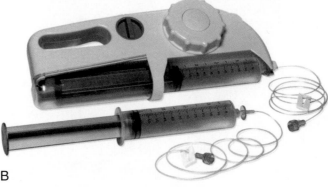

**Figure 21-16**    **A,** Syringe inserted into syringe pump. **B,** Freedom 60 syringe infusion pump system. (**A** from Elkin MK, Perry AG, Potter PA: *Nursing interventions and clinical skills,* ed. 4, St. Louis, 2007, Mosby. **B** from Repro-Med Systems, Inc., Chester, NY.)

administration are ordered by the prescriber and set on the pump. The client self-medicates by use of a control button. The pump also keeps a record of the number of times the client uses it. The display on the pump lets clients know when they are able to medicate themselves and when it is impossible to give themselves another dosage. The pump therefore has what is called a lockout interval. This is an interval during which no medications are delivered. A medication commonly administered by PCA is morphine (30 mg morphine per 30 mL). Portable PCA pumps are also available and are battery operated (see Figure 21-17, *A*).

**CAUTION**

Many infusion pumps look similar, but their functions are diverse. Because of the wide variation in infusion pumps and their function, caution is mandatory when they are used. It has been estimated that a significant number of IV medication errors result from errors in pump programming. Double-checking of programming is mandatory in the use of all infusion devices, as is client monitoring.

Nurses must be familiar with the infusion devices used at their institution; in-service education is essential in the use of all infusion devices.

TJC's (The Joint Commission's) 2005 National Patient Safety Goals established a goal designed to improve client safety when using infusion pumps. Health care organizations are required to ensure free-flow protection on all infusion devices and PCA pumps. Free-flow protection means that the tubing has a built-in mechanism similar to a clamp that is mobilized when the tubing is removed from the pump, therefore preventing flow of fluid into the client when the pump is stopped or the tubing is taken out of the infusion pump.

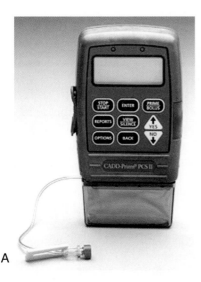
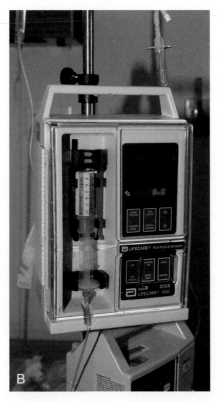

**Figure 21-17** **A,** CADD-Prizm® PCS II ambulatory battery-operated pump. **B,** Patient-controlled analgesia (PCA) infusion pump. (**A** from Smiths Medical MD, Inc., St. Paul, Minn. **B** from Elkin MK, Perry AG, Potter PA: *Nursing interventions* and clinical skills, ed. 4, St. Louis, 2007, Mosby.)

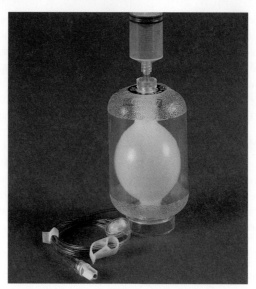

**Figure 21-18**   MedFlo® ambulatory infusion device. (From Smith & Nephew Endoscopy, Andover, Mass.)

### Infusion Devices for the Home Care Setting

Another type of infusion device is the balloon device, which is used mainly in outpatient and home care settings to administer single-dose infusion therapies. One such device is the elastometric balloon device, which is made of soft, rubberized, disposable material that inflates to a predetermined volume to hold and dispense a single dose of IV medication. Baxter manufactures this type of IV system. Med Flo, an ambulatory infusion device, is another system developed for ambulatory use. This device can be placed in a pocket to conceal it (Figure 21-18). Other infusion sets available include battery-operated pumps.

**CAUTION**

Clients must be educated about any electronic device they will use. Both devices and clients must be monitored to ascertain proper functioning.

## ■ Points to Remember

- IV orders are written by the doctor or other prescriber certified to do so (e.g., nurse practitioner, physician's assistant).
- IV orders must specify the name of the solution, medications (if any are to be added), the amount to be administered, and the infusion time.
- Several electronic devices are on the market for infusing IV solutions. Always familiarize yourself with the equipment before use.
- Follow the institution's protocol for IV administration.
- Nurses have the primary responsibility for monitoring the client during IV therapy.
- Nurses are responsible for any errors that occur in administration of IV fluids (e.g., inadequate dilution, too rapid infusion).
- Pay close attention to IV abbreviations. The letters indicate the solution components, and the numbers indicate the solution strength.
- Solution strength expressed as a percentage (%) indicates grams of solute per 100 mL of fluid.
- Principles relating to flow rate and infusion times are also applicable to parenteral nutrition solutions and blood and blood products.

**Practice Problems**

Answer the following questions as briefly as possible.

1. What does PCA stand for? _____

2. An IV initiated in a client's lower arm is called what type of line?

    _____

3. IVPB means _____..

4. A client has an IV of 1,000 mL 0.9% NS. The initials identify what type of solution?

    _____

5. A secondary line is hung _____ than the primary line.

6. Volumetric pumps infuse fluids into the vein by _____.

Identify the components and percentage strength of the following IV solutions:

7. D20W _____

8. D5W 10 mEq KCl _____

9. How many grams of dextrose does 500 mL D10W contain? _____

Calculate the amount of dextrose and/or sodium chloride in the following IV solutions:

10. 750 mL D5 NS

    dextrose _____

    NaCl _____

11. 250 mL D10W

    dextrose _____

12. 1,000 mL D5 0.33% NS

    dextrose _____

    NaCl _____

13. 500 mL D5 ½ NS

    dextrose _____

    NaCl _____

Answers on pp. 652-653

## Critical Thinking Question

**Scenario:** A client returned to the unit after surgery connected to a patient-controlled analgesia (PCA) pump. An order was written to attach a solution of 100 mL 0.9% normal saline (NS) with morphine 100 mg to the pump and infuse at a rate of 1 mg per 6 min. The ordered solution was inserted into the device and the rate set. The client had been instructed on the use of the PCA pump. The client continued to complain of severe pain on each shift despite the pump indicating that medication was being received at the set rate. The client received intermittent boluses of morphine to relieve pain.

Twenty-four hours later a nurse opened the PCA pump, found the full bag of IV solution in place, and noticed that the tubing had not been primed.

What should have been done in this situation?

_____

_____

_____

Answer on p. 654

## CHAPTER REVIEW

For each of the following IV solutions labeled *A* to *D* specify the letter of the illustration corresponding to the fluid abbreviation.

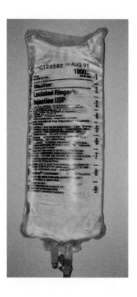

**A**

LOT                    EXP

2B2324
NDC 0338-0117-04
DIN 00061085

**1**

# Lactated Ringer's Injection USP

**2**

**3**

**1000 mL**

EACH 100 mL CONTAINS   600 mg SODIUM CHLORIDE USP
310 mg SODIUM LACTATE   30 mg POTASSIUM CHLORIDE USP
20 mg CALCIUM CHLORIDE USP   pH 6.5 (6.0 TO 7.5)   mEq/L
SODIUM 130   POTASSIUM 4   CALCIUM 2.7   CHLORIDE 109
LACTATE 28   OSMOLARITY 273 mOsmol/L (CALC)   STERILE
NONPYROGENIC   SINGLE DOSE CONTAINER   **NOT FOR USE IN THE
TREATMENT OF LACTIC ACIDOSIS**   ADDITIVES MAY BE
INCOMPATIBLE   CONSULT WITH PHARMACIST IF AVAILABLE   WHEN
INTRODUCING ADDITIVES USE ASEPTIC TECHNIQUE   MIX
THOROUGHLY   DO NOT STORE   DOSAGE   INTRAVENOUSLY AS
DIRECTED BY A PHYSICIAN   SEE DIRECTIONS   CAUTIONS
SQUEEZE AND INSPECT INNER BAG WHICH MAINTAINS PRODUCT
STERILITY   DISCARD IF LEAKS ARE FOUND   MUST NOT BE USED IN
SERIES CONNECTIONS   DO NOT ADMINISTER SIMULTANEOUSLY
WITH BLOOD   DO NOT USE UNLESS SOLUTION IS CLEAR   FEDERAL
(USA) LAW PROHIBITS DISPENSING WITHOUT PRESCRIPTION
STORE UNIT IN MOISTURE BARRIER OVERWRAP AT ROOM
TEMPERATURE (25°C/77°F) UNTIL READY TO USE   AVOID
EXCESSIVE HEAT   SEE INSERT

**4**

**5**

**6**

**7**

*Baxter*
BAXTER HEALTHCARE CORPORATION
DEERFIELD IL 60015 USA

MADE IN USA
DISTRIBUTED IN CANADA BY
BAXTER CORPORATION
TORONTO ONTARIO CANADA

Viaflex® CONTAINER
PL 146® PLASTIC

FOR PRODUCT INFORMATION
CALL 1-800-933-0303

**8**

**9**

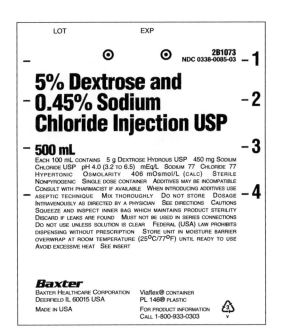

LOT       EXP

**2B1073**
NDC 0338-0085-03 — **1**

# 5% Dextrose and
# 0.45% Sodium — **2**
# Chloride Injection USP

— **500 mL** — **3**

EACH 100 mL CONTAINS 5 g DEXTROSE HYDROUS USP 450 mg SODIUM
CHLORIDE USP pH 4.0 (3.2 TO 6.5) mEq/L SODIUM 77 CHLORIDE 77
HYPERTONIC OSMOLARITY 406 mOsmol/L (CALC) STERILE
NONPYROGENIC SINGLE DOSE CONTAINER ADDITIVES MAY BE INCOMPATIBLE
CONSULT WITH PHARMACIST IF AVAILABLE WHEN INTRODUCING ADDITIVES USE — **4**
ASEPTIC TECHNIQUE MIX THOROUGHLY DO NOT STORE DOSAGE
INTRAVENOUSLY AS DIRECTED BY A PHYSICIAN SEE DIRECTIONS CAUTIONS
SQUEEZE AND INSPECT INNER BAG WHICH MAINTAINS PRODUCT STERILITY
DISCARD IF LEAKS ARE FOUND MUST NOT BE USED IN SERIES CONNECTIONS
DO NOT USE UNLESS SOLUTION IS CLEAR FEDERAL (USA) LAW PROHIBITS
DISPENSING WITHOUT PRESCRIPTION STORE UNIT IN MOISTURE BARRIER
OVERWRAP AT ROOM TEMPERATURE (25°C/77°F) UNTIL READY TO USE
AVOID EXCESSIVE HEAT SEE INSERT

***Baxter***
BAXTER HEALTHCARE CORPORATION    Viaflex® CONTAINER
DEERFIELD IL 60015 USA    PL 146® PLASTIC
MADE IN USA    FOR PRODUCT INFORMATION
       CALL 1-800-933-0303

**B**

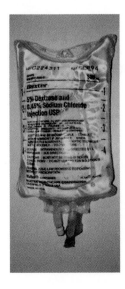

LOT       EXP

**2B0064**
NDC 0338-0017-04 **1**

# 5% Dextrose
# Injection USP **2**

**3**

**1000 mL** **4**
EACH 100 mL CONTAINS 5 g DEXTROSE HYDROUS USP
pH 4.0 (3.2 TO 6.5) OSMOLARITY 252 mOsmol/L (CALC)
STERILE NONPYROGENIC SINGLE DOSE CONTAINER ADDITIVES
MAY BE INCOMPATIBLE CONSULT WITH PHARMACIST IF AVAILABLE
WHEN INTRODUCING ADDITIVES USE ASEPTIC TECHNIQUE MIX
THOROUGHLY DO NOT STORE DOSAGE INTRAVENOUSLY AS **5**
DIRECTED BY A PHYSICIAN SEE DIRECTIONS CAUTIONS SQUEEZE
AND INSPECT INNER BAG WHICH MAINTAINS PRODUCT STERILITY
DISCARD IF LEAKS ARE FOUND MUST NOT BE USED IN SERIES
CONNECTIONS DO NOT ADMINISTER SIMULTANEOUSLY WITH BLOOD
DO NOT USE UNLESS SOLUTION IS CLEAR FEDERAL (USA) LAW **6**
PROHIBITS DISPENSING WITHOUT PRESCRIPTION STORE UNIT IN
MOISTURE BARRIER OVERWRAP AT ROOM TEMPERATURE
(25°C/77°F) UNTIL READY TO USE AVOID EXCESSIVE HEAT SEE
INSERT

**7**

***Baxter*** **8**
BAXTER HEALTHCARE CORPORATION    Viaflex® CONTAINER
DEERFIELD IL 60015 USA    PL 146® PLASTIC
MADE IN USA    FOR PRODUCT INFORMATION
       CALL 1-800-933-0303

**9**

**C**

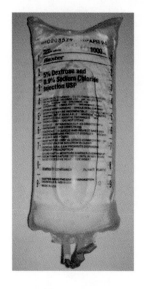

| LOT | | EXP | |
|---|---|---|---|

⊙        ⊙        **2B1064**
NDC 0338-0089-04   **1**

## 5% Dextrose and **2**
## 0.9% Sodium Chloride
## Injection USP **3**

**4**

**1000 mL**
EACH 100 mL CONTAINS   5 g DEXTROSE HYDROUS USP
900 mg SODIUM CHLORIDE USP   pH 4.0 (3.2 TO 6.5)
mEq/L   SODIUM 154   CHLORIDE 154   HYPERTONIC **5**
OSMOLARITY  560 mOsmol/L (CALC)  STERILE  NONPYROGENIC
SINGLE DOSE CONTAINER   ADDITIVES MAY BE INCOMPATIBLE
CONSULT WITH PHARMACIST IF AVAILABLE   WHEN INTRODUCING
ADDITIVES USE ASEPTIC TECHNIQUE   MIX THOROUGHLY   DO NOT
STORE   DOSAGE   INTRAVENOUSLY AS DIRECTED BY A PHYSICIAN **6**
SEE DIRECTIONS   CAUTIONS   SQUEEZE AND INSPECT INNER BAG
WHICH MAINTAINS PRODUCT STERILITY   DISCARD IF LEAKS ARE
FOUND   MUST NOT BE USED IN SERIES CONNECTIONS   DO NOT
USE UNLESS SOLUTION IS CLEAR   FEDERAL (USA) LAW PROHIBITS
DISPENSING WITHOUT PRESCRIPTION   STORE UNIT IN MOISTURE **7**
BARRIER OVERWRAP AT ROOM TEMPERATURE (25ºC/77ºF) UNTIL
READY TO USE   AVOID EXCESSIVE HEAT   SEE INSERT

**8**

*Baxter*
BAXTER HEALTHCARE CORPORATION  Viaflex® CONTAINER
DEERFIELD IL 60015 USA            PL 146® PLASTIC
MADE IN USA                       FOR PRODUCT INFORMATION
                                  CALL 1-800-933-0303

⊙        ⊙        **9**

**D**

1. D5 ½ NS _____

2. D5W _____

3. RL _____

4. D5NS _____

5. A client has a PCA in use following surgery. What is this device used to control? _____

6. When an IV medication is injected directly into the vein through a port, it is called an IV _____ or _____.

7. The two major intravenous access sites are _____ and _____.

8. A client is to receive an antibiotic IVPB. In order for the antibiotic to infuse first, how must it be hung in relation to the existing IV solution bag? _____

Calculate the amount of dextrose and/or sodium chloride in each of the following IV solutions:

9. 0.5 L D5 1/4 NS _____        10. 750 mL D5 1/2 NS _____

   dextrose _____ g                 dextrose _____ g

   NaCl _____ g                      NaCl _____ g

Answers on p. 654

 **For additional practice problems, refer to the Intravenous Calculations and Advanced Calculations sections of Drug Calculations Companion, Version 4, on Evolve.**

# Intravenous Calculations

*After reviewing this chapter, you should be able to:*
1. Calculate milliliters per hour (mL/hr)
2. Identify the two types of administration tubing
3. Identify from intravenous (IV) tubing packages the drop factor in drops per milliliter (gtt/mL)
4. Calculate IV flow rate in drops per minute (gtt/min) using a formula method and dimensional analysis
5. Calculate IV flow rate in gtt/min using a shortcut method (mL/hr and constant drop factor)
6. Calculate the flow rate for medications ordered IV over a specified time period
7. Calculate infusion times and completion times
8. Recalculate IV flow rates and determine the percentage (%) of increase or decrease
9. Calculate the rate for medications administered IV push

This chapter will present the calculations performed with intravenous therapy. As stated previously, nurses have a responsibility to make sure that clients are receiving the correct rate. Several methods are presented in the chapter to calculate IV rates: ratio and proportion, dimensional analysis, and the formula and division factor method. Let's now begin our calculations with determining IV rates in milliliters per hour (mL/hr).

## IV FLOW RATE CALCULATION

IV fluids are usually ordered to be administered at rates expressed in mL/hr. Examples: 3,000 mL in 24 hr, 1,000 mL in 8 hr. Small volumes of fluid are often used when the IV fluid contains medications such as antibiotics. Rates for IV fluids are usually expressed in drops per minute (gtt/min) when an infusion device is not used. When an infusion device is used, the rate must be expressed in mL/hr.

### Calculating Flow Rates for Volumetric Pumps in mL/hr

When a client is using an electronic infuser such as a volumetric pump, the prescriber orders the volume, and the nurse is responsible for programming the pump to deliver the ordered volume. The prescriber may order the IV volume in mL/hr; however, if not, the nurse must calculate it and program the pump.

Remember that the pump delivers volume in mL/hr, so if a decimal fraction is obtained, it must be rounded to the nearest whole number.

Solution Using Formula Method

$$x \text{ mL/hr (whole number)} = \frac{\text{Amount of solution}}{\text{Time in hours}}$$

**Example 1:**  Client with an infusion pump has an order for 3,000 mL D5W over 24 hours.

1. Think: pump is regulated in mL/hr.
2. Set up in formula:

$$x \text{ mL/hr} = \frac{3,000 \text{ mL}}{24 \text{ hr}}$$

$$x = 125 \text{ mL/hr}$$

**Answer:**    The pump would be set to deliver 125 mL/hr.

 Solution Using Ratio and Proportion

An alternative to the above formula would be to set up a ratio and proportion as follows:

$$3,000 \text{ mL} : 24 \text{ hr} = x \text{ mL} : 1 \text{ hr}$$

$$\frac{24x}{24} = \frac{3,000}{24}$$

$$x = 125 \text{ mL/hr}$$

Remember, as stated in the chapter on ratio and proportion, that a ratio and proportion can be set up in several formats. This could have been set up with the desired time for the infusion (usually 1 hr) over the total time ordered in hours, and the other side would be the hourly amount in milliliters labeled "*x*" over the total volume to be infused in milliliters:

$$\frac{1 \text{ hr}}{24 \text{ hr}} = \frac{x \text{ mL}}{3,000 \text{ mL}} \quad or \quad 1 \text{ hr} : 24 \text{ hr} = x \text{ mL} : 3,000 \text{ mL}$$

**Example 2:**  A client with an infusion pump is to receive an antibiotic in 50 mL of 0.9% NS over 30 minutes.

1. Think: The pump infuses in mL/hr. When the infusion time is less than an hour, which often occurs when antibiotics are administered, use a ratio and proportion to determine mL/hr. Remember: 1 hr = 60 min.
2. Set up proportion:

 Solution Using Ratio and Proportion

$$50 \text{ mL} : 30 \text{ min} = x \text{ mL} : 60 \text{ min}$$

$$30 \; x = 50 \times 60$$

$$\frac{30x}{30} = \frac{3,000}{30}$$

$$x = 100 \text{ mL/hr}$$

**Answer:**    The pump must be set to deliver 100 mL/hr for 50 mL to infuse within 30 minutes.

## Calculating mL/hr Using Dimensional Analysis

Calculation of mL/hr using dimensional analysis is similar to the formula method.

*Steps:*
• Identify what you are looking for, and write it to the left of the equation in a fraction format.
• Write the starting fraction using the information from the problem.

**Example 1:** Client with an infusion pump has an order for 3,000 mL of D5W over 24 hr.

Label factor: $\dfrac{x \text{ mL}}{\text{hr}} =$

Starting fraction: $\dfrac{3,000 \text{ mL}}{24 \text{ hr}}$

$$\frac{x \text{ mL}}{\text{hr}} = \frac{3,000 \text{ mL}}{24 \text{ hr}}$$

*Note:* No cancellation of units is required here.

$$x = 125 \text{ mL/hr}$$

**Example 2:** A client with an infusion pump is to receive an antibiotic in 50 mL of 0.9% NS over 30 minutes.

Notice here that the time is less than an hour. The pump delivers mL/hr. Therefore the fraction 1 hr = 60 min is added to the equation.

$$\frac{x \text{ mL}}{\text{hr}} = \frac{50 \text{ mL}}{\overset{}{\underset{1}{30 \text{ min}}}} \times \frac{\overset{2}{60 \text{ min}}}{1 \text{ hr}}$$

*Note:* Minutes are cancelled here so that you are left with mL/hr.

$$x = 100 \text{ mL/hr}$$

 **Practice Problems**

Calculate the flow rate in mL/hr.
1. 1,800 mL of D5W in 24 hr by infusion pump _____
2. 2,000 mL D5W in 24 hr by infusion pump _____
3. 500 mL RL in 12 hr by infusion pump _____
4. 100 mL 0.45% NS in 45 min by infusion pump _____
5. 1,500 mL D5RL in 24 hr by infusion pump _____
6. 750 mL D5W in 16 hr by infusion pump _____
7. 30 mL of antibiotic in 0.9% NS in 20 min by infusion pump _____

Answers on p. 654

## CALCULATING IV FLOW RATES IN gtt/min

When an electronic infusion device is *not* used, the nurse manually regulates the IV rate. To manually regulate an IV, the nurse must determine the rate in gtt/min.

IV flow rates in gtt/min are determined by the type of IV administration tubing. The drop size is regulated by the size of the tubing. (The larger the tubing, the larger the drops.) The first step in calculating IV flow rate is to identify the type of tubing and its calibration. The calibration of the tubing is printed on each IV administration package (Figure 22-1).

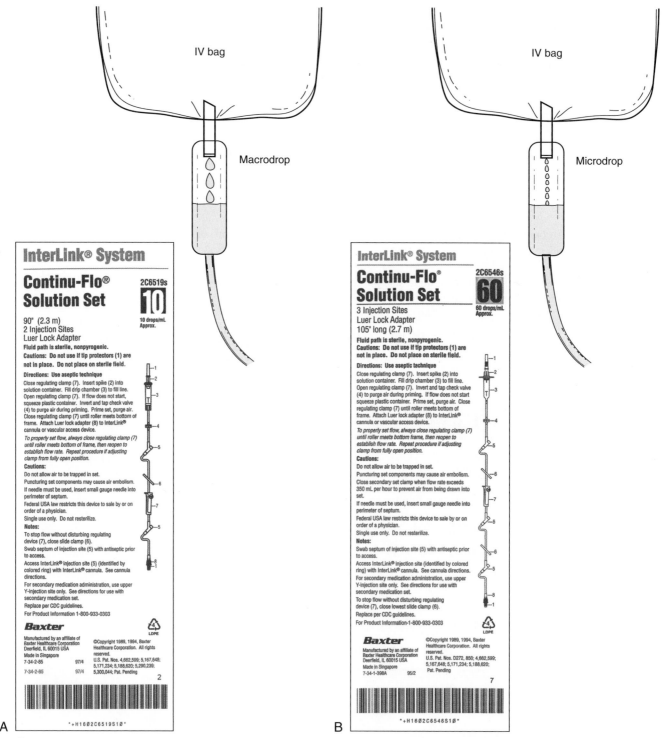

**Figure 22-1**    Administration sets. **A,** Set with drop factor of 10 (10 gtt = 1 mL). **B,** Set with drop factor of 60 (60 gtt = 1 mL).

## IV TUBING

IV tubing has a drop chamber. The nurse determines the flow rate by adjusting the clamp and observing the drop chamber to count the drops per minute (Figure 22-2). The size of the drop depends on the type of IV tubing used. The calibration of IV tubing in gtt/mL is known as the *drop factor* and is indicated on the box in which the IV tubing is packaged. This calibration, which is necessary to calculate flow rates, is shown on the packaging of IV administration sets (see Figure 22-1).

The two common types of tubing used to administer IV fluids are as follows:

### Macrodrop Tubing

Macrodrop is the standard type of tubing used for general IV administration. This type of tubing delivers a certain number of gtt/mL, as specified by the manufacturer. Macrodrop tubing delivers 10, 15, or 20 gtt equal to 1 mL. Macrodrops are large drops; therefore large amounts of fluid are administered in macrodrops (Figure 22-3, *A*).

### Microdrop Tubing

Microdrop tubing delivers tiny drops, which can be inferred from the prefix *micro*. It is used when small amounts and more exact measurements are needed, for example, in pediatrics, for the elderly, and in critical care settings. Microdrop tubing delivers 60 gtt equal to 1 mL. Because there are 60 minutes in an hour, the number of microdrops per minute is equal to the number of mL/hr. For example, if clients are receiving 100 mL/hr, they are receiving 100 microdrops/min (see Figure 22-3, *B*).

Figure 22-4 shows a comparison of calibrated drops.

## Tips for Clinical Practice

The nurse must be aware of the drop factor to accurately administer IV fluids to a client.

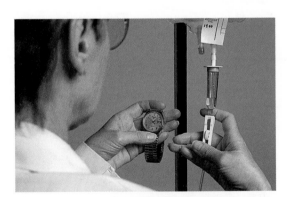

**Figure 22-2** Observing the drop chamber to count drops per minute. (From Potter PA, Perry AG: *Fundamentals of nursing,* ed. 7, St. Louis, 2009, Mosby.)

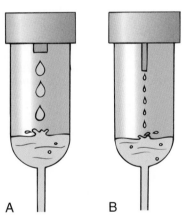

A    B

**Figure 22-3** **A,** Macrodrop chamber. **B,** Microdrop chamber. (From Clayton BD, Stock YN, Harroun RD: *Basic pharmacology for nurses,* ed. 14, St. Louis, 2007, Mosby.)

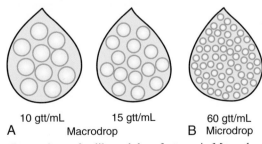

| 10 gtt/mL | 15 gtt/mL | 60 gtt/mL |
| A | Macrodrop | B Microdrop |

**Figure 22-4** Comparison of calibrated drop factors. **A,** Macrodrop. **B,** Microdrop.

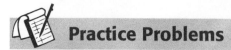  **Practice Problems**

Identify the drop factor and type of tubing for the IV tubing pictured below.

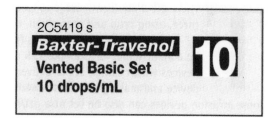

2C5419 s
**Baxter-Travenol** **10**
Vented Basic Set
10 drops/mL

8. _____

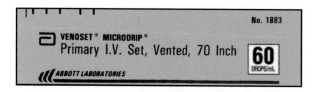

No. 1883
VENOSET® MICRODRIP®
Primary I.V. Set, Vented, 70 Inch    **60** DROPS/mL
*ABBOTT LABORATORIES*

9. _____

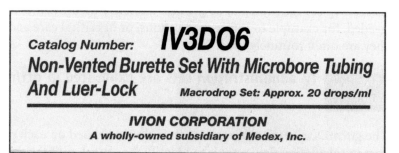

Catalog Number:    *IV3DO6*
**Non-Vented Burette Set With Microbore Tubing
And Luer-Lock**    *Macrodrop Set: Approx. 20 drops/ml*

**IVION CORPORATION**
*A wholly-owned subsidiary of Medex, Inc.*

10. _____

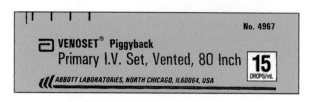

No. 4967
VENOSET® Piggyback
Primary I.V. Set, Vented, 80 Inch    **15** DROPS/mL
*ABBOTT LABORATORIES, NORTH CHICAGO, IL60064, USA*

11. _____

Answers on p. 654

- Knowing the drop factor is the *FIRST* step in accurate administration of IV fluids.
- The drop factor always appears on the package of the IV tubing.
- Macrodrops are large and deliver 10, 15, or 20 gtt/mL.
- Microdrops are small and deliver 60 gtt/mL.
- Drop factor = gtt/mL.
- To determine flow rates for an electronic infusion device (pump or controller), determine mL/hr by using the following formula:

$$x \text{ mL/hr (rounded to the nearest whole number)} = \frac{\text{Total mL ordered}}{\text{Total hr ordered}}$$

## CALCULATING FLOW RATES IN DROPS PER MINUTE USING A FORMULA

The calculation of IV flow rate in gtt/min can be done by using a formula method or dimensional analysis. Several formulas can be used; this text will focus on the most popular formula used. Calculation of the rate in gtt/min by using dimensional analysis will also be demonstrated in this chapter. The most common calculation necessary when an IV is manually regulated or an infusion device is not used involves solving to determine the rate in gtt/min.

To calculate the flow rate at which an IV is to infuse, regardless of the method used (formula or dimensional analysis), the nurse needs to know the following:
1. The volume or number of milliliters to infuse
2. The drop factor (gtt/mL) of the IV tubing
3. The time element (minutes or hours)

### Formula Method

The information is placed into a formula. Let's examine a formula that might be used. This formula is the most popular when calculating flow rate when the rate can be expressed as 60 minutes or less.

$$x \text{ gtt/min} = \frac{\text{Amount of solution (mL)} \times \text{Drop factor}}{\text{Time (min)}}$$

Before calculating, let's review some basic principles:
1. Drops per minute are always expressed in whole numbers. You cannot regulate something at a half of a drop. Because drops are expressed in whole numbers, principles of rounding off are applied; for example, 19.5 gtt = 20 gtt.
2. Carry division of the problem one decimal place to round to a whole number of drops.
3. Answers must be labeled. The label is usually drops per minute unless otherwise specified. Examples: 100 gtt/min or 17 gtt/min. To reinforce the differences in drop factor, the type of tubing is sometimes included as part of the label. Examples: 100 microgtt/min or 17 macrogtt/min.

Let's look at some sample problems and a step-by-step method of using the formula to obtain answers.

**Example 1:** Order: D5W to infuse at 100 mL/hr. Drop factor: 10 gtt/mL. At what rate in gtt/min should the IV be regulated?

1. Set up the problem, placing the information given in the correct position in the formula.

$$x \text{ gtt/min} = \frac{100 \text{ mL} \times 10 \text{ gtt/mL}}{60 \text{ min}}$$

2. Reduce where possible to make numbers smaller and easier to manage. Note that the labels are dropped when starting to perform mathematical steps.

$$x = \frac{100 \times \overset{1}{\cancel{10}}}{\underset{6}{\cancel{60}}} = \frac{100 \times 1}{6} = \frac{100}{6}$$

3. Divide $\dfrac{100}{6}$ to obtain rate in gtt/min. Carry division one decimal place and round off to the nearest whole number.

$$x = \frac{100}{6} = 16.6$$

$$x = 17 \text{ gtt/min}$$

**Answer:**   $x = 17$ gtt/min; 17 macrogtt/min

To deliver 100 mL/hr with a drop factor of 10 gtt/mL, the IV rate should be adjusted to 17 gtt/min. This answer can also be expressed with the type of tubing as part of the label, for example, 17 macrogtt/min.

**Example 2:**   Order: IV medication in 50 mL NS in 20 minutes. Drop factor: microdrop (60 gtt/mL). At what rate in gtt/min should the IV be regulated?

$$x \text{ gtt/min} = \frac{50 \text{ mL} \times \overset{3}{\cancel{60}} \text{ gtt/mL}}{\underset{1}{\cancel{20}} \text{ min}}$$

$$x = \frac{50 \times 3}{1} = \frac{150}{1}$$

$$x = 150 \text{ gtt/min}$$

**Answer:**   $x = 150$ gtt/min; 150 microgtt/min

To deliver 50 mL in 20 minutes with a drop factor of 60 gtt/mL, the IV should be adjusted to 150 gtt/min. This may sound like a lot; however, remember the type of tubing used is a microdrop.

## Dimensional Analysis Method

Let's look at calculating rate in gtt/min using the process of dimensional analysis. Remember that IV fluids are ordered in small volumes of fluid that usually contain medication or in large volumes to infuse over several hours. Let's look at the previous examples by using dimensional analysis.

**Example 1:**   Order: D5W to infuse at 100 mL/hr. Drop factor: 10 gtt/mL. At what rate in gtt/min should the IV be regulated?

1. You are calculating gtt/min, so write gtt/min to the left of the equation, followed by the equals sign (=), and label gtt/min $x$, since that is what you're looking for:

$$\frac{x \text{ gtt}}{\text{min}} =$$

2. Extract the information that contains gtt from the problem; the drop factor is 10 gtt/1 mL.

   Write this factor into the equation, placing gtt in the numerator.

$$\frac{x \text{ gtt}}{\text{min}} = \frac{10 \text{ gtt}}{1 \text{ mL}}$$

3. The next fraction is written so that the denominator matches the previous fraction (what you are looking for). Go back to the problem and you will see that the order is to infuse 100 mL in 1 hr. Enter the 1 hr as 60 min in the denominator because you are calculating gtt/min (100 mL/60 min).

$$\frac{x \text{ gtt}}{\text{min}} = \frac{10 \text{ gtt}}{1 \text{ mL}} \times \frac{100 \text{ mL}}{60 \text{ min}}$$

4. Now that you have the completed equation, cancel the units and notice that you are left with the desired gtt/min.

$$\frac{x \text{ gtt}}{\text{min}} = \frac{10 \text{ gtt}}{1 \text{ m\!L}} \times \frac{100 \text{ m\!L}}{60 \text{ min}}$$

$$x = \frac{100 \times \overset{1}{\cancel{10}}}{\underset{6}{\cancel{60}}} = \frac{100}{6}$$

$$x = 16.6 = 17 \text{ gtt/min}$$

**Answer:**   $x = 17$ gtt/min; 17 macrogtt/min

*Note:* Example 1 could have been done without changing the hourly rate to 60 min, but it would have required the addition of a 1 hr = 60 min conversion factor to the equation.

$$\frac{x \text{ gtt}}{\text{min}} = \frac{10 \text{ gtt}}{1 \text{ mL}} \times \frac{100 \text{ mL}}{1 \text{ hr}} \times \frac{1 \text{ hr}}{60 \text{ min}}$$

The next step would be to cancel the denominator/numerator mL and hr, leaving the desired gtt and min.

$$\frac{x \text{ gtt}}{\text{min}} = \frac{10 \text{ gtt}}{1 \text{ m\!L}} \times \frac{100 \text{ m\!L}}{1 \text{ h\!r}} \times \frac{1 \text{ h\!r}}{60 \text{ min}}$$

$$x = \frac{100 \times \overset{1}{\cancel{10}}}{\underset{6}{\cancel{60}}} = \frac{100}{6}$$

$$x = 16.6 = 17 \text{ gtt/min; 17 macrogtt/min}$$

Remember that reducing can make numbers smaller.

**Example 2:**   Order: An IV medication of 50 mL NS in 20 min. Drop factor: microdrop (60 gtt/mL). At what rate in gtt/min should the IV be regulated?

1. You are calculating gtt/min, so write gtt/min to the left of the equation, followed by the equals sign (=), and label gtt/min x, since that is what you're looking for:

$$\frac{x \text{ gtt}}{\text{min}} =$$

2. Extract the information that contains gtt from the problem; the drop factor is 60 gtt/1 mL. Write this factor into the equation, placing gtt in the numerator.

$$\frac{x \text{ gtt}}{\text{min}} = \frac{60 \text{ gtt}}{1 \text{ mL}}$$

3. The next fraction is written so that the denominator matches the previous fraction (what you are looking for). Go back to the problem and you will see that the order is to infuse 50 mL in 20 minutes. Enter the third fraction so that 50 mL is in the numerator and 20 minutes is in the denominator.

$$\frac{x \text{ gtt}}{\text{min}} = \frac{60 \text{ gtt}}{1 \text{ mL}} \times \frac{50 \text{ mL}}{20 \text{ min}}$$

4. Now that you have the completed equation, cancel the units and notice that you are left with the desired gtt/min.

$$\frac{x\text{ gtt}}{\text{min}} = \frac{60\text{ gtt}}{1\text{ mL}} \times \frac{50\text{ mL}}{20\text{ min}}$$

$$x = \frac{60 \times \overset{5}{\cancel{50}}}{\underset{2}{\cancel{20}}} = \frac{300}{2}$$

$$x = 150\text{ gtt/min}$$

**Answer:**    150 gtt/min; 150 microdrops/min

## Calculating Drops per Minute With Large Volumes of Fluid

Remember that IV fluids can be ordered in large volumes to infuse over several hours, for example, 1,000 mL over $x$ hr; or the large volume can be ordered by total volume to infuse and the mL/hr rate of infusion (125 mL/hr). Example: 1,000 mL D5W at a rate of 125 mL/hr. Remember that when a large volume to infuse over several hours is ordered, a preliminary step can be done to change it to mL/hr. Example: 1,000 mL D5W to infuse in 8 hr. Divide the total volume by the number of hours to get mL/hr. In this case, 1,000 mL ÷ 8 hr = 125 mL/hr. Then proceed to calculate gtt/min.

$$x\text{ mL/hr} = \frac{\text{Amount of solution (mL)}}{\text{Time (hr)}}$$

The formula method or dimensional analysis may be used to calculate gtt/min for a volume of fluid to be administered in more than 1 hour. Now let's look at some examples where a large volume of fluid will infuse over more than 1 hour.

**Example 1:**    Order: 1,000 mL D5W to infuse in 8 hr. Drop factor: 20 gtt/mL. At what rate gtt/min should IV be regulated?

 ## Solution Using the Formula Method

1. Calculate the mL/hr.

$$x\text{ mL/hr} = \frac{1,000\text{ mL}}{8\text{ hr}}$$

$$x = 125\text{ mL/hr}$$

2. Calculate the gtt/min.

$$x\text{ gtt/min} = \frac{125\text{ mL} \times 20\text{ gtt/mL}}{60\text{ min}}$$

3. Reduce.

$$x = \frac{125 \times \overset{1}{\cancel{20}}}{\underset{3}{\cancel{60}}} = \frac{125 \times 1}{3} = \frac{125}{3}$$

$$x = \frac{125}{3} = 41.6 = 42$$

$$x = 42\text{ gtt/min}$$

**Answer:**    $x = 42$ gtt/min; 42 macrogtt/min

Solution Using Dimensional Analysis

Order: 1,000 mL D5W to infuse in 8 hr. Drop factor: 20 gtt/mL. At what rate in gtt/min should IV be regulated?

1. Begin by determining mL/hr, converting the time in hours to minutes. 1 hr = 60 min. Now proceed to set up the problem in the dimensional analysis equation.
2. Enter the gtt/min being calculated first, followed by the equals sign (=).

$$\frac{x \text{ gtt}}{\min} =$$

3. Enter the drop factor (20 gtt/mL) with gtt in the numerator.

$$\frac{x \text{ gtt}}{\min} = \frac{20 \text{ gtt}}{1 \text{ mL}}$$

4. Take from the problem the amount to be administered over 1 hr (60 min) and write the fraction so that it matches the denominator of the fraction immediately before it.

$$\frac{x \text{ gtt}}{\min} = \frac{20 \text{ gtt}}{1 \text{ mL}} \times \frac{125 \text{ mL}}{60 \text{ min}}$$

5. Now that you have completed the equation, cancel the units and proceed with the mathematical process to obtain the answer.

$$\frac{x \text{ gtt}}{\min} = \frac{\overset{1}{\cancel{20}} \text{ gtt}}{1 \text{ } \cancel{mL}} \times \frac{125 \text{ } \cancel{mL}}{\underset{3}{\cancel{60}} \text{ min}}$$

$$x = \frac{125}{3} = 41.6 = 42$$

$$x = 42 \text{ gtt/min}; \ 42 \text{ macrogtt/min}$$

*Note:* The above example could have been done without changing 1 hr to 60 min; however, if it is left as 1 hr, you will need to add the additional fraction (1 hr = 60 min). With the same example, the equation would be stated as follows:

$$\frac{x \text{ gtt}}{\min} = \frac{20 \text{ gtt}}{1 \text{ mL}} \times \frac{125 \text{ mL}}{1 \text{ hr}} \times \frac{1 \text{ hr}}{60 \text{ min}}$$

Notice that the conversion factor 1 hr = 60 min is written so the numerator matches the denominator of the fraction immediately before it. To solve the equation, cancel units and proceed as follows:

$$\frac{x \text{ gtt}}{\min} = \frac{20 \text{ gtt}}{1 \text{ } \cancel{mL}} \times \frac{125 \text{ } \cancel{mL}}{1 \text{ } \cancel{hr}} \times \frac{1 \text{ } \cancel{hr}}{60 \text{ min}}$$

$$x = \frac{\overset{1}{\cancel{20}} \times 125 \times 1}{\underset{3}{\cancel{60}}} = \frac{125}{3} = 41.6 = 42$$

$$x = 42 \text{ gtt/min}; \ 42 \text{ macrogtt/min}$$

Remember that determining mL/hr before calculating gtt/min helps to keep the numbers smaller. However, using dimensional analysis also allows you to determine gtt/min without this step by writing one equation; but you would need the conversion factor 1 hr = 60 min. The equation would be stated as follows:

$$\frac{x \text{ gtt}}{\min} = \frac{20 \text{ gtt}}{1 \text{ mL}} \times \frac{1,000 \text{ mL}}{8 \text{ hr}} \times \frac{1 \text{ hr}}{60 \text{ min}}$$

Notice that the volume ordered is written to match the denominator of the fraction immediately before it and that the conversion factor 1 hr = 60 min is written so the numerator matches the denominator before it.

$$\frac{x \text{ gtt}}{\text{min}} = \frac{20 \text{ gtt}}{1 \text{ mL}} \times \frac{1,000 \text{ mL}}{8 \text{ hr}} \times \frac{1 \text{ hr}}{60 \text{ min}}$$

$$x = \frac{20 \times 1,000 \times 1}{480} = \frac{\overset{1,000}{\cancel{20,000}}}{\underset{24}{\cancel{480}}}$$

$$x = \frac{1000}{24}$$

$$x = 41.6 = 42$$

$$x = 42 \text{ gtt/min; } 42 \text{ macrogtt/min}$$

**Example 2:** Order: 1,500 mL 0.9% NS in 10 hr. Drop factor: 15 gtt/mL. At what rate in gtt/min should the IV infuse?

 **Solution Using the Formula Method**

1. Calculate mL/hr.

$$x \text{ mL/hr} = \frac{1,500 \text{ mL}}{10 \text{ hr}}$$

$$x = 150 \text{ mL/hr}$$

2. Calculate gtt/min.

$$x \text{ gtt/min} = \frac{150 \text{ mL} \times 15 \text{ gtt/mL}}{60 \text{ min}}$$

3. $$x = \frac{150 \times \overset{1}{\cancel{15}}}{\underset{4}{\cancel{60}}} = \frac{150}{4}$$

4. $$x = \frac{150}{4} = 37.5$$

**Answer:** $x = 38$ gtt/min; 38 macrogtt/min

 **Solution Using Dimensional Analysis**

Order: 1,500 mL 0.9% NS in 10 hr. Drop factor: 15 gtt/mL. At what rate in gtt/min should the IV infuse?

1. Calculate mL/hr (1,500 mL ÷ 10 hr = 150 mL/hr); convert the time in hours to minutes. Proceed using the steps outlined in Example 1.

$$\frac{x \text{ gtt}}{\text{min}} = \frac{15 \text{ gtt}}{1 \text{ mL}} \times \frac{150 \text{ mL}}{60 \text{ min}}$$

$$\frac{x \text{ gtt}}{\text{min}} = \frac{\overset{1}{\cancel{15}} \text{ gtt}}{1 \text{ mL}} \times \frac{150 \text{ mL}}{\underset{4}{\cancel{60}} \text{ min}}$$

$$x = \frac{150}{4}$$

$$x = 37.5 = 38$$

$$x = 38 \text{ gtt/min; } 38 \text{ macrogtt/min}$$

*or*

Set up the equation without changing 1 hr to 60 min.

$$\frac{x \text{ gtt}}{\text{min}} = \frac{15 \text{ gtt}}{1 \text{ mL}} \times \frac{150 \text{ mL}}{1 \text{ hr}} \times \frac{1 \text{ hr}}{60 \text{ min}}$$

$$\frac{x \text{ gtt}}{\text{min}} = \frac{15 \text{ gtt}}{1 \text{ mL}} \times \frac{150 \text{ mL}}{1 \text{ hr}} \times \frac{1 \text{ hr}}{60 \text{ min}}$$

$$x = \frac{\overset{1}{15} \times 150 \times 1}{\underset{4}{60}} = \frac{150}{4} = 37.5 = 38$$

$$x = 38 \text{ gtt/min}; \ 38 \text{ macrogtt/min}$$

*or*

Set up the equation without finding mL/hr first.

$$\frac{x \text{ gtt}}{\text{min}} = \frac{15 \text{ gtt}}{1 \text{ mL}} \times \frac{1{,}500 \text{ mL}}{10 \text{ hr}} \times \frac{1 \text{ hr}}{60 \text{ min}}$$

$$\frac{x \text{ gtt}}{\text{min}} = \frac{15 \text{ gtt}}{1 \text{ mL}} \times \frac{1{,}500 \text{ mL}}{10 \text{ hr}} \times \frac{1 \text{ hr}}{60 \text{ min}}$$

$$x = \frac{\overset{1}{15} \times 1{,}500 \times 1}{\underset{40}{600}} = \frac{1{,}500}{40} = 37.5 = 38$$

$$x = 38 \text{ gtt/min}; \ 38 \text{ macrogtt/min}$$

 **Practice Problems**

Calculate the flow rate in gtt/min using the formula method or dimensional analysis.

12. Administer D5RL at 75 mL/hr. The drop factor is 10 gtt/mL. _____

13. Administer D5 ½ NS at 30 mL/hr. The drop factor is a microdrop. _____

14. Administer RL at 125 mL/hr. The drop factor is 15 gtt/mL. _____

15. Administer 1,000 mL D5 0.33% NS in 6 hr. The drop factor is 15 gtt/mL. _____

16. An IV medication in 60 mL of 0.9% NS is to be administered in 45 min. The drop factor is a microdrop. _____

17. 1,000 mL of Ringer lactate solution (RL) is to infuse in 16 hr. The drop factor is 15 gtt/mL. _____

18. Infuse 150 mL of D5W in 2 hr. The drop factor is 20 gtt/mL. _____

19. Administer 3,000 mL D5 and ½ NS in 24 hr. The drop factor is 10 gtt/mL.    _____

20. Infuse 2,000 mL D5W in 12 hr. The drop factor is 15 gtt/mL.    _____

21. An IV medication in 60 mL D5W is to be administered in 30 minutes. The drop factor is a microdrop.    _____

Answers on pp. 654-655

## Calculation of IV Flow Rates Using a Shortcut Method

This shortcut method can be used only in settings where the IV sets have the same drop factor. Example: an institution where all the macrodrop sets deliver 10 gtt/mL. This method can also be used with microdrop sets (60 gtt/mL). It is important to note that this method can be used only if the rate of the IV infusion is expressed in mL/hr (mL/60 min). It is imperative that nurses become very familiar with the administration equipment at the institution where they work.

To use this method you must know the drop factor constant for the administration set you are using. The drop factor constant is sometimes referred to as the *division factor*. To obtain the drop factor constant (division factor) for the IV administration set being used, divide 60 by the drop factor calibration. Box 22-1 shows the constant calculated based on the drop factor for the tubing.

**Example:**    The drop factor for an IV administration set is 15 gtt/mL. To obtain the drop factor constant:

$$\frac{60}{15} = 4 \text{ (drop factor constant} = 4)$$

**RULE**

After the drop factor constant is determined, the gtt/min can be calculated in one step:

$$x \text{ gtt/min} = \frac{\text{mL/hr}}{\text{gtt factor constant}}$$

### BOX 22-1   Drop Factor Constants

| Drop Factor of Tubing | Drop Factor Constant |
|---|---|
| 10 gtt/mL | $\frac{60}{10} = 6$ |
| 15 gtt/mL | $\frac{60}{15} = 4$ |
| 20 gtt/mL | $\frac{60}{20} = 3$ |
| 60 gtt/mL | $\frac{60}{60} = 1$ |

**Practice Problems**

Calculate the drop factor constant for the following IV sets.

22. 20 gtt/mL _____

23. 10 gtt/mL _____

24. 60 gtt/mL _____

Answers on p. 655

Now that you know how to determine the drop factor constant, let's look at examples of using a shortcut method to calculate gtt/min.

**Example 1:** Administer 0.9% NS at 100 mL/hr. The drop factor is 20 gtt/mL. The drop factor constant is 3.

 Solution Using the Shortcut Method

Therefore this problem could be done by using the shortcut method once you know the drop factor constant (division factor).

$$x \text{ gtt/min} = \frac{100 \text{ mL/hr}}{3} = 33.3 = 33 \text{ gtt/min}$$

$$x = 33 \text{ gtt/min}$$

Notice that the 100 mL/hr rate divided by the drop factor constant gives the same answer.

**Answer:** 33 gtt/min; 33 macrodrops/min

 Solution Using Dimensional Analysis

Administer 0.9% NS at 100 mL/hr. The drop factor is 20 gtt/mL. The drop factor constant is 3.

**Step 1:** State mL/hr as mL/60 min.

$$\frac{x \text{ gtt}}{\min} = \frac{\overset{1}{\cancel{20}} \text{ gtt}}{1 \text{ } \cancel{mL}} \times \frac{100 \text{ } \cancel{mL}}{\underset{3}{\cancel{60}} \min}$$

*Note:* In the equation, because time is stated as 60 min, the administration set calibration (20) will be divided into 60 (min) to obtain a constant number (3). 3 is the drop factor constant for 20 gtt/mL administration set. Using the drop factor constant, you can calculate gtt/min in one step (divide mL/hr by the drop factor constant).

$$\frac{x \text{ gtt}}{\min} = \frac{\overset{1}{\cancel{20}} \text{ gtt}}{1 \text{ } \cancel{mL}} \times \frac{100 \text{ } \cancel{mL}}{\underset{3}{\cancel{60}} \min} = 33.3 = 33 \text{ gtt/min}$$

$$\text{or } 100 \text{ mL/hr} \div 3 = 33.3 = 33 \text{ gtt/min}$$

$$x = 33 \text{ gtt/min}$$

**Answer:** 33 gtt/min; 33 macrogtt/min

## NOTE

It is important to realize that with a microdrop, which delivers 60 gtt/mL, the gtt/min will be the same as mL/hr. This is because the set calibration is 60, and the drop factor constant is based on 60 minutes (1 hr); therefore the drop factor constant is 1.

**Example 2:**   Administer D5W at 125 mL/hr. The drop factor is 15 gtt/mL. The drop factor constant is 4.

### Solution Using the Shortcut Method

Calculate the gtt/min.

$$x \text{ gtt/min} = \frac{125 \text{ mL/hr}}{4} = 31.2 = 31 \text{ gtt/min}$$

$$x = 31 \text{ gtt/min}$$

**Answer:**     31 gtt/min; 31 macrogtt/min

### Solution Using Dimensional Analysis

Administer D5W at 125 mL/hr. The drop factor is 15 gtt/mL. The drop factor constant is 4.

$$\frac{x \text{ gtt}}{\text{min}} = \frac{\overset{1}{\cancel{15}} \text{ gtt}}{1 \text{ m\cancel{L}}} \times \frac{125 \text{ m\cancel{L}}}{\underset{4}{\cancel{60}} \text{ min}} = 31.2 = 31 \text{ gtt/min}$$

$$or \; 125 \text{ mL} \div 4 = 31.2 = 31 \text{ gtt/min}$$

$$x = 31 \text{ gtt/min}$$

**Answer:**     31 gtt/min; 31 macrogtt/min

**Example 3:**   Administer 0.9% NS at 75 mL/hr. The drop factor is 60 gtt/mL. The drop factor constant is 1.

### Solution Using the Shortcut Method

Calculate the gtt/min.

$$x \text{ gtt/min} = \frac{75 \text{ mL/hr}}{1} = 75 \text{ gtt/min}$$

$$x = 75 \text{ gtt/min}$$

**Answer:**     75 gtt/min; 75 microgtt/min

### Solution Using Dimensional Analysis

Administer 0.9% NS at 75 mL/hr. The drop factor is 60 gtt/mL. The drop factor constant is 1.

$$\frac{x \text{ gtt}}{\text{min}} = \frac{\overset{1}{\cancel{60}} \text{ gtt}}{1 \text{ m\cancel{L}}} \times \frac{75 \text{ m\cancel{L}}}{\underset{1}{\cancel{60}} \text{ min}} = 75 \text{ gtt/min}$$

$$x = 75 \text{ gtt/min} \; or \; 75 \div 1 = 75$$

**Answer:**   75 gtt/min; 75 microgtt/min

**Practice Problems**

Calculate the rate in gtt/min using the shortcut method.
25. Order: D5W 200 mL/hr.
    Drop factor: 10 gtt/mL                    _____

26. Order: RL 50 mL/hr.
    Drop factor: 15 gtt/mL                    _____

27. Order: 0.45% NS 80 mL/hr.
    Drop factor: 60 gtt/mL                    _____

28. Order: 0.9% NS 140 mL/hr.
    Drop factor: 20 gtt/mL                    _____

Answers on p. 656

_____

Remember that the shortcut method discussed (using the drop factor constant) can be used to calculate the gtt/min for any volume of fluid that can be stated in mL/hr or mL/60 min.

**RULE**

> The shortcut method can be used if the volume is large; however, an additional step of changing mL/hr first must be done. You can then proceed to calculate the gtt/min using the shortcut method.

_____

**Example 1:**   Order: RL 1,500 mL in 12 hr. Drop factor: 15 gtt/mL. Drop factor constant: 4.

$$1,500 \text{ mL} \div 12 = 125 \text{ mL/hr}$$

 Solution Using the Shortcut Method

Now that you have mL/hr, you can proceed with the shortcut method, using the drop factor constant.

$$x \text{ gtt/min} = \frac{125 \text{ mL}}{4} = 31.2 = 31 \text{ gtt/min}$$

$$x = 31 \text{ gtt/min}$$

**Answer:**   31 gtt/min; 31 macrogtt/min

 Solution Using Dimensional Analysis

Order: RL 1,500 mL in 12 hr. Drop factor: 15 gtt/mL. Drop factor constant: 4.

**Step 1:**   Determine mL/hr expressed as mL/60 min.

$$\frac{x \text{ gtt}}{\text{min}} = \frac{\overset{1}{\cancel{15}} \text{ gtt}}{1 \text{ mL}} \times \frac{125 \text{ mL}}{\underset{4}{\cancel{60}} \text{ min}} = \frac{125}{4} = 31.2 = 31 \text{ gtt/min}$$

$$x = 31 \text{ gtt/min}$$

**Answer:**   31 gtt/min; 31 macrogtt/min

**Example 2:**   Order: 20 mL D5W in 30 min. Drop factor: 15 gtt/mL. Drop factor constant: 4.

 Solution Using the Shortcut Method

If the volume of fluid to be infused is small, the volume and the time must each be multiplied to get mL/hr. To express this in mL/hr, you multiply by 2.

$$20 \text{ mL}/30 \text{ min} = (20 \times 2)/(2 \times 30 \text{ min}) = 40 \text{ mL/hr}$$

$$x \text{ gtt/min} = \frac{40 \text{ mL}}{4} = 10 \text{ gtt/min}$$

$$x = 10 \text{ gtt/min}$$

**Answer:**     10 gtt/min; 10 macrogtt/min

 Solution Using Dimensional Analysis

Order: 20 mL D5W in 30 min. Drop factor: 15 gtt/mL. Drop factor constant: 4.

**Step 1:**     Change 20 mL/30 min to 40 mL/hr as shown above.

**Step 2:**     Express 40 mL/hr as 40 mL/60 min.

$$\frac{x \text{ gtt}}{\text{min}} = \frac{\overset{1}{\cancel{15}} \text{ gtt}}{1 \cancel{\text{mL}}} \times \frac{40 \cancel{\text{mL}}}{\underset{4}{\cancel{60}} \text{ min}} = \frac{40}{4} = 10 \text{ gtt/min}$$

$$x = 10 \text{ gtt/min}$$

**Answer:**     10 gtt/min; 10 macrogtt/min

 **Practice Problems**

Calculate the gtt/min using the shortcut method.
29. Order: 1,000 mL D5W in 10 hr.
    Drop factor: 10 gtt/mL                    _____

30. Order: 1,500 mL RL in 12 hr.
    Drop factor: 15 gtt/mL                    _____

31. Order: 40 mL D5W in 20 min.
    Drop factor: 10 gtt/mL                    _____

Answers on p. 656

## CALCULATING IV FLOW RATES WHEN SEVERAL SOLUTIONS ARE ORDERED

IV orders are often written for different amounts or types of fluid to be given in a certain time period. These orders are frequently written for a 24-hour interval and are usually split over three shifts. IV solutions may have medications added, such as potassium chloride or multivitamins.
    Steps to calculating:
    1. Add up the total amount of fluid.
    2. Proceed as with other IV problem calculations.

*Note:* When medications such as potassium chloride and vitamins are added to IV solutions, they are generally not considered in the total volume. (At some institutions, to consider the medication in the volume it must be 10 mL or more. Always check the policy of the institution.)

**Example 1:** Order: The following IVs for 24 hours. Drop factor: 15 gtt/mL.

    a. 1,000 mL D5W with 10 mEq potassium chloride (KCl)

    b. 500 mL dextrose 5% in normal saline (D5NS) c̄ 1 ampule multivitamin (MVI)

    c. 500 mL D5W

1. Calculate mL/hr

$$x \text{ mL/hr} = \frac{2,000 \text{ mL}}{24 \text{ hr}} = 83.3 = 83 \text{ mL/hr}$$

$$x = 83 \text{ mL/hr}$$

2. Calculate gtt/min

$$x \text{ gtt/min} = \frac{83 \text{ mL} \times 15 \text{ gtt/mL}}{60 \text{ min}}$$

3. Reduce

$$x = \frac{83 \times \overset{1}{\cancel{15}}}{\underset{4}{\cancel{60}}} = \frac{83 \times 1}{4} = 20.7 = 21 \text{ gtt/min}$$

$$x = 21 \text{ gtt/min}$$

**Answer:** 21 gtt/min; 21 macrogtt/min

**Example 2:** IV orders are as follows:

    a. 1,000 mL D5W

    b. 1,000 mL normal saline (NS)

    c. 500 mL D5 and $\frac{1}{2}$ NS

Drop factor: 10 gtt/mL to infuse at 150 mL/hr.

The hourly rate is 150 mL/hr. Calculation is done based on this:

$$x \text{ gtt/min} = \frac{150 \text{ mL} \times 10 \text{ gtt/mL}}{60 \text{ min}}$$

$$x = \frac{150 \times \overset{1}{\cancel{10}}}{\underset{6}{\cancel{60}}} = \frac{150 \times 1}{6} = 25 \text{ gtt/min}$$

$$x = 25 \text{ gtt/min}$$

**Answer:** 25 gtt/min; 25 macrogtt/min

> **NOTE**
>
> This could have been done with the shortcut method by determining the drop factor constant. Calculating the IV flow rate where indicated eliminates the step of adding up the solution volumes if the hourly rate is stipulated, as shown in Example 2. The hourly rate becomes the total volume. Example 2 could also have been done with the shortcut method by determining the drop factor constant.

## Practice Problems

Calculate the flow rate in gtt/min.

32. Order: Dextrose 5% with Ringer lactate
    solution (D5RL) c̄ 20 units Pitocin for 2 L
    at 125 mL/hr. Drop factor: 15 gtt/mL    _____

33. Order: To infuse in 16 hr. Drop factor: 10 gtt/mL

    a. D5W 500 mL c̄ 10 mEq KCl

    b. D5W 1,000 mL

    c. D5W 1,000 mL c̄ 1 ampule MVI    _____

34. Order: 1,000 mL D5 0.9% NS for 3 L at
    100 mL/hr. Drop factor: microdrop.    _____

35. Order: D5W 1,000 mL + 20 mEq KCl
    for 2 L to infuse in 10 hr. Drop factor:
    15 gtt/mL    _____

Answers on p. 656

## CALCULATING INTERMITTENT IV INFUSIONS PIGGYBACK

Medications such as antibiotics can also be given by adding a secondary container of solution that contains the medication. The administration of medication by attaching it to a port on the primary line is referred to as *piggyback*. The volume of the piggyback container is usually 50 to 100 mL and should infuse over 20, 30, or 60 minutes, depending on the type and amount of medication added. If the volume of fluid in which the antibiotic is to be infused is not stated in the order, check a medication reference guide. The formula method or dimensional analysis is used to determine the rate in gtt/min at which the medication should be infused. *Note:* At some institutions the medication being added has to be 10 mL or more to be considered in the volume of IV fluid; check policy of the institution.

**Example:**    Order: Keflin 2 g IVPB (piggyback) over 30 min. The Keflin is placed in 100 mL of fluid after it is dissolved. The drop factor is 15 gtt/mL. At what rate in gtt/min should the IV be regulated?

To calculate: The 100 mL of fluid in which the medication is dissolved is used as the volume.

 Solution Using the Formula Method

$$x \text{ gtt/min} = \frac{100 \text{ mL} \times 15 \text{ gtt/mL}}{30 \text{ min}}$$

$$x = \frac{100 \times \overset{1}{\cancel{15}}}{\underset{2}{\cancel{30}}} = \frac{100 \times 1}{2} = \frac{100}{2}$$

$$x = \frac{100}{2}$$

$$x = 50 \text{ gtt/min}$$

**Answer:**    50 gtt/min; 50 macrogtt/min

The IV would be regulated at 50 gtt/min; 50 macrogtt/min.

## Solution Using Dimensional Analysis

$$\frac{x \text{ gtt}}{\text{min}} = \frac{\overset{1}{\cancel{15}} \text{ gtt}}{1 \text{ mL}} \times \frac{100 \text{ mL}}{\underset{2}{\cancel{30}} \text{ min}}$$

$$x = \frac{100}{2}$$

$$x = 50 \text{ gtt/min}$$

**Answer:**     50 gtt/min; 50 macrogtt/min

## Practice Problems

Calculate the rate in gtt/min for the following medications being administered IVPB. Use the labels where provided. (Add volume of medication being added to IV solutions, where indicated.)

36. Order: Mezlocillin 3 g IVPB in
    130 mL NS over 1 hr. Drop factor:
    15 gtt/mL                                    _____

37. Order: Erythromycin 200 mg in
    250 mL D5W to infuse over 1 hr.
    Drop factor: 10 gtt/mL                       _____

38. Order: Ampicillin 1 g is added to 50 mL D5W to infuse over 45 minutes. Drop
    factor: 10 gtt/mL. For IV reconstitute with 10 mL of diluent to get 1 g per 10 mL.
    (Consider the medication added in the volume of fluid.)

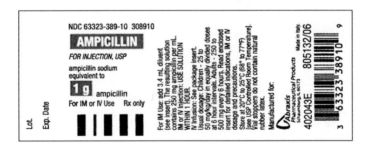

    a. How many milliliters of medication
    must be added to the solution?           _____

    b. Calculate the rate in gtt/min at which
    the IV should infuse.                     _____

> **NOTE**
>
> Electronic pumps can also be used to administer IV fluids and IV medications. The pumps are set to deliver a specific rate of flow per hour. The mechanism by which the pump works will depend on the manufacturer. Special tubing is usually required for the pump, and calculations are based on that.

39. Order: Clindamycin 900 mg in 75 mL D5W over 30 minutes. Drop factor: 10 gtt/mL

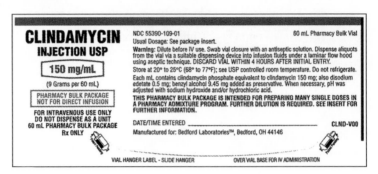

a. How many milliliters of medication must be added to the solution? _____

b. Calculate the rate in gtt/min at which the IV should infuse. _____

40. Order: Tagamet 300 mg IVPB q8hr. The medication has been added to 50 mL D5W to infuse over 30 minutes. Drop factor: 10 gtt/mL

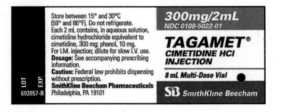

a. How many milliliters of medication must be added to the solution? _____

b. Calculate the rate in gtt/min at which the IV should infuse. _____

41. Order: Vancomycin 500 mg IVPB q24hr. The reconstituted vancomycin provides 50 mg per mL. The medication is placed in 100 mL of D5W to infuse over 60 minutes. Drop factor: 15 gtt/mL. (Consider the medication added in the volume of fluid.)

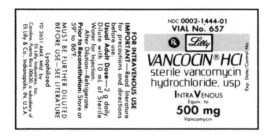

a. How many milliliters of medication must be added to the solution? _____

b. Calculate the rate in gtt/min at which the IV should infuse. _____

42. Order: Fungizone (amphotericin B) 20 mg IV Soluset (IVSS) in 300 mL D5W over 6 hr. The reconstituted material contains 50 mg per 10 mL. Drop factor: 60 gtt/per mL

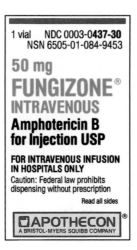

   a. How many milliliters will you add
      to the IV solution?           _____

   b. At what rate in gtt/min should the
      IV infuse?                    _____

43. Order: Septra 300 mg in 300 mL D5W over 1 hr q6h. Drop factor: 10 gtt/mL

   Available: Septra in 20-mL vial labeled 320 mg trimethoprim (16 mg per mL) and 1,600 mg sulfamethoxazole (80 mg per mL). (Calculate the dosage using trimethoprim.)

   a. How many milliliters of medication
      will be added to the IV? (Round
      answer to nearest tenth.)      _____

   b. Calculate the rate in gtt/min at
      which the IV should infuse.    _____

44. Order: Retrovir 100 mg IV q4h over 1 hr.

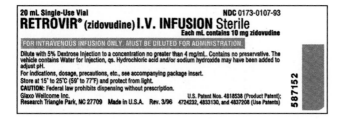

   The medication is placed in 100 mL
   of D5W. Drop factor: 10 gtt/mL
   (Consider the medication added to
   the volume of IV fluid.)           _____

Answers on pp. 657-658

## DETERMINING THE AMOUNT OF MEDICATION IN A SPECIFIC AMOUNT OF SOLUTION

Sometimes medications are added to IV solutions, and the prescriber orders a certain amount of the medication to be given in a certain time period.

**Example 1:**    The prescriber may order 20 mEq of potassium chloride to be placed in 1,000 mL of fluid to be administered at a rate of 2 mEq of potassium per hour.

 ### Solution Using Ratio and Proportion

Calculate the number of milliliters per hour of solution needed to deliver 2 mEq of potassium chloride per hour.

$$\text{What prescriber ordered}$$
$$\downarrow$$
$$20 \text{ mEq}:1,000 \text{ mL} = 2 \text{ mEq}:x \text{ mL}$$
$$\downarrow \qquad\qquad \downarrow \qquad\qquad\qquad\qquad \downarrow$$
$$\text{Total amount of medication} \quad \text{Desired volume}$$
$$\text{in volume of solution} \qquad\quad \text{of solution}$$

$$20 \text{ mEq}:1,000 \text{ mL} = 2 \text{ mEq}:x \text{ mL}$$

$$20x = 1,000 \times 2$$

$$20x = 2,000$$

$$x = \frac{2,000}{20}$$

$$x = 100 \text{ mL/hr}$$

Thus 100 mL per hour of fluid would be needed to administer 2 mEq of potassium chloride per hour.

### Solution Using Dimensional Analysis

**Step 1:**    Determine the amount of solution in milliliters per hour needed to administer 2 mEq of potassium chloride per hour. Enter mL/hr being calculated first.

$$\frac{x \text{ mL}}{\text{hr}} =$$

**Step 2:**    Enter the 1,000 mL per 20 mEq as the starting fraction.

$$\frac{x \text{ mL}}{\text{hr}} = \frac{1,000 \text{ mL}}{20 \text{ mEq}}$$

**Step 3:**    Enter the 2 mEq/1 hr rate ordered with mEq as the numerator.

$$\frac{x \text{ mL}}{\text{hr}} = \frac{1,000 \text{ mL}}{20 \text{ mEq}} \times \frac{2 \text{ mEq}}{1 \text{ hr}}$$

**Step 4:**    Cancel the units so you are left with mL/hr.

$$\frac{x \text{ mL}}{\text{hr}} = \frac{1,000 \text{ mL}}{\underset{10}{20} \text{ mEq}} \times \frac{\overset{1}{2} \text{ mEq}}{1 \text{ hr}}$$

$$x = \frac{1,000}{10}$$

$$x = 100 \text{ mL/hr}$$

100 mL/hr would deliver 2 mEq of potassium chloride per hour.

**Example 2:**   The prescriber orders 100 units of Humulin regular insulin to be added to 500 mL of 0.45% saline (½ NS) to infuse at 10 units per hour. The IV flow rate should be how many milliliters per hour?

 **Using Ratio and Proportion**

Set up a proportion with the known on one side and the unknown on the other.

$$100 \text{ units} : 500 \text{ mL} = 10 \text{ units} : x \text{ mL}$$

$$100x = 500 \times 10$$

$$100x = 5{,}000$$

$$x = \frac{5{,}000}{100}$$

$$x = 50 \text{ mL/hr}$$

For the client to receive 10 units of insulin per hour, 50 mL/hr must be administered.

 **Solution Using Dimensional Analysis**

Follow the steps outlined in Example 1.

$$\frac{x \text{ mL}}{\text{hr}} = \frac{\overset{5}{\cancel{500}} \text{ mL}}{\underset{1}{\cancel{100}} \text{ units}} \times \frac{10 \cancel{\text{ units}}}{1 \text{ hr}}$$

$$x = \frac{50}{1}$$

$$x = 50 \text{ mL/hr}$$

 **Practice Problems**

Solve the following problems using the steps indicated.

45. Order: 15 mEq of potassium chloride in 1,000 mL of D5 and ½ NS to be administered at a rate of 2 mEq/hr.

   How many mL/hr should the solution
   IV infuse at?   _____

46. Order: 10 units of Humulin regular insulin per hour. 50 units of insulin is placed in 250 mL NS.

   How many mL/hr should the
   IV infuse at?   _____

47. Order: 15 units of Humulin regular insulin per hour. 40 units of insulin is placed in 250 mL of NS.

   How many mL/hr should the
   IV infuse at?   _____

Answers on p. 658

## DETERMINING INFUSION TIMES AND VOLUMES

You may need to calculate the following:

    a. Time in hours—how long it will take a certain amount of fluid to infuse or how long it may last

    b. Volume—the total number of milliliters a client will receive in a certain time period

These unknown elements can be determined by use of the formula method or dimensional analysis.

**Formula**

$$x \text{ gtt/min} = \frac{\text{Amount of solution (mL)} \times \text{Drop factor}}{\text{Time (min)}}$$

## STEPS TO CALCULATING A PROBLEM WITH AN UNKNOWN WITH THE FORMULA METHOD

1. Take information given in the problem and place it in the formula.
2. Place an $x$ in the formula in the position of the unknown. If you are trying to determine time in hours, place $x$ in the position for minutes; once you find the minutes, divide the number of minutes by 60 (60 minutes = 1 hr) to get the number of hours. If you are trying to determine the volume the client would receive, place an $x$ in the position for amount of solution, and label $x$ mL.
3. Set up an algebraic equation so that you can solve for $x$.
4. Solve the equation.
5. Label the answer in hours or milliliters for volume.

**Sample Problem 1:**   Determining hours:

An IV is regulated at 20 microgtt/min. How many hours will it take for 100 mL to infuse?

➡ **Problem Setup in Formula Method**

If an IV is regulated at 20 microdrops, then the drop factor is a microdrop (60 gtt/mL). You cannot convert macrodrop into a microdrop and vice versa.

1. $20 \text{ microgtt/min} = \dfrac{100 \text{ mL} \times 60 \text{ gtt/mL}}{x \text{ min}}$

2. Reduce:   $\dfrac{20x}{20} = \dfrac{100 \times \overset{3}{\cancel{60}}}{\underset{1}{\cancel{20}}} = \dfrac{100 \times 3}{1}$

          $x = 300 \text{ min}$

In the sample problem you are being asked the number of hours. However, in this formula, time is in minutes, so place an $x$ in the position for minutes (60 gtt/mL is drop factor), and place the number of gtt/min in the formula. Let's now examine the problem set up in the formula.

3. Change minutes to hours:

        60 minutes = 1 hr

        Therefore $\dfrac{300 \text{ min}}{60} = 5 \text{ hr}$

        $x = 5 \text{ hr}$

*Note:* Placing 20 gtt/min over 1 does not alter the value.

$$\frac{20 \text{ microgtt/min}}{1} = \frac{100 \text{ mL} \times 60 \text{ gtt/mL}}{x \text{ min}}$$

Problem Setup in Dimensional Analysis

1. Write $x$ hr being calculated first. Now enter 1 hr = 60 min as the starting fraction, placing 1 hr as the numerator to match the hr being calculated.

$$x \text{ hr} = \frac{1 \text{ hr}}{60 \text{ min}}$$

2. Refer to the problem; the numerator min must match the denominator in the starting fraction. This is provided by the 20 microgtt/min. Place the rate as a fraction with 1 min as the numerator and 20 gtt as the denominator.

$$x \text{ hr} = \frac{1 \text{ hr}}{60 \text{ min}} \times \frac{1 \text{ min}}{20 \text{ gtt}}$$

3. Check the problem; the third fraction is entered so the numerator matches the denominator in the fraction before it. This is provided by the drop factor 60 gtt/mL. Place 60 in the numerator; and use 1 mL as the denominator.

$$x \text{ hr} = \frac{1 \text{ hr}}{60 \text{ min}} \times \frac{1 \text{ min}}{20 \text{ gtt}} \times \frac{60 \text{ gtt}}{1 \text{ mL}}$$

4. The last fraction written has to match mL in the fraction before it. The mL entry is provided by the 100 mL of fluid.

$$x \text{ hr} = \frac{1 \text{ hr}}{60 \text{ min}} \times \frac{1 \text{ min}}{20 \text{ gtt}} \times \frac{60 \text{ gtt}}{1 \text{ mL}} \times \frac{100 \text{ mL}}{1}$$

5. Cancel the units; notice that you are left with hours. Reduce if possible, and perform mathematical process.

$$x \text{ hr} = \frac{1 \text{ hr}}{\underset{1}{\cancel{60} \cancel{\text{min}}}} \times \frac{1 \cancel{\text{min}}}{\underset{1}{\cancel{20} \cancel{\text{gtt}}}} \times \frac{\overset{1}{\cancel{60} \cancel{\text{gtt}}}}{1 \cancel{\text{mL}}} \times \frac{\overset{5}{\cancel{100} \cancel{\text{mL}}}}{1}$$

$$x = 5 \text{ hr}$$

When you are calculating time intervals and the time or the answer comes out in hours and minutes, express the entire time in hours. For example, 1 hour and 30 minutes = 1.5 hr or $1\frac{1}{2}$ hr; $1\frac{1}{2}$ hr is the preferred term.

When calculating volume, proceed with the problem in the same way as calculating time interval except $x$ is placed in a different position and labeled mL.

**Sample Problem 2:** Determining volume:

An IV is regulated at 17 macrogtt/min. The drop factor is 15 gtt/mL. How much fluid volume in milliliters will the client receive in 8 hr?

 Problem Setup in Formula Method

1.
$$17 \text{ macrogtt/min} = \frac{x \text{ mL} \times 15 \text{ gtt/mL}}{480 \text{ min}}$$

2. Reduce:
$$17 = \frac{x \times \overset{1}{\cancel{15}}}{\underset{32}{\cancel{480}}}$$

$$\frac{17}{1} = \frac{x}{32}$$

3. $x = 17 \times 32 = 544$ mL

$x = 544$ mL

> **NOTE**
>
> The label is hours because that is what you were asked.

> **NOTE**
>
> Because this formula uses minutes, 8 hr was changed to minutes by multiplying 8 × 60 (60 min = 1 hr).

> **NOTE**
>
> Label on this answer is mL.

## Problem Setup in Dimensional Analysis

1. Write $x$ mL being calculated first. Now enter the drop factor as the starting fraction, placing 1 mL as the numerator to match the mL being calculated.

$$x \text{ mL} = \frac{1 \text{ mL}}{15 \text{ gtt}}$$

2. Refer to the problem; the numerator gtt must match the denominator in the starting fraction. This is provided by the IV rate; 17 macrogtt/min. Place the rate as a fraction with 17 gtt as the numerator and 1 min as the denominator.

$$x \text{ mL} = \frac{1 \text{ mL}}{15 \text{ gtt}} \times \frac{17 \text{ gtt}}{1 \text{ min}}$$

3. Refer to the problem; this fraction is entered so that it matches the denominator in the fraction before it. You could change 8 hr to minutes by using 60 min = 1 hr (8 hr = 480 min), or enter the conversion 60 min = 1 hr, since the time here is in hours. Entering 60 min = 1 hr eliminates a pre-step of converting 8 hr to minutes. Enter 60 min = 1 hr— 60 min in the numerator and 1 hr in the denominator.

If the time in the problem is converted to minutes, this eliminates the need for 60 min = 1 hr and shortens the equation by one fraction.

$$x \text{ mL} = \frac{1 \text{ mL}}{15 \text{ gtt}} \times \frac{17 \text{ gtt}}{1 \text{ min}} \times \frac{480 \text{ min}}{1}$$

$$x \text{ mL} = \frac{1 \text{ mL}}{\cancel{15} \text{ gtt}} \times \frac{17 \cancel{\text{ gtt}}}{1 \cancel{\text{ min}}} \times \frac{\cancel{480}^{32} \cancel{\text{min}}}{1}$$

$$x = \frac{17 \times 32}{1}$$

$$x = 544 \text{ mL}$$

Some of the problems illustrated in calculating an unknown may be solved without using the formula method or dimensional analysis; however, the use of one or the other is recommended.

## Practice Problems

Solve for the unknown in the following problems as indicated.

48. You find that there is 150 mL of D5W left in an IV. The IV is infusing at 60 microgtt/min. How many hours will the fluid last?   _____

49. 0.9% NS is infusing at 35 macrogtt/min. The drop factor is 15 gtt/mL. How many milliliters of fluid will the client receive in 5 hours?   _____

50. 180 mL of D5 RL is left in an IV that is infusing at 45 macrogtt/min. The drop factor is 15 gtt/mL. How many hours will the fluid last?

         _____

51. D5 ½ NS is infusing at 45 macrogtt/min. The drop factor is 15 gtt/mL. How many milliliters will the client receive in 8 hr?

         _____

52. There is 90 mL of D5 0.33% NS left in an IV that is infusing at 60 microgtt/min. The drop factor is 60 gtt/mL. How many hours will the fluid last?

         _____

Answers on pp. 658-659

## RECALCULATING AN IV FLOW RATE

Flow rates on IVs change when a client stands, sits, or is repositioned in bed, if IVs are infusing by gravity. Therefore nurses must frequently check the flow rates. IVs are generally labeled with a start and finish time, as well as markings with specific time periods. Sometimes IVs infuse ahead of schedule, or they may be behind schedule if they are not monitored closely. When this happens, the IV flow rate must be recalculated. To recalculate the flow rate the nurse uses the volume remaining and the time remaining. Recalculation may be done with uncomplicated infusions. IVs that require exact infusion rates should be monitored by an electronic infusion device.

> **CAUTION**
>
> The recalculated flow rate should not vary from the original rate by more than 25%. It is recommended that if the recalculated rate varies more than 25% from the original, the prescriber should be notified. The order may have to be revised.

When an IV is significantly ahead of or behind schedule, you may need to notify the prescriber, depending on the client's condition and the use of appropriate nursing judgment. **Always assess the client** before making any change in an IV rate. Changes depend on the client's condition. Check the institution's policy regarding the percentage of adjustment that can be made. Each situation must be individually evaluated, and appropriate action must be taken.

To determine whether the new rate calculation is greater or less than 25%, use the amount of increase or decrease divided by the original rate.

$$\frac{\text{Amount of} \uparrow \text{or} \downarrow}{\text{Original rate}} = \% \text{ of variation of original rate (round to nearest whole percent)}$$

To recalculate the IV rate, use the remaining volume and remaining time, and then proceed with calculating the gtt/min using the formula method or dimensional analysis. Refer to content in chapter if necessary.

**Example 1:** 1,000 mL of D5 RL was to infuse in 8 hr at 31 gtt/min (31 macrogtt/min). The drop factor is 15 gtt/mL. After 4 hr you notice 700 mL of fluid left in the IV. Recalculate the flow rate for the remaining solution. *Note:* The infusion is behind schedule. After 4 hr, half of the volume (or 500 mL) should have infused.

**NOTE**

Examples 1 and 2 could also be done without using the shortcut method illustrated in the examples.

 Solution Using the Shortcut Method

Time remaining: 8 hr − 4 hr = 4 hr

Volume remaining: 1,000 mL − 300 mL = 700 mL

700 mL ÷ 4 = 175 mL/hr

Drop factor is 15 gtt/mL.

Drop factor constant therefore is 4.

$$x \text{ gtt/min} = \frac{175 \text{ mL/hr}}{4}; x = 43.7 \text{ gtt/min} = 44 \text{ gtt/min}$$

**Answer:** 44 gtt/min; 44 macrogtt/min (recalculated rate). To determine the percentage of the change:

$$\frac{44 - 31}{31} = \frac{13}{31} = 0.419 = 42\%$$

 Solution Using Dimensional Analysis

Time remaining: 8 hr − 4 hr = 4 hr

Volume remaining: 700 mL

$$\frac{x \text{ gtt}}{\min} = \frac{\overset{1}{\cancel{15}} \text{ gtt}}{1 \text{ mL}} \times \frac{700 \text{ mL}}{4 \text{ hr}} \times \frac{1 \text{ hr}}{\underset{4}{\cancel{60}} \min} = 43.7 = 44 \text{ gtt/min}$$

$$x = 44 \text{ gtt/min}$$

*Note:* As shown in the earlier discussion relating to gtt/min, shortcut methods could be used in a dimensional analysis setup as well.

**Course of Action:** Assess the client; notify the prescriber. This increase could result in serious consequences if the client is seriously ill or a child. The increase is greater than 25%.

In this situation the flow rate must be increased from 31 gtt/min (31 macrogtt/min) to 44 gtt/min (44 macrogtt/min), which is more than 25% of the original. Always assess the client first to determine the client's ability to tolerate an increase in fluid. In addition to assessing the client's status, you should notify the prescriber. This same method can be used if an IV is ahead of schedule.

**Example 2:** **IV Ahead of Schedule.** An IV of 1,000 mL D5W is to infuse from 8 AM to 4 PM (8 hr). The drop factor is 10 gtt/mL. The rate is set at 20 gtt/min (20 macrogtt/min). In 5 hr you notice that 700 mL has infused. Recalculate the flow rate for the remaining solution.

 Solution Using the Shortcut Method

Time remaining: 8 hr − 5 hr = 3 hr

Volume remaining: 1,000 mL − 700 mL = 300 mL

300 mL ÷ 3 = 100 mL/hr

Drop factor is 10 gtt/mL; therefore the drop factor constant is 6.

$$x \text{ gtt/min} = \frac{100 \text{ mL/hr}}{6} = 16.6 = 17 \text{ gtt/min}$$

$$x = 17 \text{ gtt/min}$$

**Answer:** 17 gtt/min; 17 macrogtt/min

Determine the percentage of change:

$$\frac{17 - 20}{20} = \frac{-3}{20} = -0.15 = -15\%$$

 Solution Using Dimensional Analysis

Time remaining: 8 hr − 5 hr = 3 hr

Volume remaining: 1,000 mL − 700 mL = 300 mL

$$\frac{x \text{ gtt}}{\text{min}} = \frac{\overset{1}{\cancel{10}} \text{ gtt}}{1 \text{ mL}} \times \frac{\overset{100}{\cancel{300}} \text{ mL}}{\underset{1}{\cancel{3}} \text{ hr}} \times \frac{1 \text{ hr}}{\underset{6}{\cancel{60}} \text{ min}} = 16.6 = 17 \text{ gtt/min}$$

$$x = 17 \text{ gtt/min}$$

In this situation the flow rate must be decreased from 20 gtt/min (20 macrogtt/min) to 17 gtt/min (17 macrogtt/min), but this is not a change greater than 25% of the original; −15% is within the acceptable 25% of change. However, the client's condition must still be assessed to determine the ability to tolerate the change, and the prescriber may still require notification.

**Course of Action:** This is an acceptable decrease; it is less than 25%. Assess the client, adjust the rate, if allowed by institutional policy, and assess during the remainder of the infusion.

**CAUTION**

Never arbitrarily increase or decrease an IV rate without assessing a client and informing the prescriber. Increasing or decreasing the rate without thought can result in serious harm to a client. Check the policy of the institution. Avoid off-schedule IV rates by regularly monitoring the IV at least every 30 to 60 minutes.

 **Practice Problems**

For each of the problems, recalculate the IV flow rates in gtt/min rates using either method presented, determine the percentage of change, and state your course of action.

53. 500 mL of 0.9% NS was ordered to infuse in 8 hr at the rate of 16 gtt/min (16 macrogtt/min). The drop factor is 15 gtt/mL. After 5 hr, you find 250 mL of fluid left.

    a. _____ gtt/min

    b. _____ %

    c. _____ Course of action

54. 250 mL of D5W was to infuse in 3 hr at the rate of 21 gtt/min (21 macrogtt/min). Drop factor: 15 gtt/mL. With $1\frac{1}{2}$ hr remaining, you find 200 mL left.

    a. _____ gtt/min

    b. _____ %

    c. _____ Course of action

55. 1,500 mL D5 RL to infuse in 12 hr at 42 gtt/min (42 macrogtt/min). After 6 hr, 650 mL has infused. Drop factor: 20 gtt/mL.

    a. _____ gtt/min

    b. _____ %

    c. _____ Course of action

56. 1,000 mL D5 0.33% NS was to infuse in 12 hr at 28 gtt/min (28 macrogtt/min). After 4 hr, 250 mL has infused. Drop factor: 20 gtt/mL.

    a. _____ gtt/min

    b. _____ %

    c. _____ Course of action

57. 500 mL D5 0.9% NS to infuse in 5 hr at 100 gtt/min (100 microgtt/min). After 2 hr, 250 mL has infused. Drop factor: 60 gtt/mL.

    a. _____ gtt/min

    b. _____ %

    c. _____ Course of action

Answers on pp. 659-660

## CALCULATING TOTAL INFUSION TIMES

IV fluids are ordered by the prescriber for administration at a certain rate in mL/hr, such as 1,000 mL D5W to infuse at 100 mL/hr. **The nurse needs to be able to determine the number of hours that an IV solution takes to infuse.** When the nurse calculates the total time for a certain volume of solution to infuse intravenously, this is referred to as **determining total infusion time.** To calculate infusion time it is necessary for the nurse to have knowledge of the following: amount (volume) to infuse, drop rate (gtt/mL), and set calibration.

Knowing the length of time for an infusion helps the nurse monitor IV therapy and prepare for the hanging of a new solution as the one infusing is being completed. Determining infusion times helps avoid things such as a line clotting off as a result of not knowing when an IV was to be completed. A nurse who knows the infusion time can anticipate when to start a new IV infusion and when to determine lab values that may have to be obtained after a certain amount of fluid has infused.

### Calculating Infusion Time From Volume and Hourly Rate Ordered

Infusion time is determined by taking the total number of milliliters to infuse and dividing it by the rate in mL/hr at which the solution is infusing. This can also be done by using a ratio and proportion, in which the known ratio is the ordered rate in mL/hr and would be the first ratio (on one side) on the unknown ratio for total milliliters to infuse in *x* hours would be the second ratio. In addition, this can be done by using dimensional analysis.

## Formula

$$\frac{\text{Total number of mL to infuse}}{\text{mL/hr infusion rate}} = \text{Total infusion time}$$

**Example 1:** Calculate the infusion time for an IV of 1,000 mL D5W infusing at a rate of 125 mL/hr.

 Solution Using the Formula Method

1,000 mL (total number of mL to infuse)

125 mL/hr (mL/hr to infuse)

$$\frac{1{,}000 \text{ mL}}{125 \text{ mL/hr}} = 1000 \div 125 = 8 \text{ hr}$$

Infusion time = 8 hr

 Solution Using Dimensional Analysis

1. Write the hr being calculated to the left of the equals sign.

$$x \text{ hr} =$$

2. Use the problem information that contains hr, and enter it as the starting fraction (125 mL/hr). Place 1 hr in the numerator and 125 mL in the denominator.

$$x \text{ hr} = \frac{1 \text{ hr}}{125 \text{ mL}}$$

3. Refer to the problem for mL (1,000 mL to be infused). Place 1,000 mL as the next numerator to match mL in the first denominator.

$$x \text{ hr} = \frac{1 \text{ hr}}{125 \text{ mL}} = \frac{1{,}000 \text{ mL}}{1}$$

4. Cancel the units, reducing if possible; the unit hr remains and is calculated.

$$x \text{ hr} = \frac{1 \text{ hr}}{\cancel{125} \text{ } \cancel{mL}}_{1} = \frac{\overset{8}{\cancel{1000}} \text{ } \cancel{mL}}{1}$$

$$x = 8 \text{ hr}$$

**Example 2:** 1,000 mL of D5 and ½ NS is ordered to infuse at 150 mL/hr. Calculate the infusion time to the nearest hundredth.

 Solution Using the Formula Method

$$\frac{1{,}000 \text{ mL}}{150 \text{ mL/hr}} = 6.66 \text{ hr}$$

Fractions of hours can be changed to minutes: 6 represents the total number of hours; 0.66 represents a fraction of an hour and can be converted to minutes. This is done by multiplying 0.66 by 60 min (60 min = 1 hr) and then rounding off to the nearest whole number.

$$0.66 \times 60 \text{ min} = 39.6 = 40$$

Infusion time = 6 hr and 40 minutes

Solution Using Dimensional Analysis

Use the same steps as outlined in Example 1.

$$x \text{ hr} = \frac{1 \text{ hr}}{150 \text{ mL}} \times \frac{1{,}000 \text{ mL}}{1}$$

$$x = 6.66 \text{ hr}$$

Convert 0.66 hr to minutes by multiplying by 60 min (1 hr); then round off to the nearest whole number.

$$0.66 \times 60 \text{ min} = 39.6 = 40 \text{ min}$$

*or*

$$x \text{ min} = \frac{60 \text{ min}}{1 \text{ hr}} \times \frac{0.66 \text{ hr}}{1}$$

**Once infusion time has been calculated, the nurse can use this information to determine the time an IV would be completed.** For Example 2 this would be determined as follows: add the calculated infusion time to the time the infusion was started. If the IV in Example 2 was hung at 7:00 AM, add the 6 hours and 40 minutes to that time. The IV would be completed at 1:40 PM.

An easy way to do this is by using military time to determine the time it would be completed.

**Example:**    7:00 AM = 0700

After converting 7:00 AM to military time, add 6 hours and 40 minutes to arrive at your answer—1340.

$$0700 + 640 = 1340 = 1{:}40 \text{ PM}$$

*Note:* Converting traditional time to military time is covered in Chapter 9. Refer to that chapter to refresh your memory on how to do this.

 **Practice Problems**

Determine infusion time for the following IVs. State time in traditional and military time.

58.  An IV of 500 mL NS is to infuse at 60 mL/hr.

   a.  Determine the infusion time.    _____

   b.  The IV was started at 10:00 PM. When
       would the IV infusion be completed?   _____

59.  An IV of 250 mL D5W is to infuse at 80 mL/hr.

   a.  Determine the infusion time.    _____

   b.  The IV was started at 2:00 AM. When
       would the IV infusion be completed?   _____

60. 1,000 mL of D5W is to infuse at 40 mL/hr.

   a. Determine the infusion time. _____

   b. The IV was started at 2:10 PM
      on August 26. When would the
      IV infusion be completed? _____

61. An IV of 1,000 mL D5 RL is to infuse at 60 mL/hr.

   a. Determine the infusion time. _____

   b. The IV was started at 6:00 AM.
      At what time would this
      IV infusion be completed? _____

62. An IV of 500 mL D5W is to infuse at 75 mL/hr.

   a. Determine the infusion time. _____

   b. The IV was started at 2:00 PM.
      At what time would the
      IV infusion be completed? _____

Answers on p. 660

## CALCULATING INFUSION TIME WHEN RATE IN mL/hr IS NOT INDICATED FOR LARGE VOLUMES OF FLUID

There are situations in which the prescriber may order the IV solution and not indicate the rate in mL/hr. The only information may be the total number of milliliters to infuse, the flow rate (gtt/min) of the IV, and the number of gtt/mL that the tubing delivers. In this situation, before the infusion time is calculated, the following must be done:
   1. Convert gtt/min to mL/min.
   2. Convert mL/min to mL/hr.

After completing these steps, you are ready to calculate the infusion time for the IV using the same formula:

$$\frac{\text{Total number of mL to infuse}}{\text{mL/hr infusion rate}}$$

**Example:** A client is receiving 1,000 mL of RL. The IV is infusing at 21 macrogtt/min (21 gtt/min). The administration set delivers 10 gtt/mL. Calculate the infusion time.

**Step 1:** Use a ratio and proportion to change gtt/min to mL/min.

$$10 \text{ gtt}:1 \text{ mL} = 21 \text{ gtt}:x \text{ mL}$$

$$\frac{10x}{10} = \frac{21}{10}$$

$$x = 2.1 \text{ mL/min}$$

**Step 2:**    Convert mL/min to mL/hr.

$$2.1 \text{ mL/min} \times 60 \text{ min} = 126 \text{ mL/hr}$$

**Step 3:**    Determine infusion time as already shown.

a. $\dfrac{1,000 \text{ mL}}{126 \text{ mL/hr}} = 7.93 \text{ hr}$

b. $0.93 \text{ hr} \times 60 \text{ min} = 55.8 = 56 \text{ minutes}$

Infusion time = 7 hr and 56 minutes

*Note:* To determine the time the infusion would be completed, you would add the infusion time to the time the IV was started.

 ## Solution Using Dimensional Analysis

1. Write the hr being calculated first to the left of the equals sign, then write 1 hr = 60 min as the first fraction. Place 1 hr in the numerator and 60 min in the denominator.

$$x \text{ hr} = \frac{1 \text{ hr}}{60 \text{ min}}$$

2. Refer to the problem for information that contains min and place it as the second fraction, placing min in the numerator (21 gtt/min).

$$x \text{ hr} = \frac{1 \text{ hr}}{60 \text{ min}} \times \frac{1 \text{ min}}{21 \text{ gtt}}$$

3. Refer to the problem again; you need gtt to match the denominator of the second fraction. This is indicated in the drop factor (10 gtt/mL). Write the fraction with 10 gtt in the numerator and mL in the denominator.

$$x \text{ hr} = \frac{1 \text{ hr}}{60 \text{ min}} \times \frac{1 \text{ min}}{21 \text{ gtt}} \times \frac{10 \text{ gtt}}{1 \text{ mL}}$$

4. The final fraction must match the denominator of the preceeding fraction. The mL is provided by the volume of fluid to infuse (1,000 mL).

$$x \text{ hr} = \frac{1 \text{ hr}}{\underset{6}{60 \text{ min}}} \times \frac{1 \text{ min}}{21 \text{ gtt}} \times \frac{\overset{1}{10 \text{ gtt}}}{1 \text{ mL}} \times \frac{1,000 \text{ mL}}{1} = 7.93 \text{ hr}$$

$$0.93 \text{ hr} \times 60 \text{ min} = 55.8 = 56 \text{ min}$$

*or*

$$x \text{ min} = \frac{60 \text{ min}}{1 \text{ hr}} \times \frac{0.93 \text{ hr}}{1} = 55.8 = 56 \text{ min}$$

Infusion time = 7 hr and 56 min

 ## Practice Problems

Determine the infusion time for the following IVs.

63. A client is receiving 1,000 mL D5W at 25 microgtt/min. Drop factor is microdrop. _____

64. A client is receiving 250 mL of NS at 17 macrogtt/min. Drop factor: 15 gtt/mL. _____

65. A client is receiving 1,000 mL D5W.
    The IV is infusing at 30 macrogtt/min.
    Drop factor: 20 gtt/mL. _____

66. A client is receiving 1,000 mL D5W at
    20 macrogtt/min. Drop factor: 10 gtt/mL. _____

67. A client is receiving 100 mL at
    10 macrogtt/min. Drop factor: 15 gtt/mL. _____

Answers on pp. 660-661

## CALCULATING INFUSION TIME FOR SMALL VOLUMES OF FLUID

There may be times when it is necessary for the nurse to determine the infusion time for small volumes of fluid that will infuse in less than an hour. To do this the nurse must first do the following:
1. Calculate the mL/min.
2. Divide the total volume by the mL/min to obtain the infusion time. The infusion time will be in minutes.

**Example:** An IV antibiotic of 30 mL is infusing at 20 macrogtt/min. Drop factor is 10 gtt/mL. Determine the infusion time.

**Step 1:** Calculate the mL/min.

$$10 \text{ gtt} : 1 \text{ mL} = 20 \text{ gtt} : x \text{ mL}$$

$$\frac{10x}{10} = \frac{20}{10}$$

$$x = 2 \text{ mL/min}$$

**Step 2:** Divide the total volume by mL/min.

$$30 \text{ mL} \div 2 \text{ mL/min} = 15 \text{ minutes}$$

The infusion time is 15 minutes.

 Solution Using Dimensional Analysis

Place min to the left of the equals sign. (Since a small volume is being infused in less than 1 hr, the time will be in minutes.) Therefore the conversion factor 60 min = 1 hr is not necessary.

$$x \text{ min} =$$

The remaining steps are the same as for calculating infusion time for large volumes.

$$x \text{ min} = \frac{1 \text{ min}}{\underset{2}{20 \text{ gtt}}} \times \frac{\overset{1}{10 \text{ gtt}}}{1 \text{ mL}} \times \frac{30 \text{ mL}}{1}$$

$$x = \frac{30}{2} = 15 \text{ min}$$

$$x = 15 \text{ min}$$

**Answer:** The infusion time is 15 minutes.

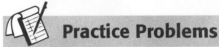

## Practice Problems

Determine the infusion times for the following:

68. An IV medication of 35 mL is infusing at 30 macrogtt/min. Drop factor: 15 gtt/mL. _____

69. An IV medication of 20 mL is infusing at 35 microgtt/min. Drop factor: 60 gtt/mL. _____

Answers on p. 661

## CHARTING IV THERAPY

At some institutions, continuous IV therapy may be charted on a special IV record or IV flow sheet. Medications that are administered intermittently by piggyback are charted on other medication sheets according to the order (e.g., standing medication sheet, p.r.n., or single, stat medication record). Forms used to chart IV therapy (whether a client is receiving IV solution that contains medications or solution without medications) vary from institution to institution. At institutions where a computerized system is used, IVs are charted directly into the computer. Appropriate assessments relating to IV sites are also charted on either a form for IV therapy or in the computer.

## LABELING SOLUTION BAGS

The markings on IV solution bags are not as precise as, for example, those on a syringe. Most IV bags are marked in increments of 50 to 100 mL. After calculating the amount of solution to infuse in 1 hour, the nurse may mark the bag to indicate where the level of fluid should be at each hour. Marking the IV bag allows the nurse to check that the fluid is infusing on time. Many institutions have commercially prepared labels for this purpose. (Figure 22-5 shows an IV with timing tape for visualizing the amount infused each hour.) The tape should indicate the start and finish times.

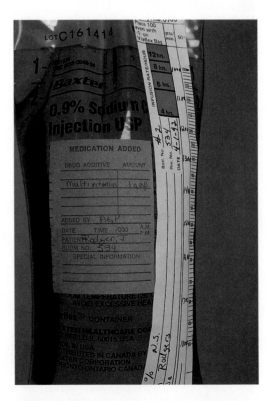

**Figure 22-5** IV solution with time taping. (From Potter PA, Perry AG: *Fundamentals of nursing,* ed. 7, St. Louis, 2009, Mosby.)

## ADMINISTRATION OF MEDICATIONS BY IV PUSH

Injection ports on IV tubing can be used for direct injection of medication with a syringe, which is called an IV push, or bolus. When medication is administered by IV push, the client experiences rapid results from the medication. Direct IV administration is used to deliver diluted or undiluted medication over a brief period (seconds or minutes). Medication literature and institutional guidelines provide the acceptable rate for IV push medication administration. Because of the rapidity of action, an error in calculation can result in a serious outcome. Medications can be administered by IV push by registered nurses who have been specially trained in this practice at some institutions.

Most IV push medications should be administered over a period of 1 to 5 minutes (can be longer). The volume of the prescribed medication should be calculated in increments of 15 to 30 seconds. This allows the use of a watch to provide accurate administration. The actual administration of IV push medications is beyond the scope of this text. For a detailed description of technique, consult a clinical skills textbook.

**CAUTION**

> Never infuse IV medications more rapidly than recommended. Carefully read literature for dilution and time for administration. IV medications are potent and rapid acting.

When administering medications by direct IV infusion, it is necessary to remember the following:
- The compatibility of the IV solution and the medication must be verified.
- The tubing will require a flush after direct administration to ensure that all the medication has been given and none remains in the tubing.
- The amount of time needed to administer a medication by direct IV infusion can be determined by using ratio and proportion or dimensional analysis. Let's look at some examples.

**Example 1:** Order: Tagamet 200 mg IV push now

Available: Tagamet 300 mg per 2 mL

The literature recommends diluting the Tagamet to a total of 20 mL. Compatible solution recommended is sodium chloride injection (0.9%). Inject over a period of not less than 2 minutes. An injection time of 5 minutes is ordered.
   a. How many mL of Tagamet will you administer?
   b. How many mL of sodium chloride must you add to obtain the desired volume?
   c. To administer the infusion in 5 minutes, how many mL should you infuse every minute?
   d. How much should you infuse every 15 seconds?

a. **Ratio and Proportion:**

$$300 \text{ mg} : 2 \text{ mL} = 200 \text{ mg} : x \text{ mL} \quad or \quad \frac{300 \text{ mg}}{2 \text{ mL}} = \frac{200 \text{ mg}}{x \text{ mL}}$$

$$\frac{300x}{300} = \frac{400}{300}$$

$$x = 1.33 = 1.3 \text{ mL}$$

**Formula Method:** $\dfrac{200 \text{ mg}}{300 \text{ mg}} \times 2 \text{ mL} = x \text{ mL}$

**Dimensional Analysis:** $x \text{ mL} = \dfrac{2 \text{ mL}}{300 \text{ mg}} \times \dfrac{200 \text{ mg}}{1}$

**Answer:** 1.3 mL Tagamet would equal 200 mg.

b. According to the literature, the total volume of the diluent and medication is 20 mL. If the literature stated to dilute in 20 mL, then the total volume would be the medication and diluent

$$
\begin{array}{r}
20 \text{ mL desired} \\
-1.3 \text{ mL dosage} \\
\hline
18.7 \text{ mL amount to add}
\end{array}
$$

c. **Ratio and Proportion:** (1 minute)

$$20 \text{ mL}:5 \text{ minutes} = x \text{ mL}:1 \text{ minute}$$

$$\frac{5x}{5} = \frac{20}{5}$$

$$x = 4 \text{ mL per minute}$$

d. **Ratio and Proportion:** (15 sec)

$$4 \text{ mL}:60 \text{ seconds} = x \text{ mL}:15 \text{ sec}$$

$$\frac{60x}{60} = \frac{60}{60}$$

$$x = 1 \text{ mL every 15 seconds}$$

**Dimensional Analysis:**

**Steps:**

1. The desired unit is mL; place it to the left of the equals sign.

$$x \text{ mL} =$$

2. Refer to the problem, and place the mL ordered as the first fraction (20 mL in 5 min); place mL in the numerator to match the mL desired.

$$x \text{ mL} = \frac{20 \text{ mL}}{5 \text{ min}}$$

3. Place 1 min in the numerator of the next fraction.

$$x \text{ mL} = \frac{\overset{4}{\cancel{20}} \text{ mL}}{\underset{1}{\cancel{5} \, \cancel{\text{min}}}} \times \frac{1 \, \cancel{\text{min}}}{1} = 4$$

$$x = 4 \text{ mL per minute}$$

**Answer:**    4 mL per minute

Notice that in this question you are asked to determine seconds. (Express 4 mL per minute as 4 mL per 60 seconds.) 60 seconds = 1 minute. The starting fraction would be 4 mL/60 sec:

$$x \text{ mL} = \frac{4 \text{ mL}}{60 \, \cancel{\text{sec}}} \times \frac{15 \, \cancel{\text{sec}}}{1}$$

$$x = \frac{60}{60} = 1$$

This could also be done using the 4 mL/min; however, you would need an additional fraction to be added to the equation. The equation would be as follows:

$$x \text{ mL} = \frac{4 \text{ mL}}{1 \, \cancel{\text{min}}} \times \frac{1 \, \cancel{\text{min}}}{60 \, \cancel{\text{sec}}} \times \frac{15 \, \cancel{\text{sec}}}{1}$$

$$x = 1 \text{ mL every 15 seconds}$$

Example 2:    Order: Ativan 3 mg IV push stat

Available: Ativan 4 mg per mL

The literature states not to exceed 2 mg/min. Determine the time to administer the medication as ordered.

    a.  How many mL of Ativan will you prepare? (Express in hundredths.)
    b.  How many min would administer the medication as ordered?

a. **Ratio and Proportion:**    $4 \text{ mg} : 1 \text{ mL} = 3 \text{ mg} : x \text{ mL}$    *or*    $\dfrac{4 \text{ mg}}{1 \text{ mL}} = \dfrac{3 \text{ mg}}{x \text{ mL}}$

$$\frac{4x}{4} = \frac{3}{4}$$

$$x = 0.75 \text{ mL}$$

**Formula Method:**    $\dfrac{3 \text{ mg}}{4 \text{ mg}} \times 1 \text{ mL} = x \text{ mL}$

**Dimensional Analysis:**    $x \text{ mL} = \dfrac{1 \text{ mL}}{4 \text{ mg}} \times \dfrac{3 \text{ mg}}{1}$

b. **Ratio and Proportion:**    $2 \text{ mg} : 1 \text{ min} = 3 \text{ mg} : x \text{ min}$    *or*    $\dfrac{2 \text{ mg}}{1 \text{ min}} = \dfrac{3 \text{ mg}}{x \text{ min}}$

$$\frac{2x}{2} = \frac{3}{2}$$

$$x = 1\frac{1}{2} \text{ min}$$

**Answer:**    $1\frac{1}{2}$ min to administer the medication as ordered

**Dimensional Analysis:**    Use the steps outlined in Example 1 to determine the time.

$$x \text{ min} = \frac{1 \text{ min}}{2 \text{ mg}} \times \frac{3 \text{ mg}}{1}$$

## Practice Problems

Calculate the IV push rate as indicated for Problems 70 to 72.
70.  Order: Valium 20 mg IV push stat at 5 mg/min for a client with seizures.

   Available: Valium 5 mg per mL

    a.  How many milliliters will be
       needed to administer the dosage?    _____

    b.  Determine the time it would take
       to infuse the dosage.    _____

    c.  How many milligrams would you
       administer every 15 seconds?    _____

71. Order: Dilantin 150 mg IV push stat.

    Available: Dilantin 250 mg per 5 mL. Literature states IV infusion not to exceed 50 mg/min.

    a. How much should you prepare to administer?  _____

    b. How much time is needed to administer the required dosage?  _____

72. Order: AquaMEPHYTON 5 mg IV push stat.

    Available: AquaMEPHYTON 10 mg per mL. The literature states that the medication should be diluted in at least 10 mL of NS and administered at a rate of 1 mg or fraction thereof per minute.

    a. How much diluent should you add to the medication?  _____

    b. How much medication should you inject every 30 seconds to infuse the medication at a rate of 1 mg/min?  _____

Answers on p. 661

## ■ Points to Remember

- Read IV labels carefully to determine whether the correct solution is being administered.
- To calculate IV flow rate in gtt/min, the nurse must have the volume of solution, the time factor for the IV to infuse, and the drop factor of the tubing.
- Drop factor is expressed as gtt/mL and indicated on the package of the IV tubing.
- Calculation of gtt/min can be done by using the formula method or dimensional analysis.

$$\text{Formula: } x \text{ gtt/min} = \frac{\text{Amount of solution (mL)} \times \text{gtt factor (gtt/mL)}}{\text{Time (min)}}$$

- Formula is used for any time period that can be expressed as 60 minutes or less.
- For time periods greater than 60 minutes find mL/hr first, and then use the formula to determine gtt/min.
- Round gtt/min to the nearest whole number (division carried one decimal place).
- A shortcut method can be used to calculate flow rates infusing in 1 hour or less, and for more than 1 hour, by determining mL/hr and determining the drop factor constant for the IV set.
- To determine the drop factor constant for any IV set, divide 60 by the calibration of the set.

### Recalculating IV Rates

- IV flow rates must be monitored by the nurse. When IV solutions are behind or ahead of schedule, the flow rate must be recalculated by using the following formula:

$$\text{Step 1: } \frac{\text{Volume (mL) remaining}}{\text{Time remaining}} = \text{recalculated mL/hr}$$

Step 2: Determine IV rate in gtt/min.
Step 3: Determine percent of variation.

- Never increase or decrease an IV flow rate without recalculating and assessing a client to determine if the change can be tolerated.
- IV flow rates should not be increased or decreased more than 25% of their original rate. Know the policy of the institution regarding recalculating IV flow rates. Check with the prescriber regarding an IV increase greater than 25%. To determine the percentage of increase and decrease, divide the amount of increase or decrease by the original rate.

**Determining Infusion Time**
- Infusion time is calculated by dividing the total volume to infuse by the rate (mL/hr) at which the solution is infusing or by dimensional analysis. To obtain the completion time for an IV, add the infusion time calculated to the time the IV was started. (Time can be stated in traditional or military time.)

**IV Push Medications**
- Medications administered by direct IV infusion must be checked for compatibility with the solution and timed properly. Never administer a medication by direct infusion at a rate faster than recommended.

## Critical Thinking Questions

**Scenario:** An elderly client has an order for 1,000 mL D5W at 100 mL/hr. The nurse assigned to the client attached IV tubing to the IV with a drop factor of 10 gtt/mL without checking the package of IV tubing. As a habit from a previous institution where she worked, the IV flow rate was calculated based on the drop factor of 20 gtt/mL. At the beginning of the next shift, the nurse making rounds noticed that the client was having difficulty breathing and seemed restless. When the nurse checked the IV rate, she discovered the rate was 33 macrogtt/min instead of 17 macrogtt/min.

a. What factors contributed to the error? _____

b. How did the IV rate contribute to the problem and why? _____

c. What should have been the action of the nurse who attached the IV tubing in relation to IV administration? _____

Answers on p. 661

## ✓ CHAPTER REVIEW

Calculate the IV flow rate in gtt/min for the following IV administrations, unless another unit of measure is stated.

1. 1,000 mL D5RL to infuse in 8 hr.
   Drop factor: 20 gtt/mL          _____

2. 2,500 mL D5NS to infuse in 24 hr.
   Drop factor: 10 gtt/mL          _____

3. 500 mL D5W to infuse in 4 hr.
   Drop factor: 15 gtt/mL          _____

4. 300 mL NS to infuse in 6 hr.
   Drop factor: 60 gtt/mL          _____

5. 1,000 mL D5W for 24 hr KVO (keep
   vein open). Drop factor: 60 gtt/mL    _____

6. 500 mL D5 and ½ NS with 20 mEq KCl
   over 12 hr. Drop factor: 20 gtt/mL    _____

7. 1,000 mL RL to infuse in 10 hr.
   Drop factor: 20 gtt/mL          _____

8. 1,500 mL NS to infuse in 12 hr.
   Drop factor: 10 gtt/mL          _____

9. A unit of whole blood (500 mL) to
   infuse in 4 hr. Drop factor: 20 gtt/mL    _____

10. A unit of packed cells (250 mL) to
    infuse in 4 hr. Drop factor: 20 gtt/mL    _____

11. 1,500 mL D5W in 8 hr.
    Drop factor: 20 gtt/mL          _____

12. 3,000 mL RL in 24 hr.
    Drop factor: 15 gtt/mL          _____

13. Infuse 2 L RL in 24 hr.
    Drop factor: 15 gtt/mL          _____

14. 500 mL D5W in 4 hr.
    Drop factor: 60 gtt/mL          _____

15. 1,000 mL D5 0.45% NS in 6 hr.
    Drop factor: 20 gtt/mL          _____

16. 250 mL D5W in 8 hr.
    Drop factor: 60 gtt/mL          _____

17. 1 L of D5W to infuse at 50 mL/hr.
    Drop factor: 60 gtt/mL          _____

18. 2 L D5RL at 150 mL/hr.
    Drop factor: 15 gtt/mL          _____

19. 500 mL D5W in 6 hr.
    Drop factor: 15 gtt/mL          _____

20. 1,500 mL NS in 12 hr.
    Drop factor: 10 gtt/mL          _____

21. 1,500 mL D5W in 24 hr.
    Drop factor: 15 gtt/mL
    _____

22. 2,000 mL D5W in 16 hr.
    Drop factor: 20 gtt/mL
    _____

23. 500 mL D5W in 8 hr.
    Drop factor: 15 gtt/mL
    _____

24. 250 mL D5W in 10 hr.
    Drop factor: 60 gtt/mL
    _____

25. Infuse 300 mL of D5W at 75 mL/hr.
    Drop factor: 60 gtt/mL
    _____

26. Infuse 125 mL/hr of D5RL.
    Drop factor: 20 gtt/mL
    _____

27. Infuse 40 mL/hr of D5W.
    Drop factor: 60 gtt/mL
    _____

28. Infuse an IV medication with a
    volume of 50 mL in 45 minutes.
    Drop factor: 60 gtt/mL
    _____

29. Infuse 90 mL/hr of NS.
    Drop factor: 15 gtt/mL
    _____

30. Infuse 150 mL/hr of D5RL.
    Drop factor: 10 gtt/mL
    _____

31. Infuse 2,500 mL of D5W in 24 hr.
    Drop factor: 15 gtt/mL
    _____

32. Infuse an IV medication in
    50 mL of 0.9% NS in 40 minutes.
    Drop factor: 10 gtt/mL
    _____

33. Infuse an IV medication in
    100 mL D5W in 30 minutes.
    Drop factor: 20 gtt/mL
    _____

34. Infuse 250 mL 0.45% NS in 5 hr.
    Drop factor: 20 gtt/mL
    _____

35. Infuse 1,000 mL of D5W at 80 mL/hr.
    Drop factor: 20 gtt/mL
    _____

36. Infuse 150 mL of D5RL in 30 minutes.
    Drop factor: 10 gtt/mL
    _____

37. Infuse Kefzol 0.5 g in 50 mL D5W
    in 30 minutes. Drop factor:
    60 gtt/mL
    _____

38. Infuse Plasmanate 500 mL over 3 hr.
    Drop factor: 10 gtt/mL
    _____

39. Infuse albumin 250 mL over 2 hr.
Drop factor: 15 gtt/mL

_____

40. The prescriber orders the following
IVs for 24 hr. Drop factor: 10 gtt/mL
   a. 1,000 mL D5W with 1 ampule
      MVI (multivitamin)
   b. 500 mL D5W
   c. 250 mL D5W

_____

41. Infuse vancomycin 1 g IVPB in
150 mL D5W in 1.5 hr. Drop factor:
60 gtt/mL

_____

42. If 2 L D5W is to infuse in 16 hr, how
many milliliters are to be administered
per hour?

_____

43. If 500 mL of RL is to infuse in 4 hr,
how many milliliters are to be
administered per hour?

_____

44. If 200 mL of NS is to infuse in 2 hr,
how many milliliters are to be
administered per hour?

_____

45. If 500 mL of D5W is to infuse in
8 hr, how many milliliters are to be
administered per hour?

_____

46. Infuse a hyperalimentation solution
of 1,100 mL in 12 hr. How many
milliliters are to be administered per
hour?

_____

47. Infuse 500 mL Intralipids IV in 6 hr.
Drop factor: 10 gtt/mL

_____

48. Infuse 3,000 mL D5W in 20 hr.
Drop factor: 20 gtt/mL

_____

49. An IV of 500 mL D5W with 200 mg
of minocycline is to infuse in 6 hr.
Drop factor: 15 gtt/mL

_____

50. An IV of D5W 500 mL was ordered
to infuse over 10 hr at a rate of
13 gtt/min (13 macrogtt/min).
Drop factor: 15 gtt/mL
After 3 hr, you notice that 300 mL of
IV solution is left. Recalculate the rate
in gtt/min for the remaining solution.    _____ gtt/min
Determine the percentage of change in
IV rate, and state your course of action.   _____ %

51. An IV of D5W 1,000 mL was ordered to infuse over 8 hr at a rate of 42 gtt/min (42 macrogtt/min).
Drop factor: 20 gtt/mL
After 4 hr, you notice that only 400 mL has infused. Recalculate the rate in gtt/min for the remaining solution.    _____ gtt/min
Determine the percentage of change, and state your course of action.    _____ %

52. An IV of 1,000 mL D5 and 1/2 NS has been ordered to infuse at 125 mL/hr.
Drop factor: 15 gtt/mL
The IV was hung at 7 AM. At 11 AM you check the IV, and there is 400 mL left. Recalculate the rate in gtt/min for the remaining solution.    _____ gtt/min
Determine the percentage of change, and state your course of action.    _____ %

53. An IV of 500 mL of 0.9% NS is to infuse in 6 hr at a rate of 14 gtt/min (14 macrogtt/min).
Drop factor: 10 gtt/mL
The IV was started at 7 AM. You check the IV at 8 AM, and 250 mL has infused. Recalculate the rate in gtt/min for the remaining solution.    _____ gtt/min
Determine the percentage of change and state your course of action.    _____ %

54. An IV of 1,000 mL D5W is to infuse in 10 hr. Drop factor: 15 gtt/mL
The IV was started at 4 AM. At 10 AM 600 mL remains in the bag. Is the IV on schedule? If not, recalculate the rate in gtt/min for the remaining solution.    _____ gtt/min
Determine the percentage of change and state your course of action.    _____ %

55. 900 mL of RL is infusing at a rate of 80 gtt/min (80 macrodrops/min).
Drop factor: 15 gtt/mL
How long will it take for the IV to infuse? (Express time in hours and minutes.)    _____

56. A client is receiving 1,000 mL of D5W at 100 mL/hr. How many hours will it take for the IV to infuse?    _____

57. 1,000 mL of D5W is infusing at
    20 gtt/min (20 macrogtt/min).
    Drop factor: 10 gtt/mL
    How long will it take for the IV to
    infuse? (Express time in hours and
    minutes.)                                    _____

58. 450 mL of NS is infusing at 25 gtt/min
    (25 macrogtt/min).
    Drop factor: 20 gtt/mL
    How many hours will it take for the
    IV to infuse?                                _____

59. 100 mL of D5W is infusing at
    10 gtt/min (10 macrogtt/min).
    The administration set delivers
    15 gtt/mL. How many hours will
    it take for the IV to infuse?                _____

60. An IV is regulated at 25 gtt/min
    (25 macrogtt/min).
    Drop factor: 15 gtt/mL
    How many milliliters of fluid will the
    client receive in 8 hr?                      _____

61. An IV is regulated at 40 gtt/min
    (40 microdrop/min).
    Drop factor: 60 gtt/mL
    How many milliliters of fluid will the
    client receive in 10 hr?                     _____

62. An IV is regulated at 30 gtt/min
    (30 macrogtt/min).
    Drop factor: 15 gtt/mL
    How many milliliters of fluid will the
    client receive in 5 hr?                      _____

63. 10 mEq of potassium chloride is
    placed in 500 mL of D5W to be
    administered at the rate of 2 mEq/hr.
    At what rate in mL/hr should the
    IV infuse?                                   _____

64. 30 mEq of potassium chloride is added
    to 1,000 mL of D5W to be administered
    at the rate of 4 mEq/hr. At what rate in
    mL/hr should the IV infuse?                  _____

65. Order: Humulin regular U-100 7 units/hr.
    The IV solution contains 50 units of
    Humulin regular insulin in 250 mL
    of 0.9% NS. At what rate in mL/hr
    should the IV infuse?                        _____

66. Order: Humulin regular U-100 18 units/hr.
    The IV solution contains 100 units of
    Humulin regular insulin in 250 mL
    of 0.9% NS. At what rate in mL/hr
    should the IV infuse?                        _____

67. Order: Humulin regular U-100 11 units/hr.
    The IV solution contains 100 units of
    Humulin regular insulin in 100 mL
    of 0.9% NS. At what rate in mL/hr
    should the IV infuse?  _____

68. Infuse gentamicin 65 mg in 150 mL
    0.9% NS IVPB over 1 hr.
    Drop factor: 10 gtt/mL
    At what rate in gtt/min should the
    IV infuse?  _____

69. Infuse ampicillin 1 g that has been diluted
    in 40 mL 0.9% NS to infuse in 40 minutes.
    Drop factor: 60 gtt/mL
    At what rate in gtt/min should the
    IV infuse?  _____

70. Administer IV medication with a
    volume of 35 mL in 30 minutes.
    Drop factor: 60 gtt/mL
    At what rate in gtt/min should the
    IV infuse?  _____

71. Administer IV medication with a
    volume of 80 mL in 40 minutes.
    Drop factor: 15 gtt/mL
    At what rate in gtt/min should the
    IV infuse?  _____

72. Administer 50 mL of an antibiotic
    in 25 minutes.
    Drop factor: 10 gtt/mL
    At what rate in gtt/min would you
    regulate the IV?  _____

73. An IV is to infuse at 65 mL/hr.
    Drop factor: 15 gtt/mL
    At what rate in gtt/min should the
    IV infuse?  _____

74. 50 mL of 0.9% NS with 1 g ampicillin
    is infusing at 50 microgtt/min (50 gtt/min).
    Drop factor: 60 gtt/mL
    Determine the infusion time.  _____

75. 500 mL RL is to infuse at a rate of
    80 mL/hr. If the IV was started at 7 PM,
    what time will the IV be completed?  _____
    State time in military and traditional
    time.  _____

76. A volume of 150 mL of NS is to
    infuse at 25 mL/hr.
    a. Calculate the infusion time.  _____
    b. The IV was started at 3:10 AM.
       What time will the IV be completed?
       State time in traditional and military
       time.  _____

77. The doctor orders 2.5 L of D5W to infuse at 150 mL/hr. Determine the infusion time. _____

78. Order: Lasix 120 mg IV stat.
    Available: 10 mg per mL. The literature states IV not to exceed 40 mg/min.
    a. How many milliliters will you prepare? _____
    b. Calculate the time required to administer the medication as ordered. _____

79. Order: Inocor 60 mg IV bolus over 2 min.
    Available: Inocor 100 mg per 20 mL
    a. How many milliliters will you prepare? _____
    b. Determine the amount that should be infused per minute. _____

80. Order: Levaquin 500 mg IVPB in 100 mL 0.9% NS q12h over 1 hr.
    Drop factor: 10 gtt/mL
    Determine rate in gtt/min. _____

81. Order: Zosyn 1.3 g in 100 mL D5W IVPB q8h to infuse over 30 min.
    Drop factor: 60 gtt/mL
    Determine rate in gtt/min. _____

82. 500 mL D5W with 30,000 units of heparin to infuse at 1,500 units per hour.
    Determine rate in mL/hr. _____

83. Order: Humulin regular U-100 20 units per hr. The IV solution contains 100 units of Humulin Regular in 500 mL of 0.9% NS.
    At what rate in mL/hr should the IV infuse? _____

84. Order: Humulin regular U-100 15 units per hr. The IV solution contains 100 units of Humulin Regular in 250 mL of 0.9% NS.
    At what rate in mL/hr should the IV infuse? _____

Answers on pp. 662-668

 **For additional practice problems, refer to the Intravenous Calculations and Advanced Calculations sections of Drug Calculations Companion, Version 4, on Evolve.**

# CHAPTER 23

# Heparin Calculations

**Objectives**

*After reviewing this chapter, you should be able to:*
1. State the importance of calculating heparin dosages accurately
2. Calculate heparin dosages being administered intravenously (mL per hr, units per hr)
3. Calculate subcutaneous dosages of heparin
4. Calculate safe heparin dosages based on weight

## HEPARIN ERRORS

Heparin has taken center stage in the media. Numerous errors have been reported relating to heparin and have attracted the attention of the health care society and the general public. Heparin is classified as a high-alert medication because it carries a significant risk of causing serious injuries or death to patients if misused. Attention has been given to unfractionated heparin, low-molecular-weight heparin, and warfarin. Cohen (2007), in the text *Medication Errors*, discusses some of the causes of error with heparin:

- Mix-ups with concentrations of heparin
- Temporary increases in heparin pump rates to give a bolus; error caused by staff forgetting to reset the pump after delivering the bolus
- Tenfold overdoses from using the abbreviation "U" for units
- Various concentrations of IV heparin bags and heparin vials being mixed up, in part because of look-alike vials and bags

These are just a few reasons for errors that have occurred with heparin. The U.S. Pharmacopoeia listed heparin as one of the top 10 medications most frequently involved in medication errors.

Because of the frequency of errors that have occurred with anticoagulants, they have received the focus of attention from ISMP (Institute for Safe Medication Practices) and The Joint Commission. The anticoagulants are among the medications that will receive targeted attention during the coming year from The Joint Commission.

The Joint Commission proposed a 2008 National Patient Safety Goal (NPSG) associated with anticoagulation therapy. The goal is to reduce the likelihood of patient harm associated with this form of therapy. The requirements will apply to all organizations that provide anticoagulation therapy. The implementation expectations began January 1, 2009. These requirements can be viewed on The Joint Commission's web site at www.jointcommission.org.

Heparin is a potent anticoagulant that prevents clot formation and blood coagulation. Heparin dosages are expressed in (USP) units. The therapeutic range for heparin is determined individually by monitoring the client's blood clotting value (activated partial thromboplastin time [APTT] measured in seconds). Heparin is considered to be most therapeutically effective when based on weight in kilograms. Heparin infusions are individualized based on the client's weight. This concept will be discussed later in the chapter. Heparin can be administered intravenously or subcutaneously; it is never administered intramuscularly because of the danger of hematomas (collections of extravasated blood trapped in tissues of skin or in an organ). When administered intravenously, heparin is ordered in units/hr or mL/hr. Usually, however, heparin is ordered on the basis of the units/hr when ordered intravenously and should be administered by an electronic infusion device. Heparin is available in single-dose and multidose vials, as well as in commercially prepared IV solutions. Heparin sodium for injection is available in several strengths (e.g., 100 units per mL; 5,000 units per mL; 20,000 units per mL). Heparin lock fluid solution, which is used for flushing, is available in 10 and 100 units per mL.

**CAUTION**

It is extremely important that the nurse be aware that heparin sodium for injection and heparin lock solution can never be used interchangeably.

Heparin used for a flush is usually concentrated to 10 units per mL or 100 units per mL. This is a different concentration of heparin than what is administered subcutaneously or intravenously.

Figure 23-1 shows the various heparin dosage strengths. The client requires continuous monitoring while receiving heparin because of the risk for hemorrhage or clots with an incorrect dosage.

## Tips for Clinical Practice

The nurse's primary responsibility is to administer the correct dosage and ensure that the dosage being administered is safe.

When in doubt regarding a dosage a client is receiving, check it with the prescriber before administering it. To avoid misinterpretation when orders are written or done by computer entry, the word *units* should not be abbreviated.

**CAUTION**

Heparin comes in different strengths; read labels carefully before administering to ensure the client's safety. Verify the dosage, vial, and amount to be given with another nurse before administering the heparin. In many institutions it is a requirement that heparin be checked by two nurses.

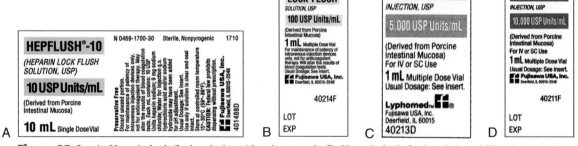

**Figure 23-1** **A,** Heparin lock flush solution, 10 units per mL. **B,** Heparin lock flush solution, 100 units per mL. **C,** 5,000 units per mL. **D,** 10,000 units per mL.

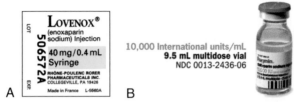

**Figure 23-2** **A,** Lovenox label. **B,** Fragmin vial. (**B** reproduced with permission by Pfizer, Inc. All rights reserved.)

Dosages of heparin are highly individualized and based on a client's coagulation time. Lovenox (enoxaparin) and Fragmin (dalteparin) are also injectable low-molecular-weight anticoagulants prescribed for prevention and treatment of deep vein thrombosis (DVT) and pulmonary emboli (PEs) after knee and hip surgery. (Figure 23-2 shows a Lovenox label and a vial of Fragmin.)

## READING HEPARIN LABELS

Always read heparin labels carefully to ensure that you have the correct concentrations. Remember that there are a number of available vial dosage strengths. Commercially prepared IV solutions are also available from pharmaceutical companies in several strengths. The dosage written in red is for the purpose of attracting attention to the fact that the bag contains heparin. The use of premixed standardized bags of intravenous fluid with heparin assists in the prevention of some dose errors with heparin. In some institutions heparin for IV use is prepared in the pharmacy in various dosage strengths. If the dosage desired is not available in a commercially prepared solution or from the pharmacy, the nurse will be responsible for preparing the solution.

**CAUTION**

Always carefully read heparin labels (three times) and the prescribed dose. Adherence to the "six rights" of medication administration is critical in preventing dosing errors with heparin.

Now let's proceed with the calculation of heparin dosages.

## CALCULATION OF SUBCUTANEOUS DOSAGES

Because of its inherent dangers and the need to ensure an accurate and exact dosage, when heparin is administered subcutaneously a tuberculin syringe is used. Heparin is also available for use in pre-packaged syringes. Institutional policies differ regarding the administration of heparin, and the nurse is responsible for knowing and following the policies. The methods of calculating presented in previous chapters are used to calculate subcutaneous (subcut) heparin, except the dosage is never rounded and is administered with a tuberculin syringe. The prescriber will order heparin in units, and an order written in any other unit of measure should be questioned before administration.

**Example:**    Order: Heparin 7,500 units subcut

Available: Heparin labeled 10,000 units per mL

What will you administer to the client?

Setup:
1. No conversion is necessary. There is no conversion for units.
2. Think—what would be a logical dosage?
3. Set up in ratio and proportion, the formula method, or dimensional analysis and solve.

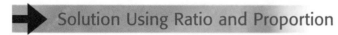
### Solution Using Ratio and Proportion

$$10{,}000 \text{ units} : 1 \text{ mL} = 7{,}500 \text{ units} : x \text{ mL}$$

*or*

$$\frac{10{,}000 \text{ units}}{1 \text{ mL}} = \frac{7{,}500 \text{ units}}{x \text{ mL}}$$

$$10{,}000x = 7{,}500$$

$$x = \frac{7{,}500}{10{,}000}$$

$$x = 0.75 \text{ mL}$$

### Solution Using the Formula Method

$$\frac{7{,}500 \text{ units}}{10{,}000 \text{ units}} \times 1 \text{ mL} = x \text{ mL}$$

$$x = 0.75 \text{ mL}$$

### Solution Using Dimensional Analysis

$$x \text{ mL} = \frac{1 \text{ mL}}{10{,}000 \text{ units}} \times \frac{7{,}500 \text{ units}}{1}$$

$$x = \frac{7{,}500}{10{,}000}$$

$$x = 0.75 \text{ mL}$$

The dosage of 0.75 mL is reasonable because the ordered dose is less than what is available. Therefore less than 1 mL will be needed to administer the dosage. This dosage can be measured accurately only with a tuberculin syringe (calibrated in tenths and hundredths of a milliliter). This dosage would not be rounded to the nearest tenth of a milliliter. A tuberculin syringe illustrating the dosage to be administered is shown in Figure 23-3.

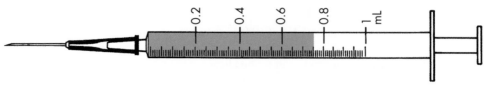

**Figure 23-3** Tuberculin syringe illustrating 0.75 mL drawn up.

## CALCULATION OF IV HEPARIN SOLUTIONS

### Using Ratio and Proportion to Calculate Units per Hour

Calculating the rate in units/hr can be done by using ratio and proportion or dimensional analysis.

**Example:** An IV solution of heparin is ordered for a client. D5W 1,000 mL containing 20,000 units of heparin is to infuse at 30 mL/hr. Calculate the dosage of heparin the client is to receive per hour.

Set up proportion:

$$20,000 \text{ units} : 1,000 \text{ mL} = x \text{ units} : 30 \text{ mL}$$

*or*

$$\frac{20,000 \text{ units}}{1,000 \text{ mL}} = \frac{x \text{ units}}{30 \text{ mL}}$$

$$1,000x = 20,000 \times 30$$

$$\frac{1,000x}{1,000} = \frac{600,000}{1,000}$$

$$x = 600 \text{ units/hr}$$

> **NOTE**
> Ratios and proportions can be stated in several formats.

### Using Dimensional Analysis to Calculate Units per Hour

**Steps:**
- Isolate units/hr being calculated first.
- Place the 20,000 units per 1,000 mL as the starting fraction with units in the numerator, to match the units in the numerator being calculated.
- Enter the 30 mL/hr rate with 30 mL as the numerator; notice that this matches the starting fraction mL denominator.
- Cancel the mL to obtain the desired unit (units/hr).
- Reduce if possible, and perform the necessary math operations.

$$\frac{x \text{ units}}{hr} = \frac{20,000 \text{ units}}{1,000 \text{ mL}} \times \frac{30 \text{ mL}}{1 \text{ hr}}$$

$$x = \frac{20 \times 30}{1}$$

$$x = \frac{600}{1}$$

$$x = 600 \text{ units/hr}$$

> **NOTE**
> Reduction is done to decrease size of numbers.

### Calculating mL/hr From Units/hr

Because heparin is ordered in units/hr and infused with an electronic infusion device, it is necessary to do calculations in mL/hr.

**CAUTION**

An infusion pump is required for all intravenous heparin drips.

**Example 1:**    Order: Infuse heparin 850 units/hr from a solution containing D5W 500 mL with heparin 25,000 units IV.

 Solution Using Ratio and Proportion

$$25{,}000 \text{ units} : 500 \text{ mL} = 850 \text{ units} : x \text{ mL}$$

*or*

$$\frac{25{,}000 \text{ units}}{500 \text{ mL}} = \frac{850 \text{ units}}{x \text{ mL}}$$

**Solve:**
$$25{,}000\, x = 500 \times 850$$

$$\frac{25{,}000x}{25{,}000} = \frac{425{,}000}{25{,}000}$$

$$x = \frac{425}{25}$$

$$x = 17 \text{ mL/hr}$$

 Solution Using Dimensional Analysis

**Steps:**
- Isolate mL/hr being calculated first.
- Enter the starting fraction 25,000 units per 500 mL, placing mL as the numerator. Notice that this will match the mL numerator of the units being calculated.
- Enter the 850 units/hr rate ordered with units in the numerator.
- Cancel units; 50 mL and hr are left.
- Reduce if possible, and perform the math operations.

$$\frac{x \text{ mL}}{\text{hr}} = \frac{\overset{1}{\cancel{500}} \text{ mL}}{\underset{50}{\cancel{25{,}000}} \text{ units}} \times \frac{850 \text{ units}}{1 \text{ hr}}$$

$$x = \frac{85\cancel{0}}{5\cancel{0}}$$

$$x = \frac{85}{5}$$

$$x = 17 \text{ mL/hr}$$

To infuse 850 units/hr from a solution of 25,000 units in D5W 500 mL, the flow rate would be 17 mL/hr.

**Example 2:**    Infuse 1,200 units of heparin per hour from a solution containing 20,000 units in 250 mL D5W.

 Solution Using Ratio and Proportion

$$20{,}000 \text{ units} : 250 \text{ mL} = 1{,}200 \text{ units} : x \text{ mL}$$

*or*

$$\frac{20{,}000 \text{ units}}{250 \text{ mL}} = \frac{1{,}200 \text{ units}}{x \text{ mL}}$$

Solve:
$$20,000x = 1,200 \times 250$$

$$\frac{20,000x}{20,000} = \frac{300,000}{20,000}$$

$$x = \frac{30}{2}$$

$$x = 15 \text{ mL/hr}$$

 ## Solution Using Dimensional Analysis

Follow the same steps outlined in Example 1.

$$\frac{x \text{ mL}}{\text{hr}} = \frac{\overset{1}{\cancel{250}} \text{ mL}}{\underset{80}{\cancel{20,000}} \text{ units}} \times \frac{1,200 \text{ units}}{1 \text{ hr}}$$

$$x = \frac{1,200}{80}$$

$$x = 15 \text{ mL/hr}$$

## CALCULATING HEPARIN DOSAGES BASED ON WEIGHT

IV heparin dosages are individualized based on a client's weight. Hospitals have protocols related to IV heparin administration. The protocols are based on the client's weight in kilograms and the client's activated partial thromboplastin time (APTT). APTT is used as the criterion to titrate the dosage, and adjustments are made accordingly. Protocols differ from one institution to another. It is imperative that nurses be familiar with the protocol at their individual institutions (see sample protocol in Figure 23-4).

The bolus or loading dosage and the infusion rate are based on the client's weight in kilograms. The bolus and infusion rate can vary among institutions. According to Clayton et al's *Basic Pharmacology for Nurses* (2007), the bolus dosage is 70 to 100 units/kg, and the infusion rate is 15 to 25 units/hr. At some institutions the weight of the client is to the nearest tenth of a kilogram, or the exact number of kilograms. Always be familiar with the values and protocol used for heparin administration at the institution.

**CAUTION**

In order for heparin to be therapeutically effective, the dosage must be accurate. A larger dosage than required can cause a client to hemorrhage, and an underdosage may not have the desired effect. Any questionable dosages should be verified with the prescriber.

| HEPARIN WEIGHT-BASED NOMOGRAM[1] | |
|---|---|
| Initial infusion rate | 14 units/kg/hr |
| aPTT < 35 sec (<1.2 × control value) | Bolus 80 units/kg, then increase rate by 4 units/kg/hr |
| aPTT 33-45 sec (1.2-1.5 × control value) | Bolus 40 units/kg, then increase rate by 2 units/kg/hr |
| *aPTT 46-70 sec (>1.5-2.3 × control value)* | *NO CHANGE* |
| aPTT 71-90 sec (>2.3-3 × control value) | Decrease infusion rate by 2 units/kg/hr |
| aPTT > 90 sec (>3 × control value) | Stop infusion for 1 hr, then decrease infusion rate by 3 units/kg/hr |
| ***Maximum initial rate not to exceed 1,000 units/hr** unless approved by Cardiology, Neurology, Hematology.* | |
| **DO NOT** bolus Heparin in **CVA or Neurosergery patients,** just use Heparin drip/infusion | |

[1]Modified from Raschke RA, et al. Ann Intern Med 1993; 119:874-881.

**FIGURE 23-4**   Heparin weight–based nomogram. (Used with permission of St. Barnabas Hospital, Bronx, NY.)

Let's work through some examples of calculation of heparin dosages based on weight. For the purpose of practice problems, the client's weight will be rounded to the nearest tenth of a kilogram.

**Example 1:**   A client weighs 160 lb. Order: Administer a bolus of heparin sodium IV.

The hospital protocol is 80 units/kg. How many units will you give?

**Step 1:**   Calculate the client's weight in kilograms.

Conversion factor:   1 kg = 2.2 lb

160 lb ÷ 2.2 = 72.72 = 72.7 kg

**Step 2:**   Calculate the heparin bolus dosage.

80 units/kg × 72.7 kg = 5,816 units

The client should receive 5,816 units IV heparin as a bolus.

**Example 2:**   A client weighs 165 lb.

Heparin infusion: Heparin 25,000 units in 1,000 mL 0.9% sodium chloride.

Bolus with heparin sodium at 80 units/kg, then initiate drip at 18 units/kg/hr.

Calculate the initial heparin bolus dosage.

Calculate the infusion rate, and determine the rate in mL/hr at which you will set the infusion device.

**Step 1:**   Calculate the client's weight in kilograms.

Conversion factor:   1 kg = 2.2 lb

165 lb ÷ 2.2 = 75 kg

**Step 2:**   Calculate the heparin bolus dosage.

80 units/kg × 75 kg = 6,000 units

The client should receive 6,000 units IV heparin as a bolus.

**Step 3:**   Calculate the infusion rate for the IV dosage.

18 units/kg/hr × 75 kg = 1,350 units/hr

**Step 4:**   Determine the rate in mL/hr at which to set the infusion device.

1,000 mL : 25,000 units = $x$ mL : 1,350 units

25,000$x$ = 1,350 × 1,000

$$\frac{25,000x}{25,000} = \frac{1,350,000}{25,000}$$

$x$ = 54 mL/hr

*or*

Formula could be used:

$$\frac{D}{H} \times Q = x$$

$$\frac{1,350 \text{ units per hr}}{25,000 \text{ units}} \times 1,000 \text{ mL} = x \text{ mL per hr}$$

$x$ = 54 mL/hr

**Practice Problems**

Calculate the units of measure indicated by the problem.

1. Order: Infuse 1,000 units/hr of heparin from a solution of 1,000 mL 0.45% NS with 25,000 units of heparin. Calculate the rate in mL/hr. _____

2. Order: Infuse D5 0.9% NS 1,000 mL with 25,000 units of heparin at 35 mL/hr. Calculate the dosage in units/hr. _____

3. Order: Infuse 750 mL D5W with 30,000 units of heparin at 25 mL/hr. Calculate the dosage in units/hr. _____

4. Order: Infuse D5W 1,000 mL with 25,000 units of heparin at 100 mL/hr. Determine the dosage in units/hr. _____

5. A client weighs 176 lb. Heparin infusion 20,000 units in 1,000 mL 0.9% sodium chloride. Order: Bolus with heparin sodium at 80 units/kg, then initiate drip at 18 units/kg/hr. (Round weight to the nearest tenth as indicated.) Calculate the following:

   a. _____ bolus dosage

   b. _____ infusion rate (initial)

   c. _____ mL/hr

Answers on pp. 668-669

**NOTE**

Any of the examples presented could be done by using dimensional analysis or a ratio and proportion, or the formula

$$\frac{D}{H} \times Q = x$$

could be used, all of which have been illustrated in other chapters, as well as this chapter.

---

## ■ Points to Remember

- Heparin is a potent anticoagulant; it is often administered intravenously but can be administered subcutaneously.
- Heparin is measured in USP units. When orders are written the word *units* is spelled out to prevent misinterpretation.
- Heparin dosages must be accurately calculated to prevent inherent dangers associated with the medication. Discrepancies in dosage should be verified with the prescriber.
- Heparin order, dosage, vial, and the amount to give should be checked by another nurse before administering.
- When subcut heparin is administered, a tuberculin syringe is used (calibrated in tenths and hundredths of a milliliter). Answers are expressed in hundredths.
- Read heparin labels carefully because heparin comes in several strengths.
- There are several IV calculations that can be done (mL/hr, units/hr).
- Heparin is commonly ordered in units/hr and infused with an electronic infusion device.
- Heparin sodium for injection and heparin lock solution cannot be used interchangeably.

- The method of calculating IV heparin dosages can also be used to calculate IV dosages for other medications. Ratio and proportion and dimensional analysis can be used as well.
- Heparin dosages are individualized according to the weight of the client in kilograms and adjusted based on the APTT.
- Protocols for IV heparin vary from institution to institution; always know and follow the institution's policy.
- Monitoring a client's APTT while he or she is receiving heparin is a **must.**

 **Critical Thinking Questions**

**Scenario:** A client has an order for heparin 3,500 units in 500 mL D5W to infuse at a rate of 40 mL/hr. The nurse prepares the IV using the heparin labeled 100 units per mL and adds 35 mL of heparin to the IV.

a. What error occurred in the preparation of the IV solution and why? _____

_____

b. What preventive measures should the nurse have taken? _____

Answers on p. 669

## ✓ CHAPTER REVIEW

For questions 1-12, calculate the dosage of heparin you will administer, and shade the dosage on the syringe provided. For questions 13 through 47, calculate the units as indicated by the problem. Use labels where provided to calculate dosages.

1. Order: Heparin 3,500 units subcut daily.

   Available:

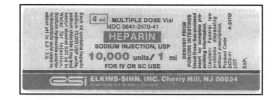

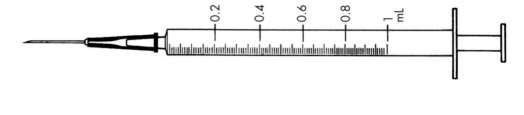

2. Order: Heparin 16,000 units subcut stat.

  Available:

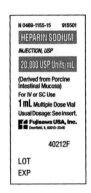

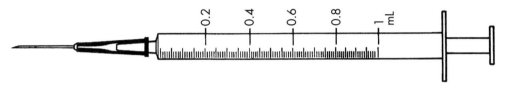

3. Order: Heparin 2,000 units subcut daily.

  Available: Heparin labeled 2,500 units per mL.

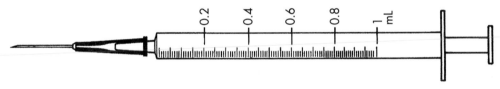

4. Order: Heparin 2,000 units subcut daily.

  Available:

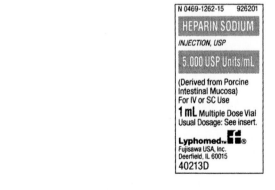

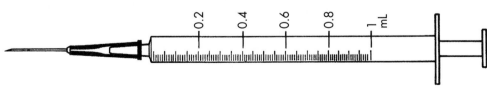

5. Order: Heparin 500 units subcut q4h.

Available:

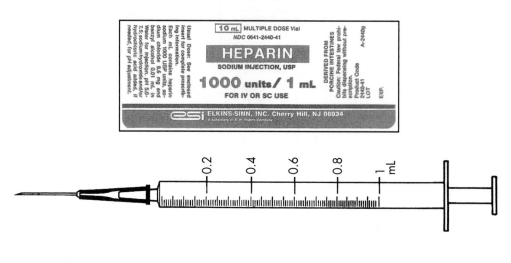

_____

6. Order: Heparin flush 10 units every shift to flush a heparin lock.

Available:

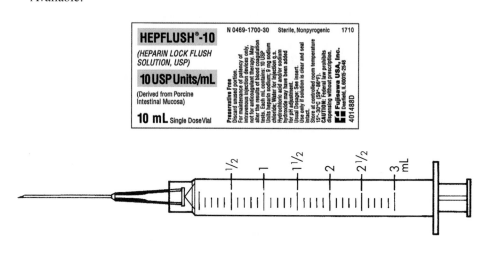

_____

7. Order: Heparin 50,000 units IV in D5W 500 mL.

Available: 10,000 units per mL.

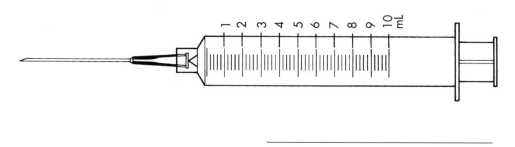

_____

8. Order: Heparin 15,000 units subcut daily.

   Available:

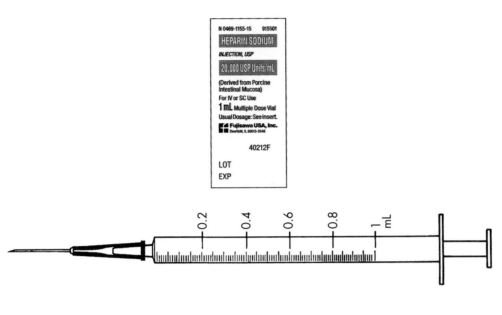

9. Order: 3,000 units of heparin to a liter of IV solution.

   Available: 2,500 units per mL.

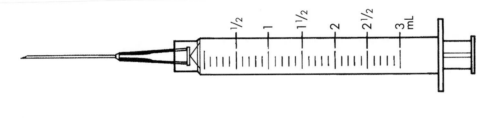

10. Order: Heparin 17,000 units subcut daily.

    Available: Heparin labeled 20,000 units per mL.

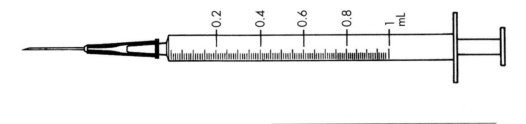

11.  Order: Heparin bolus of 8,500 units IV stat.

Available:

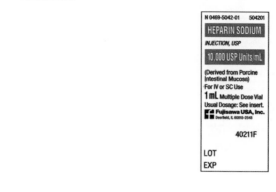

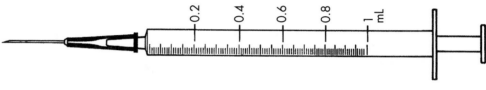

12.  Order: Heparin 2,500 units subcut q12h.

Available: Heparin labeled 10,000 units per mL.

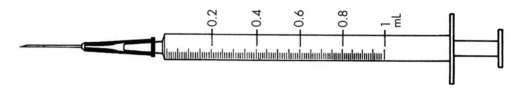

13.  Order: Heparin 2,000 units/hr IV. Available: 25,000 units of heparin in 1,000 mL of 0.9% NS.

What rate in mL/hr will deliver
2,000 units/hr?                    _____

14.  Order: Heparin 1,500 units/hr IV. Available: 25,000 units of heparin in 500 mL D5W.

What rate in mL/hr will deliver
1,500 units/hr?                    _____

15.  Order: Heparin 1,800 units/hr IV. Available: 25,000 units heparin in 250 mL D5W.

What rate in mL per hr will deliver
1,800 units/hr?                    _____

16.  Order: 40,000 units heparin in 1 L 0.9% NaCl to infuse at 25 mL/hr.

Calculate the hourly heparin dosage
(units/hr).                        _____

17. Order: Heparin 25,000 units in 250 mL D5W to infuse at 11 mL/hr.

    Calculate the hourly heparin dosage
    (units/hr).                                    _____

18. Order: Heparin 40,000 units in 500 mL D5W to infuse at 30 mL/hr.

    Calculate the hourly heparin dosage
    (units/hr).                                    _____

19. Order: Heparin 20,000 units in 500 mL D5W to infuse at 12 mL/hr.

    Calculate the hourly heparin dosage
    (units/hr).                                    _____

20. Order: Heparin 25,000 units in 500 mL D5W to infuse at 15 mL/hr.

    Calculate the hourly heparin dosage
    (units/hr).                                    _____

21. Order: 1 L of 0.9% NS with 40,000 units heparin over 24 hr. Calculate the following:

    a.  mL/hr                                      _____

    b.  units/hr                                   _____

22. Order: 1 L of D5W with 15,000 units heparin over 10 hr. Calculate the following:

    a.  mL/hr                                      _____

    b.  units/hr                                   _____

23. Order: 1 L D5W with 35,000 units of heparin at 20 mL/hr.

    Calculate the hourly heparin dosage
    (units/hr).                                    _____

24. Order: 500 mL of 0.9% NS with 10,000 units of heparin at 120 mL/hr.

    Calculate the hourly heparin dosage
    (units/hr).

                                                   _____

25. 500 mL of D5W with 25,000 units of heparin at 25 mL/hr.

    Calculate the hourly heparin dosage
    (units/hr).                                    _____

26. Order: 500 mL of D5W with 20,000 units of heparin at 40 mL/hr.

    Calculate the hourly heparin dosage
    (units/hr).                                    _____

27. Order: Infuse 1,400 units/hr of heparin IV. Available: Heparin 40,000 units in 1,000 mL of D5W.

    Calculate the rate in mL/hr.     _____

28. Order: Heparin 40,000 units IV in 1 L 0.9% NS at 1,000 units/hr.

    Calculate the rate in mL/hr.     _____

29. Order: Administer 2,000 units heparin IV every hour. Solution available is 25,000 units of heparin in 1 L 0.9% NS.

    Calculate the rate in mL/hr.     _____

Calculate the hourly dosage of heparin (units/hr).

30. A client is receiving an IV of 1,000 mL of D5W with 50,000 units of heparin infusing at 60 mL/hr.

    _____

31. A client is receiving an IV of 500 mL 0.45% NS with 25,000 units of heparin infusing at 20 mL/hr.

    _____

32. A client is receiving 500 mL of D5W with 20,000 units of heparin infusing at 20 mL/hr.

    _____

33. A client is receiving an IV of 25,000 units of heparin in 1 L of D5W infusing at 56 mL/hr.

    _____

34. A client is receiving an IV of 1,000 mL D5W with 20,000 units of heparin infusing at 45 mL/hr.

    _____

35. Order: 30,000 units of heparin in 500 mL of D5W to infuse at 25 mL/hr.     _____

36. Order: 20,000 units of heparin in 1 L of D5W to infuse at 40 mL/hr.     _____

37. Order: 40,000 units of heparin in 500 mL 0.45% NS to infuse at 25 mL/hr.     _____

38. Order: 35,000 units of heparin in 1 L of D5W to infuse at 20 mL/hr.     _____

39. Order: 25,000 units of heparin in 1 L of
    D5W to infuse at 30 mL/hr.                    _____

40. Order: 40,000 units of heparin in 1 L of
    D5W to infuse at 30 mL/hr.                    _____

41. Order: 20,000 units of heparin in 1 L of
    D5W to infuse at 80 mL/hr.                    _____

42. Order: 50,000 units of heparin in 1 L of
    D5W to infuse at 10 mL/hr.                    _____

43. Order: 20,000 units of heparin in 500 mL
    0.45% NS to infuse at 30 mL/hr.               _____

44. Order: 30,000 units of heparin in 1 L of
    D5W at 25 mL/hr.                              _____

45. A central venous line requires flushing with heparin. Which of the two labels shown
    is appropriate for a heparin flush?

_____

For problems 46-50, round the weight to the nearest tenth.

46. Order: Heparin drip at 18 units/kg.

    Available: 25,000 units of heparin in
    1,000 mL of D5W. The client weighs
    80 kg. At what rate will you set the
    infusion pump?                                _____

47. A client weighs 200 lb.

    Order: Administer a bolus of heparin
    sodium IV at 80 units/kg. How many
    units will you administer?                    _____

48. A client weighs 210 lb. Heparin IV infusion: heparin sodium 25,000 units in 1,000 mL of 0.9% NS. Order is to give a bolus with heparin sodium 80 units/kg, then initiate drip at 18 units/kg/hr.

    Calculate the following:

    a. Heparin bolus dosage                    _____

    b. Infusion rate for the IV (initial)       _____

    c. At what rate will you set the
       infusion pump?                           _____

49. A client weighs 110 lb. The hospital
    protocol is 18 units/kg/hr. How many
    units per hour will the client receive?     _____

50. A client weighs 154 lb. Heparin IV infusion: heparin sodium 20,000 units in 1,000 mL D5W. The hospital protocol is to give a bolus to the client with 80 units/kg and start drip at 14 units/kg/hr.

    Calculate the following:

    a. Heparin bolus dosage                    _____

    b. Infusion rate for the IV drip            _____ units/hr

    c. Infusion rate in mL/hr                   _____

Answers on pp. 669-673

**For additional practice problems, refer to the Advanced Calculations section of Drug Calculations Companion, Version 4, on Evolve.**

# CHAPTER 24

# Critical Care Calculations

## Objectives

*After reviewing this chapter, you should be able to:*
1. Calculate dosages in mcg/min, mcg/hr, and mg/min
2. Calculate dosages in mg/kg/hr, mg/kg/min, and mcg/kg/min

The content in this chapter may not be required as part of the nursing curriculum. It is included as a reference for nurses working in specialty areas.

This chapter will provide basic information on medicated IV drips and titration. Critically ill clients receive medications that are potent and require close monitoring. Because of the potency of the medications and their tendency to induce changes in blood pressure and heart rate, accurate calculation of dosages is essential. Medications in the critical care area can be ordered by milliliters per hour (mL/hr), drops per minute (gtt/min) (using a microdrop set), micrograms per kilogram per minute (mcg/kg/min), or milligrams per hour (mg/hr). Infusion pumps and volume control devices are usually used to administer these medications. Examples of medicated IV drips that require titration are Aramine, nitroprusside, Levophed, and epinephrine.

**Titrated medications** are added to a specific volume of fluid and then adjusted to infuse at the rate at which the desired effect is obtained. **The drugs that are titrated are potent antiarrhythmic, vasopressor, and vasodilator medications; they must be monitored very carefully by the nurse.** Because of the potency of medications used, minute changes in the infusion can cause an effect on the client. Infusion pumps are used for titration; when one is not available, a microdrip set calibrated at 60 gtt/mL must be used.

An example of an order that involves titration of medication is "Titrate sodium nitroprusside (Nipride) to maintain the client's systolic blood pressure below 140 mm Hg." The nurse may start, for example, at 3 mcg/kg/min and gradually increase the rate until the systolic blood pressure is maintained below 140 mm Hg. Each time there is a change in rate, the dosage of medication the client receives is changed; therefore it is essential that the dosage be recalculated each time the nurse changes the rate. Dosages are adjusted until the desired effect is achieved.

## Tips for Clinical Practice

Electronic infusion devices are routinely used to administer medications that are potent and require close monitoring. If an electronic infusion device, such as a volumetric pump or syringe pump, is not available, a microdrip set calibrated at 60 gtt/mL can be used.

## CALCULATING RATE IN mL/hr

Calculating the rate in mL/hr from a drug dosage ordered for IV administration is one of the most common calculations the nurse encounters. Let's look at some examples illustrating this before getting into other calculations that may be done.

**Example 1:**   A solution of Trandate (labetalol) 100 mg in100 mL D5W is to infuse at a rate of 25 mg/hr. Calculate the rate in mL/hr.

Calculate the rate in mL/hr using the solution strength available.

 ### Solution Using Ratio and Proportion

$$100 \text{ mg} : 100 \text{ mL} = 25 \text{ mg} : x \text{ mL}$$

$$100x = 100 \times 25$$

$$\frac{100x}{100} = \frac{2{,}500}{100}$$

$$x = 25 \text{ mL/hr}$$

*or*

 ### Solution Using Formula Method

$$\frac{25 \text{ mg}}{100 \text{ mg}} \times 100 \text{ mL} = x \text{ mL/hr}$$

$$x = 25 \text{ mL/hr}$$

To infuse 25 mg/hr, set the IV rate at 25 mL/hr.

 ### Solution Using Dimensional Analysis

- As shown in previous chapters involving medications in solution, the dimensional analysis equation is set up by first isolating what is being calculated. In this example it is mL/hr; therefore mL/hr is placed to the left of the equation.
- The starting fraction will be the information in the problem containing mL. (mL is placed in the numerator.)
- Set up each fraction after the starting fraction to match the previous denominator.
- Cancel the units, reduce if possible, and perform the mathematical operations.

Equation will be as follows:

$$\frac{x \text{ mL}}{\text{hr}} = \frac{100 \text{ mL}}{\underset{4}{\cancel{100} \text{ mg}}} \times \frac{\overset{1}{\cancel{25}} \text{ mg}}{1 \text{ hr}}$$

$$x = \frac{100}{4}$$

$$x = 25 \text{ mL/hr}$$

**Example 2:**   A solution of Isuprel 2 mg in 250 mL D5W is to infuse at a rate of 5 mcg/min.

**Step 1:**   Calculate the dose per hour.

$$60 \text{ min} = 1 \text{ hr}$$

$$5 \text{ mcg/min} \times 60 \text{ min/hr} = 300 \text{ mcg/hr}$$

Step 2:  Convert 300 mcg to mg to match the available strength.

$$1,000 \text{ mcg} = 1 \text{ mg}$$

$$300 \text{ mcg} = 0.3 \text{ mg}$$

Step 3:  Calculate the rate in mL/hr.

$$2 \text{ mg} : 250 \text{ mL} = 0.3 \text{ mg} : x \text{ mL}$$

$$2x = 250 \times 0.3$$

$$\frac{2x}{2} = \frac{75}{2}$$

$$x = 37.5 = 38 \text{ mL/hr}$$

To infuse 5 mcg/min, set the IV rate at 38 mL/hr.

**NOTE**

Conversions may be made from solution strength to dosage ordered, or the opposite.

## Solution Using Dimensional Analysis

*Note:* In this equation you will need two additional conversion factors, 60 min = 1 hr and 1,000 mcg = 1 mg.

$$\frac{x \text{ mL}}{\text{hr}} = \frac{\overset{125}{\cancel{250} \text{ mL}}}{\underset{1}{\cancel{2} \text{ mg}}} \times \frac{1 \cancel{mg}}{\underset{200}{\cancel{1,000} \text{ mcg}}} \times \frac{\overset{1}{\cancel{5} \text{ mcg}}}{1 \cancel{min}} \times \frac{60 \cancel{min}}{1 \text{ hr}}$$

$$x = \frac{125 \times 60}{200}$$

$$x = \frac{7,500}{200}$$

$$x = 37.5 = 38 \text{ mL/hr}$$

## Remember

Ratio and proportion can be set up by using several formats.

Now that you have seen examples of calculating the rate in mL/hr, let's look at some other calculations.

## CALCULATING CRITICAL CARE DOSAGES PER HOUR OR PER MINUTE

Example:  Infuse dopamine 400 mg in 500 mL D5W at 30 mL/hr. Calculate the dosage in mcg/min and mcg/hr.

## Solution Using Ratio and Proportion

Step 1:  $$400 \text{ mg} : 500 \text{ mL} = x \text{ mg} : 30 \text{ mL}$$

$$\text{(known)} \qquad \text{(unknown)}$$

$$500x = 400 \times 30$$

$$500x = 12,000$$

$$x = \frac{12,000}{500}$$

$$x = 24 \text{ mg/hr}$$

**Step 2:**    The next step is to convert 24 mg to mcg, because the question asked for mcg/min and mcg/hr. Change mg to mcg by using the equivalent 1,000 mcg = 1 mg. To change mg to mcg, multiply by 1,000 or, because it is a metric measure, move the decimal point three places to the right.

$$24 \text{ mg/hr} = 24{,}000 \text{ mcg/hr}$$

**Step 3:**    Now that you have the mcg/hr, the next step is to change mcg/hr to mcg/min. This is done by dividing the number of mcg/hr by 60 (60 minutes = 1 hour).

$$24{,}000 \text{ mcg/hr} \div 60 \text{ min/hr} = 400 \text{ mcg/min}$$

*(Note:* This is in mcg/min; however, these meds are usually delivered in mL/hr by pump and you would need to take calculation further. You will see problems later in this chapter changing mcg/min to mL/hr.)

 ### Solution Using Dimensional Analysis

$$\frac{x \text{ mg}}{\text{hr}} = \frac{\overset{4}{\cancel{400}} \text{ mg}}{\underset{5}{\cancel{500}} \text{ mL}} \times \frac{30 \text{ mL}}{1 \text{ hr}}$$

$$x = \frac{120}{5}$$

$$x = 24 \text{ mg/hr}$$

To determine mg/min, 24 mg ÷ 60 min/hr = 0.4 mg = 400 mcg/min

**CAUTION**

Accurate math is essential because these medications are extremely potent.

## DRUGS ORDERED IN MILLIGRAMS PER MINUTE

Drugs such as lidocaine and Pronestyl are ordered in mg/min.

**Example:**    A client is receiving Pronestyl 60 mL/hr. The solution available is Pronestyl 2 g in 500 mL D5W. Calculate the mg/hr and the mg/min the client will receive.

**Step 1:**    A conversion is necessary; g must be converted to mg. This is what you are being asked for (mg/min, mg/hr).

$$\text{Equivalent: 1 g} = 1{,}000 \text{ mg}$$

Therefore 2 g = 2,000 mg (1,000 × 2), or move decimal three places to right.

**Step 2:**    Now determine the mg/hr by setting up a proportion.

$$2{,}000 \text{ mg} : 500 \text{ mL} = x \text{ mg} : 60 \text{ mL}$$

$$500x = 2{,}000 \times 60$$

$$\frac{500x}{500} = \frac{120{,}000}{500}$$

$$x = 240 \text{ mg/hr}$$

**Step 3:**   Convert mg/hr to mg/min.

$$240 \text{ mg/hr} \div 60 \text{ min/hr} = 4 \text{ mg/min}$$

 ## Solution Using Dimensional Analysis

(*Note:* The starting factor here is the conversion factor to match the desired numerator, and mg/min is desired; the solution strength is in grams.)

$$\frac{x \text{ mg}}{\text{hr}} = \frac{1,\cancel{000}^{2} \text{ mg}}{1 \cancel{g}} \times \frac{2 \cancel{g}}{\cancel{500}_{1} \text{ mL}} \times \frac{60 \cancel{\text{ mL}}}{1 \text{ hr}}$$

$$x = \frac{240}{1}$$

$$x = 240 \text{ mg/hr}$$

To determine mg/min, 240 mg/h̶r̶ ÷ 60 min/h̶r̶ = 4 mg/min.

## CALCULATING DOSAGES BASED ON mcg/kg/min

Drugs are also ordered for clients based on dosage per kilogram per minute. These drugs include Nipride, dopamine, and dobutamine. In these problems, the weight will be rounded to the nearest tenth for calculation.

**Example:**   Order: Dopamine 2 mcg/kg/min. The solution available is 400 mg in 250 mL D5W. The client weighs 150 lb.

**Step 1:**   Convert the client's weight in pounds to kilograms.

$$2.2 \text{ lb} = 1 \text{ kg}$$

To convert the client's weight, divide 150 lb by 2.2.

$$150 \text{ lb} \div 2.2 = 68.18 \text{ kg} = 68.2 \text{ kg}$$

Note that the conversion could also be done using ratio and proportion or dimensional analysis.

**Step 2:**   Now that you have the client's weight in kilograms, determine the dosage per minute.

$$68.2 \text{ k̶g̶} \times 2 \text{ mcg/k̶g̶/min} = 136.4 \text{ mcg/min}$$

Converting mcg/min to mL/hr then would be easy using this example (conversion factor 1,000 mcg = 1 mg).

1. Convert mcg/min to mcg/hr.

$$136.4 \text{ mcg/m̶i̶n̶} \times 60 \text{ m̶i̶n̶} = 8,184 \text{ mcg/hr}$$

2. Convert mcg/hr to mg/hr.

$$8,184 \div 1,000 = 8.18 = 8.2 \text{ mg/hr}$$

3. Determine IV flow rate.

### → Solution Using Ratio and Proportion

$$400 \text{ mg} : 250 \text{ mL} = 8.2 \text{ mg} : x \text{ mL}$$

$$400x = 250 \times 8.2$$

$$\frac{400x}{400} = \frac{2{,}050}{400}$$

$$x = 5.1 = 5 \text{ mL/hr}$$

### → Solution Using Dimensional Analysis

$$\frac{x \text{ mL}}{\text{hr}} = \frac{\overset{5}{\cancel{250}} \text{ mL}}{\underset{8}{\cancel{400}} \text{ mg}} \times \frac{1 \cancel{\text{ mg}}}{1{,}000 \cancel{\text{ mcg}}} \times \frac{136.4 \cancel{\text{ mcg}}}{1 \cancel{\text{ min}}} \times \frac{60 \cancel{\text{ min}}}{1 \text{ hr}}$$

$$x = \frac{40{,}92\cancel{0}}{8{,}00\cancel{0}}$$

$$x = 5.1 = 5 \text{ mL/hr}$$

## TITRATION OF INFUSIONS

As already mentioned, critical care medications are ordered within parameters to obtain a desirable response in a client. When a solution is titrated, **the lowest dosage of the medication is set first** and increased or decreased as necessary. **The higher dosage should not be exceeded without a new order.**

**Example:**    Nipride has been ordered to titrate at 3 to 6 mcg/kg/min to maintain a client's systolic blood pressure below 140 mm Hg. The solution contains 50 mg Nipride in 250 mL D5W. The client weighs 56 kg. Determine the flow rate setting for a volumetric pump.

1. Convert to **like units.**
   Equivalent: 1,000 mcg = 1 mg
   Therefore 50 mg = 50,000 mcg

2. Calculate the concentration of solution in mcg/mL.

$$50{,}000 \text{ mcg} : 250 \text{ mL} = x \text{ mcg} : 1 \text{ mL}$$

$$\frac{250x}{250} = \frac{50{,}000}{250}$$

$$x = 200 \text{ mcg/mL}$$

   The concentration of solution is 200 mcg/mL.

3. Calculate the dosage range using the upper and lower dosages.

$$(\text{Lower dosage}) \; 3 \text{ mcg/}\cancel{\text{kg}} \times 56 \cancel{\text{ kg}} = 168 \text{ mcg/min}$$

$$(\text{Upper dosage}) \; 6 \text{ mcg/}\cancel{\text{kg}} \times 56 \cancel{\text{ kg}} = 336 \text{ mcg/min}$$

4. Convert dosage range to mL/min.

$$(\text{Lower dosage}) \ 200 \text{ mcg} : 1 \text{ mL} = 168 \text{ mcg} : x \text{ mL}$$

$$\frac{200x}{200} = \frac{168}{200}$$

$$x = 0.84 \text{ mL/min}$$

$$(\text{Upper dosage}) \ 200 \text{ mcg} : 1 \text{ mL} = 336 \text{ mcg} : x \text{ mL}$$

$$\frac{200x}{200} = \frac{336}{200}$$

$$x = 1.68 \text{ mL/min}$$

5. Convert mL/min to mL/hr.

$$(\text{Lower dosage}) \ 0.84 \text{ mL} \times 60 \text{ min} = 50.4 = 50 \text{ mL/hr (gtt/min)}$$

$$(\text{Upper dosage}) \ 1.68 \text{ mL} \times 60 \text{ min} = 100.8 = 101 \text{ mL/hr (gtt/min)}$$

A dosage range of 3 to 6 mcg/kg/min is equal to a flow rate of 50 to 101 mL/hr (gtt/min).
The client's condition has stabilized, and the flow rate is now maintained at 60 mL/hr.
What dosage will be infusing per minute?

$$200 \text{ mcg} : 1 \text{ mL} = x \text{ mcg} : 60 \text{ mL}$$

$$x = 12{,}000 \text{ mcg/hr}$$

$$12{,}000 \text{ mcg} \div 60 \text{ min} = 200 \text{ mcg/min}$$

 ## Solution Using Dimensional Analysis

1. Calculate the dosage range first.

$$(\text{Lower dosage}) \ 3 \text{ mcg/kg/min} \times 56 \text{ kg} = 168 \text{ mcg/min}$$

$$(\text{Upper dosage}) \ 6 \text{ mcg/kg/min} \times 56 \text{ kg} = 336 \text{ mcg/min}$$

2. Calculate the IV rate in mL/hr for the lower dosage.

$$\frac{x \text{ mL}}{\text{hr}} = \frac{\overset{5}{\cancel{250}} \text{ mL}}{\underset{1}{\cancel{50}} \text{ mg}} \times \frac{1 \text{ mg}}{1{,}000 \text{ mcg}} \times \frac{168 \text{ mcg}}{1 \text{ min}} \times \frac{60 \text{ min}}{1 \text{ hr}}$$

$$x = 50.4 = 50 \text{ mL/hr (gtt/min)}$$

3. Calculate the IV rate in mL/hr for the upper dosage.

$$\frac{x \text{ mL}}{\text{hr}} = \frac{\overset{5}{\cancel{250}} \text{ mL}}{\underset{1}{\cancel{50}} \text{ mg}} \times \frac{1 \text{ mg}}{1{,}000 \text{ mcg}} \times \frac{336 \text{ mcg}}{1 \text{ min}} \times \frac{60 \text{ min}}{1 \text{ hr}}$$

$$x = 100.8 = 101 \text{ mL/hr (gtt/min)}$$

A dosage range of 3 to 6 mcg/kg/min is equal to a flow rate of 50 to 101 mL/hr (gtt/min).
The client's condition has stabilized, and the IV flow rate is now maintained at
60 mL/hr. What dosage will be infusing per minute?

$$\frac{x \text{ mcg}}{\text{min}} = \frac{\overset{4}{\cancel{1{,}000}} \text{ mcg}}{1 \text{ mg}} \times \frac{50 \text{ mg}}{\underset{1}{\cancel{250}} \text{ mL}} \times \frac{60 \text{ mL}}{1 \text{ hr}} \times \frac{1 \text{ hr}}{60 \text{ min}}$$

$$x = 200 \text{ mcg/min}$$

**Practice Problems**

1. A client weighing 50 kg is to receive a Dobutrex solution of 250 mg in 500 mL D5W ordered to titrate between 2.5 and 5 mcg/kg/min.

   a. Determine the flow rate setting for
      a volumetric pump.                    _____

   b. If the IV flow rate is being maintained
      at 25 mL/hr after several titrations,
      what is the dosage infusing per minute? _____

2. Order: Epinephrine at 30 mL/hr. The solution available is 2 mg of epinephrine in 250 mL D5W. Calculate the following:

   a. mg/hr                                 _____

   b. mcg/hr                                _____

   c. mcg/min                               _____

3. Aminophylline 0.25 g is added to 500 mL D5W to infuse at 20 mL/hr. Calculate the following:

   mg/hr                                    _____

4. Order: Pitocin at 15 microgtt/min. The solution contains 10 units of Pitocin in 1,000 mL D5W.

   Calculate the number of units per hour
   the client is receiving.                 _____

5. Order: 3 mcg/kg/min of Nipride.

   Available: 50 mg of Nipride in 250 mL D5W. Client's weight is 60 kg.

   Calculate the flow rate in mL/hr that
   will deliver this dosage.                _____

6. A nitroglycerin drip is infusing at 3 mL/hr. The solution available is 50 mg of nitro-glycerin in 250 mL D5W. Calculate the following:

   a. mcg/hr                                _____

   b. mcg/min                               _____

Answers on pp. 673-674

## ■ Points to Remember

- The safest way to administer medications is by an infusion device.
- When calculating dosages to be administered without any type of electronic infusion pump, always use microdrop tubing (60 gtt = 1 mL). This is preferred because the drops are smaller, so more accurate titration is possible.
- Calculate dosages accurately. Double-checking math calculations helps ensure a proper dosage.
- Obtain an accurate weight of your client.
- Before determining the rate in mL/hr or gtt/min, calculate the dosage.
- Use a calculator whenever possible.
- Use an infusion pump for titration of IV medications in mL/hr.

## ? Critical Thinking Questions

**Scenario:** Isuprel is ordered for a client at the rate of 3 mcg/min with a solution containing Isuprel 1 mg in 250 mL D5W. The nurse performed the following calculation to determine the rate by pump in mL/hr.

- Calculated the dosage per hour:

$$3 \text{ mcg/min} \times 60 \text{ min} = 180 \text{ mcg/hr}$$

- Converted 180 mcg to milligrams to match the units in the solution strength:

$$180 \text{ mcg} = 0.018 \text{ mg}$$

- Calculated the rate in mL/hr:

$$1 \text{ mg} : 250 \text{ mL} = 0.018 \text{ mg} : x \text{ mL}$$

$$x = 250 \times 0.018$$

$$x = 4.5 = 5 \text{ mL/hr}$$

a. What error did the nurse make in her calculation to determine the rate in mL/hr?

_____

b. What could be the potential outcome of the error? _____

c. What should the rate be in mL/hr? _____

d. What preventive measures could have been taken by the nurse? _____

Answer on p. 674

## ✓ CHAPTER REVIEW

Calculate the dosages as indicated. Use the labels where provided.

1. Client is receiving Isuprel at 30 mL/hr. The solution available is 2 mg of Isuprel in 250 mL D5W. Calculate the following:

   a. mg/hr          _____

   b. mcg/hr         _____

   c. mcg/min        _____

2. Client is receiving epinephrine at 40 mL/hr. The solution available is 4 mg of epinephrine in 500 mL D5W. Calculate the following:

   a. mg/hr _____

   b. mcg/hr _____

   c. mcg/min _____

3. Infuse dopamine 800 mg in 500 mL D5W at 30 mL/hr. Calculate the dosage in mcg/hr and mcg/min.

   a. mcg/hr _____

   b. mcg/min _____

   c. Calculate the number of milliliters you will add to the IV for this dosage. _____

   Available:

   NDC 0641-**0112-25** 25 x 5 mL Single Use Vials **DOPAMINE** HCl INJECTION, USP **200 mg/5 mL** (40 mg/mL) FOR IV INFUSION ONLY — POTENT DRUG: MUST DILUTE BEFORE USING. Each mL contains dopamine hydrochloride 40 mg (equivalent to 32.3 mg dopamine base) and sodium bisulfite 10 mg in Water for Injection. pH 2.5-5.0. Sealed under nitrogen. USUAL DOSE: See package insert. Do not use if solution is discolored. Store at 15°-30°C (59°-86°F). Caution: Federal law prohibits dispensing without prescription. B-50112c — ELKINS-SINN, INC. Cherry Hill, NJ 08003-4099 A subsidiary of A. H. Robins Company

4. Infuse Nipride at 30 mL/hr. The solution available is 50 mg sodium nitroprusside in D5W 250 mL.

   Available:

   Protect from light. Exp. Lot — 2 mL Single-dose Fliptop Vial NDC 0074-3024-01 **NITROPRESS®** Sodium Nitroprusside Injection 50 mg / 2 mL Vial **(25 mg/mL)** FOR I.V. INFUSION ONLY. Monitor blood pressure before and during administration. 06-7378-2/R2-12/93 ABBOTT LABS, NORTH CHICAGO, IL 60064, USA

   Calculate the following:

   a. mcg/hr _____

   b. mcg/min _____

   c. Number of milliliters you will add to the IV for this dosage _____

5. Order: 100 mg Aramine in 250 mL D5W to infuse at 25 mL/hr. Calculate the following:

   a. mcg/hr                    _____

   b. mcg/min                   _____

6. Order: Lidocaine 2 g in 250 mL D5W to infuse at 60 mL/hr. Calculate the following:

   a. mg/hr                     _____

   b. mg/min                    _____

7. Order: Aminophylline 0.25 g to be added to 250 mL of D5W. The order is to infuse over 6 hr.

   Available:

   a. Calculate the dosage in mg/hr the
      client will receive.        _____

   b. Calculate the number of milliliters you
      will add to the IV for this dosage.  _____

8. A client is receiving Pronestyl at 30 mL/hr. The solution available is 2 g Pronestyl in 250 mL D5W. Calculate the following:

   a. mg/hr                     _____

   b. mg/min                    _____

9. Order: Pitocin (oxytocin) drip at 45 microgtt/min. The solution available is 20 units of Pitocin in 1,000 mL of D5W. Calculate the following:

   a. units/min                 _____

   b. units/hr                  _____

10. Order: 30 units Pitocin (oxytocin) in 1,000 mL D5W at 40 mL/hr.

    How many units of Pitocin is the
    client receiving per hour?     _____ units/hr

11. 30 units of Pitocin is added to 500 mL D5RL for an induction. The client is receiving 45 mL/hr.

    How many units of Pitocin is the client
    receiving per hour?            _____ units/hr

12. A client is receiving bretylium at 30 microgtt/min. The solution available is 2 g bretylium in 500 mL D5W. Calculate the following:

    a. mg/hr                                    _____

    b. mg/min                                   _____

13. A client is receiving bretylium at 45 microgtt/min. The solution available is 2 g bretylium in 500 mL D5W. Calculate the following:

    a. mg/hr                                    _____

    b. mg/min                                   _____

14. A client is receiving nitroglycerin 50 mg in 250 mL D5W. The order is to infuse 500 mcg/min.

    What flow rate in mL/hr would be
    needed to deliver this amount?              _____

15. Dopamine has been ordered to maintain a client's blood pressure; 400 mg dopamine has been placed in 500 mL D5W to infuse at 35 mL/hr.

    How many milligrams are being
    administered per hour?                      _____

16. A client is receiving Isuprel 2 mg in 250 mL D5W. The order is to infuse at 20 mL/hr. Calculate the following:

    a. mg/hr                                    _____

    b. mcg/hr                                   _____

    c. mcg/min                                  _____

17. Order: 1 g of aminophylline in 1,000 mL D5W to infuse over 10 hr.

    Calculate the dosage in mg/hr the
    client will receive.                        _____

18. A client is receiving lidocaine 2 g in 250 mL D5W. The solution is infusing at 22 mL/hr. Calculate the following:

    a. mg/hr                                    _____

    b. mg/min                                   _____

19. Order: Epinephrine 4 mg in 250 mL D5W at 8 mL/hr. Calculate the following:

    mcg/hr                                      _____

20. Order: Esmolol 2.5 g in 250 mL 0.9% NS at 30 mL/hr. Calculate the following:

    a. mg/hr                                    _____

    b. mg/min                                   _____

21. Order: Dobutamine 500 mg in 500 mL D5W to infuse at 30 mL/hr.

    Available:

    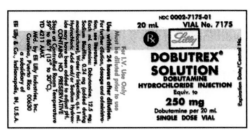

    Calculate the following:

    a. mcg/hr            _____

    b. mcg/min           _____

22. Order: 2 g/hr of 50% magnesium sulfate. The solution available is 25 g of 50% magnesium sulfate in 300 mL D5W.

    What flow rate in mL/hr would be needed
    to administer the required dose?      _____

23. Order: Dopamine 400 mg in 500 mL 0.9% NS to infuse at 200 mcg/min. A volumetric pump is being used.

    Calculate the rate in mL/hr.        _____

24. Order: Magnesium sulfate 3 g/hr.

    Available: 25 g of 50% magnesium sulfate in 300 mL D5W.

    What rate in mL/hr would be needed
    to administer the required dose?      _____

25. A client with chest pain has an order for nitroglycerin 50 mg in 250 mL D5W at 10 mcg/min.

    Calculate the IV rate in gtt/min using
    a microdrop administration set.      _____

26. Order: Nipride 50 mg in 250 mL D5W to infuse at 2 mcg/kg/min. Client's weight is 120 lb.

    Calculate the dosage per minute.     _____

27. Order: Dobutrex 250 mg in 500 mL of D5W at 3 mcg/kg/min. The client weighs 80 kg.

    What dosage in mcg/min should the
    client receive?                       _____

28. Order: Infuse 500 mL D5W with 800 mg theophylline at 0.7 mg/kg/hr. The client weighs 73.5 kg.

    How many milligrams should this client
    receive per hour?               _____

29. Order: Infuse 1 g of aminophylline in 1,000 mL of D5W at 0.7 mg/kg/hr. The client weighs 110 lb.

    a.  Calculate the dosage in mg/hr.    _____

    b.  Calculate the dosage in mg/min.    _____

    c.  Reference states no more than
        20 mg/min. Is the order safe?    _____

30. Norepinephrine (Levophed) 2 to 6 mcg/min has been ordered to maintain a client's systolic blood pressure at 100 mm Hg. The solution concentration is 2 mg in 500 mL D5W.

    Determine the flow rate setting for a
    volumetric pump.    _____

31. Esmolol is to titrate between 50 and 75 mcg/kg/min. The client weighs 60 kg. The solution strength is 5,000 mg of esmolol in 500 mL D5W.

    a.  Determine the flow rate for a
        volumetric pump.    _____

    b.  The titration rate is at 24 mL/hr.
        What is the dosage infusing per
        minute?    _____

32. Order: Dobutamine 500 mg in 250 mL D5W to infuse at 10 mcg/kg/min. The client weighs 65 kg.

    Calculate the flow rate in mL/hr (gtt/min).    _____

33. Aminophylline 0.25 g is added to 250 mL D5W. The order is to infuse over 6 hr.

    Calculate the dosage in mg/hr the
    client will receive.    _____

34. A client is receiving lidocaine 1 g in 500 mL D5W at a rate of 20 mL/hr. Calculate the following:

    a.  mg/hr    _____

    b.  mg/min    _____

35. A client is receiving Septra 300 mg in 500 mL D5W (based on trimethoprim) at a rate of 15 gtt/min (15 microgtt/min). The tubing is microdrop (60 gtt/mL). Calculate the following:

    a.  mg/min    _____

    b.  mg/hr    _____

36. Esmolol 1.5 g in 250 mL D5W has been ordered at a rate of 100 mcg/kg/min for a client weighing 102.4 kg. Determine the following:

    a.  dosage in mcg/min    _____

    b.  rate in mL/hr    _____

37. Order: Dopamine 400 mg in 500 mL D5W to infuse at 20 mL/hr. Determine the following:

    a. mg/min _____

    b. mcg/min _____

38. A client has an order for inamrinone (previously called amrinone) 250 mg in 250 mL 0.9% NS at 3 mcg/kg/min. Client's weight is 59.1 kg. Determine the flow rate in mL/hr.

    _____

39. Inocor 250 mg in 250 mL of 0.9% NS to infuse at a rate of 5 mcg/kg/min is ordered for a client weighing 165 lb. Calculate the following:

    a. mcg/min _____

    b. mcg/hr _____

    c. mL/hr _____

40. Cardizem 125 mg in 100 mL D5W to infuse at 20 mg/hr.

    Available:

    Determine the following:

    a. How many milliliters will you add to the IV? _____

    b. Determine the rate in mL/hr. (Consider the medication in the volume.) _____

41. 2 g Pronestyl in 500 mL D5W to infuse at 2 mg/min.

    Determine the rate in mL/hr. _____

Answers on pp. 675-680

**For additional practice problems, refer to the Advanced Calculations section of Drug Calculations Companion, Version 4, on Evolve.**

# CHAPTER 25

## Pediatric and Adult Dosage Calculation Based on Weight

### Objectives

*After reviewing this chapter, you should be able to:*
1. Convert body weight from pounds to kilograms
2. Convert body weight from kilograms to pounds
3. Calculate dosages based on milligram per kilogram
4. Determine whether a dosage is safe
5. Determine body surface area (BSA) using the West nomogram
6. Calculate BSA using formulas according to units of measure
7. Determine dosages using the BSA
8. Calculate the flow rates for pediatric IV therapy
9. Calculate the safe dosage ranges and determine if within normal range for medications administered IV in pediatrics

Accuracy in dosage calculation becomes even more of a priority when calculating and administering medications to infants and children. Snyderman (2008) reported that 1 in 15 hospitalized children is harmed as a result of medication errors. Snyderman stressed that the margin of error is much less in children. Cohen (2007) indicated that the rate of actual, potential, and preventable adverse drug events is three times higher for pediatric patients. Causes of errors included the following:

- Confusion between adult and pediatric formulations
- Errors with oral liquid dosage forms that are available in multiple pediatric concentrations
- Incorrect preparation of medications that require dilution
- Look-alike packaging and look-alike and sound-alike names
- Improper education of parents regarding preparation of medications and administration
- Calculation errors
- Inaccurate measuring devices (use of household teaspoons) as opposed to devices such as oral dosing devices for small volume doses

These are just a few reasons for dosing errors that occur in the administration of medications to children.

Before administering medications to children, the nurse should know whether the ordered dosage is safe. Accuracy is always important when calculating medication dosages. For infants and children, exact and careful mathematics takes on even greater importance. A miscalculation, even small discrepancies, may be dangerous because of the size, weight, and body surface area (BSA) of the infant or child. In addition, infants and children's physiological capabilities (e.g., a lessened ability to metabolize medications, immaturity of systems, differences in rate of medication absorption and excretion) differ when compared with adults. Therefore it is vital that the nurse adhere to pediatric protocols and guidelines and always use a reference to verify medication orders to ensure that medication dosages are correct.

Body weight is an important factor used to calculate medication dosages for children and adults, although it is used more frequently with children. Medications may be prescribed based on body weight or body surface area.

The safe administration of medications to infants and children requires knowledge of the methods used in calculating doses. In addition, the nurse must apply the principles of the "six rights" of medication administration (right medication, right dosage, right time, right route, right client, right documentation) when working with pediatric clients and families. Nurses are also responsible for educating the families regarding medication administration.

Dosages for infants and children are based on their unique physiological differences. The prescriber must consider weight, height, body surface area, age, and condition of the child when ordering dosages. As mentioned previously, the two methods used for calculating safe pediatric dosages are body weight (e.g., mg/kg) and body surface area (BSA, measured in square meters [$m^2$]). The body weight method is more common in pediatrics and is emphasized in this chapter, as well as the BSA. As stated previously, body weight and BSA methods are also used for adults, especially in critical care, and the calculation methods used are the same.

Although the prescriber is responsible for ordering the medication and dosage, **the nurse remains responsible for verifying the dosage to be sure it is correct and safe for administration.** If a dosage is higher than normal, it may be unsafe, and a dosage lower than normal may not have the desired therapeutic effect, which is also unsafe. It is imperative that nurses check medication labels or package inserts for specific dosage details. Other references that may be checked for more in-depth and additional information on a medication are drug formularies at the institution, the *Physician's Desk Reference (PDR),* drug reference books, and the hospital pharmacist. Various pocket-size pediatric medication handbooks are also available; one that is widely used is *The Harriet Lane Handbook* (Johns Hopkins Hospital, 2005).

The two methods currently being used to calculate pediatric dosages are as follows:
1. According to weight (milligrams per kilogram)
2. According to BSA

**CAUTION**

> To ensure safe practice, when in doubt consult a reliable source. Always double-check dosages by comparing the prescribed dose with the recommended safe dose.

Determining medication dosages according to body weight and BSA is a means of individualizing medication therapy. Although body weight and BSA are common determinants for medication dosing in children, they are also used to calculate adult medication dosages, particularly for those who are very old or grossly underweight. Body weight and BSA are also used in the administration of cancer medications. Of the two methods, the BSA method has been determined to be the most accurate for calculating dosages.

## PRINCIPLES RELATING TO BASIC CALCULATIONS

Before calculating medications for the child or infant, some guidelines are helpful to know.
1. Calculation of pediatric dosages, as with adult dosages, involves the use of ratio and proportion, the formula method, or dimensional analysis to determine the amount of medication to administer.
2. Pediatric dosages are much smaller than those for an adult. Micrograms are used a great deal. The tuberculin syringe (1-mL capacity) is used to administer very small dosages.

3. Intramuscular (IM) dosages are usually not more than 1 mL for small children and older infants; however, this can vary with the size of the child. The recommended IM dosage for small infants is not more than 0.5 mL.
4. The recommended subcutaneous (subcut) dosage for children is not more than 0.5 mL.
5. Dosages that are less than 1 mL may be measured in tenths of a milliliter, or with a tuberculin syringe in hundredths of a milliliter.
6. Medications in pediatrics generally are not rounded off to the nearest tenth but may be administered with a tuberculin syringe (measured in hundredths) to ensure accuracy.
7. All answers must be labeled.

## CALCULATION OF DOSAGES BASED ON BODY WEIGHT

Let's begin our discussion with calculation of dosages according to milligrams per kilogram (mg/kg) of body weight. Before calculating dosages according to mg/kg of body weight, it is essential that you be able to convert a child's weight. Most recommendations for medication dosages are based on weight in kilograms.

Therefore the most common conversion you will encounter involves the conversion from pounds to kilograms. To do this, remember the conversion 1 kg = 2.2 lb. Conversions of weights are presented in Chapter 9. The methods of converting presented in Chapter 8 can also be used. It is, however, essential that we review this again.

> **RULE**
>
> To convert from pounds to kilograms, use the conversion 1 kg = 2.2 lb. To convert from pounds to kilograms divide by 2.2, and express your answer to the nearest tenth.

## CONVERTING POUNDS TO KILOGRAMS

Let's do some sample problems with the conversion of weights.

**Example 1:**   Convert a child's weight of 30 lb to kilograms.

$$2.2 \text{ lb} = 1 \text{ kg} \qquad \text{(conversion factor)}$$

**NOTE**

A ratio and proportion can be written in different formats (with colons or as a fraction).

### ▶ Solution Using Ratio and Proportion

$$2.2 \text{ lb} : 1 \text{ kg} = 30 \text{ lb} : x \text{ kg}$$

$$\frac{\cancel{2.2}x}{\cancel{2.2}} = \frac{30}{2.2}$$

$$x = \frac{30}{2.2}$$

$$x = 13.63 \text{ kg} = 13.6 \text{ kg} \qquad \begin{array}{l}\text{(rounded to the}\\\text{nearest tenth)}\end{array}$$

Child's weight = 13.6 kg

### ▶ Solution Using Dimensional Analysis

$$x \text{ kg} = \frac{1 \text{ kg}}{2.2 \cancel{\text{ lb}}} \times \frac{30 \cancel{\text{ lb}}}{1}$$

$$x = \frac{30}{2.2}$$

$$x = 13.63 \text{ kg} = 13.6 \text{ kg} \qquad \begin{array}{l}\text{(rounded to the}\\\text{nearest tenth)}\end{array}$$

Child's weight = 13.6 kg

**Example 2:**   Convert an infant's weight of 14 lb and 6 oz to kilograms.

1.  Convert ounces to parts of a pound.

$$16 \text{ oz} = 1 \text{ lb} \qquad \text{(conversion factor)}$$

### Solution Using Ratio and Proportion

$$16 \text{ oz} : 1 \text{ lb} = 6 \text{ oz} : x \text{ lb}$$

$$\frac{\cancel{16}x}{\cancel{16}} = \frac{6}{16}$$

$$x = \frac{6}{16}$$

$$x = 0.37 \text{ lb} = 0.4 \text{ lb} \qquad \text{(rounded to the nearest tenth)}$$

Add the computed pounds to the total pounds as follows:

$$14 \text{ lb} + 0.4 \text{ lb} = 14.4 \text{ lb}$$

$$\text{Infant's weight} = 14.4 \text{ lb}$$

**CAUTION**

Use caution when converting ounces to a fraction of a pound. Also, after converting the ounces to pounds, remember to add the answer to the remaining whole pounds to get the total pounds. Then convert the total pounds to kilograms.

2.  Convert total pounds to kilograms.

### Solution Using Ratio and Proportion

$$2.2 \text{ lb} = 1 \text{ kg} \qquad \text{(conversion factor)}$$

$$2.2 \text{ lb} : 1 \text{ kg} = 14.4 \text{ lb} : x \text{ kg}$$

$$\frac{\cancel{2.2}x}{\cancel{2.2}} = \frac{14.4}{2.2}$$

$$x = \frac{14.4}{2.2}$$

$$x = 6.54 \text{ kg} = 6.5 \text{ kg} \qquad \text{(rounded to the nearest tenth)}$$

$$\text{Infant's weight} = 6.5 \text{ kg}$$

### Solution Using Dimensional Analysis

$$x \text{ lb} = \frac{1 \text{ lb}}{16 \cancel{\text{oz}}} \times \frac{6 \cancel{\text{oz}}}{1}$$

$$x = \frac{6}{16}$$

$$x = 0.37 \text{ lb} = 0.4 \text{ lb} \qquad \text{(rounded to the nearest tenth)}$$

$$\text{Infant's weight} = 14.4 \text{ lb}$$

$$x \text{ kg} = \frac{1 \text{ kg}}{2.2 \text{ lb}} \times \frac{14.4 \text{ lb}}{1}$$

$$x = \frac{14.4}{2.2}$$

$$x = 6.54 \text{ kg} = 6.5 \text{ kg} \qquad \text{(rounded to the nearest tenth)}$$

Infant's weight = 6.5 kg

**Example 3:**   Convert the weight of a 157-lb adult to kilograms.

$$2.2 \text{ lb} = 1 \text{ kg} \qquad \text{(conversion factor)}$$

## Solution Using Ratio and Proportion

$$2.2 \text{ lb} : 1 \text{ kg} = 157 \text{ lb} : x \text{ kg}$$

$$\frac{2.2x}{2.2} = \frac{157}{2.2}$$

$$x = \frac{157}{2.2}$$

$$x = 71.36 \text{ kg} = 71.4 \text{ kg} \qquad \text{(rounded to the nearest tenth)}$$

Adult's weight = 71.4 kg

## Solution Using Dimensional Analysis

$$x \text{ kg} = \frac{1 \text{ kg}}{2.2 \text{ lb}} \times \frac{157 \text{ lb}}{1}$$

$$x = \frac{157}{2.2}$$

$$x = 71.36 \text{ kg} = 71.4 \text{ kg} \qquad \text{(rounded to the nearest tenth)}$$

Adult's weight = 71.4 kg

 **Practice Problems**

Convert the following weights in pounds to kilograms. Round to the nearest tenth.

1. 15 lb = _____ kg    5. 71 lb = _____ kg

2. 68 lb = _____ kg    6. 133 lb = _____ kg

3. 31 lb = _____ kg    7. 8 lb 4 oz = _____ kg

4. 52 lb = _____ kg    8. 5 lb 12 oz = _____ kg

Answers on p. 680

## CONVERTING KILOGRAMS TO POUNDS

> To convert from kilograms to pounds, use the conversion 1 kg = 2.2 lb. To convert from kilograms to pounds multiply by 2.2, and express your weight to the nearest tenth.

**Example 1:**    Convert a child's weight of 24.3 kg to pounds.

$$2.2 \text{ lb} = 1 \text{ kg} \qquad \text{(conversion factor)}$$

 Solution Using Ratio and Proportion

$$2.2 \text{ lb} : 1 \text{ kg} = x \text{ lb} : 24.3 \text{ kg}$$

$$x = 24.3 \times 2.2$$

$$x = 53.46 \text{ lb} = 53.5 \text{ lb} \qquad \text{(rounded to the nearest tenth)}$$

Child's weight = 53.5 lb

 Solution Using Dimensional Analysis

$$x \text{ lb} = \frac{2.2 \text{ lb}}{1 \text{ k\!\!\!/g}} \times \frac{24.3 \text{ k\!\!\!/g}}{1}$$

$$x = 2.2 \times 24.3$$

$$x = 53.46 \text{ lb} = 53.5 \text{ lb}$$

Child's weight = 53.5 lb

**NOTE**

Any of the methods presented in Chapters 8 and 9 can be used to convert pounds to kilograms and kilograms to pounds, except decimal movement.

**Example 2:**    Convert an adult's weight of 70.2 kg to pounds.

$$2.2 \text{ lb} = 1 \text{ kg} \qquad \text{(conversion factor)}$$

 Solution Using Ratio and Proportion

$$2.2 \text{ lb} : 1 \text{ kg} = x \text{ lb} : 70.2 \text{ kg}$$

$$x = 70.2 \times 2.2$$

$$x = 154.44 \text{ lb} = 154.4 \text{ lb} \qquad \text{(rounded to the nearest tenth)}$$

Adult's weight = 154.4 lb

Solution Using Dimensional Analysis

$$x \text{ lb} = \frac{2.2 \text{ lb}}{1 \text{ k\!\!\!/g}} \times \frac{70.2 \text{ k\!\!\!/g}}{1}$$

$$x = 2.2 \times 70.2$$

$$x = 154.44 \text{ lb} = 154.4 \text{ lb} \qquad \text{(rounded to the nearest tenth)}$$

Adult's weight = 154.4 lb

**Example 3:**   Convert the weight of a 10.2-kg child to pounds.

$$2.2 \text{ lb} = 1 \text{ kg}$$   (conversion factor)

 Solution Using Ratio and Proportion

$$2.2 \text{ lb} : 1 \text{ kg} = x \text{ lb} : 10.2 \text{ kg}$$

$$x = 10.2 \times 2.2$$

$$x = 22.44 \text{ lb} = 22.4 \text{ lb}$$   (rounded to the nearest tenth)

Child's weight = 22.4 lb

 Solution Using Dimensional Analysis

$$x \text{ lb} = \frac{2.2 \text{ lb}}{1 \text{ kg}} \times \frac{10.2 \text{ kg}}{1}$$

$$x = 2.2 \times 10.2$$

$$x = 22.44 \text{ lb} = 22.4 \text{ lb}$$   (rounded to the nearest tenth)

Child's weight = 22.4 lb

 **Practice Problems**

Convert the following weights in kilograms to pounds. Round to the nearest tenth.

9.  21.3 kg = _____ lb    13.  34 kg = _____ lb

10.  17.7 kg = _____ lb    14.  71.4 kg = _____ lb

11.  22 kg = _____ lb    15.  73 kg = _____ lb

12.  15 kg = _____ lb    16.  98.3 kg = _____ lb

Answers on p. 680

**NOTE**

Decimal movement may be preferred for converting grams to kilograms; however, the other methods presented in Chapter 8 can also be used.

Infants 0 to 4 weeks old (neonates) and premature infants may also be given medications. The scale will convert the child's weight in grams, or the weight may be reported in grams, rather than kilograms. Therefore it may be necessary for the nurse to convert the weight in grams to kilograms because most dosage recommendations are commonly given in kilograms.

As discussed in the chapter on metric conversions, 1 kg = 1,000 g; therefore to convert grams to kilograms, divide by 1,000 or move the decimal point three places to the left.

**RULE**

To convert grams to kilograms use the conversion 1 kg = 1,000 g. Divide the number of grams by 1,000, or move the decimal point three places to the left. Round kilograms to the nearest tenth.

## CONVERTING GRAMS TO KILOGRAMS

**Example 1:** Convert an infant's weight of 3,000 g to kilograms.

$$1 \text{ kg} = 1,000 \text{ g} \qquad \text{(conversion factor)}$$

 Solution Using Ratio and Proportion

$$1 \text{ kg} : 1,000 \text{ g} = x \text{ kg} : 3,000 \text{ g}$$

$$\frac{1,000x}{1,000} = \frac{3,000}{1,000}$$

$$x = 3 \text{ kg}$$

Infant's weight = 3 kg

Decimal movement: 3,000 = 3 kg

 Solution Using Dimensional Analysis

$$x \text{ kg} = \frac{1 \text{ kg}}{1,000 \text{ g}} \times \frac{3,000 \text{ g}}{1}$$

$$x = \frac{3,000}{1,000}$$

$$x = 3 \text{ kg}$$

Infant's weight = 3 kg

**Example 2:** Convert an infant's weight of 1,350 g to kilograms.

$$1 \text{ kg} = 1,000 \text{ g} \qquad \text{(conversion factor)}$$

 Solution Using Ratio and Proportion

$$1 \text{ kg} : 1,000 \text{ g} = x \text{ kg} : 1,350 \text{ g}$$

$$\frac{1,000x}{1,000} = \frac{1,350}{1,000}$$

$$x = 1.35 \text{ kg} = 1.4 \text{ kg} \qquad \text{(rounded to the nearest tenth)}$$

Infant's weight = 1.4 kg

Decimal movement: 1,350 = 1.35 kg = 1.4 kg    (rounded to the nearest tenth)

 Solution Using Dimensional Analysis

$$x \text{ kg} = \frac{1 \text{ kg}}{1,000 \text{ g}} \times \frac{1,350 \text{ g}}{1}$$

$$x = \frac{1,350}{1,000}$$

$$x = 1.35 \text{ kg} = 1.4 \text{ kg} \qquad \text{(rounded to the nearest tenth)}$$

Infant's weight = 1.4 kg

**Example 3:** Convert an infant's weight of 2,700 g to kilograms.

$$1 \text{ kg} = 1,000 \text{ g} \qquad \text{(conversion factor)}$$

 Solution Using Ratio and Proportion

$$1 \text{ kg}:1,000 \text{ g} = x \text{ kg}:2,700 \text{ g}$$

$$\frac{1,000x}{1,000} = \frac{2,700}{1,000}$$

Infant's weight = 2.7 kg

Decimal movement: 2,700 = 2.7 kg

 Solution Using Dimensional Analysis

$$x \text{ kg} = \frac{1 \text{ kg}}{1,000 \text{ g}} \times \frac{2,700 \text{ g}}{1}$$

$$x = \frac{2,700}{1,000}$$

$$x = 2.7 \text{ kg}$$

Infant's weight = 2.7 kg

 **Practice Problems**

Convert the following weights in grams to kilograms. Round to the nearest tenth.

17. 4,000 g = _____ kg    20. 3,600 g = _____ kg

18. 1,450 g = _____ kg    21. 1,875 g = _____ kg

19. 2,900 g = _____ kg

Answers on p. 680

Answers on p. 680

**NOTE**

Students should know that, although a pound is an apothecary measure, a decimal may be seen when weight is expressed (e.g., 65.8 lb).

**Remember**

1. 2.2 lb = 1 kg, 1 kg = 1,000 g
2. To convert from pounds to kilograms, divide the number of pounds by 2.2. Carry the division out to the hundredths place, and round off the answer to the nearest tenth. Calculations based on body weight can be rounded off to the nearest tenth.
3. To convert from kilograms to pounds, multiply number of kilograms by 2.2 and round the answer to the nearest tenth.
4. If the child's weight is in ounces and pounds, convert the ounces to the nearest tenth of a pound, and then add the answer to pounds to get the total pounds. Convert the total pounds to kilograms, and round to the nearest tenth.
5. To convert from grams to kilograms, divide by 1,000 or move the decimal point three places to the left. Round kilograms to the nearest tenth as indicated.

Medication dosages can be calculated based on mg/kg/day, mg/lb/day, or sometimes mcg/kg. References often state the safe amount of the drug in mg/kg/day (24-hour period). Once you have determined the child's weight in kilograms, you are ready to calculate the medication dosage. Calculating the dosage involves three steps:

1. Calculation of the total daily dosage
2. Division of the daily dosage by the number of dosages to be administered
3. Use ratio and proportion, the formula method, or dimensional analysis to calculate the number of tablets or capsules or the volume to give to administer the ordered dosage

Before beginning to calculate dosages based on weight, let's review some concepts that may be used.

***Recommended dosage (also referred to as the safe dosage)***—This information comes from a reputable resource, such as a medication reference written especially for pediatrics or another medication reference book. Recommended dosages may also be indicated on the medication label under children's dosages. This is usually expressed in mg/kg for a 24-hour period to be given in one or more divided doses. This may also be seen as mcg/kg and occasionally mg/lb. Recommended dosage can also be stated as a range and referred to as safe dosage range (SDR). This is the upper and lower limits of the dosage as stated by an approved medication reference.

***Total daily dosage***—Dosage obtained by multiplying the child's weight after it is converted to kilograms with the use of a reputable medication reference: multiply child's weight in kilograms by dosage expressed as mg/kg.

***Divided dosage***—This represents the dosage a child should receive each time the medication is administered. The recommended daily dosage may be stated as mg/kg/day to be divided into a certain number of individual dosages, such as "three divided dosages," q6h, and so on. "Three divided dosages" means that the total daily dosage is divided equally and administered three times per day. q6h means the total daily dosage is divided equally and administered every 6 hours, for a total of four dosages per day (24 hr ÷ 6 hr). This is the dosage for 24 hours divided by the frequency, or the number of times, the child will receive the medication.

***Deciding if the dosage is safe***—This is done by comparing the ordered dosage with the recommended dosage. In other words, this is decided by comparing and evaluating the 24-hour ordered amount with the recommended dosage.

> **NOTE**
>
> The dosage per kilogram may be mg/kg, mcg/kg, and so on.

**Example 1:** Refer to Dilantin label.

Available:

Order: Dilantin 30 mg p.o. q8h. Child weighs 18 kg. Is the dosage safe?

Recommended dosage: 5 mg/kg/day in two or three equally divided dosages. (Notice the information written sideways on the left of the Dilantin label.)

Now that we have the dosage information and the child's weight, we can calculate the safe total daily dosage for the child. *Note:* The child's weight is in kilograms (18 kg), and the average dose range is 5 mg/kg/day. No conversion of weight is required.

**Step 1:**    Start by calculating the safe total daily dosage for this child. Multiply the recommended dosage in milligrams by the child's weight in kilograms.

$$5 \text{ mg/kg/day} \times 18 \text{ kg} = 90 \text{ mg/day}$$

The safe dosage for this child (total) is 90 mg/day.

The calculation of the safe daily dosage could also be done by setting up a ratio and proportion using the format of fractions or colons. Using this example, the setup as a ratio and proportion might be as follows:

Per day could be stated as daily or every 24 hours.

## ➡ Solution Using Ratio and Proportion

$$5 \text{ mg} : 1 \text{ kg} = x \text{ mg} : 18 \text{ kg}$$

$$x = 90 \text{ mg/day}$$

*or*

$$\frac{5 \text{ mg}}{x \text{ mg}} = \frac{1 \text{ kg}}{18 \text{ kg}}$$

$$x = 90 \text{ mg/day}$$

Calculation of the safe daily dosage could also be done using dimensional analysis. To do this, use the information regarding the recommended dosage range as the starting fraction (in this case, 5 mg/kg).

## ➡ Solution Using Dimensional Analysis

$$\frac{x \text{ mg}}{\text{day}} = \frac{5 \text{ mg}}{1 \text{ kg/day}} \times \frac{18 \text{ kg}}{1}$$

$$x = 18 \times 5$$

$$x = 90 \text{ mg/day}$$

**Step 2:**    Now determine the amount of each dosage. The dosage is to be given in three equally divided dosages. Therefore:

$$\frac{90 \text{ mg}}{3} = 30 \text{ mg per dose}$$

After calculating the safe dosage for a child, you can assess whether what the prescriber ordered is a safe dosage.

**Step 3:**    Determine if the dosage is safe. The order is 30 mg q8h. Is this a safe dosage?

$$q8h = 24 \div 8 = 3 \text{ doses}$$

30 mg $\times$ 3 = 90 mg. Compare the ordered daily dosage with the safe daily dosage you calculated in Step 1. A daily dosage of 90 mg is safe.

When dosages are compared for safety, it may be easiest to calculate how many total milligrams or micrograms are ordered. This way usually involves multiplication rather than division. This requires only one calculation, as opposed to two, and may decrease the chance of errors because fewer errors are usually made with multiplication than with division.

For example, in Example 1, the ordered dosage is 30 mg every 8 hours. 30 mg × 3 doses = 90 mg. The daily dosage of 90 mg is safe.

**Step 4:**  Use ratio and proportion, the formula method, or dimensional analysis to determine the number of capsules to administer.

Dilantin is supplied in 30-mg capsules (refer to label). The ordered dose is 30 mg per dose.

 Solution Using Ratio and Proportion

$$30 \text{ mg} : 1 \text{ cap} = 30 \text{ mg} : x \text{ caps}$$

$$\frac{30x}{30} = \frac{30}{30} \qquad x = 1 \text{ cap}$$

 Solution Using Formula Method

$$\frac{30 \text{ mg}}{30 \text{ mg}} \times 1 \text{ cap} = x \text{ caps}$$

$$x = 1 \text{ cap}$$

 Solution Using Dimensional Analysis

$$x \text{ cap} = \frac{1 \text{ cap}}{30 \text{ mg}} \times \frac{30 \text{ mg}}{1}$$

$$x = \frac{30}{30}$$

$$x = 1 \text{ cap}$$

You would give 1 cap q8h to administer the ordered dosage.

**Example 2:**  Order: Gentamicin 50 mg IVPB q8h for a child weighing 40 lb. The recommended dosage for a child is 6 to 7.5 mg/kg/day divided q8h. Is the dosage ordered safe?

**Step 1:**  First, a weight conversion is necessary because you have the child's weight in pounds and the reference is in kilograms. Convert the child's weight in pounds to kilograms and round to the nearest tenth.

 Solution Using Ratio and Proportion

$$2.2 \text{ lb} : 1 \text{ kg} = 40 \text{ lb} : x \text{ kg}$$

$$\frac{\cancel{2.2}x}{\cancel{2.2}} = \frac{40}{2.2} \qquad x = \frac{40}{2.2}$$

$$x = 18.18 \text{ kg} = 18.2 \text{ kg} \quad \text{(rounded to the nearest tenth)}$$

$$x = 18.2 \text{ kg}$$

The rounded weight is 18.2 kg.

Solution Using Dimensional Analysis

$$x \text{ kg} = \frac{1 \text{ kg}}{2.2 \text{ lb}} \times \frac{40 \text{ lb}}{1}$$

$$x = \frac{40}{2.2}$$

$$x = 18.18 \text{ kg} = 18.2 \text{ kg}$$

$$x = 18.2 \text{ kg}$$       (rounded to the nearest tenth)

The rounded weight is 18.2 kg.

**Step 2:**    Now that you have converted the weight, you can calculate the safe dosage. You must calculate and obtain a range. (The recommended dosage is 6 to 7.5 mg/kg/day.)

Therefore calculate the lower and upper ranges:

$$6 \text{ mg/kg/day} \times 18.2 \text{ kg} = 109.2 \text{ mg/day}$$

$$7.5 \text{ mg/kg/day} \times 18.2 \text{ kg} = 136.5 \text{ mg/day}$$

The safe dosage range for the child weighing 18.2 kg is 109.2 to 136.5 mg/day.

 Solution Using Dimensional Analysis

$$\frac{x \text{ mg}}{\text{day}} = \frac{6 \text{ mg}}{1 \text{ kg/day}} \times \frac{18.2 \text{ kg}}{1}$$

$$x = 18.2 \times 6$$

$$x = 109.2 \text{ mg/day}$$

$$\frac{x \text{ mg}}{\text{day}} = \frac{7.5 \text{ mg}}{\text{kg/day}} \times \frac{18.2 \text{ kg}}{1}$$

$$x = 18.2 \times 7.5$$

$$x = 136.5 \text{ mg/day}$$

The safe dosage range for the child is 109.2 mg to 136.5 mg/day.

**Step 3:**    Now divide the total daily dosage by the number of times the medication will be given in a day.

$$\text{q8h} = 24 \div 8 = 3$$

$$109.2 \text{ mg} \div 3 = 36.4 \text{ mg per dose}$$

$$136.5 \text{ mg} \div 3 = 45.5 \text{ mg per dose}$$

The dosage range is 36.4 to 45.5 mg per dosage q8h. The ordered dosage of 50 mg q8h exceeds the dosage range of 109.2 to 136.5 mg total dosage for 24 hours.

$$50 \text{ mg q8h} = 50 \text{ mg} \times 3 = 150 \text{ mg}$$

Remember that factors such as the child's medical condition might warrant a larger dose. This could be done as previously explained by looking at the total ordered dosage; in this case, it was 50 mg q8h or 50 mg × 3 doses = 150 mg. 150 mg exceeds the dosage range of 109.2 to 136.5 mg/day. Call the prescriber to verify the dosage.

**Example 3:**  Order: Dicloxacillin sodium 50 mg p.o. q6h for a child weighing 36 lb. The recommended dosage for dicloxacillin sodium for oral suspension is 12.5 mg/kg/day for children weighing less than 40 kg (88 lb) in equally divided doses q6h. Is the dosage ordered safe? If the dosage is safe, calculate the number of milliliters needed to administer the dose.

**Step 1:**  First, convert the child's weight in pounds to the nearest tenth of a kilogram.

➡ Solution Using Ratio and Proportion

$$2.2 \text{ lb} : 1 \text{ kg} = 36 \text{ lb} : x \text{ kg}$$

$$\frac{\cancel{2.2}x}{\cancel{2.2}} = \frac{36}{2.2}$$

$$x = \frac{36}{2.2}$$

$$x = 16.36 \text{ kg} = 16.4 \text{ kg} \quad \text{(rounded to the nearest tenth)}$$

To the nearest tenth, the weight is 16.4 kg.

➡ Solution Using Dimensional Analysis

$$x \text{ kg} = \frac{1 \text{ kg}}{2.2 \cancel{\text{ lb}}} \times \frac{36 \cancel{\text{ lb}}}{1}$$

$$x = \frac{36}{2.2}$$

$$x = 16.36 \text{ kg} = 16.4 \text{ kg} \quad \text{(rounded to the nearest tenth)}$$

**Step 2:**  Now that you have converted the weight to kilograms, you can calculate the safe dosage for this child.

$$12.5 \text{ mg/}\cancel{\text{kg}}\text{/day} \times 16.4 \cancel{\text{kg}} = 205 \text{ mg/day}$$

The safe dosage for a child weighing 16.4 kg is 205 mg/day.

➡ Solution Using Dimensional Analysis

$$\frac{x \text{ mg}}{\text{day}} = \frac{12.5 \text{ mg}}{\cancel{\text{kg}}\text{/day}} \times \frac{16.4 \cancel{\text{kg}}}{1}$$

$$x = 12.5 \times 16.4$$

$$x = 205 \text{ mg/day}$$

The safe dose for a child weighing 16.4 kg is 205 mg/day.

If 50 mg is ordered q6h, is this a safe dosage?

$$24 \text{ h} \div 6 \text{ h} = 4 \text{ doses per day}$$

$$50 \text{ mg} \times 4 \text{ doses} = 200 \text{ mg per day}$$

The ordered dosage is not safe; it is below the recommended dosage. According to the total milligrams ordered, which was 50 mg q6h, 50 mg × 4 doses = 200 mg/day.

Although the dosage ordered is below the recommended dosage, it would not be considered safe. It is important to realize that even when small discrepancies exist between the safe dosage and what is ordered (e.g., in this problem, the safe dosage is 205 mg and the child is receiving 200 mg), the difference, although small, can be significant. The dosage may not be sufficient to achieve the therapeutic effect. The prescriber should be notified. The discrepancy may be due to factors such as age of the child, medical condition, or other factors.

**Step 3:**   Calculate the amount of medication needed to administer the ordered dosage.

Dicloxacillin sodium oral suspension is available in a dosage strength of 62.5 mg per 5 mL. *Note:* Because the dose ordered is not safe, we will not calculate the dose in this problem.

**Example 4:**   The recommended dosage for neonates receiving ceftazidime (Tazidime) is 30 mg/kg/q12h. What is the safe daily dosage for an infant weighing 2,600 g?

**Step 1:**   Change the infant's weight in grams to kilograms. Reference expressed as mg/kg.

$$1,000 \text{ g} = 1 \text{ kg} \qquad \text{(conversion factor)}$$

$$1,000 \text{ g} : 1 \text{ kg} = 2,600 \text{ g} : x \text{ kg}$$

$$\frac{1,000x}{1,000} = \frac{2,600}{1,000}$$

$$\text{Infant's weight} = 2.6 \text{ kg}$$

Decimal movement: $2,600 = 2.6 \text{ kg}$

 **Solution Using Dimensional Analysis**

$$x \text{ kg} = \frac{1 \text{ kg}}{1,000 \text{ g}} \times \frac{2,600 \text{ g}}{1}$$

$$x = \frac{2,600}{1,000}$$

$$x = 2.6 \text{ kg}$$

**Step 2:**   Calculate the safe q12h dosage for this infant.

$$30 \text{ mg/kg q12h} \times 2.6 \text{ kg} = 78 \text{ mg/dose q12h}$$

The safe dosage for this infant is 78 mg/dosage q12h.

**Solution Using Dimensional Analysis**

$$\frac{x \text{ mg}}{\text{q12h}} = \frac{30 \text{ mg}}{1 \text{ kg/q12h}} \times \frac{2.6 \text{ kg}}{1}$$

$$x = 30 \times 2.6$$

$$x = 78 \text{ mg/dosage q12h}$$

**CAUTION**

Remember that to avoid medication errors, it is imperative to calculate a safe dosage for a child and compare it with the dosage that has been ordered. Question dosages that are significantly low and unusually high before proceeding to administer them. Remember that the nurse is legally liable for any medication administered.

When information concerning a pediatric dosage is not present on the medication label, refer to the package insert, the *PDR,* or another appropriate reference text.

## ADULT DOSAGES BASED ON BODY WEIGHT

The information that has been provided regarding the calculation of dosages for children based on weight can also be applied to adults. Let's look at an example. Refer to the partial Ticar package insert.

---

**TICAR** ®

brand of
**sterile ticarcillin disodium**
**for Intramuscular or Intravenous Administration**

**DOSAGE AND ADMINISTRATION**
Clinical experience indicates that in serious urinary tract and systemic infections, intravenous therapy in the higher doses should be used. Intramuscular injections should not exceed 2 grams per injection.
**Adults:**

| | |
|---|---|
| Bacterial septicemia | 200 to 300 mg/kg/day by I.V. infusion in divided doses every 4 or 6 hours. |
| Respiratory tract infections | (The usual dose is 3 grams given every 4 hours [18 grams/day] or 4 grams given every 6 hours |
| Skin and soft-tissue infections | [16 grams/day] depending on weight and the severity of the infection.) |
| Intra-abdominal infections | |
| Infections of the female pelvis and genital tract | |
| Urinary tract infections | |
|     Complicated: | 150 to 200 mg/kg/day by I.V. infusion in divided doses every 4 or 6 hours. |
| | (Usual recommended dosage for average [70 kg] adults: 3 grams q.i.d.) |
|     Uncomplicated: | 1 gram I.M. or direct I.V. every 6 hours. |

---

**Example:** Order: Ticar 4 g IV q6h for a client with a respiratory tract infection. Client weighs 175 lb. Notice that the recommended dosage from the package insert for a respiratory tract infection is 200 to 300 mg/kg/day q4-6h. Is the dosage ordered safe?

**Step 1:** Convert the weight in pounds to kilograms.

$$2.2 \text{ lb} = 1 \text{ kg} \qquad \text{(conversion factor)}$$

$$175 \text{ lb} \div 2.2 = 79.54 \text{ kg} = 79.5 \text{ kg} \qquad \begin{array}{l}\text{(rounded to the}\\ \text{nearest tenth)}\end{array}$$

**Step 2:** Calculate the recommended dosage.

$$200 \text{ mg/kg/day} \times 79.5 \text{ kg} = 15{,}900 \text{ mg/day}$$

$$300 \text{ mg/kg/day} \times 79.5 \text{ kg} = 23{,}850 \text{ mg/day}$$

15,900 mg to 23,850 mg/day is the recommended dosage per day.

**Step 3:** Determine the number of milligrams allowed per dosage.

$$15{,}900 \text{ mg} \div 4 = 3{,}975 \text{ mg/dosage}$$

$$23{,}850 \div 4 = 5{,}962.5 \text{ mg/dose}$$

3,975 to 5,962.5 mg/dose is allowed.

> **NOTE**
>
> The same methods shown in each step in determining a child's dosage can be applied to dosages for adults.

**Step 4:** Determine if the dosage is safe.

$$4 \text{ g} = 4{,}000 \text{ mg } (4 \times 1{,}000) = 4{,}000 \text{ mg}$$

$$4{,}000 \text{ mg} \times 4 \text{ doses} = 16{,}000 \text{ mg/day}$$

The ordered dosage of Ticar 4 g q6h is within the range of 15,900 to 23,850 mg/day and is safe.

## Practice Problems

Round weights and dosages to the nearest tenth where indicated. Use labels where provided to answer the questions.

22. A child weighs 35 lb and has an order for Keflex 150 mg p.o. q6h.

    Available:

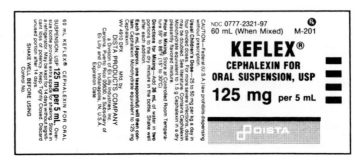

   a. What is the recommended dosage in mg/kg/day? _____

   b. What is the child's weight in kilograms to nearest tenth? _____

   c. What is the safe dosage range for this child? _____

   d. Is the dosage ordered safe? (Prove mathematically.) _____

   e. How many milliliters will you administer for each dosage? _____

23. Refer to the label. The *PDR* indicates 15 mg/kg/day q8h of kanamycin as a safe dosage. Kanamycin 200 mg IV q8h is ordered for a child weighing 35 kg.

    Available:

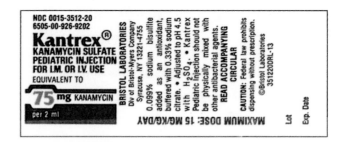

   a. What is the safe dosage for this child for 24 hours? _____

   b. What is the divided dosage? _____

   c. Is the dosage ordered safe? (Prove mathematically.) _____

24. The recommended dosage of clindamycin oral suspension is 8 to 25 mg/kg/day in four divided dosages. A child weighs 40 kg.

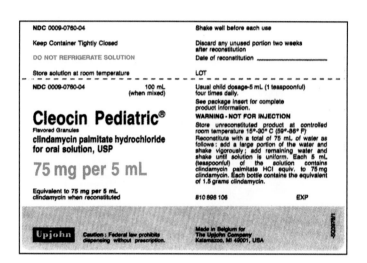

    a. What is the maximum dosage for this child in 24 hours? _____

    b. What is the divided dosage range? _____

25. Phenobarbital 10 mg p.o. q12h is ordered for a child weighing 9 lb. The recommended maintenance dosage is 3 to 5 mg/kg/day q12h.

    a. What is the child's weight in kilograms to the nearest tenth? _____

    b. What is the safe dosage range for this child? _____

    c. Is the dosage ordered safe? (Prove mathematically.) _____

    d. Phenobarbital elixir is available in a dosage strength of 20 mg per 5 mL. What will you administer for one dosage? Calculate the dosage if it is safe. _____

26. Morphine sulfate 7.5 mg subcut q4h p.r.n. is ordered for a child weighing 84 lb. The recommended maximum dose for a child is 0.1 to 0.2 mg/kg/dose.

Available:

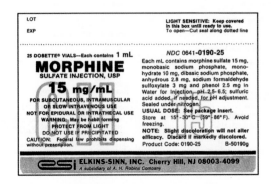

a. What is the child's weight in kilograms to the nearest tenth? _____

b. What is the safe dosage range for this child? _____

c. Is the dosage ordered safe? (Prove mathematically.) _____

d. How many milliliters will you administer for one dosage? _____

27. The recommended dosage of Dilantin is 4 to 8 mg/kg/day q12h. Dilantin 15 mg p.o. q12h is ordered for a child weighing 11 lb.

Available:

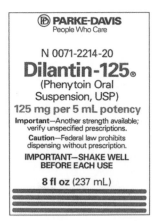

a. What is the child's weight in kilograms? _____

b. What is the safe dosage range for this child? _____

c. Is the dosage ordered safe? (Prove mathematically.) _____

d. How many milliliters will you administer for one dosage? _____

28. The recommended initial dosage of mercaptopurine is 2.5 mg/kg/day p.o. The child weighs 44 lb.

    a. What is the child's weight in kilograms? _____

    b. What is the initial safe daily dosage for this child? _____

29. For a child the recommended dosage of IV vancomycin is 40 mg/kg/day. Vancomycin 200 mg IV q6h is ordered for a child weighing 38 lb.

    **8:12**
    **VIALS**
    # VANCOCIN® HCl
    **STERILE VANCOMYCIN HYDROCHLORIDE, USP**
    **INTRAVENOUS**

    **PA 8289 AMP**

    **DOSAGE AND ADMINISTRATION**
    A concentration of no more than 10 mg/mL is recommended. An infusion of 10 mg/min or less is associated with fewer infusion-related events (*see* Adverse Reactions).
    *Patients With Normal Renal Function*
    *Adults*—The usual daily intravenous dose is 2 g divided either as 500 mg every 6 hours or 1 g every 12 hours. Each dose should be administered over a period of at least 60 minutes. Other patient factors, such as age or obesity, may call for modification of the usual daily intravenous dose.
    *Children*—The total daily intravenous dosage of Vancocin HCl, calculated on the basis of 40 mg/kg of body weight, can be divided and incorporated into the child's 24-hour fluid requirement. Each dose should be administered over a period of at least 60 minutes.
    *Infants and Neonates*—In neonates and young infants, the total daily intravenous dosage may be lower. In both neonates and infants, an initial dose of 15 mg/kg is suggested, followed by 10 mg/kg every 12 hours for neonates in the 1st week of life and every 8 hours thereafter up to the age of 1 month. Close monitoring of serum concentrations of vancomycin may be warranted in these patients.

    a. What is the child's weight in kilograms to the nearest tenth? _____

    b. What is the safe dosage for this child in 24 hours? _____

    c. What is the divided dosage? _____

    d. Is the dosage ordered safe? (Prove mathematically.) _____

30. A 16-lb child has an order for amoxicillin 125 mg p.o. q8h.

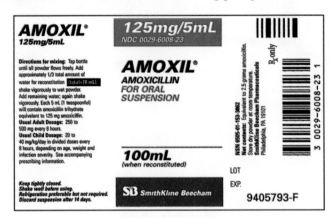

   a. What is the recommended dosage
      in mg/kg/day?    _____

   b. What is the child's weight in
      kilograms to the nearest tenth?    _____

   c. What is the safe range of dosage
      for this child in 24 hours?    _____

   d. Is the dosage ordered safe?    _____

31. A 44-lb child has an order for Ilosone oral suspension 250 mg p.o. q6h. The usual
dosage for children under 50 lb is 30 to 50 mg/kg/day in divided dosages q6h, and
for children over 20 lb, 250 mg q6h.

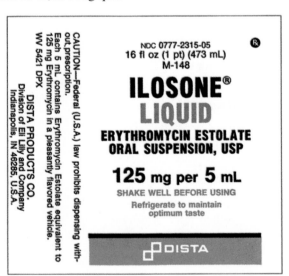

   a. What is the child's weight in
      kilograms?    _____

   b. What is the range of dosages
      safe for this child in 24 hours?    _____

   c. Is the dosage ordered safe?
      (Prove mathematically.)    _____

32. Refer to the Fungizone insert to calculate the dosage for an adult weighing 66.3 kg with good cardiorenal function. _____

1 vial NDC 0003-**0437-30**
NSN 6505-01-084-9453

**50 mg**
**FUNGIZONE**®
**INTRAVENOUS**
**Amphotericin B**
**for Injection USP**

**FOR INTRAVENOUS INFUSION**
**IN HOSPITALS ONLY**
Caution: Federal law prohibits
dispensing without prescription

Read all sides

☐**APOTHECON**®
A BRISTOL-MYERS SQUIBB COMPANY

Partial Insert for Fungizone (Amphotericin B)

**DOSAGE AND ADMINISTRATION**
**CAUTION: Under no circumstances should a total daily dose of 1.5 mg/kg be exceeded. Amphotericin B overdoses can result in cardio-respiratory arrest (see OVERDOSAGE).**
FUNGIZONE Intravenous should be administered by *slow* intravenous infusion. Intravenous infusion should be given over a period of approximately 2 to 6 hours (depending on the dose) observing the usual precautions for intravenous therapy (see PRECAUTIONS, General). The recommended concentration for intravenous infusion is 0.1 mg/mL (1 mg/10 mL).
Since patient tolerance varies greatly, the dosage of amphotericin B must be individualized and adjusted according to the patient's clinical status (e.g., site and severity of infection, etiologic agent, cardio-renal function, etc.).
A single intravenous **test dose** (1 mg in 20 mL of **5%** dextrose solution) administered over 20-30 minutes may be preferred. The patient's temperature, pulse, respiration, and blood pressure should be recorded every 30 minutes for 2 to 4 hours.
In patients with **good cardio-renal function** and a **well tolerated test dose**, therapy is usually initiated with a daily dose of 0.25 mg/kg of body weight. However, in those patients having **severe and rapidly progressive fungal infection**, therapy may be initiated with a daily dose of 0.3 mg/kg of body weight. In patients with **impaired cardio-renal function** or a **severe reaction to the test dose**, therapy should be initiated with smaller daily doses (i.e., 5 to 10 mg).

33. A 200-lb adult is to be treated with Ticar for a complicated urinary tract infection. The recommended dosage is 150 to 200 mg/kg/day IV in divided dosages every 4 or 6 hours.

    a. What is the adult's weight in kilograms to the nearest tenth? _____

    b. What is the daily dosage range in grams for this client? _____

34. A child weighs 12 lb, 6 oz. The recommended dosage of V-Cillin oral solution for a child is 15 to 50 mg/kg/day in four divided doses.

    a. What is the child's weight in kilograms to the nearest tenth? _____

    b. What is the safe daily dosage range for this child? _____

Answers on pp. 680-682

---

## ■ Points to Remember

- To convert pounds to kilograms divide by 2.2; express answer to nearest tenth.
- To convert kilograms to pounds multiply by 2.2; express answer to nearest tenth.
- To convert grams to kilograms divide by 1,000; round to the nearest tenth as indicated.
- To calculate dosages the weight must be converted to the reference.
- To calculate the dosage based on weight, do the following:
  1. Determine the weight in kilograms if needed.
  2. Multiply the weight in kilograms by the dosage stated.
  3. Divide the total daily dosage by the number of dosages needed to administer.
  4. Calculate the number of tablets or the volume to administer for each dosage by use of ratio and proportion, the formula method, or dimensional analysis.

- When the recommended dosage is given as a range, calculate based on the low and high values for each dosage.
- Question any discrepancies in dosages ordered and remember that factors such as age, weight, and medical conditions can cause the differences. Ask the prescriber to clarify the order when a discrepancy exists. Small discrepancies can be significant. Dosages that exceed the recommended dosage are not safe, and a dosage less than recommended is also unsafe because it may not achieve the intended therapeutic effect.
- Use appropriate resources to determine the safe range for a child's dosage. Compare the safe dosage with the dosage ordered to decide if the dosage is safe.

## CALCULATING PEDIATRIC DOSAGE USING BODY SURFACE AREA

A child's body surface area (BSA) is determined by comparing a child's weight and height with what is considered average or the norm. BSA is used to calculate dosages for infants and children and selected adult populations. Pediatric dosages are prescribed based on the child's BSA. The BSA is determined from the height and weight of a child and the use of the West nomogram (Figure 25-1).

This information is then applied to a formula for dosage calculation. Remember that all children are not the same size at the same age; therefore the West nomogram can be used to determine the BSA of a child. The West nomogram is not easy to use, although it is still employed in some institutions. The nomogram can be used to calculate the BSA for both children and adults for heights up to 240 cm (95 inches) and weights up to 80 kg (180 lb). The West nomogram is the most well-known BSA chart (see Figure 25-1). It is possible to determine the BSA from weight alone, if the child is of normal height and weight. BSA is expressed in meters squared ($m^2$).

## READING THE WEST NOMOGRAM CHART

Refer to Figure 25-1. It is important to note that the increments of measurement and the spaces on the BSA nomogram are not consistent. **Always read the numbers to determine what the calibrations are measuring.** For example, refer to the column for children of normal height and weight (second column from left); the calibrations between 15 and 20 lb are 1-lb increments. However, if you look at the bottom of the scale representing surface area in square meters, there are four calibrations between 0.10 and 0.15. Each line, therefore, is read as 0.11, 0.12, 0.13, etc. If the child is of a normal height and weight for his or her age, the BSA can be determined from weight alone. Notice the boxed column listing weight on the left and surface in square meters on the right; this is used when a child is of normal height for his or her weight. For example, a child weighing 70 lb has a BSA of 1.10 $m^2$. If you look on the nomogram for a child who weighs 10 lb and use the nomogram column of normal height for weight, you will see that a 10-lb child has a BSA of 0.27 $m^2$. Using the nomogram for a child weighing 70 lb and having a normal height for weight reveals that this child would have a BSA of 1.10 $m^2$.

**CAUTION**

The increments and the spaces on the BSA nomogram are not consistent. Be certain that you read the numbers and the calibration values between them correctly.

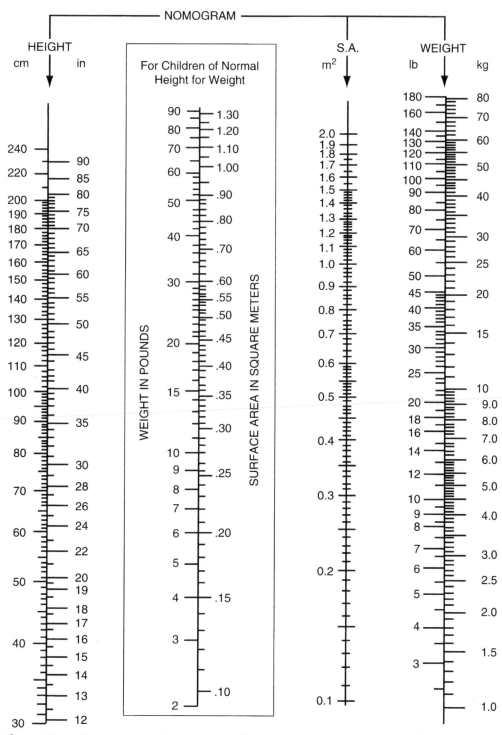

**Figure 25-1** West nomogram for estimation of body surface area. (Nomogram modified with data from Kliegman R, Behrman RE, Jenson HB, Stanton BF: *Nelson textbook of pediatrics,* ed. 18, Philadelphia, 2007, Saunders.)

**Practice Problems**

Refer to the nomogram and determine the BSA (expressed in square meters) for the following children of normal height and weight.

35.  For a child weighing 30 lb                    _____

36.  For a child weighing 42 lb                    _____

37.  For a child weighing 52 lb                    _____

38.  For a child weighing 44 lb                    _____

39.  For a child weighing 11 lb                    _____

40.  For a child weighing 20 lb                    _____

Answers on p. 682

In addition to being determined based on weight, the BSA can also be calculated by using both height and weight. If you refer to the chart, you will notice the columns for height and weight. This chart includes weight in both pounds and kilograms and height in both centimeters and inches.

For children who are not of normal height for their weight, the scales at the far left (height) and far right (weight) are used. Notice that both of these scales have two measurements: centimeters and inches for height and pounds and kilograms for weight. To find the BSA, place a ruler extending from the height column on the left to the weight column on the far right. The estimated BSA for the child is where the line intersects the SA (surface area) column. For example, by using the far right and left scales, you will find that a child who weighs 50 lb and is 36 inches tall has a BSA of 0.8 m$^2$.

 **Practice Problems**

Using the nomogram, calculate the following BSAs.

41.  A child who is 90 cm long and weighs 50 lb        _____

42.  A child who is 60 cm long and weighs 10 lb        _____

43.  A child who is 100 cm long and weighs 10 kg       _____

44.  A child who is 30 inches long and weighs 20 lb    _____

45.  A child who weighs 60 lb and is 39 inches tall    _____

46.  A baby who weighs 13 lb and is 19 inches long     _____

47.  A child who weighs 30 lb and is 32 inches tall    _____

48.  A child who weighs 13 kg and is 65 cm tall        _____

49.  A child who is 90 cm long and weighs 40 lb        _____

50.  A child who is 19 inches long and weighs 5 lb     _____

Answers on p. 682

# CALCULATING BODY SURFACE AREA USING A FORMULA

BSA is used in calculating dosages for children and adults, often to determine dosages for medications such as chemotherapeutic agents that are used in the treatment of cancer. As already shown, BSA can be calculated by using the tool called the West nomogram; however, it is a tool that requires practice to use and can result in an error if the ruler is just slightly off the line.

To calculate BSA the client's height and weight are used (adults and children). Instead of using the West nomogram one can calculate the BSA with two tools:

1. Calculator
2. Formula

Calculators are increasingly being used for determination of critical care dosages and in pediatric units where extensive calculations may be required. It has been determined that the safest way to calculate a BSA is to use a formula and a calculator that can perform square roots ($\sqrt{\phantom{x}}$). The formula used is based on the units in which the measurements are obtained (e.g., kilograms, centimeters, pounds, inches).

## Formula for Calculating BSA From Kilograms and Centimeters

*STEPS*

1. Multiply the weight in kilograms by height in centimeters.
2. Divide the product obtained in Step 1 by 3,600.
3. Enter the square root sign into the calculator.
4. Round the final BSA in square meters to the nearest hundredth.

**NOTE**

This formula uses metric measures.

### Formula

$$\text{Metric BSA (m}^2) = \sqrt{\frac{\text{Weight (kg)} \times \text{Height (cm)}}{3,600}}$$

**Example 1:**   Calculate the BSA for a child who weighs 23 kg and whose height is 128 cm. Express BSA to the nearest hundredth.

$$\sqrt{\frac{23 \text{ (kg)} \times 128 \text{ (cm)}}{3,600}} = \sqrt{0.817}$$

$$\sqrt{0.817} = 0.903 = 0.9 \text{ m}^2$$

The BSA was calculated as follows: $23 \times 128 \div 3,600 = 0.817$, then the square root ($\sqrt{\phantom{x}}$) was entered. The final BSA in square meters was rounded to the nearest hundredth.

**Example 2:**   Calculate the BSA for an adult who weighs 100 kg and whose height is 180 cm. Express BSA to the nearest hundredth.

$$\sqrt{\frac{100 \text{ (kg)} \times 180 \text{ (cm)}}{3,600}} = \sqrt{5}$$

$$\sqrt{5} = 2.236 = 2.24 \text{ m}^2$$

## Formula for Calculating Body Surface Area From Pounds and Inches

The formula is the same with the exception of the number used in the denominator, which is 3,131, and the measurements used are household units.

### Formula

$$\text{Household BSA (m}^2) = \sqrt{\frac{\text{Weight (lb)} \times \text{Height (in)}}{3,131}}$$

**Example 1:**   Calculate the BSA for a child who weighs 25 lb and is 32 inches tall. Express the BSA to the nearest hundredth.

$$\sqrt{\frac{25 \text{ (lb)} \times 32 \text{ (in)}}{3,131}} = \sqrt{0.255}$$

$$\sqrt{0.255} = 0.504 = 0.5 \text{ m}^2$$

**Example 2:**   Calculate the BSA for an adult who weighs 143.7 lb and is 61.2 inches tall. Express the BSA to the nearest hundredth.

$$\sqrt{\frac{143.7 \text{ (lb)} \times 61.2 \text{ (in)}}{3,131}} = \sqrt{2.808}$$

$$\sqrt{2.808} = 1.675 = 1.68 \text{ m}^2$$

 **Practice Problems**

Determine the BSA for each of the following clients using a formula. Express the BSA to the nearest hundredth.

51. An adult whose weight is 95.5 kg and height is 180 cm                                    _____

52. A child whose weight is 10 kg and height is 70 cm                                          _____

53. A child whose weight is 4.8 lb and height is 21 inches                                        _____

54. An adult whose weight is 170 lb and height is 67 inches                                        _____

55. A child whose weight is 92 lb and height is 35 inches                                          _____

56. A child whose weight is 24 kg and height is 92 cm                                            _____

Answers on p. 683

**CAUTION**   Always check a dosage against BSA in square meter recommendations using appropriate resources, for example, the PDR, medication inserts, or a pediatric medication handbook.

Medications, particularly chemotherapy agents, often provide the recommended dosage according to BSA in square meters.

**Example:**   Cisplatin is an antineoplastic agent. The recommended pediatric/adult IV dosage for bladder cancer is 50 to 70 mg/m² every 3 to 4 weeks. For carmustine, which is used to treat Hodgkin disease and brain tumors, the recommended IV dosage for an adult is 150 to 200 mg/m².

### ■ Points to Remember

- The formula method to calculate BSA is more accurate than use of the nomogram.
- The formulas used to calculate BSA are as follows:

$$\text{Metric BSA (m}^2) = \sqrt{\frac{\text{Weight (kg)} \times \text{Height (cm)}}{3,600}}$$

$$\text{Household BSA (m}^2) = \sqrt{\frac{\text{Weight (lb)} \times \text{Height (in)}}{3,131}}$$

**Determining BSA With a Formula Requires Use of a Calculator**
- Multiply height × weight (cm × kg, or lb × inches).
- Divide by 3,600 or 3,131, depending on the units of measure (divide by 3,600 if measures are in metric units [cm, kg] and by 3,131 if measures are in household units [inches, lb]).
- Enter the $\sqrt{\phantom{x}}$ (square root sign) to arrive at BSA in square meters.
- Round square meters to hundredths (two decimal places).

## DOSAGE CALCULATION BASED ON BODY SURFACE AREA

If you know the child's BSA, the dosage is calculated by multiplying the recommended dosage by the child's BSA (m²).

**Example 1:** The recommended dosage is 3 mg per m². The child has a BSA of 1.2 m².

$$1.2 \; \text{m}^2 \times \frac{3 \; \text{mg}}{\text{m}^2} = 3.6 \; \text{mg}$$

 Solution Using Dimensional Analysis

$$x \; \text{mg} = \frac{3 \; \text{mg}}{\text{m}^2} \times \frac{1.2 \; \text{m}^2}{1}$$

$$x = 1.2 \times 3$$

$$x = 3.6 \; \text{mg}$$

**Example 2:** The recommended dose is 30 mg per m². The child has a BSA of 0.75 m².

$$0.75 \; \text{m}^2 \times \frac{30 \; \text{mg}}{\text{m}^2} = 22.5 \; \text{mg}$$

 Solution Using Dimensional Analysis

$$x \; \text{mg} = \frac{30 \; \text{mg}}{\text{m}^2} \times \frac{0.75 \; \text{m}^2}{1}$$

$$x = 30 \times 0.75$$

$$x = 22.5 \; \text{mg}$$

To do the calculation with dimensional analysis, use the recommended dosage given to convert the BSA to dosage in milligrams, as the first fraction.

## CALCULATING USING THE FORMULA

A child's BSA is expressed in square meters (m²) and inserted into the formula below.

**Formula**

$$\frac{\text{BSA of child (m}^2)}{1.7\ (\text{m}^2)} \times \text{Adult dosage} = \text{Estimated child's dosage}$$

**RULE**

If only the recommended dosage for an adult is cited, then the formula is used to calculate the child's dosage. The formula uses the average adult dosage, the average adult BSA (1.7 m²), and the child's BSA in square meters.

**Example 1:** The prescriber has ordered a medication for which the average adult dosage is 125 mg. What will the dosage be for a child with a BSA of 1.4 m²?

$$\frac{1.4\ \text{m}^2}{1.7\ (\text{m}^2)} \times 125\ \text{mg} = 102.94\ \text{mg} = 102.9\ \text{mg (round to the nearest tenth)}$$

**Example 2:** The adult dosage for a medication is 100 to 300 mg. What will the dosage range be for a child with a BSA of 0.5 m²?

$$\frac{0.5\ \text{m}^2}{1.7\ (\text{m}^2)} \times 100 = 29.41\ \text{mg} = 29.4\ \text{mg (round to nearst tenth)}$$

$$\frac{0.5\ \text{m}^2}{1.7\ (\text{m}^2)} \times 300 = 88.23\ \text{mg} = 88.2\ \text{mg (round to nearst tenth)}$$

The dosage range is 29.4 to 88.2 mg.

 **Practice Problems**

Using the West nomogram chart when indicated, calculate the child's dosage for the following medications. Express your answer to the nearest tenth.

57. The child's height is 32 inches, and weight is 25 lb. The recommended adult dosage is 25 mg.

   a. What is the child's BSA?  _____

   b. What is the child's dosage?  _____

58. The child's height is 100 cm and weight is 10 kg. The adult dosage is 200 to 400 mg.

   a. What is the child's BSA?  _____

   b. What is the child's dosage range?  _____

59. The normal adult dosage of a medication is 5 to 15 mg. What will the dosage range be for a child whose BSA is 1.5 m²?  _____

60. 5 mg of a medication is ordered for a child with a BSA of 0.8 m². The average adult dosage is 20 mg. Is this a correct dosage? (Prove mathematically.)  _____

61. 7 mg of a medication is ordered for a child with a BSA of 0.9 m$^2$. The average adult dosage is 25 mg. Is this correct? (Prove mathematically.)

_____

62. An antibiotic for which the average adult dosage is 250 mg is ordered for a child with a BSA of 1.5 m$^2$. What will the child's dosage be?

_____

63. The recommended adult dosage of a medi-child is 20 to 30 mg. The child has a BSA of 0.74 m$^2$. What will the child's dosage range be?

_____

64. 8 mg of a medication is ordered for a child who has a BSA of 0.67 m$^2$. The average adult dosage is 20 mg. Is the dosage correct? (Prove mathematically.)

_____

65. The child has a BSA of 0.94 m$^2$. The recommended adult dosage of a medication is 10 to 20 mg. What will the child's dosage range be?

_____

66. The child's weight is 20 lb and height is 30 inches. The adult dosage of a medication is 500 mg.

    a. What is the child's BSA?

    _____

    b. What is the child's dosage?

    _____

67. The recommended adult dosage for an antibiotic is 500 mg 4 times a day. The child's BSA is 1.3 m$^2$. What will the child's dosage be?

_____

68. The child's weight is 30 lb and height is 28 inches. The adult dosage of a medication is 25 mg.

    a. What is the child's BSA?

    _____

    b. What is the child's dosage?

    _____

69. The child's BSA is 0.52 m$^2$. The average adult dosage for a medication is 15 mg. What will the child's dosage be?

_____

70. The recommended adult dosage for a medication is 150 mg. The child's BSA is 1.1 m$^2$. What will the child's dosage be?

_____

Answers on pp. 683-684

## ■ Points to Remember

- BSA is determined from the West nomogram by using the child's height and weight and is expressed in square meters.
- The BSA can also be determined by using a formula and calculator. The formula used depends on the units in which measurements are obtained.

$$\text{Metric BSA (m}^2) = \sqrt{\frac{\text{Weight (kg)} \times \text{Height (cm)}}{3{,}600}}$$

$$\text{Household BSA (m}^2) = \sqrt{\frac{\text{Weight (lb)} \times \text{Height (in)}}{3{,}131}}$$

- The normal height and weight column on the West nomogram is used only when the child's height and weight are within normal limits.
- Read the numbers and calibration values between them on the West nomogram.
- When you know the child's BSA, the dosage is determined by multiplying the BSA by the recommended dosage. (This is used when the recommended dosage is written by using the average dosage per square meter.) Dimensional analysis can also be used with the recommended dosage as the equivalent fraction.
- To determine whether a child's dosage is safe, a comparison must be made between what is ordered and the calculation of the dosage based on BSA.
- The formula for calculating a child's dosage when the average adult dosage per adult mean BSA (1.7 m²) is known is written as follows:

$$\frac{\text{BSA of child (m}^2)}{1.7 \ (\text{m}^2)} \times \text{Adult dosage} = \text{Estimated child's dosage}$$

- If a dosage seems to be unsafe, consult the prescriber before administering the dose.

## IV THERAPY AND CHILDREN
### Pediatric IV Administration

Administration of IV fluids to children is very specific because of their physiological development. Microdrop sets are used for infants and small children; electronic devices are used to control the rate of delivery. The rate of infusion for infants and children must be carefully monitored. The IV drop rate must be slow for small children to prevent complications such as cardiac failure because of fluid overload. Various IV devices decrease the size of the drop to "mini" or "micro" drop or 1/60 mL, thus delivering 60 minidrops or microdrops per milliliter. IV medications may be administered to a child over a period of time (several hours) or on an intermittent basis. For intermittent medication administration, several methods of delivery are used, including the following:

*Small-volume IV bags*—These may be used if the child has a primary IV line in place. A secondary tubing set is attached to a small-volume IV bag, and the piggyback method is used.

*Calibrated burettes*—These are often referred to by their trade names: Buretrol, Volutrol, or Soluset. (Figure 25-2 shows a typical system that consists of a calibrated chamber that can hold 100 to 150 mL of fluid.) The burette is calibrated in small increments that allow exact measurements of small volumes. Medication is added to the IV fluid in the chamber for a prescribed dilution of volume (see Figure 25-2).

An electronic controller or pump may also be used to administer intermittent IV medications. When used, the electronic device sounds an alarm when the Buretrol chamber is empty. Buretrols may also be used in the adult setting for clients with fluid restrictions.

**CAUTION**

IV infusions should be monitored as frequently as every hour. A solution to flush the IV tubing is administered after the medication.

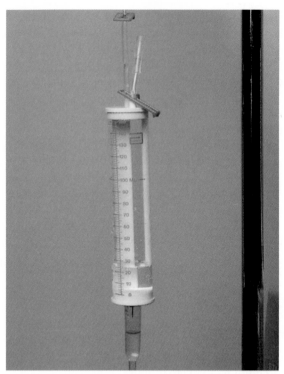

**Figure 25-2**   Volume-controlled device (burette). (From Potter PA, Perry AG: *Fundamentals of nursing,* ed. 7, St. Louis, 2009, Mosby).

Regardless of the method used for medication administration in children, **a solution to flush the IV tubing is administered after the medication.** The purpose of the flush is to make sure the medication has cleared the tubing and the total dosage has been administered. Most institutions flush with normal saline solution as opposed to heparin. The amount of fluid used varies according to the length of the tubing from the medication source to the infusion site. **When IV medications are diluted for administration, the policy for including medication volume as part of the volume specified for dilution varies from institution to institution, as does the amount of flush. When flow rates (gtt/min, mL/hr) are calculated, it varies from institution to institution as to whether the flush is included. The nurse is responsible for checking the protocol at the institution to ensure that the correct procedure is followed.**

*Note:* In the sample calculations that follow, a 15-mL volume will be used as a flush unless otherwise specified, and the medication volume will be considered as part of the total dilution volume. The flush will not be considered in the total volume.

**CAUTION**

An excessively high concentration of an IV medication can cause vein irritation and potentially life-threatening effects. Dilution calculation is essential for the nurse.

## CALCULATING IV MEDICATIONS BY BURETTE

A calibrated burette can be used to administer medications by using a roller clamp rather than a pump. In this case it is necessary to use the formula presented in Chapter 22 or dimensional analysis and calculate gtt/min. Remember, burettes are volume control devices and have a drop factor of 60 gtt/mL.

$$x \text{ gtt/min} = \frac{\text{Total volume (mL)} \times \text{drop factor (gtt/mL)}}{\text{Time in minutes}}$$

**NOTE**

In doing the calculations, the total volume will include adding the medication to the diluent to calculate the gtt/min.

**Example:** An antibiotic dose of 100 mg in 2 mL is to be diluted in 20 mL of D5W to infuse over 30 minutes. A 15-mL flush follows. The administration set is a microdrop (burette).

**Step 1:** Read the drug label, and determine what volume the 100 mg is contained in. This is 2 mL.

**Step 2:** Allow 18 mL of D5W to run into the burette, and then add the 2 mL containing the 100 mg of medication. Roll the burette between your hands to allow medication to mix thoroughly. (2 mL + 18 mL = 20 mL for volume)

**Step 3:** Determine the flow rate necessary to deliver the medication plus the flush in 30 minutes.

Total volume is 20 mL. Infusion time is 30 minutes.

$$x \text{ gtt/min} = \frac{20 \text{ mL (diluted medication)} \times 60 \text{ gtt/mL}}{30 \text{ min}}$$

$$x = \frac{20 \times \overset{2}{\cancel{60}}}{\underset{1}{\cancel{30}}} = 40 \text{ gtt/min}$$

$$x = 40 \text{ gtt/min}$$

**Answer:** $x = 40$ gtt/min; 40 microgtt/min

> **NOTE**
>
> Reducing numbers can make them smaller and easier to deal with. If the flush is considered with the intermittent medication, note that the total volume will be diluted drug + flush, and then proceed with calculation (gtt/min, mL/hr).

### ➡ Solution Using Dimensional Analysis

To calculate gtt/min (refer to steps in Chapter 22 if necessary):

$$\frac{x \text{ gtt}}{\min} = \frac{\overset{20}{\cancel{60}} \text{ gtt}}{1 \text{ mL}} \times \frac{\overset{2}{\cancel{20}} \text{ mL}}{\underset{\underset{1}{3}}{\cancel{30}} \min}$$

$$x = \frac{40}{1}$$

$$x = 40 \text{ gtt/min}; 40 \text{ microgtt/min}$$

**Step 4:** Adjust the IV flow rate to deliver 40 microgtt/min (40 gtt/min).

**Step 5:** Label the burette with the medication name, dosage, and medication infusing label.

**Step 6:** When administration of the medication is completed, add the 15-mL flush, and continue to infuse at 40 microgtt/min. Replace the label with a "flush infusing" label.

> **NOTE**
>
> Always think and remember that volume control sets are microdrop and mL/hr = gtt/min when the drop factor is 60 gtt/mL.

**Step 7:** When the flush is completed, restart the primary line and remove the flush infusing label. Document the medication according to institution policy on the medication administration record (MAR) or in the computer and the volume of fluid on the intake and output (I&O) sheet according to agency policy.

## Tips for Clinical Practice

To express the volume of gtt/min in mL/hr, remember that a microdrop administration set delivers 60 gtt/mL; therefore gtt/min = mL/hr. In this case if the gtt/min = 40, then the mL/hr = 40.

As already mentioned, the burette can be used along with an electronic controller or pump. When used as previously stated, the electronic device will sound an alarm each time the burette empties. Let's examine the calculation necessary if the burette is used along with the pump or a controller. Calculations where the burette is used with a pump or controller are done in mL/hr. Let's use the same example shown previously to illustrate the difference in calculation steps.

**Example:** An antibiotic dose of 100 mg in 2 mL is to be diluted in 20 mL of D5W to infuse over 30 minutes. A 15-mL flush follows. An infusion controller is used, and the tubing is a microdrop burette.

The same Steps 1 and 2 as shown in the previous example for burette only are followed.

**Step 1:** Calculate the flow rate for this microdrop.

Total volume is 20 mL; the flush is not considered in the volume.

**Step 2:** Total volume is 20 mL. Infusion time is 30 minutes. Use a ratio and proportion or dimensional analysis to calculate the rate in mL/hr.

> **NOTE**
>
> When medication has infused, add the 15-mL flush and continue to infuse at 40 mL/hr; replace the label with a "flush infusing" label. Once the flush is finished, restart the primary IV or disconnect from lock. Remove the "flush infusing" label. Document the medication according to institution policy (MAR or in computer) and on the I&O sheet according to institution policy.

 **Solution Using Ratio and Proportion**

$$20 \text{ mL}:30 \text{ minutes} = x \text{ mL}:60 \text{ minutes}$$

$$30x = 60 \times 20$$

$$\frac{30x}{30} = \frac{1{,}20\cancel{0}}{3\cancel{0}} = 40 \text{ mL/hr}$$

$$x = 40 \text{ mL/hr}$$

**Answer:** Set the controller to infuse at 40 mL/hr.

 **Solution Using Dimensional Analysis**

To calculate mL/hr (refer to steps in Chapter 22 if necessary):

**Example 1:**

$$\frac{x \text{ mL}}{\text{hr}} = \frac{20 \text{ mL}}{\cancel{30} \text{ min}_1} \times \frac{\overset{2}{\cancel{60}} \text{ min}}{1 \text{ hr}}$$

$$x = \frac{40}{1}$$

$$x = 40 \text{ mL/hr}$$

**Example 2:** An antibiotic dose of 150 mg in 1 mL is to be diluted in 35 mL NS to infuse over 45 minutes. A 15-mL flush follows. A volumetric pump will be used.

Total volume is 35 mL. Infusion time is 45 minutes. Calculate mL/hr rate.

$$35 \text{ mL}:45 \text{ minutes} = x \text{ mL}:60 \text{ minutes}$$

$$45x = 35 \times 60$$

$$\frac{45x}{45} = \frac{2{,}100}{45} = 46.6 = 47 \text{ mL/hr}$$

$$x = 47 \text{ mL/hr}$$

> **NOTE**
>
> As shown in Chapter 22, the shortcut method using the drop factor constant could be used. Ratio and proportion can be stated by using several formats.

**Answer:** Set the pump to infuse at 47 mL/hr.

Solution Using Dimensional Analysis

$$\frac{x \text{ mL}}{\text{hr}} = \frac{35 \text{ mL}}{\overset{}{\underset{3}{45 \text{ min}}}} \times \frac{\overset{4}{60 \text{ min}}}{1 \text{ hr}}$$

$$x = \frac{140}{3} = 46.6 = 47 \text{ mL}$$

$$x = 47 \text{ mL/hr}$$

Set the pump to infuse at 47 mL/hr.

 **Practice Problems**

Determine the volume of solution that must be added to the burette in the following problems. Then determine the flow rate in gtt/min for each IV using a microdrop and indicate mL/hr for a controller.

71. An IV medication dosage of 500 mg is ordered to be diluted to 30 mL and infuse over 50 minutes with a 15 mL flush to follow. The dosage of medication is contained in 3 mL. Determine the following:

    a. Dilution volume          _____

    b. Rate in gtt/min          _____

    c. Rate in mL/hr          _____

72. The volume of a 20 mg dosage of medication is 2 mL. Dilute to 15 mL, and administer over 45 minutes with a 15 mL flush to follow. Determine the following:

    a. Dilution volume          _____

    b. Rate in gtt/min          _____

    c. Rate in mL/hr          _____

Answers on p. 684

## DETERMINING WHETHER IV DOSE IS SAFE FOR CHILDREN

As seen earlier in this chapter, medications can be calculated based on mg/kg or body surface area (BSA). IV dosages for children are calculated on that basis as well. The IV medication can be assessed to determine if it is within normal range as well. The safe daily dosage is calculated and then compared with the order.

To determine whether an IV dosage for a child is safe, consult an appropriate medication resource for the recommended dosage. Remember to carefully read the reference to determine if the medication is calculated according to BSA in square meters (common with chemotherapy drugs), micrograms, or units per day or per hour. When a dosage is within the normal limits, calculate and administer the dosage. If a dosage is not within the normal limits, consult the prescriber before administering the medication. *Note:* If the order is based on the child's BSA and the BSA is not known, you will need to use the West nomogram or the formula presented and determine the BSA. Let's look at some examples.

**Example 1:** A child's BSA is 0.8 m², and the order is for 1.8 mg of a medication in 100 mL D5W at 10 AM. The recommended dosage is 2 mg/m².

**Step 1:** As previously shown in this chapter, if BSA is known, calculate the dosage for the child by multiplying the recommended dosage by the BSA. The recommended dosage is 2 mg/m², and the child's BSA is 0.8 m².

$$0.8 \text{ m}^2 \times 2 \text{ mg/m}^2 = 1.6 \text{ mg}$$

**Step 2:** Determine if dosage is within the normal range.

The safe dosage is 1.6 mg for this child, but 1.8 mg is ordered. Notify the prescriber before administering the dosage. *Note:* The dosage in this example can also be determined by using dimensional analysis.

 Solution Using Dimensional Analysis

$$x \text{ mg} = \frac{2 \text{ mg}}{\text{m}^2} \times \frac{0.8 \text{ m}^2}{1}$$
$$x = 1.6 \text{ mg}$$

**Example 2:** A child weighing 10 kg has an order for IV Solu-Medrol 125 mg IV q6h for 48 hours. The recommended dosage is 30 mg/kg/day IV and can be replicated q4-6h for 48 hours.

**Step 1:** Determine the dosage for the child.

$$10 \text{ kg} \times 30 \text{ mg/kg/day} = 300 \text{ mg/day}$$

**Step 2:** Determine if dosage ordered is within normal range.

The dosage: 125 mg q6h (4 doses).

$$125 \text{ mg} \times 4 = 500 \text{ mg/day}$$

Check with the prescriber; the dosage is more than what the child should receive. *Note:* The dosage in this example can also be determined by using dimensional analysis.

 Solution Using Dimensional Analysis

$$\frac{x \text{ mg}}{\text{kg}} = \frac{30 \text{ mg}}{1 \text{ kg/day}} \times \frac{10 \text{ kg}}{1}$$
$$x = 300 \text{ mg/day}$$

 **Practice Problems**

Determine the normal dosage range for the following problems to the nearest tenth. State your course of action.

73. A child weighing 17 kg has an order for an IV of 250 mL D5W containing 2,500 units of medication, which is to infuse at 50 mL/hr. The recommended dosage for the medication is 10 to 25 units/kg/hr. Determine whether the dosage ordered is within normal limits. _____

74. A child with a BSA of 0.75 m$^2$ has an order for 84 mg IV of a medication in 100 mL D5W q12h. The recommended dosage is 100 to 250 mg/m$^2$/day in two divided doses. Determine whether the dosage ordered is within normal limits. _____

Answers on p. 684

## ■ Points to Remember

### IV Therapy and Children

- Pediatric IV medications are diluted for administration. It is important to know the institution's policy as to whether the medication volume is included as part of the total dilution volume.
- A flush is used after administration of IV medications in children. The volume of the flush will vary depending on the length of the IV tubing from the medication source.
- Check the institution's policy as to whether the volume of the flush is added to the diluted medication volume.
- Pediatric medication administration requires frequent assessment.
- Use an appropriate reference to calculate the normal dosage range for IV administration, and then compare it with the dosage ordered to determine whether it is within normal range.

## PEDIATRIC ORAL AND PARENTERAL MEDICATIONS

Several methods have been presented to determine dosages for children in this chapter. It is important, however, to bear in mind that although the dosage may be determined according to weight, BSA, and so on, the dosage to administer is calculated by using the same methods as for adults (ratio and proportion, the formula method, or dimensional analysis). It is important to remember the following differences with children's dosages.

### Remember

1. Dosages are smaller for children than for adults.
2. Most oral drugs for infants and small children come in liquid form to facilitate swallowing.
3. The oral route is preferred; however, when necessary, medications are administered by the parenteral route.
4. Not more than 1 mL is injected IM for small children and older infants; small infants should not receive more than 0.5 mL by IM injection.
5. Parenteral dosages are frequently administered with a tuberculin syringe.

**CAUTION**

When in doubt, always double-check pediatric dosages with another person to decrease the chance of an error. Never assume! Think before administering.

**Critical Thinking Questions**

**Scenario:** According to the *Harriet Lane Handbook,* the recommended dosage for a child for ibuprofen as an antipyretic is 5-10 mg/kg/dose q6-8h p.o. The 7 month old weighs 18½ lb. The prescriber ordered 20 mg p.o. q6h for a temperature above 102° F. The infant's temperature is 102.8° F, and the nurse is preparing to administer the medication. The nurse believes the dosage is low but administers the medication based on the dosage being safe because it is below the safe dosage range. Several hours have passed, and the infant's temperature continues to increase.

a. What is the required single dosage for this infant?    _____

b. What should the nurse's actions have been and why?    _____

c. What preventive measures could have been taken by
   the nurse in this situation?    _____

Answers on p. 684

## CHAPTER REVIEW

Read the dosage information or label given for the following problems. Express body weight conversion to the nearest tenth where indicated and dosages to the nearest tenth.

1. Lasix 10 mg IV stat is ordered for a
   child weighing 22 lb. The recommended
   initial dose is 1 mg/kg. Is the dosage
   ordered safe? (Prove mathematically.)    _____

2. Amoxicillin 150 mg p.o. q8h is ordered for an infant weighing 23 lb.

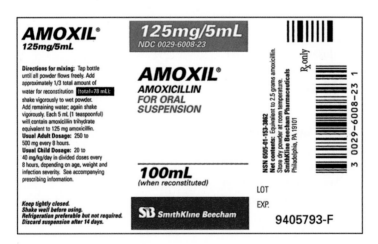

a. What is the child's weight in
   kilograms to the nearest tenth?    _____

b. What is the recommended dosage
   range?    _____

c. What is the divided dosage range?    _____

d. Is the dosage ordered safe?
   (Prove mathematically.)    _____

3. Furadantin oral suspension 25 mg p.o. q6h is ordered for a child weighing 17 kg. Recommended dosage is 2.2 to 3.2 mg/lb/day.

Available:

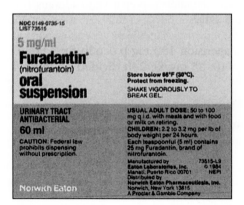

a. What is the child's weight in pounds to the nearest tenth?  _____

b. What is the dosage range for this child?  _____

c. Is the dosage ordered safe? (Prove mathematically.)  _____

d. How many milliliters must be given per dosage to administer the ordered dosage? Calculate the dose if the order is safe.  _____

4. Dicloxacillin 100 mg p.o. q6h is ordered for a child weighing 35 kg. The recommended dosage is 12.5 mg/kg/day in equally divided dosages q6h for children weighing less than 40 kg. Is the dosage ordered safe? (Prove mathematically.)  _____

5. Vibramycin 75 mg p.o. q12h is
   ordered for a child weighing 30 lb.
   Refer to the following label, and
   determine if this is a safe dosage.
   (Prove mathematically.) _____

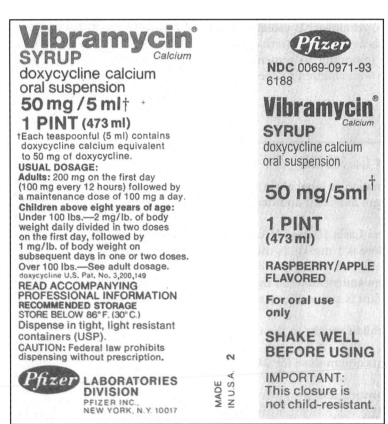

6. Oxacillin oral solution 250 mg p.o. q6h
   is ordered for a child weighing 42 lb. The
   recommended dosage is 50 mg/kg/day
   in equally divided dosages q6h. Is
   the dosage ordered safe? (Prove
   mathematically.) _____

7. Cleocin suspension 150 mg p.o. q8h is
   ordered for a child weighing 36 lb. The
   recommended dosage is 10 to 25 mg/kg/day
   divided q6-8h. Is the dosage ordered
   safe? (Prove mathematically.) _____

8. Keflex suspension 250 mg p.o. q6h is ordered for a child weighing 66 lb. The usual
   pediatric dosage is 25 to 50 mg/kg/day in four divided dosages. Available: Keflex
   suspension 125 mg per 5 mL.

   a. Is the dosage ordered safe?
      (Prove mathematically.) _____

   b. How many milliliters would you need
      to administer one dosage? Calculate
      the dose if the order is safe. _____

9. Streptomycin sulfate 400 mg IM q12h is ordered for a child weighing 35 kg. The recommended dosage is 20 to 40 mg/kg/day divided q12h IM.

    a. Is the dosage ordered safe? (Prove mathematically.)     _____

    b. A 1-g vial of streptomycin sulfate is available in powdered form with the following instructions: Dilution with 1.8 mL of sterile water will yield 400 mg per mL. How many milliliters will you need to administer the ordered dosage? Calculate the dosage if the order is safe.     _____

10. A child weighs 46 lb and has a mild infection. Gantrisin oral suspension 250 mg p.o. q6h is ordered. The recommended dosage is 120 mg/kg/day in four equally divided dosages. Is the dosage ordered safe? (Prove mathematically.)     _____

11. The recommended dosage for neonates receiving ceftazidime (Tazidime) is 30 mg/kg q12h. The neonate weighs 3,500 g.

    a. What is the neonate's weight in kilograms to the nearest tenth?     _____

    b. What is the safe dosage for this neonate?     _____

12. A child weighs 14 kg. The usual dosage range of Velosef is 50 to 100 mg/kg/day in equally divided dosages four times a day.

    a. What will the daily dosage range be for a child weighing 14 kg?     _____

    b. What is the divided dosage range for this child?     _____

    c. Velosef 250 mg IV q6h has been ordered. Is this a safe dosage? (Prove mathematically.)     _____

13. The recommended dosage for Mithracin for the treatment of testicular tumors is 25 to 30 mcg/kg. A client weighs 190 lb.

    a. What is the client's weight in kilograms to the nearest tenth?     _____

    b. What is the dosage range in milligrams for this client? (Round to the nearest tenth.)     _____

Using the nomogram on p. 559, determine the BSA and calculate each child's dosage by using the formula. Express dosages to the nearest tenth.

14. The child's height is 30 inches, and weight is 20 lb. The adult dosage of an antibiotic is 500 mg.

    a. What is the BSA?                    _____

    b. What is the child's dosage?         _____

15. The child's height is 32 inches, and weight is 27 lb. The adult dosage for a medication is 25 mg.

    a. What is the BSA?                    _____

    b. What is the child's dosage?         _____

16. The child's height is 120 cm, and weight is 40 kg. The adult dosage for a medication is 250 mg.

    a. What is the BSA?                    _____

    b. What is the child's dosage?         _____

17. The child's height is 50 inches, and weight is 75 lb. The adult dosage for a medication is 30 mg.

    a. What is the BSA?                    _____

    b. What is the child's dosage?         _____

18. The child's height is 50 inches, and weight is 70 lb. The adult dosage for a medication is 150 mg.

    a. What is the BSA?                    _____

    b. What is the child's dosage?         _____

Determine the child's dosage for the following medications. Express answers to the nearest tenth.

19. The adult dosage of a medication is 50 mg. What will the dosage be for a child with a BSA of 0.7 m$^2$?         _____

20. The adult dosage of a medication is 10 to 20 mg. What will the dosage range be for a child whose BSA is 0.66 m$^2$?         _____

21. The adult dosage of a medication is 2,000 units. What will the dosage be for a child with a BSA of 0.55 m$^2$?         _____

22. The adult dosage of a medication is 200 to 250 mg. What will the dosage range be for a child with a BSA of 0.55 m$^2$?         _____

23. The adult dosage of a medication is 150 mg.
What will the dosage be for a child
with a BSA of 0.22 m²?   _____

Calculate the child's dosage in the following problems. Determine if the prescriber's order
is correct. If the order is incorrect, give the correct dosage. Express answers to the nearest
tenth.

24. A child with a BSA of 0.49 m² has an
order for 25 mg of a medication. The adult
dosage is 60 mg.   _____

25. A child with a BSA of 0.32 m² has an
order for 4 mg of a medication. The adult
dosage is 10 mg.   _____

26. A child with a BSA of 0.68 m² has
an order for 50 mg of a medication. The
adult dosage is 125 to 150 mg.   _____

27. A child with a BSA of 0.55 m² has
an order for 5 mg of a medication. The
adult dosage is 25 mg.   _____

28. A child with a BSA of 1.2 m² has
an order for 60 mg of a medication. The
adult dosage is 75 to 100 mg.   _____

Using the formula method for calculating BSA, determine the BSA in the following clients
and express answers to the nearest hundredth.

29. A 15-year-old who weighs 100 lb and is 55 inches tall   _____

30. An adult who weighs 60.9 kg and is 130 cm tall   _____

31. A child who weighs 55 lb and is 45 inches tall   _____

32. A child who weighs 60 lb and is 35 inches tall   _____

33. An adult who weighs 65 kg and is 132 cm tall   _____

34. A child who weighs 24 lb and is 28 inches tall   _____

35. An infant who weighs 6 kg and is 55 cm long   _____

36. A child who weighs 42 lb and is 45 inches tall   _____

37. An infant who weighs 8 kg and is 70 cm long   _____

38. An adult who weighs 74 kg and is 160 cm tall   _____

Calculate the dosages to be given. Use labels where provided.

39. Order: Azidothymidine 7 mg p.o. q6h.

    Available: Azidothymidine 10 mg per mL   _____

40. Order: Epivir 150 mg p.o. b.i.d.

    Available:

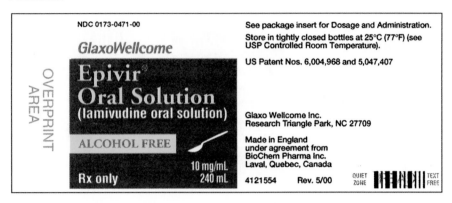

41. Order: Digoxin 0.1 mg p.o. daily.

    Available:

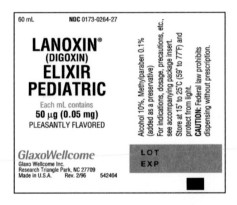

42. Order: Retrovir 80 mg p.o. q8h.

    Available:

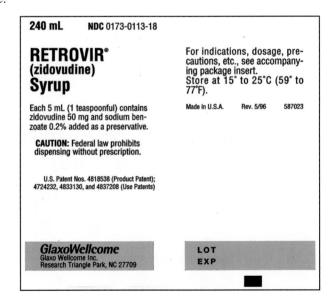

43. Order: Augmentin 250 mg p.o. q6h.

    Available:

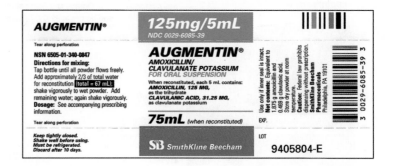

_____

44. Order: Tegretol 0.25 g p.o. t.i.d.

    Available:

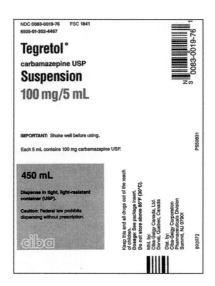

_____

45. Order: Amoxicillin 100 mg p.o. t.i.d.

    Available:

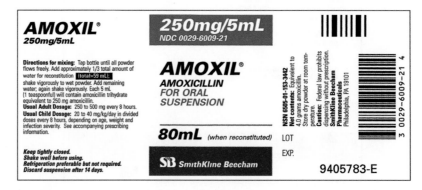

_____

Calculate the dosages below. Use the labels where provided. Calculate to the nearest hundredth where necessary.

46. Order: Gentamicin 7.3 mg IM q12h.

    Available: 20 mg per 2 mL

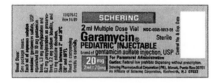

    _____

47. Order: Atropine 0.1 mg subcut stat.

    Available: Atropine 400 mcg per mL    _____

48. Order: Ampicillin 160 mg IM q12h.

    Available: Ampicillin 250 mg per mL    _____

49. Order: Morphine 3.5 mg subcut q6h p.r.n. for pain.

    Available:

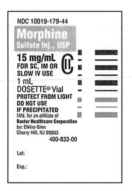

    _____

50. Order: Nebcin (tobramycin sulfate) 60 mg IV q8h.

    Available:

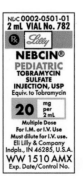

    _____

Calculate the dosages to be given. Round answers to the nearest tenth as indicated (express answers in milliliters).

51. Order: Tylenol 0.4 g p.o. q4h p.r.n. for temp greater than 101° F.

    Available: Tylenol elixir labeled
    160 mg per 5 mL                                 _____

52. Order: Methotrexate 35 mg IM daily once a week (on Tuesdays).

    Available:

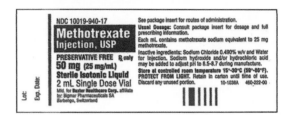

    _____

53. Order: Clindamycin 100 mg IV q6h.

    Available:

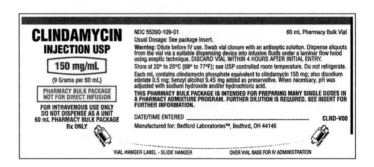

    _____

54. Order: Procaine penicillin 150,000 units IM q12h.

    Available: Procaine penicillin
    300,000 units per mL                             _____

55. Order: Amikacin 150 mg IV q8h.

    Available:

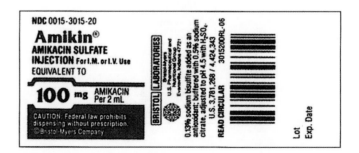

    _____

56. Order: Dilantin 62.5 mg p.o. b.i.d.

    Available: Dilantin oral suspension
    labeled 125 mg per 5 mL　　_____

57. Order: Meperidine 20 mg IM q4h p.r.n.

    Available:

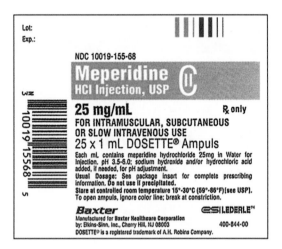

_____

58. Order: Erythromycin 300 mg p.o. q6h.

    Available: Erythromycin oral suspension
    labeled 200 mg per 5 mL　　_____

59. Order: Proventil 3 mg p.o. b.i.d.

    Available:

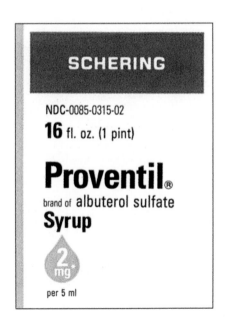

_____

60. Order: Tetracycline 250 mg p.o. q6h.

   Available: Tetracycline oral suspension
   labeled 125 mg per 5 mL _____

61. Order: Theophylline (Elixophyllin) 40 mg p.o. q.i.d.

   Available:

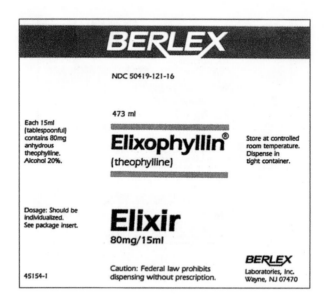

   _____

62. Order: Ferrous sulfate 45 mg p.o. every day.

   Available: Ferrous sulfate drops
   15 mg per 0.6 mL _____

63. Order: Methylprednisolone 14 mg IV q6h.

   Available:

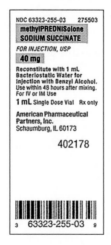

   _____

64. Order: Famotidine 20 mg p.o. b.i.d.

   Available: Famotidine 8 mg per mL.  _____

65. Order: Furosemide 75 mg IV b.i.d.

   Available:

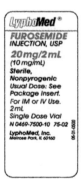

   _____

Round weights and dosages to the nearest tenth as indicated.

66. Order: Ceclor (cefaclor) 180 mg p.o. q8h. The infant weighs 10 lb. The recommended dosage is 20 mg/kg/day in three divided doses.

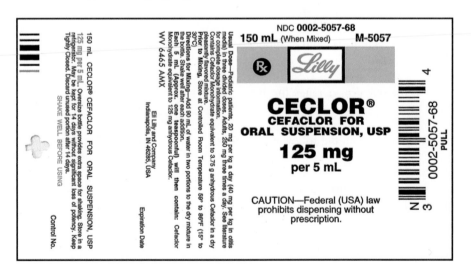

   a. Is the dosage ordered safe?  _____

   b. How many milliliters will you need
      to administer the dosage? Calculate
      the dose to administer if the dosage
      is safe.  _____

67. Order: Biaxin 200 mg p.o. q12h for a child weighing 45 lb.

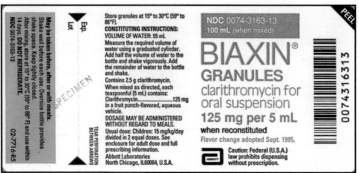

    Is the dosage ordered safe?    _____

68. Order: Amprenavir 650 mg p.o. t.i.d. for a child weighing 66 lb. The recommended dosage is 22.5 mg/kg up to three times a day.

    Is the dosage ordered safe?    _____

69. Order: Lamivudine (3TC) 120 mg p.o. b.i.d. for a child weighing 65 lb. The recommended dosage is 4 mg/kg twice a day.

    a.  What is the safe dosage for this child?    _____

    b.  Is the dosage ordered safe?    _____

70. Order: Minoxidil for a child weighing 31 lb. The recommended dosage range is 0.25 to 1 mg/kg/day.

    What is the safe dosage range for this child?    _____

Determine the dosage in the following problems. Round dosages to the nearest tenth as indicated.

71. The recommended dose for Oncovin (vincristine) is 2 mg per $m^2$. The child has a BSA of 0.8 $m^2$.    _____

72. The recommended dose for acyclovir is 250 mg per $m^2$. The child has a BSA of 0.82 $m^2$.    _____

73. The recommended dose for bleomycin in an adult with Hodgkin disease is 10 to 20 units per $m^2$. The adult has a BSA of 1.83 $m^2$. Give the dosage range.    _____

Determine the flow rate in gtt/min for each IV using a microdrip, then indicate mL/hr for a controller. (Consider the medication volume as part of the total dilution volume as shown in the chapter.)

74. A child is to receive 10 units of a medication. The dosage of 10 units is contained in 1 mL. Dilute to 30 mL, and infuse in 20 minutes. A 15-mL flush is to follow. Medication is placed in a burette. Determine the rate in:

    a. gtt/min        _____

    b. mL/hr          _____

75. A child is to receive 80 mg of a medication. The dosage of 80 mg is contained in 2 mL. Dilute to 80 mL, and infuse in 60 minutes. A 15-mL flush is to follow. Medication is placed in a burette. Determine the rate in:

    a. gtt/min        _____

    b. mL/hr          _____

76. A dosage of 250 mg in 5 mL has been ordered diluted to 40 mL and infused in 45 minutes. A 15-mL flush follows. Medication is placed in a burette. Determine the rate in:

    a. gtt/min        _____

    b. mL/hr          _____

Determine the normal dosage range for the following problems to the nearest tenth. State your course of action.

77. A child weighing 23 kg has an order for 500 mg of a medication in 100 mL D5W q12h. The normal daily dosage range is 40 to 50 mg/kg. Determine if the dosage ordered is within normal range, and state your course of action.        _____

78. A child weighing 20 kg has an order for 2 mg IV of a medication at 10 AM in 100 mL D5W. The normal daily dosage is 0.05 mg/kg. Determine if the dosage ordered is within normal range, and state your course of action.        _____

79. A child weighing 15 kg has an order for 55 mcg of a medication IV q12h. The dosage range is 6 to 8 mcg/kg/day q12h. Determine if the dosage ordered is within normal range and state your course of action.        _____

Answers on pp. 685-691

 **For additional practice problems, refer to the Pediatric Calculations section of Drug Calculations Companion, Version 4, on Evolve.**

Solve the following calculation problems. Remember to apply the principles learned in the text relating to dosages. Use labels where provided. Shade in the dosage on the syringe where indicated.

1. Order: Augmentin 300 mg p.o. q8h.

   Available:

   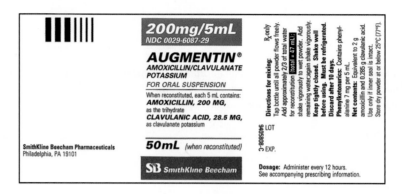

   _____

2. Order: Procan SR 1 g p.o. q6h for a client with atrial fibrillation.

   Available: Procan SR tablets 500 mg.   _____

3. Order: Lanoxicaps 0.2 mg p.o. every day.

   Available:

   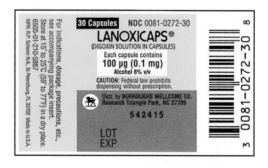

   _____

4. Order: Septra DS 1 tab p.o. q12h for 14 days.

Available:

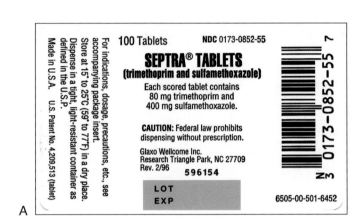 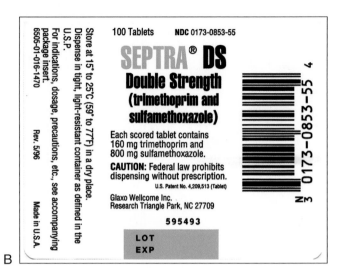

a. Indicate by letter which tablets you
   would choose to administer to the
   client based on the order.         _____

b. State why.                         _____

5. Order: Corvert 1 mg IV stat for a client with atrial arrhythmia; repeat in
   10 minutes if arrhythmia does not terminate.

Available:

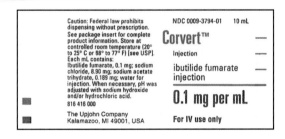

_____

6. Order: Heparin 6,500 units subcut daily. (Express your answer in hundredths.)

Available:

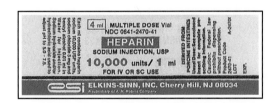

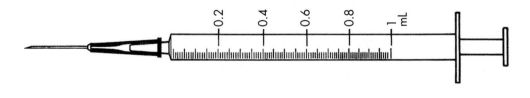

_____

7. Order: Cipro 0.75 g IV q12h for 7 days.

   Available:

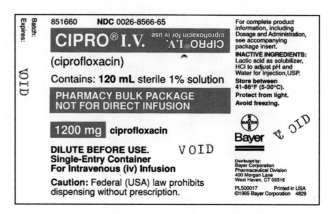

8. Order: Amphotericin B 75 mg in 1,000 mL D5W to infuse over 6 hr daily. The reconstituted solution contains 50 mg per 10 mL.

   Available:

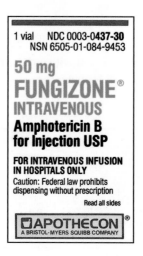

   a. How many milliliters will you add to the IV solution?

   b. The IV is to infuse in 6 hr. The administration set delivers 10 gtt/mL. At what rate in gtt/min should the IV infuse?

9. The recommended dose of Retrovir for adults with symptomatic HIV infection is 1 mg/kg infused over 1 hour q4h. Determine dosage for a client weighing 110 lb.

10. Order: Epivir 0.3 g p.o. every day.

    Available:

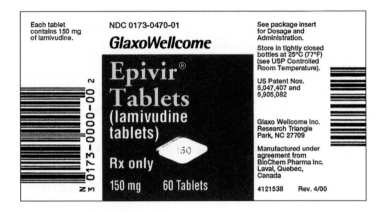

    How many tablets will you administer? _____

11. Order: Tazicef 0.25 g IV q12h.

    Available:

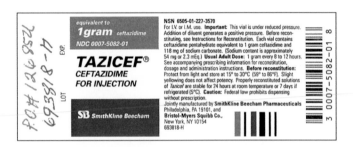

Directions for reconstitution state the following for IV infusion: 1-g vial, add 10 mL sterile water to provide 95 mg per mL; 2-g vial, add 10 mL sterile water to provide 180 mg per mL.

    a. Using the label provided, what concentration will you prepare? _____

    b. How many milliliters will you administer? _____

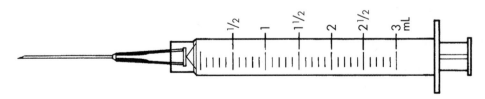

12. Order: Thorazine 75 mg p.o. b.i.d.

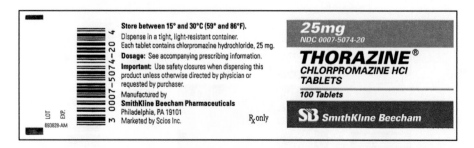

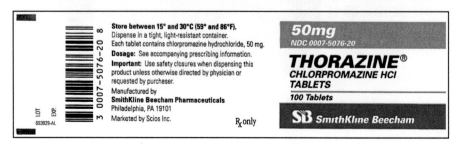

How many of which tablets would
be best to administer to the client?                    _____

13. Order: Transfuse 1 unit packed red
blood cells (250 mL) over 3 hr. The
administration set delivers 20 gtt/mL.
At what rate in gtt/min should the
IV infuse?                                              _____

14. Order: Lactated Ringer solution
1,000 mL to infuse at 80 mL/hr.
The administration set delivers
15 gtt/mL. At what rate in gtt/min
should the IV infuse?                                  _____

15. A client is receiving 500 mg of
Flagyl IVPB q8h. The Flagyl has
been placed in 100 mL D5W to
infuse over 45 minutes. The
administration set delivers
10 gtt/mL. At what rate in gtt/min
should the IV infuse?                                  _____

16. Calculate the infusion time for an
IV of 1,000 mL of D5NS infusing
at 60 mL/hr. Express time in hours
and minutes.                                           _____

17. The prescriber orders Septra Suspension 60 mg p.o. q12h for a child weighing 12 kg. The pediatric drug reference states that Septra Suspension contains trimethoprim (TMP) 40 mg and sulfamethoxazole (SMZ) 200 mg in 5 mL oral suspension, and the safe dosage of the medication is based on trimethoprim. The safe dosage is 6 to 12 mg/kg/day of TMP given q12h. Is the dosage ordered safe?     _____

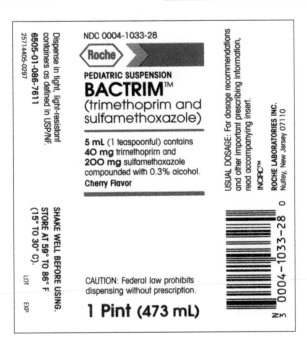

18. A medicated IV of 100 mL is to infuse at a rate of 50 mL/hr.

   a. Determine the infusion time.     _____

   b. The IV was started at 10:00 AM. When will it be completed? (State time in military and traditional time.)     _____

19. A client is to receive 10 mcg/min nitroglycerin IV. The concentration of solution is 50 mg in 250 mL D5W. What should the flow rate be (in mL/hr) to deliver 10 mcg/min?     _____

20. Order: Humulin Regular U-100 6 units and Humulin NPH U-100 16 units subcut at 7:30 AM.

What is the total volume you will
administer?  _____

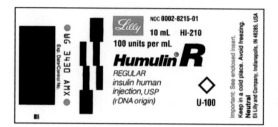 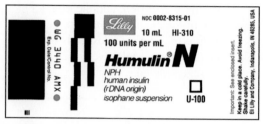

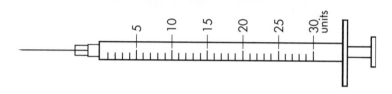

21. A dosage of 500 mg in a volume of 3 mL is to be diluted to 55 mL to infuse over 50 minutes. A 20-mL flush is to follow.

a. What is the dilution volume?  _____

b. At what rate in gtt/min should the IV infuse? (Administration set is a microdrop.)  _____

c. Indicate the rate in mL/hr.  _____

22. Order: Zocor 40 mg p.o. daily.

Available:

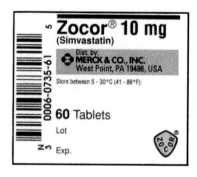 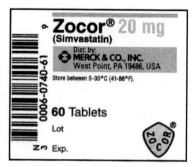

Which strength of Zocor would you
administer and why?  _____

23. Calculate the body surface area (BSA),
    using the formula, for a child who weighs
    102 lb and is 51 inches tall. Calculate
    the BSA to the nearest hundredth. _____

24. Zovirax IV is to be administered to a child who has herpes simplex
    encephalitis. The child weighs 13.6 kg and is 60 cm tall. The recommended
    dosage is 500 mg/m². Use the formula to calculate the BSA.

    Available:

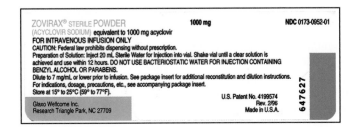

    a. What is the BSA? (Express your
       answer to the nearest hundredth.) _____

    b. What will the dosage be? _____

    c. The reconstituted Zovirax provides
       50 mg per mL. Calculate the number
       of milliliters to administer. _____

25. Order: Capoten 50 mg p.o. t.i.d. Hold if systolic blood pressure (SBP) less than 100.

    Available:

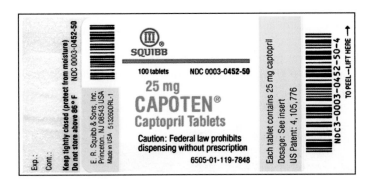

    a. How many tablets will you give? _____

    b. The client's blood pressure is 90/60.
       What should the nurse do? _____

26. Prepare the following strength solution:
    2/5 strength Ensure Plus 250 mL. _____

27. Order: 400 mL of Pulmocare over 6 hr by nasogastric tube. The feeding is placed in an enteral infusion pump. Determine rate in mL/hr. Round your answer to nearest whole number.)

    _____

28. A medication of 1 g in 4 mL is to be diluted to 70 mL and infused over 50 minutes. A 15-mL flush follows. Medication is placed in a burette. Determine the following:

    a. gtt/min          _____

    b. mL/hr           _____

29. A child weighing 21.4 kg has an order for 500 mg of a medication in 100 mL D5W q12h. The normal daily dosage range is 40 to 50 mg/kg. Determine if the dosage is within normal range, and state your course of action.

    _____

30. Calculate the amount of dextrose and NaCl in 2 L of D5 $\frac{1}{4}$ NS.

    a. Dextrose        _____ g

    b. Sodium chloride _____ g

31. 500 mL D5W was to infuse in 3 hours at 28 gtt/min (28 macrogtt/min). The drop factor is 10 gtt/mL. After 1$\frac{1}{2}$ hours, you notice 175 mL has infused.

    a. Recalculate the IV flow rate.      _____

    b. Determine the percentage of change.  _____

    c. State your course of action.       _____

32. 1,000 mL D5R/L was to infuse in 8 hours at 31 gtt/min (31 macrogtt/min). After 4 hours, you notice 600 mL has infused. The administration set delivers 15 gtt/mL.

    a. Recalculate the IV flow rate.      _____

    b. Determine the percentage of change.  _____

    c. State your course of action.       _____

33. Order: Infuse D5W 500 mL with 20,000 units heparin at 25 mL/hr. Determine the following:

    _____ units/hr

34. Order: Phenergan (promethazine) 25 mg IV push before surgery. The literature states: Do not give at rate above 25 mg/min.

    Available:

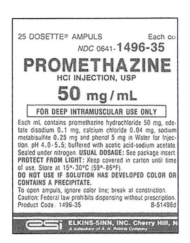

    a. How many milliliters will you prepare? _____

    b. What is the number of minutes the
       medication should be administered? _____

35. Order: Morphine sulfate 80 mg in 250 mL of IV fluid to infuse at a rate of 20 mL/hr.

    Determine the dosage in mg/hr the
    client is receiving. _____

36. Order: Cardizem 25 mg IV over 2 minutes.

    Available:

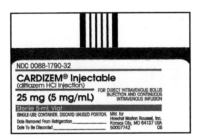

    a. How many milliliters will you
       add to the IV? _____

    b. How many milliliters will you
       infuse per minute? _____

37. Order: Levodopa 0.75 g p.o. t.i.d.

    Available: Tablets labeled 250 mg.

    How many tablets will be needed for
    10 days of therapy? _____

38. Order: Lanoxin (digoxin) tablets 0.375 mg p.o. stat.

    Available: Scored tablets labeled 125 mcg, 250 mcg, and 500 mcg.

    a.  Which Lanoxin tablet(s) will you
        use to prepare the dosage?            _____

    b.  How many tablets should the
        client receive?                       _____

39. Order: Infergen 12 mcg subcut stat.

    Available: Infergen 15 mcg per 0.5 mL.

    How many milliliters will you
    administer?                               _____

40. Order: Urokinase 125,000 units IV stat.

    Available:

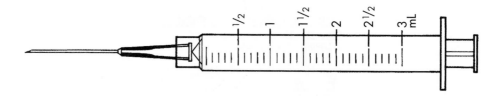

    a.  How many milliliters will you
        administer?                           _____

    b.  Shade the dosage in on the
        syringe provided.

For problems 41-43, round weight to the nearest tenth as indicated.

41. The heparin protocol at an institution is: Bolus client with 80 units/kg of body
    weight and start drip at 14 unit/kg/hr. Using the heparin protocol, determine the fol-
    lowing for a client weighing 242 lb. (Round weight and dosage to the nearest tenth
    as indicated.)

    a.  Heparin bolus dosage              _____

    b.  Infusion rate for the heparin
        IV drip                          _____

42. Order: 20 units/kg/hr heparin IV. The client weighs 88 kg.

    How many units will the client
    receive per hour?　　　　　　　　_____

43. Order: 20,000 units heparin IV in 250 mL to infuse at 25 units/kg/hr. Client weighs
    184 lb.

    How many units per hour will the
    client receive?　　　　　　　　_____

44. Order: Digoxin 0.375 mg IV push (infused slowly over 5 minutes).

    Available: Digoxin 0.25 mg per mL

    a. How many milliliters should you
       administer?　　　　　　　　_____

    b. At what rate in mL/min should the
       IV infuse?　　　　　　　　_____

45. Order: Morphine 8 mg IV q4h p.r.n. (infusion not to exceed 10 mg/4 min).

    Available:

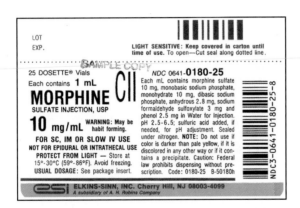

    a. How many milliliters will you
       administer?　　　　　　　　_____

    b. How many minutes will it take
       for the IV to infuse?　　　　_____

Answers on pp. 692-695

 **For another Comprehensive Post-Test, refer to Drug Calculations
Companion, Version 4, on Evolve.**

# Answer Key

## ANSWERS TO PRE-TEST FOR UNIT ONE

1. ix, $\overline{ix}$, IX
2. xvi, $\overline{xvi}$, XVI
3. xxiii, $\overline{xxiii}$, XXIII
4. xss, $\overline{xss}$
5. xxii, $\overline{xxii}$, XXII
6. $11\frac{1}{2}$
7. 12
8. 18
9. 24
10. 6

11. $\frac{2}{3}$
12. $\frac{1}{4}$
13. $\frac{1}{75}$
14. $\frac{4}{5}$
15. $\frac{4}{6} = \frac{2}{3}$
16. 2
17. $5\frac{1}{3}$

18. $\frac{23}{45}$
19. $4\frac{13}{42}$
20. $18\frac{2}{3}$
21. 0.9
22. 0.3
23. 0.7
24. 0.9
25. $\frac{7}{8}$

26. $\frac{11}{12}$
27. 87.45
28. 5.008
29. 40.112
30. 47.77
31. 1,875
32. 23.7
33. 36.8
34. 0.674
35. 0.38
36. 0.6

37. $x = 12$
38. $x = 2$
39. $x = 3$
40. $x = 0.5$ or $\frac{1}{2}$
41. 0.4
42. 0.7
43. 1.5
44. 0.74
45. 0.83
46. 1.23

| | Percent | Decimal | Ratio | Fraction | |
|---|---|---|---|---|---|
| 47. | 6% | 0.06 | 3 : 50 | $\frac{3}{50}$ | |
| 48. | 35% | 0.35 | 7 : 20 | $\frac{7}{20}$ | 51. 4.75 |
| | | | | | 52. 5 |
| 49. | 525% | 5.25 | 21 : 4 | $5\frac{1}{4}$ | 53. 0.33% |
| | | | | | 54. 20% |
| 50. | 1.5% | 0.015 | 3 : 200 | $\frac{3}{200}$ | 55. 18.29% |

## CHAPTER 1

### Answers to Practice Problems

1. xv, $\overline{xv}$, XV
2. xiii, $\overline{xiii}$, XIII
3. xxviii, $\overline{xxviii}$, XXVIII
4. xi, $\overline{xi}$, XI
5. xvii, $\overline{xvii}$, XVII
6. 14
7. 29
8. 4
9. 19
10. 34

### Answers to Chapter Review

1. vi, $\overline{vi}$, VI
2. xxx, $\overline{xxx}$, XXX
3. iss, $\overline{iss}$, iss
4. xxvii, $\overline{xxvii}$, XXVII
5. xii, $\overline{xii}$, XII
6. xviii, $\overline{xviii}$, XVIII
7. xx, $\overline{xx}$, XX
8. iii, $\overline{iii}$, III
9. xxi, $\overline{xxi}$, XXI
10. xxvi, $\overline{xxvi}$, XXVI

11. $7\frac{1}{2}$
12. 19
13. 15
14. 30
15. $\frac{1}{2}$
16. 3
17. 22
18. 16
19. 5
20. 27

# CHAPTER 2
## Answers to Practice Problems

1. LCD $= 30$; therefore $\dfrac{6}{30}$ has the lesser value.

2. LCD $= 8$; therefore $\dfrac{6}{8}$ has the lesser value.

3. $\dfrac{1}{150}$ has the lesser value; the denominator (150) is larger.

4. $\dfrac{6}{18}$ has the lesser value; the numerator (6) is smaller.

5. $\dfrac{3}{5}$ has the lesser value; the numerator (3) is smaller.

6. $\dfrac{1}{8}$ has the lesser value; the numerator (1) is smaller.

7. $\dfrac{1}{40}$ has the lesser value; the denominator (40) is larger.

8. $\dfrac{1}{300}$ has the lesser value; the denominator (300) is larger.

9. $\dfrac{4}{24}$ has the lesser value; the numerator (4) is smaller.

10. LCD $= 6$; therefore $\dfrac{1}{6}$ has the lesser value.

11. LCD $= 72$; therefore $\dfrac{6}{8}$ has the higher value.

12. LCD $= 6$; therefore $\dfrac{7}{6}$ has the higher value.

13. LCD $= 72$; therefore $\dfrac{6}{12}$ has the higher value.

14. $\dfrac{1}{6}$ has the higher value; the denominator (6) is smaller.

15. $\dfrac{1}{75}$ has the higher value; the denominator (75) is smaller.

16. $\dfrac{6}{5}$ has the higher value; the numerator (6) is larger.

17. LCD $= 24$; therefore $\dfrac{4}{6}$ has the higher value.

18. $\dfrac{8}{9}$ has the higher value; the numerator (8) is larger.

19. $\dfrac{1}{10}$ has the higher value; the denominator (10) is smaller.

20. $\dfrac{6}{15}$ has the higher value; the numerator (6) is larger.

---

21. $\dfrac{10 \div 5}{15 \div 5} = \dfrac{2}{3}$

22. $\dfrac{7 \div 7}{49 \div 7} = \dfrac{1}{7}$

23. $\dfrac{64 \div 2}{128 \div 2} = \dfrac{32}{64} = \dfrac{1}{2}$

24. $\dfrac{100 \div 2}{150 \div 2} = \dfrac{50}{75} = \dfrac{2}{3}$

25. $\dfrac{20 \div 4}{28 \div 4} = \dfrac{5}{7}$

26. $\dfrac{14 \div 2}{98 \div 2} = \dfrac{7}{49} = \dfrac{1}{7}$

27. $\dfrac{10 \div 2}{18 \div 2} = \dfrac{5}{9}$

28. $\dfrac{24 \div 12}{36 \div 12} = \dfrac{2}{3}$

29. $\dfrac{10 \div 10}{50 \div 10} = \dfrac{1}{5}$

30. $\dfrac{9 \div 9}{27 \div 9} = \dfrac{1}{3}$

31. $\dfrac{9 \div 9}{9 \div 9} = \dfrac{1}{1} = 1$

32. $\dfrac{15 \div 15}{45 \div 15} = \dfrac{1}{3}$

33. $\dfrac{124 \div 31}{155 \div 31} = \dfrac{4}{5}$

34. $\dfrac{12 \div 6}{18 \div 6} = \dfrac{2}{3}$

35. $\dfrac{36 \div 4}{64 \div 4} = \dfrac{9}{16}$

36. $3\dfrac{3}{5}$

37. $4\dfrac{2}{7}$

38. $1\dfrac{5}{8}$

39. $2\dfrac{11}{12}$

40. $1\dfrac{3}{25}$

41. $\dfrac{29}{25}$

42. $\dfrac{34}{8}$

43. $\dfrac{9}{2}$

44. $\dfrac{27}{8}$

45. $\dfrac{79}{5}$

46. $1\dfrac{1}{2}$

47. $2\dfrac{19}{24}$

48. $7\dfrac{1}{6}$

49. $8\dfrac{1}{15}$

50. $22\dfrac{5}{6}$

51. $\dfrac{19}{21}$

52. $1\dfrac{31}{40}$

53. $\dfrac{11}{16}$

54. $\dfrac{1}{12}$

55. $\dfrac{1}{24}$

56. $\dfrac{8}{15}$

57. $\dfrac{18}{125}$

58. $\dfrac{3}{50}$

59. $7\dfrac{7}{32}$

60. $\dfrac{5}{27}$

61. $1\dfrac{13}{20}$

62. $\dfrac{1}{30}$

63. 15

64. 1

65. $2\dfrac{2}{19}$

## Answers to Chapter Review

1. $1\frac{2}{8} = 1\frac{1}{4}$

2. $7\frac{2}{4} = 7\frac{1}{2}$

3. $3\frac{4}{6} = 3\frac{2}{3}$

4. $2\frac{3}{4}$

5. $4\frac{3}{14}$

6. $6\frac{7}{10}$

7. $4\frac{1}{2}$

8. $2\frac{1}{5}$

9. $4\frac{4}{15}$

10. $7\frac{9}{13}$

11. $\frac{5}{2}$

12. $\frac{59}{8}$

13. $\frac{43}{5}$

14. $\frac{65}{4}$

15. $\frac{16}{5}$

16. $\frac{13}{5}$

17. $\frac{84}{10}$

18. $\frac{37}{4}$

19. $\frac{51}{4}$

20. $\frac{47}{7}$

21. LCD $= 30$; $1\frac{13}{30}$

22. LCD $= 24$; $\frac{13}{24}$

23. LCD $= 4$; $\frac{88}{4} = 22$

24. LCD $= 10$; $\frac{7}{10}$

25. LCD $= 36$; $\frac{234}{36} = 6\frac{18}{36} = 6\frac{1}{2}$

26. $\frac{1}{9}$

27. LCD $= 4$; $\frac{3}{4}$

28. $2\frac{2}{4} = 2\frac{1}{2}$

29. LCD $= 30$; $\frac{19}{30}$

30. LCD $= 4$; $1$

31. LCD $= 20$; $\frac{11}{20}$

32. LCD $= 24$; $\frac{7}{24}$

33. LCD $= 6$; $\frac{17}{6} = 2\frac{5}{6}$

34. LCD $= 15$; $\frac{19}{15} = 1\frac{4}{15}$

35. LCD $= 21$; $\frac{5}{21}$

36. $\frac{4}{36} = \frac{1}{9}$

37. $9\frac{11}{32}$

38. $14$

39. $10$

40. $27$

41. $\frac{10}{16} = \frac{5}{8}$

42. $\frac{2}{30} = \frac{1}{15}$

43. $\frac{12}{120} = \frac{1}{10}$

44. $\frac{7}{27}$

45. $\frac{50}{75} = \frac{2}{3}$

46. $\frac{42}{75} = \frac{14}{25}$

47. $\frac{2}{3}$

48. $2$

49. $1\frac{25}{50} = 1\frac{1}{2}$

50. $7\frac{1}{2}$

51. $\frac{28}{72} = \frac{7}{18}$

52. $1\frac{25}{50} = 1\frac{1}{2}$

53. $\frac{8}{6} = \frac{4}{3} = 1\frac{1}{3}$

54. $\frac{15}{300} = \frac{1}{20}$

55. $1$

56. $\frac{14}{16}, \frac{7}{16}, \frac{5}{16}, \frac{3}{16}, \frac{1}{16}$

57. $\frac{5}{6}, \frac{5}{8}, \frac{5}{12}, \frac{5}{32}, \frac{5}{64}$

58. $\frac{2}{5}$ of water remains

59. $\frac{1}{5}$ the dosage

60. $\frac{1}{6}$ of Ensure remains

61. 24 tablets

62. 280 mL

63. $2\frac{1}{4}$ lb

64. 84 hours

65. $4\frac{1}{12}$ ounces

# CHAPTER 3

## Answers to Practice Problems

1. eight and thirty-five hundredths

2. eleven and one thousandth

3. four and fifty-seven hundredths

4. five and seven ten thousandths

5. ten and five tenths

6. one hundred sixty-three thousandths

7. 0.4

8. 84.07

9. 0.07

10. 2.23

11. 0.05

12. 0.009

13. 0.5

14. 2.87

15. 0.375

16. 0.175

17. 7.35

18. 0.087

19. 18.4

20. 40.449

21. 3.95

22. 3.87

23. 2.92

24. 43.1

25. 0.035

26. 5.88

27. 0.04725

28. 0.9125

29. 9,650

30. 1.78

31. 100.8072

32. 4

33. 1.16

34. 70.88

35. 30.46

36. 0.59

37. 3.6

38. 1

39. 2

40. 3.55

41. 0.61

42. 0.74

43. 0.0005

44. 0.00004

45. 584

46. 500

47. 0.75

48. 0.555

49. 0.5

50. $\dfrac{3}{4}$

51. $\dfrac{1}{2000}$

52. $\dfrac{1}{25}$

## Answers to Chapter Review

1. 0.444

2. 0.8

3. 1.5

4. 0.2

5. 0.725

6. 9.783

7. 28.9

8. 2.743

9. 5.12

10. 2.5

11. 6.33

12. 1.5

13. 1.5

14. 15

15. 31.2

16. 0.94

17. 1.8

18. 0.1

19. 1.43

20. 0.15

21. 0.125

22. 0.06

23. 6.5

24. $1\dfrac{1}{100}$

25. $\dfrac{13}{200}$

26. 0.175 mg

27. 0.08 mg

28. 0.125 mg

29. 4.5 mg

30. 1.2 mg

31. 0.8

32. 565

33. 849

34. 23.4

35. 0.2

36. 0.65

37. 0.38

38. 0.52

39. 0.98

40. 0.35

41. 4.248

42. 0.567

43. 2.325

44. 7.839

45. 5.833

46. 4.55 L

47. 1.6 mg/dL

48. 3.05 kg

49. 0.1 mg

50. 0.352 g

51. False

52. True

53. No, 0.7 mg is outside the allowable limits of the safe dosage range of 0.175 mg to 0.35 mg. It is twice the allowable maximum dosage.

54. 0.4

55. 0.085

## CHAPTER 4
## Answers to Practice Problems

1. 1 : 100

2. 1 : 3

3. 1 : 2

4. 1 : 1,000

5. $\dfrac{15}{2}$, 15 : 2

6. 100 mg : 0.5 mL, 0.5 mL : 100 mg, 100 mg/0.5 mL, 0.5 mL/100 mg

7. 0.25 mg : 1 tab, 1 tab: 0.25 mg, 0.25 mg/1 tab, 1 tab/0.25 mg

8. 1 g : 10 mL, 10 mL : 1 g, 1 g/10 mL, 10 mL/1 g

9. 500 mg : 1 cap, 1 cap : 500 mg, 500 mg/1 cap, 1 cap/500 mg

10. $x = 9.6$

11. $x = 3$

12. $x = 2.4$

13. $x = 7.5$

14. $x = 18$

## Answers to Chapter Review

1. 2 : 3
2. 1 : 9
3. 3 : 4
4. 1 : 5
5. 1 : 2
6. 1 : 5
7. $\dfrac{3}{7}$
8. $\dfrac{2}{3}$
9. $\dfrac{1}{7}$
10. $1\dfrac{1}{3}$
11. $\dfrac{3}{4}$
12. $x = 5$
13. $x = 2$
14. $x = 4$
15. $x = 3.33$
16. $x = 4.5$
17. $x = 0.8$
18. $x = 1.33$

19. $x = 0.16$
20. $x = 0.1$
21. $x = 8$
22. $x = 22.5$
23. $x = 1.25$
24. $x = 0.6$
25. $x = 0.09$
26. 1,000 units : 1 mL *or* 1 mL : 1,000 units

$$\dfrac{1{,}000 \text{ units}}{1 \text{ mL}} \quad or \quad \dfrac{1 \text{ mL}}{1{,}000 \text{ units}}$$

27. 0.2 mg : 1 tab *or* 1 tab : 0.2 mg

$$\dfrac{0.2 \text{ mg}}{1 \text{ tab}} \quad or \quad \dfrac{1 \text{ tab}}{0.2 \text{ mg}}$$

28. 250 mg : 1 cap *or* 1 cap : 250 mg

$$\dfrac{250 \text{ mg}}{1 \text{ cap}} \quad or \quad \dfrac{1 \text{ cap}}{250 \text{ mg}}$$

29. 125 mg : 5 mL *or* 5 mL : 125 mg

$$\dfrac{125 \text{ mg}}{5 \text{ mL}} \quad or \quad \dfrac{5 \text{ mL}}{125 \text{ mg}}$$

30. 40 mg : 1 mL *or* 1 mL : 40 mg

$$\dfrac{40 \text{ mg}}{1 \text{ mL}} \quad or \quad \dfrac{1 \text{ mL}}{40 \text{ mg}}$$

31. 1,000 mcg : 2 mL *or* 2 mL : 1,000 mcg

$$\dfrac{1{,}000 \text{ mcg}}{2 \text{ mL}} \quad or \quad \dfrac{2 \text{ mL}}{1{,}000 \text{ mcg}}$$

32. 1 g : 3.6 mL *or* 3.6 mL : 1 g

$$\dfrac{1 \text{ g}}{3.6 \text{ mL}} \quad or \quad \dfrac{3.6 \text{ mL}}{1 \text{ g}}$$

33. 0.4 mg : 1 tab *or* 1 tab : 0.4 mg

$$\dfrac{0.4 \text{ mg}}{1 \text{ tab}} \quad or \quad \dfrac{1 \text{ tab}}{0.4 \text{ mg}}$$

34. 1 g : 1 cap *or* 1 cap : 1 g

$$\dfrac{1 \text{ g}}{1 \text{ cap}} \quad or \quad \dfrac{1 \text{ cap}}{1 \text{ g}}$$

35. 0.5 mg : 1 mL *or* 1 mL : 0.5 mg

$$\dfrac{0.5 \text{ mg}}{1 \text{ mL}} \quad or \quad \dfrac{1 \text{ mL}}{0.5 \text{ mg}}$$

36. 1 : 2,000
37. 1 : 400
38. 1 : 50
39. 1 : 5,000
40. 1 : 60

## CHAPTER 5

### Answers to Practice Problems

1. 50 g
2. 100 g
3. 12.5 g
4. 50 g
5. 7.5 g
6. 1%
7. 0.5%
8. 0.25%
9. $\dfrac{1}{100}$
10. $\dfrac{1}{50}$
11. $\dfrac{1}{2}$
12. $\dfrac{4}{5}$
13. $\dfrac{3}{100}$
14. 0.1
15. 0.35
16. 0.5

17. 0.14
18. 0.86
19. 1 : 4
20. 11 : 100
21. 3 : 4
22. 9 : 200
23. 1 : 250
24. 40%
25. 275%
26. 50%

27. 25%
28. 70%
29. 4%
30. 75%
31. 10%
32. 1%
33. 50%
34. 18
35. 15
36. 1%

37. 10%
38. 4%
39. 25.26
40. 0.42
41. 123.75
42. 62.5%
43. 25%
44. 0.17
45. 41.67%

## Answers to Chapter Review

| Percent | Ratio | Fraction | Decimal |
|---|---|---|---|
| 1. 52% | 13 : 25 | $\frac{13}{25}$ | 0.52 |
| 2. 71% | 71 : 100 | $\frac{71}{100}$ | 0.71 |
| 3. 7% | 7 : 100 | $\frac{7}{100}$ | 0.07 |
| 4. 2% | 1 : 50 | $\frac{1}{50}$ | 0.02 |
| 5. 6% | 3 : 50 | $\frac{3}{50}$ | 0.06 |
| 6. 38% | 3 : 8 | $\frac{3}{8}$ | 0.38 |
| 7. 61% | 61 : 100 | $\frac{61}{100}$ | 0.61 |
| 8. 0.7% | 7 : 1,000 | $\frac{7}{1,000}$ | 0.007 |
| 9. 5% | 1 : 20 | $\frac{1}{20}$ | 0.05 |
| 10. 2.5% | 1 : 40 | $\frac{1}{40}$ | 0.025 |

11. 4.8 oz
12. 56
13. 13.3%
14. 0.83%
15. 37.5
16. 25%
17. 0.25%
18. 4 : 25
19. 9 : 20
20. 400 mL
21. 9 oz
22. 99 mL
23. 20%
24. 7 lb
25. 4.4 oz
26. 23% protein, 4% fat
27. 92.3%
28. 30%
29. 357.5 mg
30. 7.7 mg

# ANSWERS TO POST-TEST FOR UNIT ONE

1. v, $\bar{v}$, V
2. xvii, $\overline{xvii}$, XVII
3. xxvii, $\overline{xxvii}$, XXVII
4. xxix, $\overline{xxix}$, XXIX
5. xxx, $\overline{xxx}$, XXX
6. $6\frac{1}{2}$
7. 24
8. 19
9. 25
10. 15
11. $1\frac{1}{3}$
12. $\frac{2}{3}$
13. $\frac{3}{7}$
14. $\frac{2}{3}$
15. $1\frac{3}{5}$
16. $1\frac{4}{21}$

17. $1\frac{2}{9}$
18. $25\frac{1}{3}$
19. $1\frac{22}{35}$
20. $1\frac{17}{36}$
21. 1.1
22. 0.1
23. 0.1
24. 0.9
25. $\frac{2}{3}$
26. $\frac{3}{4}$
27. 37.7
28. 17.407
29. 105.7
30. 32.94
31. 84.8
32. 22.5
33. 0.5

34. 0.85
35. 3.002
36. 0.493
37. $x = 4$
38. $x = 2.5$ *or* $2\frac{1}{2}$
39. $x = 0.1$ *or* $\frac{1}{10}$

40. $x = 4$
41. 0.6
42. 1
43. 1.4
44. 0.68
45. 0.83
46. 1.22

| Percent | Decimal | Ratio | Fraction |
|---|---|---|---|
| 47. 10% | 0.1 | 1 : 10 | $\frac{1}{10}$ |
| 48. 60% | 0.6 | 3 : 5 | $\frac{3}{5}$ |
| 49. $66\frac{2}{3}$% | 0.67 | 67 : 100 | $\frac{67}{100}$ |
| 50. 25% | 0.25 | 1 : 4 | $\frac{1}{4}$ |

51. 18
52. 18.75
53. 66 2/3% *or* 66.7% *or* 67%
54. 0.25%
55. 38.46% *or* 38.5% *or* 39%

56. 1 : 80
57. 1 : 20
58. 1 : 300
59. 1 : 80
60. 1 : 1,000

## CHAPTER 6

### Answers to Practice Problems

1. 0.3 g
2. 6,000 mcg
3. 700 mL
4. 0.18 mg
5. 20 mcg
6. 4,500 mL
7. 4,200 mg
8. 900 mg
9. 3.25 L
10. 0.042 kg
11. 0.529 g
12. 0.645 mg
13. 347,000 mL
14. 238,000,000 mcg
15. 3.5 L
16. 40 g
17. 658,000 g
18. 0.051 L
19. 1,600 mcg
20. 0.028 L

### Answers to Chapter Review

1. gram (g), liter (L), meter (m)
2. kilogram (kg)
3. 0.001 L
4. a. L (liter), mL (milliliter)
   b. g (gram), mg (milligram), mcg (microgram), kg (kilogram)
5. 1 g
6. 1,000 mL
7. 1 mg
8. 1 L
9. L
10. mcg
11. mL
12. g
13. kg
14. thousand times
15. the thousandth part of
16. 0.6 g
17. 50 kg
18. 0.4 mg
19. 0.04 L
20. 4.2 mcg
21. 0.005 g
22. 0.06 g
23. 2.6 mL
24. 100 mL
25. 0.03 mL
26. 0.95 mg
27. 58,500 mL
28. 0.13 L
29. 276,000 mg
30. 0.55 L
31. 56,500 mL
32. 0.205 kg
33. 25 g
34. 1,000 mL
35. 15 mg
36. 0.25 mg
37. 8,000 g
38. 2,000 L
39. 5,000 mL
40. 750 mL
41. 330 mg
42. 0.75 g
43. 6,280 g
44. 0.0365 g
45. 0.0022 g
46. 0.4 kg
47. 24 mL
48. 0.1 g
49. 150,000 mg
50. 0.085 mg
51. 1,250 mL
52. 50 mcg
53. 0.12 g
54. 0.475 L
55. 4,500 mg
56. 0.5 g
57. 4 kg
58. Lasix 20 mg
59. Gentamicin 1.5 mL
60. Ampicillin 500 mg

## CHAPTER 7

### Answers to Practice Problems

1. oz
2. gr
3. pt
4. 15 mL
5. 10 mL
6. 3 tbs
7. oz 8
8. oz 3
9. oz 10
10. gr $^1/_2$, gr $\overline{ss}$, gr ss
11. 1 T, 1 tbs (varies)
12. 5 cups

### Answers to Chapter Review

1. gr $8\frac{1}{2}$, gr viiiss
2. oz 8, 8 oz
3. qt
4. pt
5. gr $\frac{1}{125}$
6. 2 oz, oz 2
7. 5 oz, oz 5
8. weight
9. 1 g
10. 60
11. oz 16, 16 oz
12. oz 32, 32 oz
13. 900 mg (gr 15 = 1 g)
14. gtt
15. tablespoon
16. teaspoon
17. 5 mL
18. 30 mL
19. 8 oz
20. 15 mL
21. 16 oz
22. 32 oz

## CHAPTER 8
### Answers to Practice Problems

1. 0.6 L
2. 16 mg
3. 4,000 g
4. 0.003 mg
5. 0.0003 g
6. 10 g
7. 1,900 mL
8. 0.0005 kg
9. 70 mcg
10. 0.65 L
11. 40 mg
12. 0.00012 kg
13. 0.18 g
14. 1.7 L
15. 15,000 g
16. 3,500 mg
17. 160 g
18. 4 mL
19. 0.001 L
20. 0.008 g
21. 500 mg
22. 0.3 kg
23. 0.025 g
24. 65,000 g
25. 6 mcg
26. 0.5 L
27. 4,000 g
28. 1,400 mL
29. oz $1\frac{1}{2}$, $1\frac{1}{2}$ oz
30. 4,500 mcg
31. 105 mL
32. 6,500 mL
33. 0.06 kg
34. 0.6 g
35. 736 mcg
36. 1.6 L
37. 15 mL
38. 180 mg
39. 0.025 mg
40. 0.0052 kg
41. 27.27 kg
42. gr 1/4
43. 150 mL
44. 300 mg
45. 210 mL
46. 1/4 qt
47. 3 tbs
48. 3 g
49. 90 mg
50. 4 tsp
51. 330 mg
52. 4,000 mL
53. 158.4 lb *or* $158\frac{2}{5}$ lb
54. 0.48 mg
55. 2,400 mL
56. 700 mL
57. 550 mL
58. 900 mL
59. 81 mL/hr
60. 31 mL/hr
61. 42 mL/hr
62. 52 mL/hr
63. 875 mL
64. 0.875 L
65. 125 mL

### Answers to Chapter Review

1. 7 mg
2. 0.001 g
3. 6 kg
4. 0.005 L
5. 450 mL
6. oz $2\frac{1}{2}$, $2\frac{1}{2}$ oz
7. 0.2 mg
8. gr $\frac{1}{60}$
9. 120 mg
10. 1,500 mL
11. gr ss, gr $\overline{ss}$, gr $\frac{1}{2}$
12. 1,600 mL
13. 103.4 lb *or* $103\frac{2}{5}$ lb
14. 0.003 L
15. 34.09 kg
16. 8 mg
17. 2,250 mL
18. 30 mg
19. 0.4 mg
20. 6.172 kg
21. 40 tsp
22. 46.36 kg
23. 0.204 kg
24. 1,500 mL
25. 0.2 mg
26. 48,600 mL
27. 700 mL
28. 195 mL
29. 20 mL
30. 240 mg (gr i = 60 mg)
31. 30 mL
32. $13\frac{1}{2}$ t
33. gr $\frac{3}{4}$
34. 3 g
35. 600 mL
36. 150 mg
37. 22.5 mg
38. 600 mg (gr i = 60 mg)
39. 8.8 lb *or* $8\frac{4}{5}$ lb
40. 3,250 mcg
41. oz $\frac{1}{3}$
42. 0.5 mg
43. 6,653 mg
44. 4,000 mg
45. 0.036 g
46. 800 mg
47. gr 135 or gr cxxxv
48. gr $\frac{1}{120}$
49. 2 L
50. 245 mL
51. 1,310 mL
52. 540 mL
53. 720 mL
54. 270 mL
55. 870 mL
56. 105 mL
57. 180 mL
58. 725 mL
59. 450 mL
60. 925 mL
61. 63 mL/hr
62. 27 mL/hr
63. 88 mL/hr
64. 375 mL
65. 275 mL
66. 1.75 L
67. 0.125 mg
68. $2\frac{1}{2}$ cups
69. 50 oz, oz 50
70. 1,100 mL

## CHAPTER 9
### Answers to Practice Problems

1. 39.2° F
2. 38.3° C
3. 100.6° F
4. 38.5° C
5. 99.5° F
6. 68° F to 77° F
7. 38.3° C
8. −13.9° C
9. 98.6° F
10. 7.8° C
11. 4 in
12. 4.5 cm
13. 375 mm
14. 51.25 cm
15. 37 cm
16. 2.6 in
17. 250 cm
18. 12.8 in
19. 15.2 in
20. 50 cm
21. 2.9 kg
22. 5.5 kg
23. 4.7 kg
24. 3.5 kg
25. 9.1 kg

| | | | | |
|---|---|---|---|---|
| 26. 29.1 kg | 32. 216 lb | 37. 1030 | 42. 1330 | 47. 12:59 PM |
| 27. 10 kg | 33. 22.9 lb | 38. 2010 | 43. 2:07 AM | 48. 0445 |
| 28. 55 kg | 34. 76.8 lb | 39. 1745 | 44. 5:43 PM | 49. 0800 |
| 29. 38.6 kg | 35. 12.8 lb | 40. 0016 | 45. 12:04 AM | 50. 7:15 AM |
| 30. 44 lb | 36. 0730 | 41. 0620 | 46. 2:40 AM | 51. 3:30 PM |
| 31. 101.2 lb | | | | |

## Answers to Chapter Review

| | | | | |
|---|---|---|---|---|
| 1. 38.6° C | 16. 21.1° C | 30. 10 cm | 44. 19.8 lb | 58. 4:50 PM |
| 2. 25° C | 17. 103.3° F | 31. 366 mm | 45. 123.4 lb | 59. 1:45 PM |
| 3. 59° F to 86° F | 18. 18° C | 32. 15.5 cm | 46. 31.8 kg | 60. 9:22 PM |
| 4. 97.7° F | 19. 95° F | 33. 14 in | 47. 4.1 cm | 61. 0520 |
| 5. 42.8° F | 20. 10° C | 34. 53.75 cm | 48. 218.2 lb | 62. 2400 |
| 6. 100° F | 21. 103.6° F | 35. 50 mm | 49. 16 in | (0000 used in military) |
| 7. 28.9° C | 22. 30° C | 36. 28.6 kg | 50. 406 mm | 63. 0005 |
| 8. 366.8° F | 23. 105.8° F | 37. 68.2 kg | 51. 3.2 kg | 64. 1630 |
| 9. 39.2° F | 24. 45 cm | 38. 35.5 kg | 52. 4.2 kg | 65. 1335 |
| 10. 31.1° C | 25. 12.4 in | 39. 36.8 kg | 53. 4.9 kg | 66. AM |
| 11. 14° F | 26. 445 mm | 40. 12.3 kg | 54. 3.9 kg | 67. PM |
| 12. −17.8° C | 27. 80 cm | 41. 170.1 lb | 55. 2.4 kg | 68. 0300 |
| 13. 39.3° C | 28. 30 mm | 42. 15.4 lb | 56. 12:32 AM | 69. 3:20 AM |
| 14. 84.2° F | 29. 79 mm | 43. 9.9 lb | 57. 2:20 AM | 70. 0140 |
| 15. 222.8° F | | | | |

# CHAPTER 10

## Answers to Practice Problems

1. metric, apothecary, and house-hold
2. elderly and children
3. route
4. smaller
5. souffle
6. topical
7. assessment, nursing diagnosis, planning, implementation, evaluation, teaching
8. critical thinking
9. calibrated
10. buccal

## Answers to Chapter Review

1. medication, dosage, client, route, time, documentation
2. two, client's (patient's) room number
3. three
4. after
5. parenteral, oral, inhalation, insertion, topical, percutaneous, intranasal
6. 30 mL or 1 oz
7. False
8. oral syringe
9. milliliters (mL)
10. 30 mL
11. medication-related problems
12. Institute for Safe Medication Practices
13. The Joint Commission
14. intranasal
15. heparin, insulin, morphine, neuromuscular drugs, chemotherapy drugs

# CHAPTER 11

## Answers to Practice Problems

1. after meals
2. hour
3. every twelve hours, every 12 hours
4. twice daily, twice a day
5. when necessary/required, as needed
6. Give or administer zidovudine 200 milligrams orally (by mouth) every 4 hours.
7. Give or administer procaine penicillin G 400,000 units by intravenous injection every 8 hours.
8. Give or administer gentamicin sulfate 45 milligrams by intravenous piggyback injection every 12 hours.
9. Give or administer regular Humulin insulin 5 units by subcutaneous injection before meals at 7:30 AM and at bedtime.
10. Give or administer vitamin B$_{12}$ 1,000 micrograms by intramuscular injection every other day.
11. Give or administer Prilosec 20 milligrams orally (by mouth) twice a day (two times a day).
12. Give or administer Tofranil 75 milligrams orally (by mouth) at bedtime.
13. Give or administer Restoril 30 milligrams orally (by mouth) at bedtime.
14. Give or administer Mylanta 30 milliliters orally (by mouth) every 4 hours when necessary (when required).
15. Give or administer Synthroid 200 micrograms orally (by mouth) daily.

## Answers to Chapter Review

1. name of the client
2. date and time the order was written
3. name of the medication
4. dosage of medication
5. route by which medication is to be administered
6. time and/or frequency of administration
7. signature of the person writing the order
8. twice a day (twice daily, two times a day)
9. as desired
10. subcutaneous
11. with
12. before meals
13. four times a day
14. twice a week
15. elixir
16. syrup
17. nothing by mouth
18. sublingual
19. p.c. *or* pc
20. t.i.d. *or* tid
21. I.M. *or* IM
22. q.8.h. *or* q8h
23. supp
24. I.V. *or* IV
25. s.o.s. *or* sos
26. $\bar{s}$
27. stat *or* STAT
28. ung *or* oint
29. mEq
30. p.r. *or* pr

31. Give or administer Methergine 0.2 milligrams orally (by mouth) every 4 hours for 6 doses.
32. Give or administer digoxin 0.125 milligrams orally (by mouth) once a day.
33. Give or administer regular Humulin insulin 14 units by subcutaneous injection daily at 7:30 AM.
34. Give or administer Demerol 50 milligrams by intramuscular injection and atropine 0.4 milligrams by intramuscular injection on call to the operating room.
35. Give or administer ampicillin 500 milligrams orally (by mouth) immediately and then 250 milligrams orally (by mouth) four times a day thereafter.
36. Give or administer Lasix 40 milligrams by intramuscular injection immediately (at once).
37. Give or administer Librium 50 milligrams orally (by mouth) every 4 hours when necessary (when required) for agitation.
38. Give or administer Tylenol 650 milligrams orally (by mouth) every 4 hours when necessary (when required) for pain.
39. Give or administer Mylicon 80 milligrams orally (by mouth) after meals and at bedtime.
40. Give or administer folic acid 1 milligram orally (by mouth) every day.
41. Give or administer Nembutal 100 milligrams orally (by mouth) at bedtime when necessary (when required).
42. Give or administer aspirin 10 grains orally (by mouth) every 4 hours when necessary (when required) for temperature greater than 101° F.
43. Give or administer Dilantin 100 milligrams orally (by mouth) three times a day.
44. Give or administer Minipress 2 milligrams orally (by mouth) two times a day. Hold for systolic blood pressure less than 120.
45. Give or administer Compazine 10 milligrams by intramuscular injection every 4 hours when necessary (when required) for nausea or vomiting.
46. Give or administer ampicillin 1 gram by intravenous piggyback injection every 6 hours for 4 doses.

47. Give or administer heparin 5,000 units by subcutaneous injection every 12 hours.

48. Give or administer Dilantin suspension 200 milligrams every morning and 300 milligrams by nasogastric tube at bedtime.

49. Give or administer Benadryl 50 milligrams orally (by mouth) immediately (at once).

50. Give or administer vitamin $B_{12}$ 1,000 micrograms by intramuscular injection three times a week.

51. Give or administer milk of magnesia 30 milliliters orally (by mouth) at bedtime when necessary (when required) for constipation.

52. Give or administer Septra 1 double-strength tablet orally (by mouth) daily.

53. Apply or administer neomycin ophthalmic 1% ointment to the right eye three times a day.

54. Give or administer Carafate 1 gram by nasogastric tube four times a day.

55. Give or administer morphine sulfate 15 milligrams by subcutaneous injection immediately (at once) and 10 milligrams by subcutaneous injection every 4 hours when necessary (when required) for pain.

56. Give or administer ampicillin 120 milligrams by intravenous Soluset every 6 hours for 7 days.

57. Give or administer prednisone 10 milligrams orally (by mouth) every other day.

58. route of administration

59. frequency of administration

60. dosage of medication (drug)

61. name of medication (drug)

62. dosage of medication (drug) and route of administration

63. Notify the prescriber that the order is incomplete; route is missing from the order; do not administer, order not legal. Never assume.

64. Inderal 20 mg po daily. Adequate spacing is needed among drug name, dosage, and unit of measure. Could be misread as 120 mg, which is 6 times the dosage ordered.

65. Lasix 10 mg po bid. Trailing zeros could cause dosage to be interpreted as 100 mg.

66. Humulin Regular Insulin 4 units IV stat. The abbreviation for units here could be misread as a zero. Write out units.

67. Haldol 0.5 mg po tid. Omission of the zero before the decimal point could result in the dosage being read as 5 mg, which would be 10 times the dosage ordered.

## CHAPTER 12

### Answers to Practice Problems

1. True
2. False
3. True
4. client, medication (drug), dosage, dose (amount), route, time, documentation
5. nurse
6. automated dispensing cabinet (ADC). Sometimes referred to as computer-controlled dispensing system
7. override, verification
8. False
9. documentation
10. computer prescriber order entry

### Answers to Practice Exercise 1 (Reading of Medication Record, Figure 12-1)

Questions relating to this assignment not in chapter.

| Date 4/2/11 | Medication | Dosage | Route | Time |
|---|---|---|---|---|
| 1. | Keflex | 250 mg | p.o. | 9 AM |
| 2. | Keflex | 250 mg | p.o. | 1 PM |
| 3. | MVI | 1 tab | p.o. | 9 AM |
| 4. | Colace | 100 mg | p.o. | 9 AM |

| Date 4/3/11 | Medication | Dosage | Route | Time |
|---|---|---|---|---|
| 1. | Keflex | 250 mg | p.o. | 5 PM |
| 2. | Keflex | 250 mg | p.o. | 9 PM |
| 3. | Colace | 100 mg | p.o. | 5 PM |

### Answers to Chapter Review

1. hospital, institution, or health care facility
2. No, b.i.d. means the order will be given two times in 24 hours, whereas a q2h order would be given 12 times in 24 hours.
3. to ensure dispensing and administration of the correct medication to the right client
4. electronic medication administration record
5. traditional time, military time (international time)

**Answers to Chapter Review Exercise 1 (Figure 12-7)**

## ST. BARNABAS HOSPITAL
### BRONX, NY 10457

### DEPARTMENT OF NURSING
### MEDICATION ADMINISTRATION RECORD

| DIAGNOSIS: |
| --- |
| Pancreatitis |

| ALLERGIC TO: | NKDA | DATE 4/9/11 |
| --- | --- | --- |

Addressograph or printed label with client identification.

LEGEND
Omitted doses (use red pen):
Document in Medication Omission Record

1. NPO    3. I.V. Out    5. Other
2. Off-unit    4. Pt. Refused

Page ____ of ____

| ORDER DATE / EXP DATE | STANDING MEDICATION / MED-DOSE-FREQ-ROUTE | DATE 2011 / HOUR | 4/9 INIT. | 4/10 INIT. | 4/11 INIT. | 4/12 INIT. | 4/13 INIT. | 4/14 INIT. | 4/15 INIT. | 4/16 INIT. | 4/17 INIT. |
| --- | --- | --- | --- | --- | --- | --- | --- | --- | --- | --- | --- |
| RN. INIT. DM — 4/9/11 / 5/9/11 | Norvasc 5 mg PO daily / hold for SBP less than 100 | 9A / B/P | | | | | | | | | |
| RN. INIT. DM — 4/9/11 / 5/9/11 | Thiamine 100 mg PO / daily | 9A | | | | | | | | | |
| RN. INIT. DM — 4/9/11 / 4/16/11 | Heparin 5,000 units subcut / q12h | 9A / site / 9P / site | | | | | | | | | |
| RN. INIT. DM — 4/9/11 / 5/9/11 | FeSO4 325 mg PO / tid | 9A / 1P / 5P | | | | | | | | | |
| RN. INIT. | | | | | | | | | | | |

INJECTION CODES:
RT = RIGHT THIGH    RA = RIGHT ARM    ▲ RAB = UPPER RIGHT ABDOMEN    ▲ LAB = UPPER LEFT ABDOMEN
LT = LEFT THIGH    LA = LEFT ARM    ▼ RAB = LOWER RIGHT ABDOMEN    ▼ LAB = LOWER LEFT ABDOMEN

Used with permission of St. Barnabas Hospital, Bronx, New York.

## Answers to Chapter Review Exercise 2 (Figure 12-8)

### ST. BARNABAS HOSPITAL
BRONX, NY 10457

DEPARTMENT OF NURSING
MEDICATION ADMINISTRATION RECORD

| DIAGNOSIS: |
|---|
| Pancreatitis |

| ALLERGIC TO: | DATE |
|---|---|
| NKDA | 4/10/11 |

Addressograph or printed label
with client identification

| ORDER DATE / EXP DATE | REORDER DATE / EXP DATE | P.R.N. MEDICATION / MED-DOSE-FREQ-ROUTE | | | | | | | | | | |
|---|---|---|---|---|---|---|---|---|---|---|---|---|
| DM R.N. INIT. 4/10/11 | | Percocet 2 tabs | DATE | 4/10 | / | / | / | / | / | / | / | / |
| | | PO q4h prn for | TIME | 2p | | | | | | | | |
| | | pain X 3 days | SITE | PO | | | | | | | | |
| REORD INIT. 4/13/11 | | | INIT. | DM | | | | | | | | |
| DM R.N. INIT. 4/10/11 | | Tylenol 650 mg | DATE | / | / | / | / | / | / | / | / | / |
| | | PO q4h prn for | TIME | | | | | | | | | |
| | | Temp greater than 101° F | SITE | | | | | | | | | |
| REORD INIT. 4/17/11 | | | INIT. | | | | | | | | | |
| R.N. INIT. | | | DATE | / | / | / | / | / | / | / | / | / |
| | | | TIME | | | | | | | | | |
| | | | SITE | | | | | | | | | |
| REORD INIT. | | | INIT. | | | | | | | | | |
| R.N. INIT. | | | DATE | / | / | / | / | / | / | / | / | / |
| | | | TIME | | | | | | | | | |
| | | | SITE | | | | | | | | | |
| REORD INIT. | | | INIT. | | | | | | | | | |
| R.N. INIT. | | | DATE | / | / | / | / | / | / | / | / | / |
| | | | TIME | | | | | | | | | |
| | | | SITE | | | | | | | | | |
| REORD INIT. | | | INIT. | | | | | | | | | |

### INITIAL IDENTIFICATION

| | INITIAL | PRINT NAME, TITLE | | INITIAL | PRINT NAME, TITLE | | INITIAL | PRINT NAME, TITLE |
|---|---|---|---|---|---|---|---|---|
| 1 | DM | Deborah C. Morris RN | 1 | | | 1 | | |
| 2 | | | 2 | | | 2 | | |
| 3 | | | 3 | | | 3 | | |
| 4 | | | 4 | | | 4 | | |

Used with permission of St. Barnabas Hospital, Bronx, New York.

# CHAPTER 13

## Answers to Practice Problems

1. Trade name: Augmentin
   Generic name: amoxicillin/clavulanate potassium
   Form: oral suspension
   Dosage strength: 125 mg per 5 mL
   Total volume: 100 mL (when reconstituted)
2. Trade name: Vistaril
   Generic name: hydroxyzine hydrochloride
   Form: injectable liquid
   Dosage strength: 50 mg per mL
   Total volume: 10 mL
3. Dosage strength: 100 mg per capsule
   Total amount in container: 1,000 capsules

4. Trade name: Gleevec
   Generic name: imatinib mesylate
   Dosage strength: 400 mg per tab
   Total amount in container: 30 tablets (tabs)
   Storage: See package insert. Store at 25° C (77° C); excursions permitted to 15° to 30° C.
5. Trade name: Coumadin
   Form: tablets
   Dosage strength: $2^{1}/_{2}$ mg per tablet
   NDC number: 0056-0176-90
   Total amount in container: 1,000 tablets (tabs)

## Answers to Chapter Review

1. Trade name: Coumadin
   Generic name: warfarin sodium
   Form: tablets (tabs)
   Dosage strength: 5 mg per tablet
   Total amount in container: 100 tablets (tabs)
   Warning: highly potent anticoagulant. Serious bleeding results from overdosage. Do not use or dispense before reading directions and warnings in accompanying product information.
2. Trade name: Lanoxin
   Generic name: digoxin
   Form: injectable liquid
   Total volume: 2 mL
   Dosage strength: 250 mcg per mL, 500 mcg per 2 mL
3. Trade name: Cialis
   Generic name: tadalafil
   Form: tablets (tabs)
   Dosage strength: 10 mg per tablet (tab)
   Total amount in container: 30 tablets (tabs)
   Storage: Store at 25° C (77° F). See insert.
4. Trade name: Synthroid
   Generic name: levothyroxine sodium
   Form: tablets (tabs)
   Dosage strength: 50 mcg per tablet, 0.05 mg per tablet
   Total amount in container: 100 tablets (tabs)
5. Trade name: none stated
   Generic name: potassium chloride
   Drug manufacturer: Lyphomed
   Form: injectable liquid
   Dosage strength: 2 mEq per mL or 40 mEq per 20 mL

6. Trade name: Fortovase
   Generic name: saquinavir
   Form: capsules; soft gelatin capsules
   Dosage strength: 200 mg per capsule (caps)
   Total amount in container: 180 capsules (caps)
   Usual dosage: See accompanying package insert.
   Alert: Find out about medicines that should not be taken with Fortovase.
7. Trade name: none stated
   Generic name: streptomycin sulfate
   Form: powder (injectable liquid once reconstituted)
   Directions for mixing: The dry powder is dissolved by adding 9 mL water USP or sodium chloride for injection.
   Dosage strength after reconstitution: 400 mg per mL.
   Storage: In dry form store below 86° F (30° C). Protect reconstituted solution from light, may store at room temperature for 4 weeks.
8. Generic name: morphine sulfate
   Form: oral solution
   NDC number: 0054-8585
   Dosage strength: 10 mg per 5 mL
   Warning: may be habit forming
   Controlled substance schedule: 2
   Total volume: 5 mL

9. Trade name: Diovan

   Generic name: valsartan

   Form: tablets

   Dosage strength: 40 mg per tablet (tab)

   Storage: Store at 25° C (77° F); excursions permitted to 15° to 30° C (59° to 86° F) (see USP controlled room temperature). Protect from moisture. Dispense in tight container (USP).

10. Trade name: Zantac

    Generic name: ranitidine hydrochloride

    Form: injectable liquid

    Dosage strength: 25 mg per mL

11. Trade name: Cipro

    Generic name: ciprofloxacin hydrochloride

    Total amount in container: 50 tablets (tabs)

    Form: tablets

    Dosage strength: 750 mg per tablet

12. Trade name: Fungizone

    Generic name: amphotericin B

    Form: powder (injectable liquid once reconstituted)

    Drug manufacturer: Apothecon

13. Trade name: Depo-Provera

    Generic name: medroxyprogesterone acetate

    Form: injectable suspension

    Dosage strength: 150 mg per mL

    Directions for use: Contraceptive (intramuscular use only); shake vigorously before using.

    NDC number: 0009-7376-01

14. Trade name: Depo-Provera

    Generic name: medroxyprogesterone acetate

    Dosage strength: 400 mg per mL

    Directions for use: For intramuscular use only; shake vigorously immediately before each use.

15. Form: sublingual tablets

    Dosage strength: 2,500 mcg per tablet (tab)

    Suggested use: as a dietary supplement

    Total amount in container: 90 tablets (tabs)

16. Generic name: ibutilide fumarate

    Form: injectable liquid (intravenous infusion only)

    Dosage strength: 0.1 mg per mL

    Directions for use: for IV use only

17. Trade name: none stated

    Generic name: hydromorphone hydrochloride

    Directions for use: IM, SC,* or slow IV use

    Form: injectable liquid

    Dosage strength: 2 mg per mL

    Total volume: 20 mL

    Warning: may be habit forming

18. Trade name: Zocor

    Generic name: simvastatin

    Dosage strength: 10 mg per tablet (tab)

    NDC number: 0006-0735-61

19. Generic name: diltiazem HCl

    Form: sustained-release capsules

    Dosage strength: 60 mg per capsule (caps)

20. Trade name: Ativan

    Dosage strength: 0.5 mg per tablet

    Total amount in container: 100 tablets

    Controlled substance schedule: 4

21. Trade name: Epogen

    Generic name: epoetin alfa

    Total volume: 2 mL

    Dosage strength: 10,000 units per mL, 20,000 units per 2 mL

    Storage: Store at 2° to 8° C.

22. Trade name: none stated

    Generic name: atropine sulfate

    Dosage strength: 0.5 mg per 5 mL, 0.1 mg per mL

    Total volume: 5 mL

23. Trade name: Glucophage

    Generic name: metformin hydrochloride

    Form: tablets

    Dosage strength: 500 mg per tablet (tab)

    Total amount in container: 500 tablets

24. Generic name: methylphenidate hydrochloride

    Dosage strength: 5 mg per tablet (tab)

    Instructions to pharmacist: Dispense in a tight, light-resistant container as defined in the USP with a child-resistant closure.

25. Trade name: Easprin

    Form: delayed-release, enteric-coated tablets

    Total amount in container: 100 delayed-release, enteric-coated tablets

---

*Note:* SC is older abbreviation used for subcutaneous. Correct abbreviation is subcut.

26. Trade name: Meclomen

    Generic name: meclofenamate sodium

    Form: capsules

    Dosage strength: 50 mg per capsule (cap)

27. Trade name: Bumex

    Generic name: bumetanide

    Form: injectable liquid

    Dosage strength: 0.5 mg per 2 mL; 0.25 mg per mL

    Directions for use: for intramuscular or intravenous use

28. Total volume: 1,000 mL

    Form: oral solution

    Dosage strength: 10 g per 15 mL

    Storage: store at controlled room temperature: 15° to 30° C (59° to 86° F). Do not freeze.

29. Trade name: Halcion

    Generic name: triazolam

    Dosage strength: 0.125 mg per tablet (tab)

    Total amount in container: 10 tablets

30. Trade name: Celebrex

    Generic name: celecoxib

    Form: capsules

    Dosage strength: 100 mg per capsule (cap)

31. Trade name: none stated

    Generic name: nitroglycerin

    Form: extended-release capsules

    Dosage strength: 9 mg per extended-release capsule (cap)

    Storage information: store at controlled room temperature: 15° to 30° C (59° to 86° F).

32. Trade name: Biaxin

    Generic name: clarithromycin

    Form: granules

    Dosage strength (when reconstituted oral suspension): 125 mg per 5 mL

    Total volume when mixed: 100 mL

33. by mouth, p.o.

34. 5 mg of hydrocodone bitartrate and 500 mg of acetaminophen

35. 100 tablets

36. B (Percocet)

37. 4.5 mg of oxycodone hydrochloride and 325 mg of aspirin. Percocet contains 5 mg of oxycodone hydrochloride and 325 mg of acetaminophen.

38. Percodan (it contains aspirin)

39. 10%

40. 100 mg per mL

# CHAPTER 14

## Answers to Practice Problems

1. Less than 1 tab

2. More than 1 tab

3. Less than 1 tab

4. Less than 1 tab

5. More than 1 tab

6. $\dfrac{5 \text{ mg}}{1 \text{ tab}} = \dfrac{7.5 \text{ mg}}{x \text{ tab}}$

   $\dfrac{5x}{5} = \dfrac{7.5}{5}$

   *or*

   5 mg : 1 tab = 7.5 mg : $x$ tab

   $\dfrac{5x}{5} = \dfrac{7.5}{5}$

   $x = \dfrac{7.5}{5}$

   $x = 1.5$ tabs or $1\dfrac{1}{2}$ tabs. 5 mg is less than 7.5 mg; therefore you will need more than 1 tab to administer the dosage.

7. Equivalent: 60 mg = gr 1 (gr $\dfrac{3}{4}$ = 45 mg)

   $\dfrac{30 \text{ mg}}{1 \text{ tab}} = \dfrac{45 \text{ mg}}{x \text{ tab}}$

   $\dfrac{30x}{30} = \dfrac{45}{30}$

   $x = \dfrac{45}{30}$

   *or*

   30 mg : 1 tab = 45 mg : $x$ tab

   $\dfrac{30x}{30} = \dfrac{45}{30}$

   $x = \dfrac{45}{30}$

   $x = 1.5$ tabs or $1\dfrac{1}{2}$ tabs. 45 mg is more than 30; therefore you need more than 1 tab to administer the dosage.

8. Equivalent: 60 mg = gr 1

$$\text{gr } 1\frac{1}{2} = 90 \text{ mg}$$

$$\frac{100 \text{ mg}}{1 \text{ cap}} = \frac{90 \text{ mg}}{x \text{ cap}}$$

$$\frac{100x}{100} = \frac{90}{100}$$

$$x = \frac{90}{100}$$

*or*

$$100 \text{ mg} : 1 \text{ cap} = 90 \text{ mg} : x \text{ cap}$$

$$\frac{100x}{100} = \frac{90}{100}$$

$$x = \frac{90}{100}$$

$x = 1$ cap. It would be impossible to administer 0.9 of a capsule. A 10% margin of difference is allowed between what is ordered and what is administered. When this 10% safety margin is used, no more than 110 mg and no less than 90 mg may be given. The prescriber ordered gr $1\frac{1}{2}$ (90 mg). The capsules available are 100 mg. Capsules are not divisible. Administering 1 cap is within the 10% margin of difference allowed.

9. 
$$\frac{0.5 \text{ mg}}{1 \text{ mL}} = \frac{0.25 \text{ mg}}{x \text{ mL}}$$

$$\frac{0.5x}{0.5} = \frac{0.25}{0.5}$$

$$x = \frac{0.25}{0.5}$$

*or*

$$0.5 \text{ mg} : 1 \text{ mL} = 0.25 \text{ mg} : x \text{ mL}$$

$$\frac{0.5x}{0.5} = \frac{0.25}{0.5}$$

$$x = \frac{0.25}{0.5}$$

$x = 0.5$ mL, 0.25 mg is less than 0.5 mg; you will need less than 1 mL to administer the dosage.

10. 
$$\frac{125 \text{ mg}}{5 \text{ mL}} = \frac{100 \text{ mg}}{x \text{ mL}}$$

$$\frac{125x}{125} = \frac{500}{125}$$

$$x = \frac{500}{125}$$

*or*

$$125 \text{ mg} : 5 \text{ mL} = 100 \text{ mg} : x \text{ mL}$$

$$\frac{125x}{125} = \frac{500}{125}$$

$$x = \frac{500}{125}$$

$x = 4$ mL. 100 mg is less than 125 mg; therefore you will need less than 5 mL to administer the dosage.

11. 
$$\frac{40 \text{ mEq}}{10 \text{ mL}} = \frac{20 \text{ mEq}}{x \text{ mL}}$$

$$\frac{40x}{40} = \frac{200}{40}$$

$$40 \text{ mEq} : 10 \text{ mL} = 20 \text{ mEq} : x \text{ mL}$$

*or*

$$\frac{40x}{40} = \frac{200}{40}$$

$$x = \frac{200}{40}$$

$x = 5$ mL. 20 mEq is less than 40 mEq; you will need less than 10 mL to administer the dosage.

12. 
$$\frac{10,000 \text{ units}}{1 \text{ mL}} = \frac{5,000 \text{ units}}{x \text{ mL}}$$

$$\frac{10,000x}{10,000} = \frac{5,000}{10,000}$$

$$x = \frac{5,000}{10,000}$$

*or*

$$10,000 \text{ units} : 1 \text{ mL} = 5,000 \text{ units} : x \text{ mL}$$

$$\frac{10,000x}{10,000} = \frac{5,000}{10,000}$$

$$x = \frac{5,000}{10,000}$$

$x = 0.5$ mL, 10,000 units is more than 5,000 units; therefore you will need less than 1 mL to administer the dosage.

13. 
$$\frac{80 \text{ mg}}{2 \text{ mL}} = \frac{50 \text{ mg}}{x \text{ mL}}$$

$$\frac{80x}{80} = \frac{100}{80}$$

$$x = \frac{100}{80}$$

*or*

$$80 \text{ mg} : 2 \text{ mL} = 50 \text{ mg} : x \text{ mL}$$

$$\frac{80x}{80} = \frac{100}{80}$$

$$x = \frac{100}{80}$$

$x = 1.25 = 1.3$ mL. 50 mg is less than 80 mg; therefore you will need less than 2 mL to administer the dosage.

14. Equivalent: 1,000 mg = 1 g (0.5 g = 500 mg)

$$\frac{250 \text{ mg}}{1 \text{ cap}} = \frac{500 \text{ mg}}{x \text{ cap}}$$

$$\frac{250x}{250} = \frac{500}{250}$$

*or*

250 mg : 1 cap = 500 mg : x cap

$$\frac{250x}{250} = \frac{500}{250}$$

$$x = \frac{500}{250}$$

x = 2 caps. 500 mg is more than 250 mg; therefore you will need more than 1 cap to administer the dosage.

15. $$\frac{125 \text{ mg}}{5 \text{ mL}} = \frac{400 \text{ mg}}{x \text{ mL}}$$

$$\frac{125x}{125} = \frac{2,000}{125}$$

$$x = \frac{2,000}{125}$$

*or*

125 mg : 5 mL = 400 mg : x mL

$$\frac{125x}{125} = \frac{2,000}{125}$$

$$x = \frac{2,000}{125}$$

x = 16 mL. 400 mg is larger than 125 mg; therefore you will need more than 5 mL to administer the dosage.

16. $$\frac{80 \text{ mg}}{1 \text{ mL}} = \frac{50 \text{ mg}}{x \text{ mL}}$$

$$\frac{80x}{80} = \frac{50}{80}$$

$$x = \frac{50}{80}$$

*or*

80 mg : 1 mL = 50 mg : x mL

$$\frac{80x}{80} = \frac{50}{80}$$

$$x = \frac{50}{80}$$

x = 0.62 = 0.6 mL. 50 mg is less than 80 mg; therefore you will need less than 1 mL to administer the dosage.

17. $$\frac{\text{gr } \frac{1}{2}}{1 \text{ mL}} = \frac{\text{gr } 1}{x \text{ mL}}$$

$$\frac{\frac{1}{2}x}{\frac{1}{2}} = \frac{1}{\frac{1}{2}}$$

$$x = 1 \div \frac{1}{2} = 1 \times \frac{2}{1}$$

$$\frac{2}{1} = 2$$

*or*

gr $\frac{1}{2}$ : 1 mL = gr 1 : x mL

$$\frac{\frac{1}{2}x}{\frac{1}{2}} = \frac{1}{\frac{1}{2}}$$

$$x = 1 \div \frac{1}{2} = 1 \times \frac{2}{1}$$

$$\frac{2}{1} = 2$$

x = 2 mL. gr $\frac{1}{2}$ is less than gr 1; therefore you will need more than 1 mL to administer the dosage.

18. $$\frac{\text{gr } 5}{1 \text{ tab}} = \frac{\text{gr } 15}{x \text{ tab}}$$

$$\frac{5x}{5} = \frac{15}{5}$$

*or*

gr 5 : 1 tab = gr 15 : x tab

$$\frac{5x}{5} = \frac{15}{5}$$

$$x = \frac{15}{5}$$

x = 3 tabs. gr 15 is more than gr 5; therefore you will need more than 1 tab to administer the dosage.

Copyright © 2010, 2006, 2002, 1998, 1994 by Mosby, Inc. All rights reserved.

19. Equivalent: 1,000 mg = 1 g (0.24 g = 240 mg)

$$\frac{80 \text{ mg}}{7.5 \text{ mL}} = \frac{240 \text{ mg}}{x \text{ mL}}$$

$$\frac{80x}{80} = \frac{1,800}{80}$$

$$x = \frac{1,800}{80}$$

*or*

80 mg : 7.5 mL = 240 mg : $x$ mL

$$\frac{80x}{80} = \frac{1,800}{80}$$

$$x = \frac{1,800}{80}$$

$x$ = 22.5 mL. 240 mg is more than 80 mg; therefore you would need more than 7.5 mL to administer the dosage.

20.
$$\frac{10 \text{ g}}{15 \text{ mL}} = \frac{20 \text{ g}}{x \text{ mL}}$$

$$\frac{10 \, x}{10} = \frac{300}{10}$$

$$x = \frac{300}{10}$$

*or*

10 g : 15 mL = 20 g : $x$ mL

$$\frac{10x}{10} = \frac{300}{10}$$

$$x = \frac{300}{10}$$

$x$ = 30 mL. 20 g is more than 10 g; therefore you would need more than 15 mL to administer the dosage.

21.
$$\frac{0.5 \text{ mg}}{2 \text{ mL}} = \frac{0.125 \text{ mg}}{x \text{ mL}}$$

$$\frac{0.5 \, x}{0.5} = \frac{0.25}{0.5}$$

*or*

0.5 mg : 2 mL = 0.125 mg : $x$ mL

$$\frac{0.5x}{0.5} = \frac{0.25}{0.5}$$

$$x = \frac{0.25}{0.5}$$

$x$ = 0.5 mL, 0.125 mg is less than 0.5 mg; therefore you will need less than 2 mL to administer the dosage.

22.
$$\frac{0.25 \text{ mg}}{1 \text{ mL}} = \frac{0.75 \text{ mg}}{x \text{ mL}}$$

$$\frac{0.25x}{0.25} = \frac{0.75}{0.25}$$

*or*

0.25 mg : 1 mL = 0.75 mg : $x$ mL

$$\frac{0.25x}{0.25} = \frac{0.75}{0.25}$$

$$x = \frac{0.75}{0.25}$$

$x$ = 3 mL. 0.75 mg is more than 0.25 mg; therefore you will need more than 1 mL to administer the dosage.

23.
$$\frac{125 \text{ mg}}{5 \text{ mL}} = \frac{375 \text{ mg}}{x \text{ mL}}$$

$$\frac{125x}{125} = \frac{375 \times 5}{125}$$

*or*

125 mg : 5 mL = 375 mg : $x$ mL

$$\frac{125x}{125} = \frac{375 \times 5}{125}$$

$$x = \frac{1,875}{125}$$

$x$ = 15 mL. 375 mg is more than 125 mg; therefore you will need more than 5 mL to administer the dosage.

24.
$$\frac{7,500 \text{ units}}{1 \text{ mL}} = \frac{10,000 \text{ units}}{x \text{ mL}}$$

$$\frac{7,500x}{7,500} = \frac{10,000}{7,500}$$

*or*

7,500 units : 1 mL = 10,000 units : $x$ mL

$$\frac{7,500x}{7,500} = \frac{10,000}{7,500}$$

$$x = \frac{10,000}{7,500}$$

$x$ = 1.33 = 1.3 mL. 10,000 units is more than 7,500 units; therefore you will need more than 1 mL to administer the dosage.

25. 
$$\frac{0.3 \text{ mg}}{1 \text{ tab}} = \frac{0.45 \text{ mg}}{x \text{ tab}}$$

$$\frac{0.3x}{0.3} = \frac{0.45}{0.3}$$

*or*

$$0.3 \text{ mg} : 1 \text{ tab} = 0.45 \text{ mg} : x \text{ tab}$$

$$\frac{0.3x}{0.3} = \frac{0.45}{0.3}$$

$$x = \frac{0.45}{0.3}$$

$x = 1.5$ tabs or $1\frac{1}{2}$ tabs. 0.45 mg is more than 0.3 mg; therefore you will need more than 1 tab to administer the dosage.

## NOTE

For questions 26-40 and Chapter Review Parts I and II, answers only are provided. Refer to setup for problems 1-25 if needed.

| | | | | |
|---|---|---|---|---|
| 26. 1.2 mL | 29. 2 mL | 32. 2.2 mL | 35. 0.6 mL | 38. 3.3 mL |
| 27. 1.9 mL | 30. 1.1 mL | 33. 2 mL | 36. 0.8 mL | 39. 0.9 mL |
| 28. 0.7 mL | 31. 1.7 mL | 34. 2.2 mL | 37. 5 mL | 40. 1.6 mL |

## Answers to Chapter Review Part I

| | | | | |
|---|---|---|---|---|
| 1. 1 tab | 9. 1 tab | 19. 1 tab | 27. 1 tab | 35. 2 caps |
| 2. 1 cap | 10. 1 tab | 20. 2 tabs | 28. 2 tabs | 36. 3 caps |
| 3. 2 tabs | 11. 2 caps | 21. 0.5 tab *or* $\frac{1}{2}$ tab | 29. $1\frac{1}{2}$ tabs *or* 1.5 tabs | 37. 3 tabs |
| 4. 2 tabs | 12. 1 tab | | | 38. $1\frac{1}{2}$ tabs *or* 1.5 tabs |
| 5. 2 tabs | 13. 2 caps | 22. 1 tab | 30. 2 tabs | |
| 6. 0.5 tab *or* $\frac{1}{2}$ tab | 14. 2 caps | 23. 2 caps | 31. 3 tabs | 39. $\frac{1}{2}$ tab *or* 0.5 tab |
| | 15. 2 tabs | 24. 2 caps | 32. 2 tabs | |
| | 16. 1 tab | 25. 1 cap | 33. 2 tabs | 40. 1 tab |
| 7. 1 tab | 17. 2 caps | 26. 3 tabs | 34. 2 caps | |
| 8. 2 tabs | 18. 2 caps | | | |

## Answers to Chapter Review Part II

| | | | | |
|---|---|---|---|---|
| 41. 4 mL | 49. 0.67 mL | 57. 0.5 mL | 65. 30 mL | 73. 6.7 mL |
| 42. 20 mL | 50. 7.5 mL | 58. 0.5 mL | 66. 40 mL | 74. 8 mL |
| 43. 1.3 mL | 51. 1 mL | 59. 0.7 mL | 67. 10 mL | 75. 1.2 mL |
| 44. 20 mL | 52. 0.5 mL | 60. 4 mL | 68. 1 mL | 76. 0.8 mL |
| 45. 0.7 mL | 53. 2 mL | 61. 6 mL | 69. 16.7 mL | 77. 0.3 mL |
| 46. 2.3 mL | 54. 10 mL | 62. 6.3 mL | 70. 45 mL | 78. 0.25 mL |
| 47. 1 mL | 55. 0.75 mL | 63. 0.8 mL | 71. 1.3 mL | 79. 10 mL |
| 48. 1 mL | 56. 1.1 mL | 64. 20 mL | 72. 1.4 mL | 80. 12.5 mL |

# CHAPTER 15

## Answers to Practice Problems

1. $\dfrac{0.4 \text{ mg}}{0.2 \text{ mg}} \times 1 \text{ tab} = x \text{ tab}$

$$x = \dfrac{0.4}{0.2}$$

$x = 2$ tabs. 0.4 mg is greater than 0.2 mg; therefore you will need more than 1 tab to administer the dosage.

2. Equivalent: 1,000 mg = 1 g (0.75 g = 750 mg)

$\dfrac{750 \text{ mg}}{250 \text{ mg}} \times 1 \text{ cap} = x \text{ cap}$

$$x = \dfrac{750}{250}$$

$x = 3$ caps. 750 mg is larger than 250 mg; therefore you will need more than 1 cap to administer the dosage.

3. $\dfrac{90 \text{ mg}}{60 \text{ mg}} \times 1 \text{ tab} = x \text{ tab}$

$$x = \dfrac{90}{60}$$

$x = 1.5$ or $1\dfrac{1}{2}$ tabs. 90 mg is larger than 60 mg; therefore you will need more than 1 tab to administer the dosage.

4. $\dfrac{7.5 \text{ mg}}{2.5 \text{ mg}} \times 1 \text{ tab} = x \text{ tab}$

$$x = \dfrac{7.5}{2.5}$$

$x = 3$ tabs. 7.5 mg is larger than 2.5 mg; therefore you will need more than 1 tab to administer the dosage.

5. Equivalent: 1,000 mcg = 1 mg (0.05 mg = 50 mcg)

$\dfrac{50 \text{ mcg}}{25 \text{ mcg}} \times 1 \text{ tab} = x \text{ tab}$

$$x = \dfrac{50}{25}$$

$x = 2$ tabs. 50 mcg is larger than 25 mcg; therefore you will need more than 1 tab to administer the dosage.

6. Equivalent: 1,000 mcg = 1 mg (0.4 mg = 400 mcg)

$\dfrac{400 \text{ mcg}}{200 \text{ mcg}} \times 1 \text{ tab} = x \text{ tab}$

$$x = \dfrac{400}{200}$$

$x = 2$ tabs. 400 mcg is more than the dosage available; therefore you will need more than one tab to administer the dosage.

7. $\dfrac{1,000 \text{ mg}}{500 \text{ mg}} \times 1 \text{ tab} = x \text{ tab}$

$$x = \dfrac{1,000}{500}$$

$x = 2$ tabs. 1,000 mg is more than 500 mg; therefore you will need more than 1 tab to administer the dosage.

8. Equivalent: 1,000 mg = 1 g (0.6 g = 600 mg)

$\dfrac{600 \text{ mg}}{600 \text{ mg}} \times 1 \text{ cap} = x \text{ cap}$

$$x = \dfrac{600}{600}$$

$x = 1$ cap. 0.6 g = 600 mg. 600-mg tabs are available; therefore give 1 cap to administer the dosage.

9. Equivalent: 1,000 mcg = 1 mg (1.25 mg = 1,250 mcg)

$\dfrac{1,250 \text{ mcg}}{625 \text{ mcg}} \times 1 \text{ tab} = x \text{ tab}$

$$x = \dfrac{1,250}{625}$$

$x = 2$ tabs. 1,250 mcg is more than 625 mcg; therefore you will need more than one tab to administer the dosage.

10. $\dfrac{10 \text{ mg}}{15 \text{ mg}} \times 1 \text{ mL} = x \text{ mL}$

$$x = \dfrac{10}{15}$$

$x = 0.66 = 0.7$ mL. 10 mg is less than 15 mg; you will need less than 1 mL to administer the dosage.

11. $\dfrac{400 \text{ mg}}{200 \text{ mg}} \times 5 \text{ mL} = x \text{ mL}$

$$x = \frac{2,000}{200}$$

$x = 10$ mL. 400 mg is more than 200 mg; therefore you will need more than 5 mL to administer the dosage.

12. $\dfrac{15 \text{ mEq}}{20 \text{ mEq}} \times 10 \text{ mL} = x \text{ mL}$

$$x = \frac{150}{20}$$

$x = 7.5$ mL. 15 mEq is less than 20 mEq; therefore you will need less than 10 mL to administer the dosage.

13. $\dfrac{125 \text{ mg}}{250 \text{ mg}} \times 5 \text{ mL} = x \text{ mL}$

$$x = \frac{625}{250}$$

$x = 2.5$ mL. 125 mg is less than 250 mg; therefore you will need less than 5 mL to administer the dosage.

14. $\dfrac{0.025 \text{ mg}}{0.05 \text{ mg}} \times 5 \text{ mL} = x \text{ mL}$

$$x = \frac{0.125}{0.05}$$

$x = 2.5$ mL. 0.025 mg is less than 0.05 mg; therefore you will need less than 5 mL to administer the dosage.

15. $\dfrac{375 \text{ mg}}{125 \text{ mg}} \times 5 \text{ mL} = x \text{ mL}$

$$x = \frac{1,875}{125}$$

$x = 15$ mL. 375 mg is more than 125 mg; therefore you will need more than 5 mL to administer the dosage.

## Answers to Chapter Review

**NOTE**

For Chapter Review Problems, only answers are shown. If needed, review setup of problems in Practice Problems 1-15.

1. 1 tab
2. 1 tab
3. 2 caps
4. 2 tabs
5. 2 caplets
6. $1\frac{1}{2}$ tabs *or* 1.5 tabs
7. 1 cap
8. 1 cap
9. 2 caps
10. 2 tabs
11. $1\frac{1}{2}$ tabs *or* 1.5 tabs

12. 2 caps
13. 1 tab
14. 3 tabs
15. 2 caps (extended)
16. 0.7 mL
17. 1 mL
18. 0.4 mL
19. 12 mL
20. 10 mL
21. 11.3 mL
22. 0.6 mL
23. 2 mL
24. 1.8 mL

25. 10 mL
26. 0.8 mL
27. 2 mL
28. 0.6 mL
29. 0.8 mL
30. 0.5 mL
31. 0.3 mL
32. 1 mL
33. 2 mL
34. 3.2 mL
35. 5 mL
36. 1 tab
37. 1 tab

38. 2 caps (pulvules)
39. 5 mL
40. 1 tab
41. 2 tabs
42. 1.3 mL
43. 2 mL
44. 3 mL
45. 2 tabs
46. 2 tabs
47. 2 tabs
48. 30 mL
49. 12 mL
50. 2.5 mL

51. 1 tab
52. 2 tabs
53. $1\frac{1}{2}$ tabs *or* 1.5 tabs
54. 28 mL
55. 0.5 mL
56. 3 tabs
57. 2 tabs *or* 2 film tabs
58. 1 tab
59. 0.8 mL
60. 2 tabs (extended release)

## CHAPTER 16

### Answers to Practice Problems

**NOTE**

The following problems could be set up without placing 1 under a value; placing a 1 under the value as shown in the setup for problems 1-20 does not alter the value of the number.

1. $\text{gr } x = \dfrac{\text{gr } 1}{60 \text{ mg}} \times \dfrac{15 \text{ mg}}{1}$

2. $x \text{ mg} = \dfrac{60 \text{ mg}}{\text{gr } 1} \times \dfrac{\text{gr v}}{1}$

3. $x \text{ mg} = \dfrac{1 \text{ mg}}{1,000 \text{ mcg}} \times \dfrac{400 \text{ mcg}}{1}$

4. $x \text{ mL} = \dfrac{15 \text{ mL}}{1 \text{ tbs}} \times \dfrac{2 \text{ tbs}}{1}$

5. $x \text{ mg} = \dfrac{1,000 \text{ mg}}{1 \text{ g}} \times \dfrac{0.007 \text{ g}}{1}$

6. $x \text{ mL} = \dfrac{1,000 \text{ mL}}{1 \text{ L}} \times \dfrac{0.5 \text{ L}}{1}$

7. $x \text{ g} = \dfrac{1 \text{ g}}{1,000 \text{ mg}} \times \dfrac{529 \text{ mg}}{1}$

8. $x \text{ L} = \dfrac{1 \text{ L}}{1,000 \text{ mL}} \times \dfrac{1,600 \text{ mL}}{1}$

9. $x \text{ lb} = \dfrac{2.2 \text{ lb}}{1 \text{ kg}} \times \dfrac{46.4 \text{ kg}}{1}$

10. $x \text{ inch} = \dfrac{1 \text{ inch}}{2.5 \text{ cm}} \times \dfrac{5 \text{ cm}}{1}$

11. $x \text{ mL} = \dfrac{1.5 \text{ mL}}{0.4 \text{ g}} \times \dfrac{0.3 \text{ g}}{1}$

12. $x \text{ mL} = \dfrac{1 \text{ mL}}{15 \text{ mg}} \times \dfrac{60 \text{ mg}}{\text{gr } 1} \times \dfrac{\text{gr } 1/4}{1}$

13. $x \text{ cap} = \dfrac{1 \text{ cap}}{500 \text{ mg}} \times \dfrac{1,000 \text{ mg}}{1 \text{ g}} \times \dfrac{1 \text{ g}}{1}$

14. $x \text{ mL} = \dfrac{5 \text{ mL}}{400 \text{ mg}} \times \dfrac{400 \text{ mg}}{1}$

15. $x \text{ mL} = \dfrac{1 \text{ mL}}{25 \text{ mg}} \times \dfrac{150 \text{ mg}}{1}$

16. $x \text{ tab} = \dfrac{1 \text{ tab}}{250 \text{ mg}} \times \dfrac{1,000 \text{ mg}}{1 \text{ g}} \times \dfrac{0.5 \text{ g}}{1}$

17. $x \text{ tab} = \dfrac{1 \text{ tab}}{0.25 \text{ mg}} \times \dfrac{0.125 \text{ mg}}{1}$

18. $x \text{ mL} = \dfrac{5 \text{ mL}}{125 \text{ mg}} \times \dfrac{300 \text{ mg}}{1}$

19. $x \text{ mL} = \dfrac{5 \text{ mL}}{125 \text{ mg}} \times \dfrac{1,000 \text{ mg}}{1 \text{ g}} \times \dfrac{1 \text{ g}}{1}$

20. $x \text{ mL} = \dfrac{1 \text{ mL}}{150 \text{ mg}} \times \dfrac{1,000 \text{ mg}}{1 \text{ g}} \times \dfrac{0.3 \text{ g}}{1}$

**NOTE**

Placing a 1 under the value does not alter the value of the number.

### Answers to Chapter Review

1. $x \text{ tab} = \dfrac{1 \text{ tab}}{25 \text{ mg}} \times \dfrac{50 \text{ mg}}{1}$

   $x = \dfrac{50}{25}$

   $x = 2 \text{ tabs}$

2. $x \text{ mL} = \dfrac{15 \text{ mL}}{\overset{}{\underset{2}{30}} \text{ mEq}} \times \dfrac{\overset{2}{20} \text{ mEq}}{1}$

   $x = \dfrac{15 \times 2}{3}$

   $x = \dfrac{30}{3}$

   $x = 10 \text{ mL}$

3. $x \text{ mL} = \dfrac{1 \text{ mL}}{15 \text{ mg}} \times \dfrac{20 \text{ mg}}{1}$

   $x = \dfrac{20}{15}$

   $x = 1.3 \text{ mL}$

4. $x \text{ mL} = \dfrac{1 \text{ mL}}{225 \text{ mg}} \times \dfrac{1,000 \text{ mg}}{1 \text{ g}} \times \dfrac{0.5 \text{ g}}{1}$

   $x = \dfrac{1 \times 1,000}{225} \times 0.5 = \dfrac{500}{225}$

   $x = 2.2 \text{ mL}$

5. $x$ tab $= \dfrac{1 \text{ tab}}{12.5 \text{ mg}} \times \dfrac{25 \text{ mg}}{1}$

$x = \dfrac{25}{12.5}$

$x = 2$ tabs

6. $x$ mL $= \dfrac{1 \text{ mL}}{100 \text{ mg}} \times \dfrac{80 \text{ mg}}{1}$

$x = \dfrac{80}{100}$

$x = 0.8$ mL

7. $x$ mL $= \dfrac{1 \text{ mL}}{10,000 \text{ units}} \times \dfrac{6,500 \text{ units}}{1}$

$x = \dfrac{6,500}{10,000}$

$x = 0.65$ mL

8. $x$ mL $= \dfrac{4 \text{ mL}}{0.6 \text{ g}} \times \dfrac{1 \text{ g}}{1,000 \text{ mg}} \times \dfrac{300 \text{ mg}}{1}$

$x = \dfrac{4 \times 300}{0.6 \times 1,000} = \dfrac{1,200}{600}$

$x = 2$ mL

9. $x$ tab $= \dfrac{1 \text{ tab}}{150 \text{ mg}} \times \dfrac{\overset{2}{300} \text{ mg}}{1}$
   $\phantom{x tab = \dfrac{1}{\underset{1}{150}}}$

$x = \dfrac{2}{1}$

$x = 2$ tabs

10. $x$ mL $= \dfrac{1 \text{ mL}}{62.5 \text{ mg}} \times \dfrac{175 \text{ mg}}{1}$

$x = \dfrac{175}{62.5}$

$x = 2.8$ mL

11. $x$ tab $= \dfrac{1 \text{ tab}}{400 \text{ mg}} \times \dfrac{1,000 \text{ mg}}{1 \text{ g}} \times \dfrac{0.4 \text{ g}}{1}$

$x = \dfrac{1,000 \times 0.4}{400}$

$x = \dfrac{400}{400}$

$x = 1$ tab

12. $x$ tab $= \dfrac{1 \text{ tab}}{250 \text{ mg}} \times \dfrac{\overset{4}{1,000} \text{ mg}}{1 \text{ g}} \times \dfrac{0.5 \text{ g}}{1}$
   $\phantom{x tab = \dfrac{1}{\underset{1}{250}}}$

$x = \dfrac{4 \times 0.5}{1}$

$x = \dfrac{2}{1}$

$x = 2$ tab (film tab)

13. $x$ tab $= \dfrac{1 \text{ tab}}{0.5 \text{ mg}} \times \dfrac{0.5 \text{ mg}}{1}$

$x = \dfrac{0.5}{0.5}$

$x = 1$ tab

14. $x$ mL $= \dfrac{1 \text{ mL}}{80 \text{ mg}} \times \dfrac{200 \text{ mg}}{1}$

$x = \dfrac{200}{80}$

$x = 2.5$ mL

15. $x$ mL $= \dfrac{1 \text{ mL}}{10 \text{ mg}} \times \dfrac{25 \text{ mg}}{1}$

$x = \dfrac{25}{10}$

$x = 2.5$ mL

*or*

$x$ mL $= \dfrac{5 \text{ mL}}{50 \text{ mg}} \times \dfrac{25 \text{ mg}}{1}$

$x = \dfrac{5 \times 25}{50}$

$x = \dfrac{125}{50}$

$x = 2.5$ mL

16. $x$ mL $= \dfrac{1 \text{ mL}}{25 \text{ mg}} \times \dfrac{15 \text{ mg}}{1}$

$x = \dfrac{15}{25}$

$x = 0.6$ mL

*or*

$x$ mL $= \dfrac{10 \text{ mL}}{250 \text{ mg}} \times \dfrac{15 \text{ mg}}{1}$

$x = \dfrac{10 \times 15}{250}$

$x = \dfrac{150}{250}$

$x = 0.6$ mL

17. $x \text{ mL} = \dfrac{1 \text{ mL}}{2 \text{ mEq}} \times \dfrac{15 \text{ mEq}}{1}$

$x = \dfrac{15}{2}$

$x = 7.5 \text{ mL}$

*or*

$x \text{ mL} = \dfrac{15 \text{ mL}}{30 \text{ mEq}} \times \dfrac{15 \text{ mEq}}{1}$

$x = \dfrac{15 \times 15}{30}$

$x = \dfrac{225}{30}$

$x = 7.5 \text{ mL}$

18. $x \text{ mL} = \dfrac{1 \text{ mL}}{50 \text{ mg}} \times \dfrac{60 \text{ mg}}{1}$

$x = \dfrac{60}{50}$

$x = 1.2 \text{ mL}$

19. $x \text{ mL} = \dfrac{5 \text{ mL}}{375 \text{ mg}} \times \dfrac{1,000 \text{ mg}}{1 \text{ g}} \times \dfrac{0.4 \text{ g}}{1}$

$x = \dfrac{5,000 \times 0.4}{375}$

$x = \dfrac{2,000}{375}$

$x = 5.33 \text{ mL} = 5.3 \text{ mL}$ (to the nearest tenth)

20. $x \text{ tab} = \dfrac{1 \text{ tab}}{0.05 \text{ mg}} \times \dfrac{0.075 \text{ mg}}{1}$

$x = \dfrac{0.075}{0.05}$

$x = 1.5$ tabs or $1\frac{1}{2}$ tabs ($1\frac{1}{2}$ tabs preferred for administrative purposes.)

21. $x \text{ mL} = \dfrac{1,000 \text{ mL}}{1 \text{ qt}} \times \dfrac{3 \text{ qt}}{1}$

$x = \dfrac{1,000 \times 3}{1}$

$x = \dfrac{3,000}{1}$

$x = 3,000 \text{ mL}$

22. $x \text{ kg} = \dfrac{1 \text{ kg}}{2.2 \text{ lb}} \times \dfrac{79 \text{ lb}}{1}$

$x = \dfrac{79}{2.2}$

$x = 35.9 \text{ kg}$ (to the nearest tenth)

23. $x \text{ mg} = \dfrac{1 \text{ mg}}{1,000 \text{ mcg}} \times \dfrac{5 \text{ mcg}}{1}$

$x = \dfrac{5}{1,000}$

$x = 0.005 \text{ mg}$

24. $x \text{ L} = \dfrac{1 \text{ L}}{1,000 \text{ mL}} \times \dfrac{2,400 \text{ mL}}{1}$

$x = \dfrac{2,400}{1,000}$

$x = 2.4 \text{ L}$

25. $x \text{ cm} = \dfrac{2.5 \text{ cm}}{1 \text{ in}} \times \dfrac{8 \text{ in}}{1}$

$x = \dfrac{2.5 \times 8}{1}$

$x = 20 \text{ cm}$

26. $x \text{ mg} = \dfrac{1 \text{ mg}}{1,000 \text{ mcg}} \times \dfrac{1.25 \text{ mcg}}{1}$

$x = \dfrac{1.25}{1,000}$

$x = 0.00125 \text{ mg}$

27. $x \text{ oz} = \dfrac{1 \text{ oz}}{30 \text{ mL}} \times \dfrac{240 \text{ mL}}{1}$

$x = \dfrac{240}{30}$

$x = 8 \text{ oz}$

28. $x \text{ mcg} = \dfrac{1,000 \text{ mcg}}{1 \text{ mg}} \times \dfrac{1.75 \text{ mg}}{1}$

$x = \dfrac{1,000 \times 1.75}{1}$

$x = 1,750 \text{ mcg}$

29. $x \text{ L} = \dfrac{1 \text{ L}}{1,000 \text{ mL}} \times \dfrac{125 \text{ mL}}{1}$

$x = \dfrac{125}{1,000}$

$x = 0.125 \text{ L}$

30. $x \text{ mL} = \dfrac{1,000 \text{ mL}}{1 \text{ L}} \times \dfrac{8.5 \text{ L}}{1}$

$x = \dfrac{1,000 \times 8.5}{1}$

$x = 8,500 \text{ mL}$

31. $140\frac{1}{2}$ lb is written as 140.5 lb to solve

$$x \text{ kg} = \frac{1 \text{ kg}}{2.2 \text{ lb}} \times \frac{140.5 \text{ lb}}{1}$$

$$x = \frac{140.5}{2.2}$$

$$x = 63.86 \text{ kg} = 63.9 \text{ kg (to nearest tenth)}$$

32. $x \text{ tbs} = \frac{1 \text{ tbs}}{15 \text{ mL}} \times \frac{127.5 \text{ mL}}{1}$

$$x = \frac{127.5}{15}$$

$$x = 8\frac{1}{2} \text{ tbs}$$

33. $x \text{ mL} = \frac{30 \text{ mL}}{1 \text{ oz}} \times \frac{25 \text{ oz}}{1}$

$$x = \frac{30 \times 25}{1}$$

$$x = 750 \text{ mL}$$

34. $x \text{ in} = \frac{1 \text{ in}}{2.5 \text{ cm}} \times \frac{36 \text{ cm}}{1}$

$$x = \frac{36}{2.5}$$

$$x = 14.4 \text{ in}$$

35. $x \text{ cm} = \frac{1 \text{ cm}}{10 \text{ mm}} \times \frac{50 \text{ mm}}{1}$

$$x = \frac{50}{10}$$

$$x = 5 \text{ cm}$$

# CHAPTER 17

## Answers to Practice Problems

The answers to the practice problems include the rationale for the answer where indicated. Where necessary, the methods for calculation of the dosage are shown as well.

**NOTE**

Unless stated, no conversion is required to calculate dosage. In problems that required a conversion before calculating the dosage, the problem setup shown illustrates the problem after appropriate conversions have been made.

1. 0.025 mg = 25 mcg

   50 mcg : 1 tab = 25 mcg : $x$ tab

   *or*

   $\frac{25 \text{ mcg}}{50 \text{ mcg}} \times 1 \text{ tab} = x \text{ tab}$

   Answer: 0.5 or $\frac{1}{2}$ tab. This is an acceptable answer, because the tabs are scored. (For administration purposes state as $\frac{1}{2}$ tab.) Note that the problem could have been done without converting by using the dosage indicated on the label in mg. This would net the same answer.

   0.05 mg : 1 tab = 0.025 mg : $x$ tab

   0.025 mg/0.05 × 1 tab = $x$ tab

2. 25 mg : 1 cap = 50 mg : $x$ cap

   *or*

   $\frac{50 \text{ mg}}{25 \text{ mg}} \times 1 \text{ cap} = x \text{ cap}$

   Answer: 2 caps. The dosage ordered is greater than what is available; therefore you will need more than 1 cap to administer the dosage.

3. Conversion is necessary: 1,000 mg = 1 g.

   Therefore 1 g = 1,000 mg.

   500 mg : 1 tab = 1,000 mg : $x$ tab

   *or*

   $\frac{1,000 \text{ mg}}{500 \text{ mg}} \times 1 \text{ tab} = x \text{ tab}$

   Answer: 2 tabs. The dosage ordered is greater than what is available; therefore you will need more than 1 tab to administer the dosage.

4. It would be best to administer one of the 5-mg tablets and one of the 2.5 mg ($2\frac{1}{2}$ mg) tablets (5 mg + 2.5 mg = 7.5 mg).

5. a.  125-mcg tablet is the appropriate strength to use (0.125 mg = 125 mcg).

   b.  1 tab. Even though the tablets are scored, one half of 500 mcg would still be twice the dosage desired.

$$125 \text{ mcg} : 1 \text{ tab} = 125 \text{ mcg} : x \text{ tab}$$

*or*

$$\frac{125 \text{ mcg}}{125 \text{ mcg}} \times 1 \text{ tab} = x \text{ tab}$$

   Answer: 1 tab

6. a.  500-mg caps would be appropriate to use.

   b.  2 caps (500 mg each). 1,000 mg = 1 g; therefore 2 caps of 500 mg each would be the least number of capsules. Using the 250-mg strength capsules would require 4 caps.

   c.  2 caps q6h = 8 caps. Multiplying the number of caps needed by the number of days gives you the number of capsules required.

   8 (number of caps per day) × 7 (number of days) = 56 (total caps needed)

$$500 \text{ mg} : 1 \text{ cap} = 1,000 \text{ mg} : x \text{ cap}$$

$$\frac{1,000 \text{ mg}}{500 \text{ mg}} \times 1 \text{ cap} = x \text{ cap}$$

$$x = 2 \text{ caps}$$

7.  $5 \text{ mg} : 1 \text{ tab} = 10 \text{ mg} : x \text{ tab}$

$$\frac{10 \text{ mg}}{5 \text{ mg}} \times 1 \text{ tab} = x \text{ tab}$$

   Answer: 2 tabs. The dosage ordered is greater than what is available; therefore you will need more than 1 tab to administer the dosage.

8. a.  $1\frac{1}{2}$ tabs; the tablets are scored. (State as $1\frac{1}{2}$ tabs for administration purposes.)

$$10 \text{ mg} : 1 \text{ tab} = 15 \text{ mg} : x \text{ tab}$$

$$\frac{15 \text{ mg}}{10 \text{ mg}} \times 1 \text{ tab} = x \text{ tab}$$

$$x = 1\frac{1}{2} \text{ tab}$$

   b.  15 mg × 3 (t.i.d.) = 45 mg/day. The total number of milligrams received for 3 days is 135 mg.

$$45 \text{ mg} \times 3 = 135 \text{ mg}$$

9.  0.075 mg = 75 mcg

$$50 \text{ mcg} : 1 \text{ tab} = 75 \text{ mcg} : x \text{ tab}$$

*or*

$$\frac{75 \text{ mcg}}{50 \text{ mcg}} \times 1 \text{ tab} = x \text{ tab}$$

   Answer: 1.5 or $1\frac{1}{2}$ tabs, since the tabs are scored.

   (State as $1\frac{1}{2}$ for administration purposes.)

10. 1.3 g = 1,300 mg

$$650 \text{ mg} : 1 \text{ tab} = 1,300 \text{ mg} : x \text{ tab}$$

*or*

$$\frac{1,300 \text{ mg}}{650 \text{ mg}} \times 1 \text{ tab} = x \text{ tab}$$

   Answer: 2 tabs. The dosage ordered is more than what is available; therefore you will need more than 1 tab to administer the dosage.

11.  $30 \text{ mg} : 1 \text{ cap} = 90 \text{ mg} : x \text{ cap}$

*or*

$$\frac{90 \text{ mg}}{30 \text{ mg}} \times 1 \text{ cap} = x \text{ cap}$$

   Answer: 3 caps. The dosage ordered is greater than what is available. You will need more than 1 cap to administer the dosage.

12.  $100 \text{ mg} : 1 \text{ tab} = 200 \text{ mg} : x \text{ tab}$

*or*

$$\frac{200 \text{ mg}}{100 \text{ mg}} \times 1 \text{ tab} = x \text{ tab}$$

   Answer: 2 tabs. The dosage ordered is greater than what is available; therefore you will need more than 1 tab to administer the dosage.

13. a.  2 caps (1 g = 1,000 mg)

   500 mg × 2 = 1,000 mg.

   Answer: 2 caps.

   b.  1 cap (500 mg = 0.5 g)

   1 cap of 500 mg

   Initial dosage: $500 \text{ mg} : 1 \text{ cap} = 1,000 \text{ mg} : x \text{ cap}$

*or*

$$\frac{1000 \text{ mg}}{500 \text{ mg}} \times 1 \text{ cap} = x \text{ cap}$$

   Answer: 2 caps

   Daily dosage: $500 \text{ mg} : 1 \text{ cap} = 500 \text{ mg} : x \text{ cap}$

*or*

$$\frac{500 \text{ mg}}{500 \text{ mg}} \times 1 \text{ cap} = x \text{ cap}$$

14. $125 \text{ mg} : 1 \text{ tab} = 250 \text{ mg} : x \text{ tab}$

*or*

$$\frac{250 \text{ mg}}{125 \text{ mg}} \times 1 \text{ tab} = x \text{ tab}$$

Answer: 2 tabs. The dosage ordered is more than what is available; therefore you will need more than 1 tab to administer the dosage.

15. Conversion is necessary.

$$\text{gr } 1\frac{1}{2} = 90 \text{ mg}$$

a. 30-mg tablets

b. Three 30-mg tablets. This strength will allow the client to take three tabs to achieve the desired dosage, as opposed to six 15 mg tabs. This dosage is logical, because the maximum number of tablets administered is generally three.

$30 \text{ mg} : 1 \text{ tab} = 90 \text{ mg} : x \text{ tab}$

*or*

$$\frac{90 \text{ mg}}{30 \text{ mg}} \times 1 \text{ tab} = x \text{ tab}$$

Answer: three 30 mg tabs

16. a. The best strength to use is 1.5 mg. This would allow the client to swallow the least amount.

$1.5 \text{ mg} : 1 \text{ tab} = 3 \text{ mg} : x \text{ tab}$

*or*

$$\frac{3 \text{ mg}}{1.5 \text{ mg}} \times 1 \text{ tab} = x \text{ tab}$$

b. Answer: Two 1.5-mg tabs would be the least number of tablets; 0.75 mg would require the client to swallow 4 tabs to receive the dosage ($0.75 \times 4 = 3$).

17. $50 \text{ mg} : 1 \text{ tab} = 100 \text{ mg} : x \text{ tab}$

*or*

$$\frac{100 \text{ mg}}{50 \text{ mg}} \times 1 \text{ tab} = x \text{ tab}$$

Answer: You need 2 tabs to administer 100 mg. 2 tabs t.i.d. (3 times a day) = 6 tabs × 3 days = 18 tabs.

18. It would be best to administer one 80-mg tablet and one 40-mg tablet ($80 + 40 = 120$ mg). This would be the least number of tablets.

19. $10 \text{ mg} : 1 \text{ tab} = 20 \text{ mg} : x \text{ tab}$

*or*

$$\frac{20 \text{ mg}}{10 \text{ mg}} \times 1 \text{ tab} = x \text{ tab}$$

Answer: 2 tabs. The dosage ordered is larger than the available dosage; therefore more than 1 tab will be required.

20. $0.5 \text{ mg} : 1 \text{ tab} = 1 \text{ mg} : x \text{ tab}$

*or*

$$\frac{1 \text{ mg}}{0.5 \text{ mg}} \times 1 \text{ tab} = x \text{ tab}$$

$$x = 2 \text{ tabs}$$

Answer: 2 tabs. The dosage ordered is more than what is available; therefore you will need more than 1 tab to administer the dosage.

21. $1 \text{ mg} : 1 \text{ cap} = 3 \text{ mg} : x \text{ cap}$

*or*

$$\frac{3 \text{ mg}}{1 \text{ mg}} \times 1 \text{ cap} = x \text{ cap}$$

Answer: 3 caps. They are administered in whole numbers. The answer is logical. The maximum number of tablets or capsules administered is generally three.

22. Conversion is required. Equivalent: 1,000 mg = 1 g; therefore 0.6 g = 600 mg

$600 \text{ mg} : 1 \text{ tab} = 600 \text{ mg} : x \text{ tab}$

*or*

$$\frac{600 \text{ mg}}{600 \text{ mg}} \times 1 \text{ tab} = x \text{ tab}$$

Answer: 1 tab. 0.6 mg = 600 mg, which is equal to 1 tab.

23. Choose the 6-mg tab and give 1 tab, which allows the client to swallow the least number of tabs without dividing tabs.

$6 \text{ mg} : 1 \text{ tab} = 6 \text{ mg} : x \text{ tab}$

*or*

$$\frac{6 \text{ mg}}{6 \text{ mg}} \times 1 \text{ tab} = x \text{ tab}$$

Answer: one 6-mg tab

24. Conversion is required. Equivalent: 1,000 mg = 1 g; therefore 0.2 g = 200 mg.

$100 \text{ mg} : 1 \text{ tab} = 200 \text{ mg} : x \text{ tab}$

*or*

$$\frac{200 \text{ mg}}{100 \text{ mg}} \times 1 \text{ tab} = x \text{ tab}$$

Answer: 2 tabs. The dosage ordered is larger than what is available; therefore more than 1 tab is needed to administer the dosage.

25. $10 \text{ mg} : 1 \text{ tab} = 20 \text{ mg} : x \text{ tab}$

*or*

$$\frac{20 \text{ mg}}{10 \text{ mg}} \times 1 \text{ tab} = x \text{ tab}$$

Answer: 2 tabs. The dosage ordered is more than what is available. You will need more than 1 tab to administer the dosage.

26.    50 mg : 1 tab = 100 mg : $x$ tab

*or*

$\dfrac{100 \text{ mg}}{50 \text{ mg}} \times 1 \text{ tab} = x \text{ tab}$

Answer: 2 tabs. The dosage ordered is more than what is available. You will need more than 1 tab to administer the dosage.

27.    200 mg : 1 tab = 400 mg : $x$ tab

*or*

$\dfrac{400 \text{ mg}}{200 \text{ mg}} \times 1 \text{ tab} = x \text{ tab}$

Answer: 2 tabs. The dosage ordered is more than what is available. You will need more than 1 tab to administer the dosage.

28.    75 mg : 1 cap = 150 mg : $x$ cap

*or*

$\dfrac{150 \text{ mg}}{75 \text{ mg}} \times 1 \text{ cap} = x \text{ cap}$

Answer: 2 caps. The dosage ordered is more than what is available. You will need more than 1 cap to administer the dosage.

29. Change 1 g to 1,000 mg (1,000 mg = 1 g)

500 mg : 1 tab = 1,000 mg : $x$ tab

*or*

$\dfrac{1,000 \text{ mg}}{500 \text{ mg}} \times 1 \text{ tab} = x \text{ tab}$

Answer: 2 tabs. The dosage ordered is greater than what is available. You will need more than 1 tab to administer the dosage.

30.    30 mg : 1 cap = 60 mg : $x$ cap

*or*

$\dfrac{60 \text{ mg}}{30 \text{ mg}} \times 1 \text{ cap} = x \text{ cap}$

Answer: 2 caps. The dosage ordered is more than what is available. You will need more than 1 cap to administer the dosage.

31. It would be best to administer one 75-mcg tablet and one 25 mcg tablet for a total of 100 mcg. This would be the least number of tablets (75 mcg + 25 mcg = 100 mcg).

32.    12.5 mg : 1 tab = 25 mg : $x$ tab

*or*

$\dfrac{25 \text{ mg}}{12.5 \text{ mg}} \times 1 \text{ tab} = x \text{ tab}$

Answer: 2 tabs. The dosage ordered is more than what is available. You will need more than 1 tab to administer the dosage.

33.    0.5 mg : 1 tab = 0.25 mg : $x$ tab

*or*

$\dfrac{0.25 \text{ mg}}{0.5 \text{ mg}} \times 1 \text{ tab} = x \text{ tab}$

Answer: 0.5 tab or $\dfrac{1}{2}$ tab. This is an acceptable answer because the tablet is scored. (State answer as $\dfrac{1}{2}$ tab for administration purposes.)

34. Conversion is necessary: 1,000 mg = 1 g; therefore 0.25 g = 250 mg

250 mg : 1 tab = 250 mg : $x$ tab

*or*

$\dfrac{250 \text{ mg}}{250 \text{ mg}} \times 1 \text{ tab} = x \text{ tab}$

Answer: 1 tab. 0.25 g = 250 mg, which is equal to 1 tab.

35. Label indicates 0.025 mg = 25 mcg.

25 mcg : 1 tab = 25 mcg : $x$ tab

*or*

$\dfrac{25 \text{ mcg}}{25 \text{ mcg}} \times 1 \text{ tab} = x \text{ tab}$

Answer: 1 tab. 0.025 mg is equal to 25 mcg. Therefore only 1 tab is needed to administer the dosage.

36.    325 mg : 1 tab = 650 mg : $x$ tab

*or*

$\dfrac{650 \text{ mg}}{325 \text{ mg}} \times 1 \text{ tab} = x \text{ tab}$

Answer: 2 tabs. The dosage ordered is greater than what is available; you will need more than 1 tab to administer the dosage.

37. Conversion is necessary. 1,000 mg = 1 g; therefore 0.2 g = 200 mg.

100 mg : 1 cap = 200 mg : $x$ cap

*or*

$\dfrac{200 \text{ mg}}{100 \text{ mg}} \times 1 \text{ cap} = x \text{ cap}$

Answer: 2 caps. The dosage ordered is greater than what is available. You will need more than 1 cap to administer the dosage.

38.    400 mg : 1 tab = 800 mg : $x$ tab

*or*

$\dfrac{800 \text{ mg}}{400 \text{ mg}} \times 1 \text{ tab} = x \text{ tab}$

Answer: 2 tabs. The dosage ordered is greater than what is available. You will need more than 1 tab to administer the dosage.

39.     30 mg : 1 tab = 60 mg : $x$ tab

*or*

$$\frac{60 \text{ mg}}{30 \text{ mg}} \times 1 \text{ tab} = x \text{ tab}$$

Answer: 2 tabs. The dosage ordered is greater than what is available. You will need more than 1 tab to administer the dosage.

40. Conversion: 1,000 mg = 1 g. Therefore 0.03 g = 30 mg.

       10 mg : 1 tab = 30 mg : $x$ tab

*or*

$$\frac{30 \text{ mg}}{10 \text{ mg}} \times 1 \text{ tab} = x \text{ tab}$$

Answer: 3 tabs. The dosage ordered is greater than what is available. You will need more than 1 tab to administer the dosage. Three tablets is the maximum number of tablets that should generally be given.

41.     80 mg : 1 cap = 160 mg : $x$ cap

*or*

$$\frac{160 \text{ mg}}{80 \text{ mg}} \times 1 \text{ cap} = x \text{ cap}$$

Answer: 2 caps. The dosage ordered is greater than what is available. You will need more than 1 cap to administer the dosage.

## NOTE

The setup shown for problems that required conversions reflect conversion of what the prescriber ordered to what is available. Unless stated in problems 42-70, no conversion is required to calculate the dosage.

42.     50 mg : 15 mL = 100 mg : $x$ mL

*or*

$$\frac{100 \text{ mg}}{50 \text{ mg}} \times 15 \text{ mL} = x \text{ mL}$$

Answer: 30 mL. In order to administer the dosage required, more than 15 mL will be necessary. The dosage ordered is two times larger than what the available strength is.

43.     125 mg : 5 mL = 100 mg : $x$ mL

*or*

$$\frac{100 \text{ mg}}{125 \text{ mg}} \times 5 \text{ mL} = x \text{ mL}$$

Answer: 4 mL. The dosage ordered is less than the available strength; therefore less than 5 mL will be needed to administer the required dosage.

44.     40 mEq : 15 mL = 40 mEq : $x$ mL

*or*

$$\frac{40 \text{ mEq}}{40 \text{ mEq}} \times 15 \text{ mL} = x \text{ mL}; \quad \frac{40 \text{ mEq}}{40 \text{ mEq}} = \frac{x \text{ mL}}{15 \text{ mL}}$$

Answer: 15 mL. The dosage ordered is contained in 15 mL of the medication.

45.     80 mg : 15 mL = 120 mg : $x$ mL

*or*

$$\frac{120 \text{ mg}}{80 \text{ mg}} \times 15 \text{ mL} = x \text{ mL}$$

Answer: 22.5 mL. The dosage ordered is more than the available strength; therefore you will need more than 15 mL to administer the dosage.

46.     200 mg : 5 mL = 250 mg : $x$ mL

*or*

$$\frac{250 \text{ mg}}{200 \text{ mg}} \times 5 \text{ mL} = x \text{ mL}$$

Answer: 6.3 mL. The dosage ordered is greater than the available strength; therefore more than 5 mL will be needed to administer the required dosage. The answer to the nearest tenth is 6.3 mL.

47.     125 mg : 5 mL = 100 mg : $x$ mL

*or*

$$\frac{100 \text{ mg}}{125 \text{ mg}} \times 5 \text{ mL} = x \text{ mL}$$

Answer: 4 mL. The amount ordered is less than the available strength; therefore less than 5 mL will be needed to administer the required dosage.

48. Use the microgram equivalent to calculate the dosage.

$$50 \text{ mcg} : 1 \text{ mL} = 125 \text{ mcg} : x \text{ mL}$$

*or*

$$\frac{125 \text{ mcg}}{50 \text{ mcg}} \times 1 \text{ mL} = x \text{ mL}$$

Answer: 2.5 mL. (2.5 mL is metric and stated with decimal.) The dosage ordered is larger than the available strength; therefore you will need more than 1 mL to administer the dosage.

49.    $$1 \text{ mg} : 5 \text{ mL} = 4 \text{ mg} : x \text{ mL}$$

*or*

$$\frac{4 \text{ mg}}{1 \text{ mg}} \times 5 \text{ mL} = x \text{ mL}$$

Answer: 20 mL. The dosage ordered is more than the available strength; therefore you will need more than 5 mL to administer the required dosage.

50. Conversion is required. Equivalent: 1,000 mg = 1 g. Therefore 0.5 g = 500 mg.

$$125 \text{ mg} : 5 \text{ mL} = 500 \text{ mg} : x \text{ mL}$$

*or*

$$\frac{500 \text{ mg}}{125 \text{ mg}} \times 5 \text{ mL} = x \text{ mL}$$

Answer: 20 mL. The dosage ordered is four times larger than the available strength; therefore more than 5 mL will be needed to administer the dosage.

51.    $$20 \text{ mg} : 5 \text{ mL} = 60 \text{ mg} : x \text{ mL}$$

$$\frac{20x}{20} = \frac{300}{20}$$

*or*

$$\frac{60 \text{ mg}}{20 \text{ mg}} \times 5 \text{ mL} = x \text{ mL}$$

Answer: 15 mL. The dosage ordered is more than the available strength. You will need more than 5 mL to administer the dosage.

52.    $$30 \text{ mg} : 1 \text{ mL} = 150 \text{ mg} : x \text{ mL}$$

*or*

$$\frac{150 \text{ mg}}{30 \text{ mg}} \times 1 \text{ mL} = x \text{ mL}$$

Answer: 5 mL. The dosage ordered is five times larger than the available strength. You will need more than 1 mL to administer the required dosage.

53.    $$12.5 \text{ mg} : 5 \text{ mL} = 25 \text{ mg} : x \text{ mL}$$

*or*

$$\frac{25 \text{ mg}}{12.5 \text{ mg}} \times 5 \text{ mL} = x \text{ mL}$$

Answer: 10 mL. The dosage needed is two times more than the available strength; therefore you will need more than 5 mL to administer the required dosage.

54. The label indicates that 5 mL = 300 mg of the medication.

$$300 \text{ mg} : 5 \text{ mL} = 600 \text{ mg} : x \text{ mL}$$

*or*

$$\frac{600 \text{ mg}}{300 \text{ mg}} \times 5 \text{ mL} = x \text{ mL}$$

a. 10 mL. The dosage ordered is two times more than the available strength. You will need more than 5 mL to administer the required dosage.

b. Two containers are needed. One container contains 300 mg.

55.    $$2 \text{ mg} : 1 \text{ mL} = 10 \text{ mg} : x \text{ mL}$$

*or*

$$\frac{10 \text{ mg}}{2 \text{ mg}} \times 1 \text{ mL} = x \text{ mL}$$

Answer: 5 mL. The dosage ordered is five times greater than the available strength. More than 1 mL will be needed to administer the required dosage.

56. Conversion is required. Equivalent: 1,000 mg = 1 g. Therefore 0.5 g = 500 mg.

$$62.5 \text{ mg} : 5 \text{ mL} = 500 \text{ mg} : x \text{ mL}$$

*or*

$$\frac{500 \text{ mg}}{62.5 \text{ mg}} \times 5 \text{ mL} = x \text{ mL}$$

Answer: 40 mL. The dosage ordered is larger than the available strength. You will need more than 5 mL to administer the required dosage.

57.    $$200,000 \text{ units} : 5 \text{ mL} = 500,000 \text{ units} : x \text{ mL}$$

*or*

$$\frac{500,000 \text{ units}}{200,000 \text{ units}} \times 5 \text{ mL} = x \text{ mL}$$

Answer: 12.5 mL. The amount ordered is greater than the strength available. You will need more than 5 mL to administer the required dosage.

58. Conversion is required. Equivalent: 1 g = 1,000 mg.

$$125 \text{ mg} : 5 \text{ mL} = 1,000 \text{ mg} : x \text{ mL}$$

*or*

$$\frac{1,000 \text{ mg}}{125 \text{ mg}} \times 5 \text{ mL} = x \text{ mL}; \quad \frac{1000 \text{ mg}}{125 \text{ mg}} = \frac{x \text{ mL}}{5 \text{ mL}}$$

Answer: 40 mL. The dosage ordered is more than the strength available. You will need more than 5 mL to administer the dosage.

59.    $$16 \text{ mg} : 5 \text{ mL} = 24 \text{ mg} : x \text{ mL}$$

*or*

$$\frac{24 \text{ mg}}{16 \text{ mg}} \times 5 \text{ mL} = x \text{ mL}; \quad \frac{24 \text{ mg}}{16 \text{ mg}} = \frac{x \text{ mL}}{5 \text{ mL}}$$

Answer: 7.5 mL. The dosage ordered is greater than the available strength. You will need more than 5 mL to administer the required dosage.

60.    $325 \text{ mg} : 10.15 \text{ mL} = 650 \text{ mg} : x \text{ mL}$

*or*

$$\frac{650 \text{ mg}}{325 \text{ mg}} \times 10.15 \text{ mL} = x \text{ mL}$$

Answer: 20.3 mL. The dosage ordered is two times more than the available strength. You will need more than 10.15 mL to administer the required dosage.

61.    $300 \text{ mg} : 5 \text{ mL} = 400 \text{ mg} : x \text{ mL}$

*or*

$$\frac{400 \text{ mg}}{300 \text{ mg}} \times 5 \text{ mL} = x \text{ mL}$$

Answer: 6.66 = 6.7 mL to the nearest tenth. The dosage ordered is more than the available strength. You will need more than 5 mL to administer the dosage.

62.    $10 \text{ mg} : 1 \text{ mL} = 150 \text{ mg} : x \text{ mL}$

*or*

$$\frac{150 \text{ mg}}{10 \text{ mg}} \times 1 \text{ mL} = x \text{ mL}$$

Answer: 15 mL. The dosage ordered is greater than the available strength; therefore you will need more than 1 mL to administer the required dosage.

63. Conversion is necessary. 1,000 mg = 1 g; therefore 0.3 g = 300 mg.

$$50 \text{ mg} : 5 \text{ mL} = 300 \text{ mg} : x \text{ mL}$$

*or*

$$\frac{300 \text{ mg}}{50 \text{ mg}} \times 5 \text{ mL} = x \text{ mL}$$

Answer: 30 mL. The dosage ordered is greater than the available strength; therefore you will need more than 5 mL to administer the required dosage.

64.    $100,000 \text{ units} : 1 \text{ mL} = 200,000 \text{ units} : x \text{ mL}$

*or*

$$\frac{200,000 \text{ units}}{100,000 \text{ units}} \times 1 \text{ mL} = x \text{ mL}$$

Answer: 2 mL. The dosage ordered is greater than the available strength; therefore you will need more than 1 mL to administer the required dosage.

65.    $80 \text{ mg} : 1 \text{ mL} = 600 \text{ mg} : x \text{ mL}$

*or*

$$\frac{600 \text{ mg}}{80 \text{ mg}} \times 1 \text{ mL} = x \text{ mL}$$

Answer: 7.5 mL. The dosage ordered is greater than the available strength; therefore you will need more than 1 mL to administer the required dosage.

66. Conversion is necessary. 1,000 mg = 1 g; therefore 0.25 g = 250 mg.

$$125 \text{ mg} : 5 \text{ mL} = 250 \text{ mg} : x \text{ mL}$$

*or*

$$\frac{250 \text{ mg}}{125 \text{ mg}} \times 5 \text{ mL} = x \text{ mL}$$

Answer: 10 mL. The dosage ordered is greater than the available strength; therefore you will need more than 5 mL to administer the dosage.

67.    $200 \text{ mg} : 5 \text{ mL} = 200 \text{ mg} : x \text{ mL}$

*or*

$$\frac{200 \text{ mg}}{200 \text{ mg}} \times 5 \text{ mL} = x \text{ mL}$$

Answer: 5 mL. The dosage ordered is equivalent to the available strength. Label indicates 200 mg = 5 mL.

68.    $20 \text{ mg} : 5 \text{ mL} = 30 \text{ mg} : x \text{ mL}$

*or*

$$\frac{30 \text{ mg}}{20 \text{ mg}} \times 5 \text{ mL} = x \text{ mL}$$

Answer: 7.5 mL. The dosage ordered is greater than the available strength; therefore you will need more than 5 mL to administer the required dosage.

69.    $15 \text{ mg} : 1 \text{ mL} = 150 \text{ mg} : x \text{ mL}$

*or*

$$\frac{150 \text{ mg}}{15 \text{ mg}} \times 1 \text{ mL} = x \text{ mL}$$

Answer: 10 mL. The dosage ordered is 10 times more than the available strength; therefore you will need more than 1 mL to administer the required dosage.

70.    $20 \text{ mg} : 1 \text{ mL} = 30 \text{ mg} : x \text{ mL}$

*or*

$$\frac{30 \text{ mg}}{20 \text{ mg}} \times 1 \text{ mL} = x \text{ mL}$$

Answer: 1.5 mL, the dosage ordered is greater than the available strength; therefore you will need more than 1 mL to administer the required dosage.

## Answers to Critical Thinking Questions

1.
   a. 6 tablets
   b. Question the order before administering. Double-check your calculation with another nurse. If order is correct, check with the pharmacy regarding available dosage strengths for the medication. Check a reliable and reputable medication reference for the usual dosage and action of this medication.
   c. Any calculation that requires you to administer more than the maximum number of tablets or capsules, which is usually three (3), to achieve a single dose should be questioned and calculation rechecked. An unusual number of tablets or capsules should alert the nurse to a possible error in prescribing, transcribing, or calculation.

2.
   a. After checking a reliable and reputable drug resource for the usual dosage, contact the pharmacy regarding the available dosage strengths for the medication.
   b. The dosage ordered would require that the tablets be broken to administer the dosage. The tablets are unscored and should not be broken. Unscored tablets will not break evenly, and there is no way to determine the dosage being administered. Breaking an unscored tablet could lead to the administration of an unintended dosage.

3.
   a. The right medication
   b. In preparing the medication the nurse did not read the label carefully and administered Percodan, the wrong medication, which has a similar spelling to Percocet. By not reading the label carefully the nurse did not notice that combination medications contain more than one medication; in this case Percodan contained aspirin. Percocet contained Tylenol.
   c. A medication error occurred because the wrong medication was administered. The client was allergic to aspirin and could have had a reaction from mild to a severe anaphylactic reaction (dyspnea, airway obstruction, shock, and in some cases death).
   d. The error could have been prevented by carefully reading the medication label three times while preparing the medication. The nurse must use caution when administering medications that look alike or that have similar spellings. Tablets or capsules that contain more than one medication must be read carefully. (Percocet contains acetaminophen [Tylenol] and Percodan contains aspirin.)

## NOTE

Refer to problems 1-69 for setup of problems if needed.

## Answers to Chapter Review

1. 3 tabs
2. 20 mL
3. 2 tabs
4. 3 tabs
5. 2 tabs
6. 12.5 mL
7. 2 tabs
8. 2 tabs
9. $\frac{1}{2}$ tab
10. 2 tabs
11. 2 mL
12. 15 mL
13. $\frac{1}{2}$ tab

14. 20.3 mL
15. 20 mL
16. 28.1 mL
17. 3 tabs
18. 2 tabs
19. 2 tabs
20. 6.3 mL
21. 1 0.3-mg tab and 1 0.2-mg tab
22. 1 tab
23. 2 tabs
24. 30 mL
25. 2 caps
26. a. 2 tabs

   b. 8 tabs
27. 2 tabs (1 10-mg tab, 1 20-mg tab)
28. 2 tabs
29. 12.5 mL
30. 1 40-mg tab
31. 7.5 mL
32. 2 tabs
33. $2\frac{1}{2}$ tabs
34. 3 40-mg caps
35. 12.5 mL
36. 2 tabs
37. 2 tabs

38. 2 tabs
39. 20 mL
40. 1 tab
41. 2 tabs: 1 7.5-mg tab, 1 2.5-mg tab
42. 2 tabs
43. 10 mL
44. 1 tab
45. 2 tabs
46. 4 mL
47. 2 caps
48. 10 mL
49. 1 tab
50. 2 tabs

## CHAPTER 18

### Answers to Practice Problems

**NOTE**

Problems requiring conversion reflect conversion of what the prescriber ordered to what is available.

1.
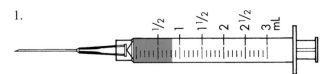

3.
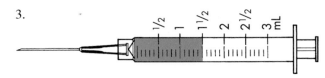

2.
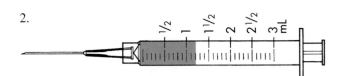

4.
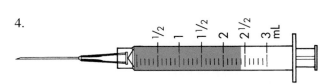

5. 1.4 mL

6. 1 mL

7. 0.9 mL

8. 0.4 mL

9. 4.4 mL

10. 7 mL

11. 3.2 mL

12. a. 20 mL

    b. 25 mg per mL;
       500 mg per 20 mL
       is also correct.

    c. 10 mL

13. a. 10 mL

    b. 0.1 mg per mL

    c. IV use only

14. a. 10 mL

    b. 25 mg per mL

    c. 2 mL

15. a. 20 mL

    b. 100 mg per mL

    c. 0.5 mL

16. a. 10 mL

    b. 400 mcg per mL,
       0.4 mg per mL

    c. IM, subcut, IV

17. a. 20 mL

    b. 2 mg per mL

    c. 2

18. a. 2.5 mL

    b. 10 mg per mL

19. a. 10 mL

    b. 80 mg per mL

20. a. 200 mg per 100 mL,
       2 mg per mL

    b. IV infusion only

21. a. 10 mL

    b. 10 mg per 10 mL,
       1 mg per mL

22. a. 2.5 mL

    b. 1 g per 2.5 mL,
       400 mg per mL

    c. IM use only

23. a. 20 mL

    b. 2 mEq per mL

24. a. 50 mL

    b. 1 mEq per mL

25. a. 10 mL

    b. 1,000 units per mL

26. a. 10 mL

    b. 100 units per mL

27. a. 2 mL

    b. 10,000 units per
       mL, 20,000 units
       per 2 mL

28.    $5 \text{ mg} : 1 \text{ mL} = 10 \text{ mg} : x \text{ mL}$

*or*

$$\frac{10 \text{ mg}}{5 \text{ mg}} \times 1 \text{ mL} = x \text{ mL}$$

Answer: 2 mL. The dosage ordered is more than the available strength; therefore you will need more than 1 mL to administer the dosage.

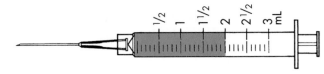

29.    $10 \text{ mg} : 1 \text{ mL} = 5 \text{ mg} : x \text{ mL}$

*or*

$$\frac{5 \text{ mg}}{10 \text{ mg}} \times 1 \text{ mL} = x \text{ mL}$$

Answer: 0.5 mL. The dosage ordered is less than the available strength; therefore you will need less than 1 mL to administer the dosage. Answer stated as decimal (0.5 mL); mL is a metric measure.

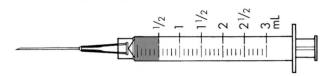

30.    $2 \text{ mg} : 2 \text{ mL} = 1 \text{ mg} : x \text{ mL}$

*or*

$$\frac{1 \text{ mg}}{2 \text{ mg}} \times 2 \text{ mL} = x \text{ mL}$$

Answer: 1 mL. The dosage ordered is less than the available strength; therefore you will need less than 2 mL to administer the dosage.

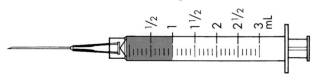

31.    $5 \text{ mg} : 1 \text{ mL} = 8 \text{ mg} : x \text{ mL}$

*or*

$$\frac{8 \text{ mg}}{5 \text{ mg}} \times 1 \text{ mL} = x \text{ mL}$$

Answer: 1.6 mL. The dosage ordered is more than the available strength; therefore you will need more than 1 mL to administer the dosage.

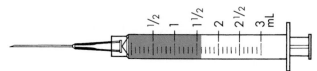

32.    Conversion is required. Equivalent: 1,000 mcg = 1 mg. Therefore 0.05 mg = 50 mcg.

$100 \text{ mcg} : 1 \text{ mL} = 50 \text{ mcg} : x \text{ mL}$

*or*

$$\frac{50 \text{ mcg}}{100 \text{ mcg}} \times 1 \text{ mL} = x \text{ mL}$$

Answer: 0.5 mL. The dosage ordered is less than what is available. Therefore you will need less than 1 mL to administer the dosage. Milliliter (mL) is metric, and answer is expressed as decimal.

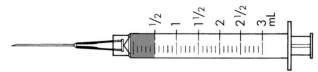

33.    Demerol:

$75 \text{ mg} : 1 \text{ mL} = 50 \text{ mg} : x \text{ mL}$

*or*

$$\frac{50 \text{ mg}}{75 \text{ mg}} \times 1 \text{ mL} = x \text{ mL}$$

Answer: 0.66 mL = 0.7 mL. The dosage ordered is less than the available strength. Therefore less than 1 mL would be required to administer the dosage.

Vistaril:

$50 \text{ mg} : 1 \text{ mL} = 25 \text{ mg} : x \text{ mL}$

*or*

$$\frac{25 \text{ mg}}{50 \text{ mg}} \times 1 \text{ mL} = x \text{ mL}$$

Answer: 0.5 mL. The dosage ordered is less than the available strength. Therefore you will need less than 1 mL to administer the dosage. The total number of milliliters you will prepare to administer is 1.2 mL. This dosage is measurable on the small hypodermics. These two medications are often administered in the same syringe (0.7 mL Demerol + 0.5 mL Vistaril = 1.2 mL).

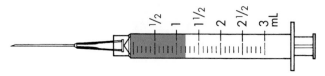

34.    $5 \text{ mg} : 1 \text{ mL} = 5 \text{ mg} : x \text{ mL}$

*or*

$$\frac{5 \text{ mg}}{5 \text{ mg}} \times 1 \text{ mL} = x \text{ mL}$$

Answer: 1 mL. The dosage required is contained in 1 mL. Therefore you will need 1 mL to administer the dosage.

Alternate solution:

$50 \text{ mg} : 10 \text{ mL} = 5 \text{ mg} : x \text{ mL}$

*or*

$$\frac{5 \text{ mg}}{50 \text{ mg}} \times 10 \text{ mL} = x \text{ mL}$$

This setup still gives an answer of 1 mL.

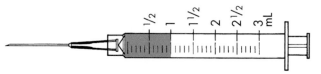

35.    $20,000 \text{ units} : 1 \text{ mL} = 5,000 \text{ units} : x \text{ mL}$

*or*

$$\frac{5,000 \text{ units}}{20,000 \text{ units}} \times 1 \text{ mL} = x \text{ mL}$$

Answer: 0.25 mL. The dosage ordered is less than the available strength. Therefore you will need less than 1 mL to administer the dosage. This dosage can be measured accurately on the 1-mL (tuberculin) syringe, because it is measured in hundredths of a milliliter. The dosage you are administering is 0.25 mL, which is $\dfrac{25}{100}$.

36. Conversion is required. Equivalent: 60 mg = gr 1.

Therefore gr $\frac{1}{4}$ = 15 mg.

$$15 \text{ mg} : 1 \text{ mL} = 15 \text{ mg} : x \text{ mL}$$

*or*

$$\frac{15 \text{ mg}}{15 \text{ mg}} \times 1 \text{ mL} = x \text{ mL}$$

Answer: 1 mL. The label indicates that the dosage ordered is contained in 1 mL.

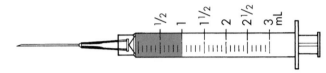

37.  $$10 \text{ mg} : 1 \text{ mL} = 20 \text{ mg} : x \text{ mL}$$

*or*

$$\frac{20 \text{ mg}}{10 \text{ mg}} \times 1 \text{ mL} = x \text{ mL}$$

Answer: 2 mL. The dosage ordered is more than the available strength. Therefore you will need more than 1 mL to administer the required dosage (if dosage strength used is 10 mg per mL as indicated on the label).

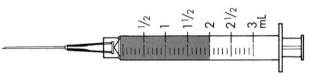

Alternate solution:

$$40 \text{ mg} : 4 \text{ mL} = 20 \text{ mg} : x \text{ mL}$$

*or*

$$\frac{20 \text{ mg}}{40 \text{ mg}} \times 4 \text{ mL} = x \text{ mL}$$

This setup still gives an answer of 2 mL.

## Answers to Critical Thinking Questions

a. The right medication. Hydroxyzine and hydralazine have similar names but are two different medications.

b. Not reading the medication labels carefully and comparing them with the order, or medication administration record (MAR).

c. Hydralazine is an antihypertensive and could cause a fatal drop in the client's blood pressure.

d. Carefully comparing the medication label and dosage with the order or MAR three times while preparing the medication. Perhaps if the nurse had consulted a reliable drug reference it may have alerted the nurse to the fact that hydralazine is used to treat hypertension and hydroxyzine is used for anxiety, which is what the medication was prescribed for.

## Answers to Chapter Review

1. Conversion is required. Equivalent: 1,000 mg = 1 g. Therefore 0.3 g = 300 mg.

$$150 \text{ mg} : 1 \text{ mL} = 300 \text{ mg} : x \text{ mL}$$

*or*

$$\frac{300 \text{ mg}}{150 \text{ mg}} \times 1 \text{ mL} = x \text{ mL}$$

Answer: 2 mL. The dosage ordered is more than the dosage strength available; therefore you will need more than 1 mL to administer the dosage.

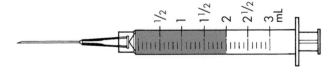

2.  $$0.1 \text{ mg} : 1 \text{ mL} = 0.2 \text{ mg} : x \text{ mL}$$

*or*

$$\frac{0.2 \text{ mg}}{0.1 \text{ mg}} \times 1 \text{ mL} = x \text{ mL}$$

Alternate solution:

$$0.5 \text{ mg} : 5 \text{ mL} = 0.2 \text{ mg} : x \text{ mL}$$

*or*

$$\frac{0.2 \text{ mg}}{0.5 \text{ mg}} \times 5 \text{ mL} = x \text{ mL}$$

This setup still gives an answer of 2 mL.

Answer: 2 mL. The dosage ordered is more than the dosage strength available per mL; therefore you will need more than 1 mL to administer the dosage.

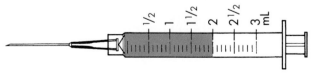

3. Conversion is required. Equivalent: 1,000 mg = 1 g. Therefore 0.5 g = 500 mg.

$$225 \text{ mg} : 1 \text{ mL} = 500 \text{ mg} : x \text{ mL}$$

*or*

$$\frac{500 \text{ mg}}{225 \text{ mg}} \times 1 \text{ mL} = x \text{ mL}$$

Answer: 2.2 mL. The dosage ordered is more than the available strength; therefore you will need more than 1 mL to administer the dosage. The dosage 2.2 mL was rounded off to the nearest tenth of a milliliter. The small hypodermics are marked in tenths of a milliliter.

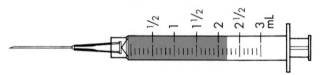

4. No conversion is required. Label indicates dosage in micrograms.

$$500 \text{ mcg} : 2 \text{ mL} = 100 \text{ mcg} : x \text{ mL}$$

*or*

$$\frac{100 \text{ mcg}}{500 \text{ mcg}} \times 2 \text{ mL} = x \text{ mL}$$

Answer: 0.4 mL. The dosage ordered is less than the available strength. The dosage required would be less than 2 mL.

Alternated solution:

$$250 \text{ mcg} : 1 \text{ mL} = 100 \text{ mcg} : x \text{ mL}$$

*or*

$$\frac{100 \text{ mcg}}{250 \text{ mcg}} \times 1 \text{ mL} = x \text{ mL}$$

This would net the same answer, 0.4 mL.

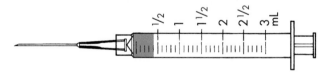

5. $$10 \text{ mg} : 1 \text{ mL} = 4 \text{ mg} : x \text{ mL}$$

*or*

$$\frac{4 \text{ mg}}{10 \text{ mg}} \times 1 \text{ mL} = x \text{ mL}$$

Answer: 0.4 mL. The dosage ordered is less than the available strength; therefore less than 1 mL is required to administer the dosage.

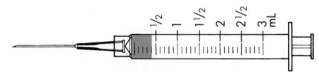

6. $$1,200,000 \text{ units} : 2 \text{ mL} = 1,200,000 \text{ units} : x \text{ mL}$$

*or*

$$\frac{1,200,000 \text{ units}}{1,200,000 \text{ units}} \times 2 \text{ mL} = x \text{ mL}$$

Answer: 2 mL. The dosage ordered is contained in 2 mL; therefore you will need 2 mL to administer the dosage.

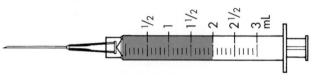

7. $$125 \text{ mg} : 2 \text{ mL} = 100 \text{ mg} : x \text{ mL}$$

*or*

$$\frac{100 \text{ mg}}{125 \text{ mg}} \times 2 \text{ mL} = x \text{ mL}$$

Answer: 1.6 mL. The amount ordered is less than the available strength; therefore you will need less than 2 mL to administer the required dosage.

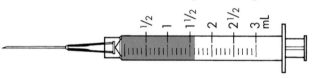

8. $$0.2 \text{ mg} : 1 \text{ mL} = 0.4 \text{ mg} : x \text{ mL}$$

*or*

$$\frac{0.4 \text{ mg}}{0.2 \text{ mg}} \times 1 \text{ mL} = x \text{ mL}$$

Answer: 2 mL. The dosage ordered is more than the available strength; therefore you will need more than 1 mL to administer the required dosage.

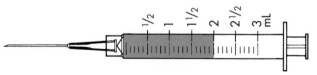

9. $$10,000 \text{ units} : 1 \text{ mL} = 8,000 \text{ units} : x \text{ mL}$$

*or*

$$\frac{8,000 \text{ units}}{10,000 \text{ units}} \times 1 \text{ mL} = x \text{ mL}$$

Answer: 0.8 mL. The dosage ordered is less than the available strength. You will need less than 1 mL to administer the dosage.

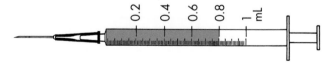

10.     250 mg : 5 mL = 200 mg : $x$ mL

*or*

$$\frac{200 \text{ mg}}{250 \text{ mg}} \times 5 \text{ mL} = x \text{ mL}$$

Answer: 4 mL. The dosage ordered is less than the available strength; therefore you will need less than 5 mL to administer the dosage.

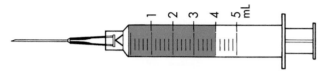

11.     10 mg : 1 mL = 10 mg : $x$ mL

*or*

$$\frac{10 \text{ mg}}{10 \text{ mg}} \times 1 \text{ mL} = x \text{ mL}$$

Answer: 1 mL. The dosage ordered is the same as the available strength; therefore you will need 1 mL to administer the dosage.

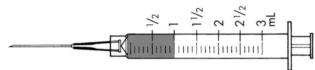

12. Conversion is not required. Label indicates dosage in mg and gr; use the metric equivalent, therefore will need to convert.

$$\text{gr } \frac{1}{2} = 30 \text{ mg.}$$

30 mg : 1 mL = 15 mg : $x$ mL

*or*

$$\frac{15 \text{ mg}}{30 \text{ mg}} \times 1 \text{ mL} = x \text{ mL}$$

Answer: 0.5 mL. The dosage ordered is less than the available strength; therefore you will need less than 1 mL to administer the dosage. (The preferred answer is 0.5 mL. mL is a metric measure.)

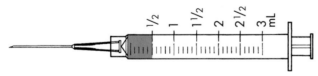

13.     50 mg : 1 mL = 25 mg : $x$ mL

*or*

$$\frac{25 \text{ mg}}{50 \text{ mg}} \times 1 \text{ mL} = x \text{ mL}$$

Answer: 0.5 mL. The dosage ordered is less than the available strength; therefore you will need less than 1 mL to administer the dosage. (The preferred answer is 0.5 mL. mL is a metric measure.)

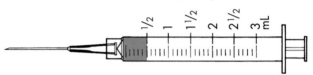

14.     2 mg : 1 mL = 1.5 mg : $x$ mL

*or*

$$\frac{1.5 \text{ mg}}{2 \text{ mg}} \times 1 \text{ mL} = x \text{ mL}$$

Answer: 0.8 mL. 0.75 mL is rounded to nearest tenth. The dosage ordered is less than the available strength. You will need less than 1 mL to administer the dosage.

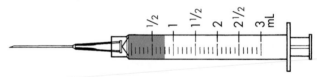

15.     40 mg : 1 mL = 50 mg : $x$ mL

*or*

$$\frac{50 \text{ mg}}{40 \text{ mg}} \times 1 \text{ mL} = x \text{ mL}$$

Answer: 1.3 mL. 1.25 mL is rounded to nearest tenth. The dosage ordered is more than the available strength per mL. You will need more than 1 mL to administer the dosage.

Alternate solution:

80 mg : 2 mL = 50 mg : $x$ mL

*or*

$$\frac{50 \text{ mg}}{80 \text{ mg}} \times 2 \text{ mL} = x \text{ mL}$$

This setup still gives an answer of 1.3 mL.

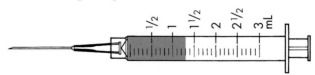

16. $\quad 0.5 \text{ mg} : 5 \text{ mL} = 0.2 \text{ mg} : x \text{ mL}$

*or*

$$\frac{0.2 \text{ mg}}{0.5 \text{ mg}} \times 5 \text{ mL} = x \text{ mL}$$

Answer: 2 mL. The dosage ordered is less than the available strength. You will need less than 5 mL to administer the dosage.

Alternate solution:

$\quad 0.1 \text{ mg} : 1 \text{ mL} = 0.2 \text{ mg} : x \text{ mL}$

*or*

$$\frac{0.2 \text{ mg}}{0.1 \text{ mg}} \times 1 \text{ mL} = x \text{ mL}$$

This setup will still give an answer of 2 mL.

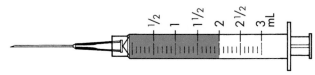

17. $\quad 5 \text{ mg} : 1 \text{ mL} = 3 \text{ mg} : x \text{ mL}$

*or*

$$\frac{3 \text{ mg}}{5 \text{ mg}} \times 1 \text{ mL} = x \text{ mL}$$

Answer: 0.6 mL. The dosage ordered is less than the available strength. You will need less than 1 mL to administer the dosage.

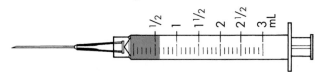

18. $250 \text{ mg} : 2 \text{ mL} = 400 \text{ mg} : x \text{ mL}$

*or*

$$\frac{400 \text{ mg}}{250 \text{ mg}} \times 2 \text{ mL} = x \text{ mL}$$

Answer: 3.2 mL. The dosage ordered is more than the available strength. You will need more than 2 mL to administer the dosage.

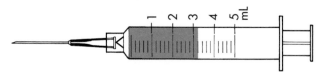

19. Use the dosage indicated on the label in mg; no conversion required.

$\quad 0.4 \text{ mg} : 1 \text{ mL} = 0.2 \text{ mg} : x \text{ mL}$

*or*

$$\frac{0.2 \text{ mg}}{0.4 \text{ mg}} \times 1 \text{ mL} = x \text{ mL}$$

Answer: 0.5 mL. The dosage ordered is less than the available strength. You will need less than 1 mL to administer the dosage.

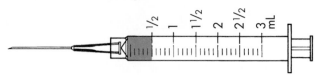

20. Conversion is required. Equivalent: 1,000 mcg = 1 mg. Therefore 200 mcg = 0.2 mg.

$\quad 0.2 \text{ mg} : 1 \text{ mL} = 0.2 \text{ mg} : x \text{ mL}$

*or*

$$\frac{0.2 \text{ mg}}{0.2 \text{ mg}} \times 1 \text{ mL} = x \text{ mL}$$

Answer: 1 mL. Because 200 mcg = 0.2 mg, you will need 1 mL to administer the required dosage.

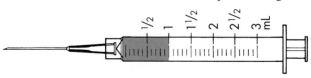

21. $\quad 10,000 \text{ units} : 1 \text{ mL} = 2,500 \text{ units} : x \text{ mL}$

*or*

$$\frac{2,500 \text{ units}}{10,000 \text{ units}} \times 1 \text{ mL} = x \text{ mL}$$

Answer: 0.25 mL. The dosage ordered is less than the available strength. You will need less than 1 mL to administer the dosage.

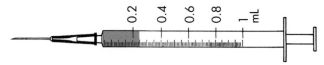

22. $\quad 50 \text{ mg} : 1 \text{ mL} = 35 \text{ mg} : x \text{ mL}$

*or*

$$\frac{35 \text{ mg}}{50 \text{ mg}} \times 1 \text{ mL} = x \text{ mL}$$

Answer: 0.7 mL. The dosage ordered is less than the available strength. You will need less than 1 mL to administer the required dosage.

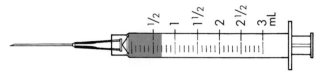

23.     100 mg : 1 mL = 60 mg : $x$ mL

*or*

$$\frac{60 \text{ mg}}{100 \text{ mg}} \times 1 \text{ mL} = x \text{ mL}$$

Answer: 0.6 mL. The dosage ordered is less than the available strength. You will need less than 1 mL to administer the required dosage.

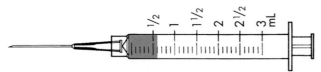

24.     300,000 units : 1 mL = 400,000 units : $x$ mL

*or*

$$\frac{400,000 \text{ units}}{300,000 \text{ units}} \times 1 \text{ mL} = x \text{ mL}$$

Answer: 1.3 mL. 1.33 mL is rounded to the nearest tenth. The dosage ordered is more than the available strength. You will need more than 1 mL to administer the required dosage.

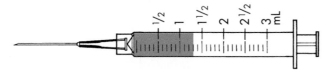

25.     0.5 mg : 2 mL = 0.4 mg : $x$ mL

*or*

$$\frac{0.4 \text{ mg}}{0.5 \text{ mg}} \times 2 \text{ mL} = x \text{ mL}$$

Answer: 1.6 mL. The dosage ordered is less than the available strength. You will need less than 2 mL to administer the required dosage.

Alternate solution:

    0.25 mg : 1 mL = 0.4 mg : $x$ mL

*or*

$$\frac{0.4 \text{ mg}}{0.25 \text{ mg}} \times 1 \text{ mL} = x \text{ mL}$$

This setup still gives the answer of 1.6 mL.

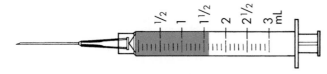

26.     500 mg : 2 mL = 100 mg : $x$ mL

*or*

$$\frac{100 \text{ mg}}{500 \text{ mg}} \times 2 \text{ mL} = x \text{ mL}$$

Answer: 0.4 mL. The dosage ordered is less than the available strength. You will need less than 2 mL to administer the required dosage.

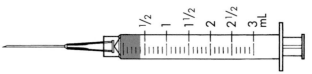

27.     300 mg : 1 mL = 500 mg : $x$ mL

*or*

$$\frac{500 \text{ mg}}{300 \text{ mg}} \times 1 \text{ mL} = x \text{ mL}$$

Answer: 1.7 mL. 1.66 mL is rounded to the nearest tenth. The dosage ordered is more than the available strength. You will need more than 1 mL to administer the dosage.

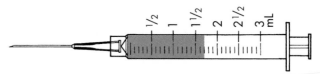

28.     4 mg : 1 mL = 2 mg : $x$ mL

*or*

$$\frac{2 \text{ mg}}{4 \text{ mg}} \times 1 \text{ mL} = x \text{ mL}$$

Answer: 0.5 mL. [Stated as a decimal (0.5); mL is a metric measure.] The dosage ordered is less than the available strength. Therefore you will need less than 1 mL to administer the dosage.

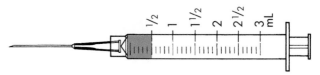

29.     25 mg : 1 mL = 75 mg : $x$ mL

*or*

$$\frac{75 \text{ mg}}{25 \text{ mg}} \times 1 \text{ mL} = x \text{ mL}$$

Answer: 3 mL. The dosage ordered is greater than the available strength. Therefore you will need more than 1 mL to administer the dosage.

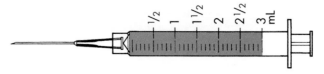

30.     50 mg : 1 mL = 120 mg : x mL

*or*

$$\frac{120 \text{ mg}}{50 \text{ mg}} \times 1 \text{ mL} = x \text{ mL}$$

Answer: 2.4 mL. The dosage ordered is greater than the available strength. Therefore you will need more than 1 mL to administer the dosage.

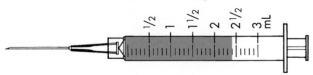

31.     2,000 units : 1 mL = 3,000 units : x mL

*or*

$$\frac{3,000 \text{ units}}{2,000 \text{ units}} \times 1 \text{ mL} = x \text{ mL}$$

Answer: 1.5 mL. The dosage ordered is greater than the available strength. Therefore you will need more than 1 mL to administer the dosage. (The answer is 1.5 mL; mL is a metric measure.)

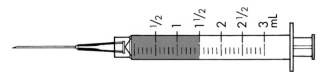

32.     25 mg : 1 mL = 50 mg : x mL

*or*

$$\frac{50 \text{ mg}}{25 \text{ mg}} \times 1 \text{ mL} = x \text{ mL}$$

Answer: 2 mL. The dosage ordered is greater than the available strength. Therefore you will need more than 1 mL to administer the dosage.

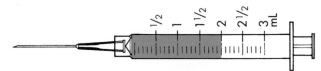

33.     40 mg : 0.4 mL = 30 mg : x mL

*or*

$$\frac{30 \text{ mg}}{40 \text{ mg}} \times 0.4 \text{ mL} = x \text{ mL}$$

Answer: 0.3 mL. The dosage ordered is less than the available strength. You will need less than 0.4 mL to administer the dosage.

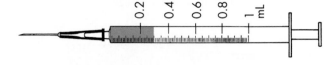

34. Conversion is required. Equivalent: 1,000 mg = 1 g. Therefore 0.3 g = 300 mg.

    300 mg : 2 mL = 300 mg : x mL

*or*

$$\frac{300 \text{ mg}}{300 \text{ mg}} \times 2 \text{ mL} = x \text{ mL}$$

Answer: 2 mL. The label indicates that the dosage ordered, 300 mg, is contained in a volume of 2 mL.

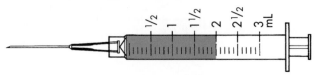

35.     5 mg : 1 mL = 7.5 mg : x mL

*or*

$$\frac{7.5 \text{ mg}}{5 \text{ mg}} \times 1 \text{ mL} = x \text{ mL}$$

Answer: 1.5 mL. (State the answer as a decimal; mL is a metric measure.) The dosage ordered is greater than the available strength. Therefore you will need more than 1 mL to administer the dosage.

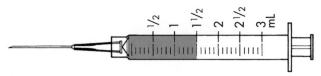

36.     30 mg : 1 mL = 24 mg : x mL

*or*

$$\frac{24 \text{ mg}}{30 \text{ mg}} \times 1 \text{ mL} = x \text{ mL}$$

Answer: 0.8 mL. The dosage ordered is less than the available strength. Therefore you will need less than 1 mL to administer the dosage.

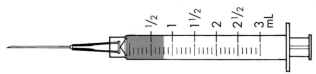

37.     130 mg : 1 mL = 100 mg : x mL

*or*

$$\frac{100 \text{ mg}}{130 \text{ mg}} \times 1 \text{ mL} = x \text{ mL}$$

Answer: 0.8 mL. 0.76 is rounded to the nearest tenth. The dosage ordered is less than the available strength. Therefore you will need less than 1 mL to administer the dosage.

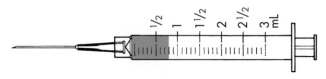

38.     6 mg : 1 mL = 12 mg : $x$ mL

*or*

$$\frac{12 \text{ mg}}{6 \text{ mg}} \times 1 \text{ mL} = x \text{ mL}$$

Answer: 2 mL. The dosage ordered is greater than the available strength. Therefore you will need more than 1 mL to administer the dosage.

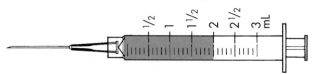

39. Conversion is required. Equivalent: 1,000 mg = 1 g. Therefore 0.25 g = 250 mg.

   25 mg : 1 mL = 250 mg : $x$ mL

*or*

$$\frac{250 \text{ mg}}{25 \text{ mg}} \times 1 \text{ mL} = x \text{ mL}$$

Alternate solution:

   500 mg : 20 mL = 250 mg : $x$ mL

*or*

$$\frac{250 \text{ mg}}{500 \text{ mg}} \times 20 \text{ mL} = x \text{ mL}$$

This setup will still give an answer of 10 mL.

Answer: 10 mL. The dosage ordered is greater than the available strength. Therefore you will need more than 1 mL to administer the dosage.

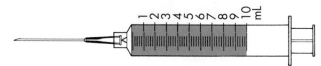

40. Conversion is required. Equivalent: 1,000 mg = 1 g. Therefore 0.5 g = 500 mg.

   500 mg : 1 mL = 500 mg : $x$ mL

*or*

$$\frac{500 \text{ mg}}{500 \text{ mg}} \times 1 \text{ mL} = x \text{ mL}$$

Answer: 1 mL. The dosage ordered, 500 mg, is contained in a volume of 1 mL.

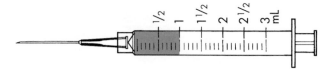

41.     100 mg : 1 mL = 150 mg : $x$ mL

*or*

$$\frac{150 \text{ mg}}{100 \text{ mg}} \times 1 \text{ mL} = x \text{ mL}$$

Answer: 1.5 mL. (Answer stated as a decimal; mL is a metric measure.) The dosage ordered is greater than the available strength; therefore you will need more than 1 mL to administer the dosage.

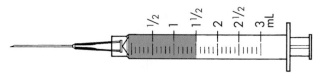

42. Demerol:

   100 mg : 1 mL = 65 mg : $x$ mL

*or*

$$\frac{65 \text{ mg}}{100 \text{ mg}} \times 1 \text{ mL} = x \text{ mL}$$

Answer: 0.65 = 0.7 mL. The dosage ordered is less than the available strength. Therefore less than 1 mL would be required to administer the dosage.

Promethazine:

   50 mg : 1 mL = 25 mg : $x$ mL

*or*

$$\frac{25 \text{ mg}}{50 \text{ mg}} \times 1 \text{ mL} = x \text{ mL}$$

Answer: 0.5 mL. The dosage ordered is less than the strength available; therefore you will need less than 1 mL to administer the required dosage. These two medications are often administered in the same syringe (0.7 mL of Demerol + 0.5 mL of promethazine = 1.2 mL).

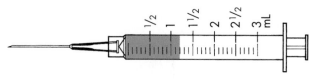

43.     4 mg : 1 mL = 9 mg : $x$ mL

*or*

$$\frac{9 \text{ mg}}{4 \text{ mg}} \times 1 \text{ mL} = x \text{ mL}$$

Answer: 2.25 mL = 2.3 mL. The dosage ordered is greater than the available strength. You would need more than 1 mL to administer the dosage.

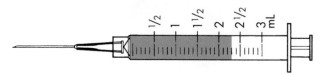

44. 50 mcg : 1 mL = 60 mcg : x mL

*or*

$$\frac{60 \text{ mcg}}{50 \text{ mcg}} \times 1 \text{ mL} = x \text{ mL}$$

Answer: 1.2 mL. The dosage ordered is greater than the available strength. You will need more than 1 mL to administer the dosage.

Alternate solution:

100 mcg : 2 mL = 60 mcg : x mL

*or*

$$\frac{60 \text{ mcg}}{100 \text{ mcg}} \times 2 \text{ mL} = x \text{ mL}$$

This setup will still give an answer of 1.2 mL.

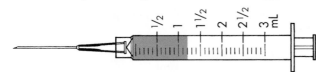

45. 20 mg : 1 mL = 10 mg : x mL

*or*

$$\frac{10 \text{ mg}}{20 \text{ mg}} \times 1 \text{ mL} = x \text{ mL}$$

Answer: 0.5 mL. (Stated as 0.5 mL; mL is a metric measure.) The dosage ordered is less than the available strength. You will need less than 1 mL to administer the dosage.

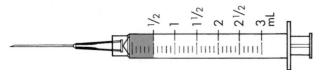

46. 10 mg : 1 mL = 4 mg : x mL

*or*

$$\frac{4 \text{ mg}}{10 \text{ mg}} \times 1 \text{ mL} = x \text{ mL}$$

Answer: 0.4 mL. The dosage ordered is less than the available strength. You will need less than 1 mL to administer the dosage.

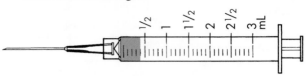

47. 300 mcg : 1 mL = 175 mcg : x mL

*or*

$$\frac{175 \text{ mcg}}{300 \text{ mcg}} \times 1 \text{ mL} = x \text{ mL}$$

Answer: 0.58 = 0.6 mL. The dosage ordered is less than the available strength. You will need less than 1 mL to administer the dosage.

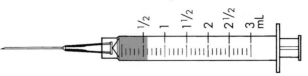

Alternate solution:

480 mcg : 1.6 mL = 175 mcg : x mL

*or*

$$\frac{175 \text{ mcg}}{480 \text{ mcg}} \times 1.6 \text{ mL} = x \text{ mL}$$

This setup would give the same answer of 0.58 mL = 0.6 mL.

## CHAPTER 19

### Answers to Practice Problems

1. 1 g per vial (1 gram per vial)
2. 3.5 mL
3. none stated
4. 250 mg per mL
5. 1 hr
6. 2 mL

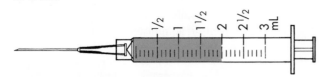

7. 500 mg per vial
8. 1.5 mL

9. none stated (use an approved diluent)
10. 280 mg per mL
11. 24 hours (1 day)
12. 7 days (1 week)
13. 1.4 mL

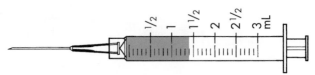

14. 1 g per vial (1 gram per vial)
15. sterile water for injection
16. 2 mL

17. 1 g per 2.6 mL
18. 1.3 mL

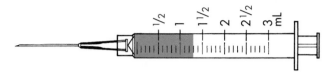

19. 1 g per vial (1 gram per vial)
20. IM or IV (intravenous) use
21. 9.6 mL

22. IV diluent specified in the accompanying package insert
23. 100 mg per mL
24. 2.1 mL
25. 1% Lidocaine hydrochloride injection or sterile water for injection
26. 10 mL

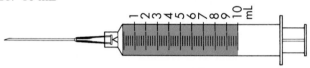

27. 5 mL; 1 tsp
28. water
29. 125 mg per 5 mL
30. Refrigerate and keep tightly closed.
31. 1,000 mg (1 g) per vial
32. 20 mL
33. sterile water for injection
34. 50 mg per mL
35. IV infusion only
36. 140 mL
37. 200 mL
38. 200 mg per 5 mL
39. 10 days (refrigerated)
40. 500 mg per vial
41. 4.8 mL
42. sterile water for injection
43. 100 mg per mL

44. IV infusion only
45. 1 g per vial
46. 2.5 mL
47. sterile water for injection
48. 330 mg per mL
49. 24 hr
50. 24 mL
51. distilled water *or* purified water
52. 50 mg per 5 mL; 10 mg per mL
53. Store suspension at 5° to 25° C (41° to 77° F). Protect from freezing.
54. 20,000,000 units
55. 500,000 units per mL
56. 1,000,000 units per mL— This strength is closest to what is ordered.
57. 2 mL
58. 7 days (1 week)

59. 5,000,000 units
60. 500,000 units per mL
61. 1.4 mL
62. refrigerator
63. 7 days (1 week)
64. 250,000 units per mL
65. 7 days (1 week)
66. 1 g (1 gram) per vial
67. 3 mL
68. sterile water for injection
69. 280 mg per mL
70. 10 mL
71. 95 mg per mL
72. $\dfrac{480 \text{ mL}}{8 \text{ hr}} = 60 \text{ mL/hr}$
73. $\dfrac{1,600 \text{ mL}}{24 \text{ hr}} = 66.6 = 67 \text{ mL/hr}$

74. 300 mL qid = 300 mL × 4 = 1,200 mL

$$\tfrac{2}{3} \times 1,200 \text{ mL} = x \text{ mL}$$

$$\frac{2,400}{3} = x$$

$x$ = 800 mL of formula needed

1,200 mL − 800 mL = 400 mL (water)

Therefore you will add 400 mL of water to 800 mL of Sustacal to make 1,200 mL of $\tfrac{2}{3}$-strength Sustacal.

75. 1 oz = 30 mL; therefore 16 oz = 480 mL

$$\tfrac{3}{4} \times 480 \text{ mL} = x \text{ mL} \quad or \quad \tfrac{3}{4} \times 16 \text{ oz} = x \text{ oz}$$

$$\frac{1,440}{4} = x \qquad\qquad \frac{48}{4} = x$$

$$x = 12 \text{ oz}$$

$x$ = 12 oz (360 mL) of formula needed.

16 oz (480 mL) − 12 oz (360 mL) = 4 oz water (120 mL). You would need 360 mL of formula and 120 mL of water.

## NOTE

For question using ounces, give answer in ounces.

76. 1 oz = 30 mL      20 oz = 600 mL

$$\tfrac{1}{2} \times 600 \text{ mL} = x \text{ mL} \quad or \quad \tfrac{1}{2} \times 20 \text{ oz} = x \text{ oz}$$

$$\frac{600}{2} = x \qquad\qquad \frac{20}{2} = x$$

$$x = 10 \text{ oz}$$

$x$ = 300 mL; you need 10 oz of Ensure.

600 mL (20 oz) − 300 mL (10 oz) Ensure = 300 mL (10 oz of water)

Answer: 10 oz Ensure + 10 oz water = 20 oz $\tfrac{1}{2}$-strength Ensure.

## Answers to Critical Thinking Questions

1. a. The wrong dosage was administered because the nurse chose the incorrect dilution instructions. The dilution instructions used were for IV instead of IM.

   b. The concentration for IM should have been made (add 3 mL of diluents to give a concentration of 280 mg per mL).

   c. The nurse added 10.6 mL of a diluent and made the concentration for IV administration 95 mg per mL.

   d. The client received three times the dose of medication IM (0.9 mL). Interchanging dilution instructions for IV and IM administration can have serious outcomes ranging from irritation of muscles to formation of a sterile abscess.

   e. This type of error could have been prevented by the nurse by reading the label carefully for the correct amount of diluents for the route ordered. Nurses must always check the route ordered and follow the directions that correspond to that route. The dilution instructions for IV and IM should never be interchanged.

## NOTE

For problems where conversion is indicated, answers are shown with order converted to what is available. Calculations could also be performed using dimensional analysis.

## Answers to Chapter Review

1. a. 2 mL

   b. 225 mg per mL

   c. $225 \text{ mg} : 1 \text{ mL} = 250 \text{ mg} : x \text{ mL}$

   $$\frac{225x}{225} = \frac{250}{225}$$

   $$x = 1.11 = 1.1 \text{ mL}$$

   *or*

   $$\frac{250 \text{ mg}}{225 \text{ mg}} \times 1 \text{ mL} = x \text{ mL}$$

   d. Answer: 1.1 mL. The dosage ordered is more than the available strength. You will need more than 1 mL to administer the dosage.

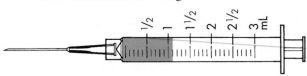

2. $1 \text{ g} : 10 \text{ mL} = 1 \text{ g} : x \text{ mL}$

   $$\frac{10}{1} = x \quad x = 10 \text{ mL}$$

   *or*

   $$\frac{1 \text{ g}}{1 \text{ g}} \times 10 \text{ mL} = x \text{ mL}$$

   $$\frac{10}{1} = x$$

   a. Answer: 10 mL. The dosage ordered is equal to the volume of the reconstituted solution. Large volumes of IV solution may be administered; therefore 10 mL IV is acceptable.

b.

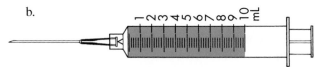

3. a. 11.5 mL

   b. 250 mg per 1.5 mL

   c. $250 \text{ mg} : 1.5 \text{ mL} = 300 \text{ mg} : x \text{ mL}$

   $$\frac{250x}{250} = \frac{450}{250}$$

   $$x = 1.8 \text{ mL}$$

   *or*

   $$\frac{300 \text{ mg}}{250 \text{ mg}} \times 1.5 \text{ mL} = x \text{ mL}$$

   d. Answer: 1.8 mL. The dosage ordered is greater than the available strength; you will need more than 1.5 mL to administer the dosage.

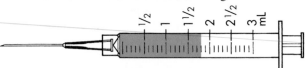

4. $3 \text{ g} : 30 \text{ mL} = 1.5 \text{ g} : x \text{ mL}$

   $$\frac{3x}{3} = \frac{45}{3}$$

   $$x = 15 \text{ mL}$$

   *or*

   $$\frac{1.5 \text{ g}}{3 \text{ g}} \times 30 \text{ mL} = x \text{ mL}$$

   $$\frac{1.5 \times 30}{3} = x, \quad \frac{45}{3} = x$$

   Answer: 15 mL. The dosage ordered is less than the available strength. You will need less than 30 mL to administer the dosage; 15 mL IV can be administered.

5. a. 38 mL

   b. water

   c. 125 mg per 5 mL

   $$125 \text{ mg} : 5 \text{ mL} = 300 \text{ mg} : x \text{ mL}$$

   $$\frac{125x}{125} = \frac{1,500}{125}$$

   $$x = 12 \text{ mL}$$

   *or*

   $$\frac{300 \text{ mg}}{125 \text{ mg}} \times 5 \text{ mL} = x \text{ mL}$$

   d. Answer: 12 mL. The dosage ordered is more than the available strength. You will need more than 5 mL to give the dosage. 12 mL p.o. can be administered; sometimes large volumes are administered p.o.

   e. 10 days

6. a. 500,000 units per mL

   b. 1.8 mL

   c. $500,000 \text{ units} : 1 \text{ mL} = 600,000 \text{ units} : x \text{ mL}$

   $$\frac{500,000x}{500,000} = \frac{600,000}{500,000}$$

   $$x = \frac{6}{5}$$

   $$x = 1.2 \text{ mL}$$

   *or*

   $$\frac{600,000 \text{ units}}{500,000 \text{ units}} \times 1 \text{ mL} = x \text{ mL}$$

   d. Answer: 1.2 mL. The dosage ordered is more than what is available; therefore you will need more than 1 mL to administer the dosage.

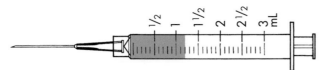

7. a. 250 mg per 2 mL

   b. $250 \text{ mg} : 2 \text{ mL} = 200 \text{ mg} : x \text{ mL}$

   $$\frac{250x}{250} = \frac{400}{250}$$

   $$x = 1.6 \text{ mL}$$

   *or*

   $$\frac{200 \text{ mg}}{250 \text{ mg}} \times 2 \text{ mL} = x \text{ mL}$$

   Answer: 1.6 mL. The dosage ordered is less than what is available; therefore you will need less than 2 mL to administer the dosage.

   c.

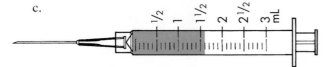

8. a. 1 g per vial

   b. bacteriostatic water for injection with benzyl alcohol

   c. $62.5 \text{ mg} : 1 \text{ mL} = 175 \text{ mg} : x \text{ mL}$

   $$\frac{62.5x}{62.5} = \frac{175}{62.5}$$

   $$x = 2.8 \text{ mL}$$

   *or*

   $$\frac{175 \text{ mg}}{62.5 \text{ mg}} \times 1 \text{ mL} = x \text{ mL}$$

   Alternate solution:

   Convert 175 mg to grams. 1 g = 1,000 mg.

   $$175 \text{ mg} = 0.175 \text{ g}.$$

   $$1 \text{ g} : 16 \text{ mL} = 0.175 \text{ g} : x \text{ mL}$$

   *or*

   $$\frac{0.175 \text{ g}}{1 \text{ g}} \times 16 \text{ mL} = x \text{ mL}$$

   This setup would still give an answer of 2.8 mL.

   Answer: 2.8 mL. When mixed according to directions the dosage is 62.5 mg per mL. You will need more than 1 mL to administer the dosage ordered.

   d.

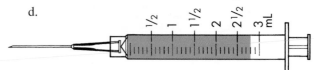

9. a. 78 mL

   b. 125 mg per 5 mL

   c. 20 mL

   $$125 \text{ mg} : 5 \text{ mL} = 500 \text{ mg} : x \text{ mL}$$

   $$\frac{125x}{125} = \frac{2,500}{125}$$

   $$x = 20 \text{ mL}$$

   *or*

   $$\frac{500 \text{ mg}}{125 \text{ mg}} \times 5 \text{ mL} = x \text{ mL}$$

   Answer: 20 mL. The dosage ordered is more than the available strength. You will need more than 5 mL to give the dosage. Since it is a p.o. liquid and sometimes large volumes are administered, 20 mL p.o. can be administered.

10. Conversion is required. Equivalent: 1,000 mg = 1 g; therefore 1.2 g = 1,200 mg.

   a. $500 \text{ mg} : 1 \text{ mL} = 1,200 \text{ mg} : x \text{ mL}$

   $$\frac{500x}{500} = \frac{1,200}{500}$$

   $$x = 2.4 \text{ mL}$$

   *or*

   $$\frac{1,200 \text{ mg}}{500 \text{ mg}} \times 1 \text{ mL} = x \text{ mL}$$

b. Answer: 2.4 mL. The dosage ordered is greater than the available strength; therefore you will need more than 1 mL to administer the dosage.

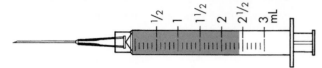

11. a. 250 mg per mL

A conversion is required.

1,000 mg = 1 g; therefore 0.5 g = 500 mg

250 mg : 1 mL = 500 mg : x mL

$$\frac{250x}{250} = \frac{500}{250}$$

$$x = 2 \text{ mL}$$

*or*

$$\frac{500 \text{ mg}}{250 \text{ mg}} \times 1 \text{ mL} = x \text{ mL}$$

b. Answer: 2 mL. The dosage ordered is more than the available strength; therefore you will need more than 1 mL to administer the dosage.

c.

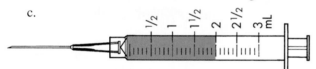

12. a. 55 mL

b. 125 mg per 5 mL

c.    125 mg : 5 mL = 350 mg : x mL

$$\frac{125x}{125} = \frac{1,750}{125}$$

$$x = 14 \text{ mL}$$

*or*

$$\frac{350 \text{ mg}}{125 \text{ mg}} \times 5 \text{ mL} = x \text{ mL}$$

Answer: 14 mL. The dosage ordered is more than the available strength. Therefore you will need more than 5 mL to administer the dosage.

13. a. 20 mL

b. 50 mg per mL

c. Conversion: 1,000 mg = 1 g; therefore 2.4 g = 2,400 mg

$$50 \text{ mg} : 1 \text{ mL} = 2,400 \text{ mg} : x \text{ mL}$$

*or*

$$\frac{2,400 \text{ mg}}{50 \text{ mg}} \times 1 \text{ mL} = x \text{ mL}$$

Answer: 48 mL. The dosage ordered is more than the available strength; therefore you will need more than 1 mL to administer the dosage and three vials.

14. a.    500,000 units : 1 mL = 400,000 units : x mL

*or*

$$\frac{400,000 \text{ units}}{500,000 \text{ units}} \times 1 \text{ mL} = x \text{ mL}$$

Answer: 0.8 mL. The dosage ordered is less than the available strength; therefore you will need less than 1 mL to administer the dosage. *Note:* 500,000 units per mL was used because it is closest to the ordered dose.

b.

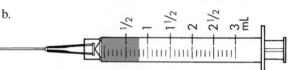

15. a.    280 mg : 1 mL = 250 mg : x mL

*or*

$$\frac{250 \text{ mg}}{280 \text{ mg}} \times 1 \text{ mL} = x \text{ mL}$$

Answer: 0.89 = 0.9 mL rounded to the nearest tenth. The dosage ordered is less than the available strength; therefore you will need less than 1 mL to administer the dosage.

b.

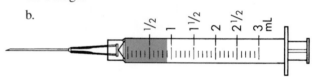

16. a.    1 g : 2.6 mL = 0.5 g : x mL

*or*

$$\frac{0.5 \text{ g}}{1 \text{ g}} \times 2.6 \text{ mL} = x \text{ mL}$$

Answer: 1.3 mL. The dosage ordered is one half of the available strength; therefore you will need less than 2.6 mL to administer the dosage.

b.

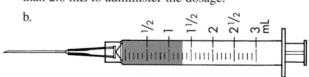

17. Conversion is required. Equivalent: 1,000 mg = 1 g; therefore 0.4 g = 400 mg.

a.    95 mg : 1 mL = 400 mg : x mL

*or*

$$\frac{400 \text{ mg}}{95 \text{ mg}} \times 1 \text{ mL} = x \text{ mL}$$

Answer: 4.2 mL. 4.21 mL is rounded to the nearest tenth. The dosage ordered is greater than the available strength; you will need more than 1 mL to administer the dosage. (Syringe is calibrated in 0.2 increments.)

b.

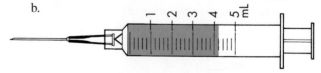

18. Conversion is required. Equivalent: 1,000 mg = 1 g; therefore 0.5 g = 500 mg.

    a. 10 mL

    b. 50 mg per mL

    c.  50 mg : 1 mL = 500 mg : $x$ mL

    $$x = 10 \text{ mL}$$

    *or*

    $$\frac{500 \text{ mg}}{50 \text{ mg}} \times 1 \text{ mL} = x \text{ mL}$$

    Answer: 10 mL. The dosage ordered is greater than the available strength; therefore you will need more than 1 mL to administer the dosage.

    d.

    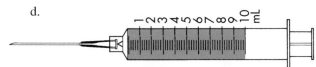

19. Conversion is required. Equivalent: 1,000 mcg = 1 mg; therefore 0.05 mg = 50 mcg.

    a.  40 mcg : 1 mL = 50 mcg : $x$ mL

    $$\frac{40x}{40} = \frac{50}{40}$$

    $$x = 1.3 \text{ mL}$$

    *or*

    $$\frac{50 \text{ mcg}}{40 \text{ mcg}} \times 5 \text{ mL} = x \text{ mL}$$

    Answer: 1.3 mL. 1.25 mL is rounded to the nearest tenth. The dosage ordered is less than the available strength; therefore you will need less than 5 mL to administer the dosage.

    b.

    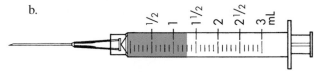

20. Conversion is required. Equivalent: 1,000 mg = 1 g; therefore 0.25 g = 250 mg.

    a.  50 mg : 1 mL = 250 mg : $x$ mL

    $$\frac{50x}{50} = \frac{250}{50}$$

    $$x = 5 \text{ mL}$$

    *or*

    $$\frac{250 \text{ mg}}{50 \text{ mg}} \times 1 \text{ mL} = x \text{ mL}$$

    Answer: 5 mL. The dosage ordered is more than the available strength; therefore you will need more than 1 mL to administer the dosage.

b.

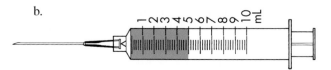

21.  100 mg : 5 mL = 200 mg : $x$ mL

    *or*

    $$\frac{200 \text{ mg}}{100 \text{ mg}} \times 5 \text{ mL} = x \text{ mL}$$

    Answer: 10 mL. The dosage ordered is greater than the available strength; therefore you will need more than 5 mL to administer the dosage.

22. Conversion is required. Equivalent: 1,000 mg = 1 g; therefore 2 g = 2,000 mg.

    200 mg : 1 mL = 2,000 mg : $x$ mL

    *or*

    $$\frac{2,000 \text{ mg}}{200 \text{ mg}} \times 1 \text{ mL} = x \text{ mL}$$

    a. Answer: 10 mL. The dosage ordered is more than what is available; therefore you will need more than 1 mL to administer the dosage.

    b.

    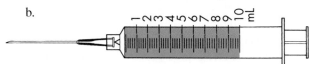

23. Conversion is required. Equivalent: 1,000 mg = 1 g; therefore 2 g = 2,000 mg.

    160 mg : 1 mL = 2,000 mg : $x$ mL

    *or*

    $$\frac{2,000 \text{ mg}}{160 \text{ mg}} \times 1 \text{ mL} = x \text{ mL}$$

    Answer: 12.5 mL. The dosage ordered is more than the available strength; therefore you will need more than 1 mL to administer the dosage.

24.  250 mg : 1 mL = 300 mg : $x$ mL

    *or*

    $$\frac{300 \text{ mg}}{250 \text{ mg}} \times 1 \text{ mL} = x \text{ mL}$$

    a. Answer: 1.2 mL. The dosage ordered is more than the available strength; therefore you will need more than 1 mL to administer the dosage.

    b.

    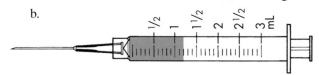

25. Conversion is required. Equivalent: 1,000 mg = 1 g; therefore 1 g = 1,000 mg.

    a. 20 mL

    b.     50 mL : 1 mL = 1,000 mg : $x$ mL

    $$\frac{50x}{50} = \frac{1,000}{50}$$

    $$x = 20 \text{ mL}$$

    *or*

    $$\frac{1,000 \text{ mg}}{50 \text{ mg}} \times 1 \text{ mL} = x \text{ mL}$$

    Answer: 20 mL. The dosage ordered is more than the available strength; therefore you will need more than 1 mL to administer the dosage.

26. a. 60 mL

    b. 100 mL

    c.     200 mg : 5 mL = 375 mg : $x$ mL

    $$\frac{200x}{200} = \frac{1,875}{200}$$

    $$x = 9.4 \text{ mL}$$

    *or*

    $$\frac{375 \text{ mg}}{200 \text{ mg}} \times 5 \text{ mL} = x \text{ mL}$$

    Answer: 9.4 mL. 9.37 mL is rounded to the nearest tenth. The dosage ordered is greater than the available strength; therefore you will need more than 5 mL to administer the dosage.

27. a. 152 mL

    b. 40.5 g per vial

    c. Conversion is required. 1,000 mg = 1 g; 2.25 g = 2,250 mg

    $$200 \text{ mg} : 1 \text{ mL} = 2,250 \text{ mg} : x \text{ mL}$$

    $$\frac{200x}{200} = \frac{2,250}{200}$$

    $$x = 11.3 \text{ mL}$$

    *or*

    $$\frac{2,250 \text{ mg}}{200 \text{ mg}} \times 1 \text{ mL} = x \text{ mL}$$

    Answer: 11.3 mL. 11.25 mL rounded to the nearest tenth. The dosage ordered is greater than the available strength; therefore more than 1 mL is needed to administer the dosage.

28.     2 g : 10 mL = 1.5 g : $x$ mL

    $$\frac{2x}{2} = \frac{15}{2}$$

    $$x = 7.5 \text{ mL}$$

    *or*

    $$\frac{1.5 \text{ g}}{2 \text{ g}} \times 10 \text{ mL} = x \text{ mL}$$

    Answer: 7.5 mL. The dosage ordered is less than what is available; therefore you will need less than 10 mL to administer the dosage.

29. a.     1 g : 2 mL = 1 g : $x$ mL

    $$x = 2 \text{ mL}$$

    *or*

    $$\frac{1 \text{ g}}{1 \text{ g}} \times 2 \text{ mL} = x \text{ mL}$$

    b. Answer: 2 mL. When mixed according to directions, the solution gives 1 g in 2 mL; therefore you will need to give 2 mL to administer the ordered dosage.

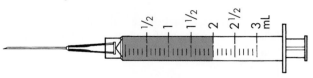

30.     3 g : 8 mL = 1.5 g : $x$ mL

    *or*

    $$\frac{1.5 \text{ g}}{3 \text{ g}} \times 8 \text{ mL} = x \text{ mL}$$

    Answer: 4 mL. The dosage ordered is less than the available strength; therefore you will need less than 8 mL to administer the dosage. (Ordered dosage is half of the available strength.)

31.     40 mg : 5 mL = 20 mg : $x$ mL

    $$\frac{40x}{40} = \frac{100}{40}$$

    $$x = 2.5 \text{ mL}$$

    *or*

    $$\frac{20 \text{ mg}}{40 \text{ mg}} \times 5 \text{ mL} = x \text{ mL}$$

    Answer: 2.5 mL. The dosage ordered is less than the available strength; you will need less than 5 mL to administer the dosage.

32. a. 30 mL

    b. 40 mg per mL

    c.     40 mg : 1 mL = 250 mg : $x$ mL

    $$\frac{40x}{40} = \frac{250}{40}$$

    $$x = 6.3 \text{ mL}$$

    *or*

    $$\frac{250 \text{ mg}}{40 \text{ mg}} \times 1 \text{ mL} = x \text{ mL}$$

    Answer: 6.3 mL. 6.25 mL rounded to the nearest tenth. The dosage ordered is more than what is available; therefore you need more than 1 mL to administer the dosage.

33. a. 10 mL
    b. sterile water for injection without a bacteriostatic agent
    c. 5 mg per mL
    d.      5 mg : 1 mL = 45.5 mg : $x$ mL

    *or*

    $$\frac{45.5 \text{ mg}}{5 \text{ mg}} \times 1 \text{ mL} = x \text{ mL}$$

    Answer: 9.1 mL. The dosage ordered is more than the available strength; therefore you need more than 1 mL to administer the dosage.

34. a. 10 mL
    b. 100 mg per mL
    c.      100 mg : 1 mL = 850 mg : $x$ mL

    *or*

    $$\frac{850 \text{ mg}}{100 \text{ mg}} \times 1 \text{ mL} = x \text{ mL}$$

    Answer: 8.5 mL. The dosage ordered is greater than what is available; therefore you will need more than 1 mL to administer the dosage.

35. a. 2.5 mL
    b. 325 mg per mL
    c. Conversion is required. Equivalent:
       1 g = 1,000 mg.
           325 mg : 1 mL = 1,000 mg : $x$ mL

    *or*

    $$\frac{1,000 \text{ mg}}{325 \text{ mg}} \times 1 \text{ mL} = x \text{ mL}$$

    Answer: 3.07 = 3.1 mL rounded to the nearest tenth. The dosage ordered is greater than what is available; therefore you will need more than 1 mL to administer the dosage.

36. 1 oz = 30 mL; 12 oz = 360 mL

    $$\frac{1}{4} \times 360 \text{ mL} = x \text{ mL}$$

    $$\frac{360}{4} = x$$

    $$x = 90 \text{ mL}$$

    *or*

    $$\frac{1}{4} \times 12 \text{ oz} = x \text{ oz}$$

    $$\frac{12}{4} = x$$

    $$x = 3 \text{ oz}$$

    $x$ = 90 mL; you need 3 oz of Ensure.
    360 mL (12 oz) − 90 mL (3 oz) Ensure = 270 mL (9 oz of water)
    Answer: 3 oz Ensure + 9 oz water = 12 oz ¼ strength Ensure.

37. *Note:* 6 oz q4h = 6 feedings; 6 oz × 6 = 36 oz
    1 oz = 30 mL; therefore 36 oz = 1,080 mL

    $$\frac{2}{3} \times 1,080 \text{ mL} = x \text{ mL}$$

    $$\frac{2,160}{3} = x$$

    $x$ = 720 mL of the formula (Isomil) needed
    1,080 mL − 720 mL = 360 mL (water)
    Answer: You add 360 mL (12 oz) of water to 720 mL (24 oz) of Isomil to make 1,080 mL of ⅔ strength Isomil (12 oz water + 24 oz of Isomil).

38. $$\frac{1,200 \text{ mL}}{16 \text{ hr}} = 75 \text{ mL/hr}$$

39. 4 oz q4h would be 24 oz
    ⅛ × 24 oz = 3 oz, or 90 mL Ensure
    24 oz − 3 oz = 21 oz
    1 oz = 30 mL (21 oz × 30 = 630 mL); 21 oz or 630 mL of water would be added to make ⅛ strength.

# CHAPTER 20

## Answers to Practice Problems

1. Humalog, rapid acting (fast acting)
2. Novolin R Regular, rapid acting (fast acting)
3. Lantus, long acting
4. Humulin N, NPH, intermediate acting
5. 22 units
6. 41 units
7.

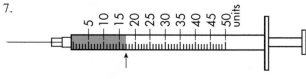

8.

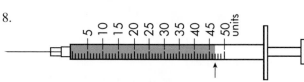

9. 40 units

10. 27 units
11. 53 units
12. 14 units
13.

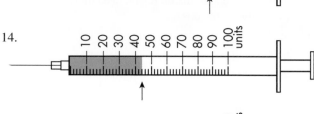

14.

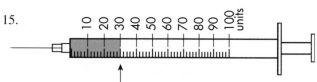

15.

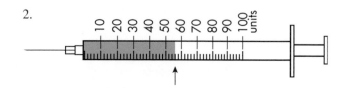

## Answers to Critical Thinking Questions

1. a. Failure to clarify an insulin order when the type of insulin was not specified and the dosage was not clear because the U for units was used. U almost closed caused the "U" to be mistaken for "0."

   b. The right medication, the right dosage.

   c. The client received 10 times the dose of an insulin (regular) that was not ordered. Regular insulin is short acting, and NPH is intermediate acting and was desired. Administering the insulin would likely cause a dangerously low glucose level (hypoglycemia). Results could be tremors, confusion, sweating, and death. This incident constitutes malpractice.

   d. The error could have been prevented by remembering that all the essential components of an insulin order should have been in the order (name of insulin, number of units to be administered, route, frequency, and strength). When one element is missing, never assume. The order should have been clarified

with the prescriber. Further, the dosage should have been double-checked with another nurse. In addition, units should have been written out in the order to avoid misinterpretation of "U" as a zero (0). Many insulin errors occur when the nurse fails to clarify an incomplete order or misinterprets the dosage when units is abbreviated.

2. a. The nurse should have injected the 14 units of air into the NPH vial and then injected 10 units of air into the regular vial and drawn up the 10 units of regular insulin first. First regular, then NPH. Another nurse should have been present during the mixing and to verify the dosage drawn.

   b. Contamination of insulins. Regular (rapid acting) is drawn up first to prevent it from becoming contaminated with the intermediate-acting insulin. This can also result in reversing the doses of the two insulins being drawn up and result in incorrect insulin dosages.

## Answers to Chapter Review

1.

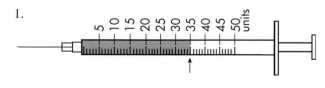

2.

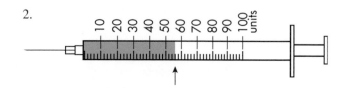

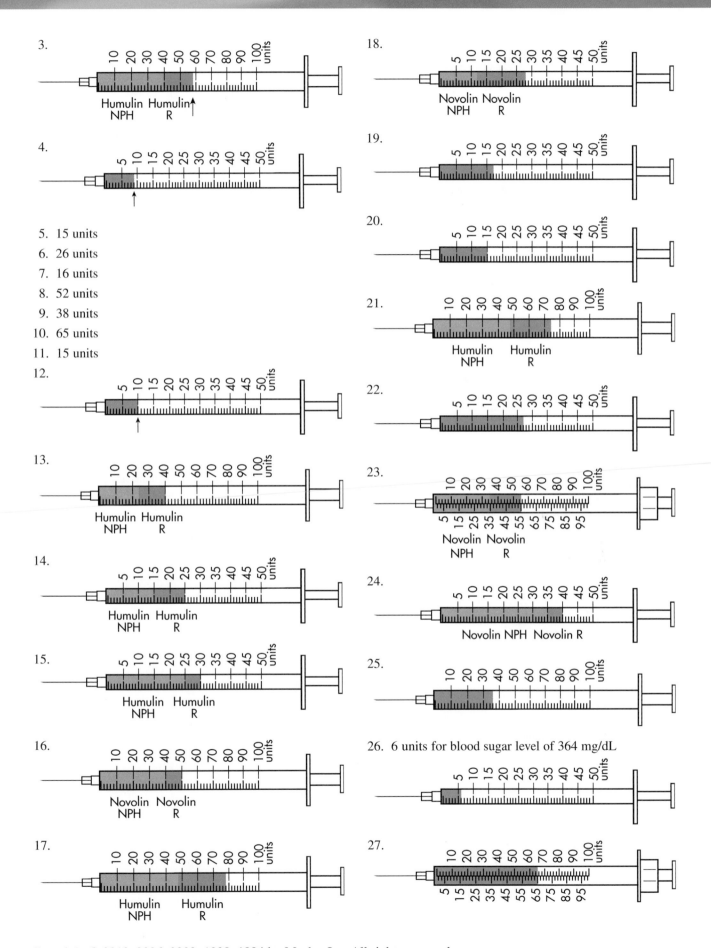

3.

4.

5. 15 units
6. 26 units
7. 16 units
8. 52 units
9. 38 units
10. 65 units
11. 15 units

12.

13.

14.

15.

16.

17.

18.

19.

20.

21.

22.

23.

24.

25.

26. 6 units for blood sugar level of 364 mg/dL

27.

28.

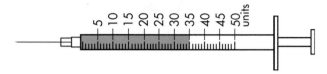

29.

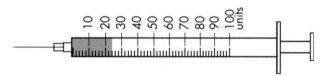

30.

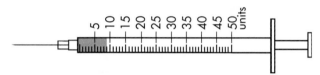

31.

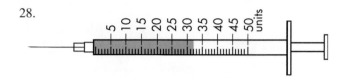

32.

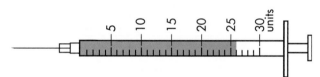

33.

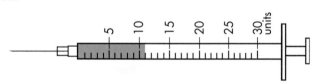

34.

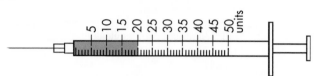

35.

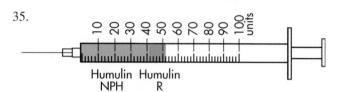

Humulin   Humulin
  NPH          R

36.

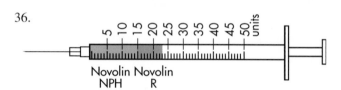

Novolin  Novolin
  NPH        R

37.

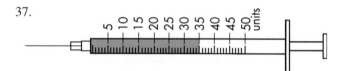

38.

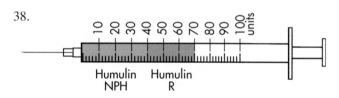

Humulin        Humulin
  NPH                R

39.  10 unit blood sugar 354 mg/dL

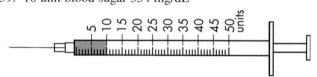

## CHAPTER 21

### Answers to Practice Problems

1.  patient-controlled analgesia

2.  peripheral

3.  intravenous piggyback

4.  0.9% normal saline

5.  higher

6.  pressure

7.  20% dextrose in water

8.  5% dextrose in water with 10 mEq potassium chloride (KCl)

9.  50 g

10. Dextrose: $5 \text{ g} : 100 \text{ mL} = x \text{ g} : 750 \text{ mL}$

$$\frac{100x}{100} = \frac{3{,}750}{100}$$

$$x = 37.5 \text{ g dextrose}$$

*or*

$$\frac{5 \text{ g}}{100 \text{ mL}} = \frac{x \text{ g}}{750 \text{ mL}}$$

NaCl: $0.9 \text{ g} : 100 \text{ mL} = x \text{ g} : 750 \text{ mL}$

$$\frac{100x}{100} = \frac{675}{100}$$

$$x = 6.75 \text{ g NaCl}$$

*or*

$$\frac{0.9 \text{ g}}{100 \text{ mL}} = \frac{x \text{ g}}{750 \text{ mL}}$$

11. $10 \text{ g} : 100 \text{ mL} = x \text{ g} : 250 \text{ mL}$

$$\frac{100x}{100} = \frac{2{,}500}{100}$$

$$x = 25 \text{ g dextrose}$$

*or*

$$\frac{10 \text{ g}}{100 \text{ mL}} = \frac{x \text{ g}}{250 \text{ mL}}$$

12. Dextrose: $5 \text{ g} : 100 \text{ mL} = x \text{ g} : 1{,}000 \text{ mL}$

$$\frac{100x}{100} = \frac{5{,}000}{100}$$

$$x = 50 \text{ g dextrose}$$

*or*

$$\frac{5 \text{ g}}{100 \text{ mL}} = \frac{x \text{ g}}{1{,}000 \text{ mL}}$$

NaCl: $0.33 \text{ g} : 100 \text{ mL} = x \text{ g} : 1{,}000 \text{ mL}$

$$\frac{100x}{100} = \frac{330}{100}$$

$$x = 3.3 \text{ g NaCl}$$

*or*

$$\frac{0.33 \text{ g}}{100 \text{ mL}} = \frac{x \text{ g}}{1{,}000 \text{ mL}}$$

13. Dextrose: $5 \text{ g} : 100 \text{ mL} = x \text{ g} : 500 \text{ mL}$

$$\frac{100x}{100} = \frac{2{,}500}{100}$$

$$x = 25 \text{ g dextrose}$$

*or*

$$\frac{5 \text{ g}}{100 \text{ mL}} = \frac{x \text{ g}}{500 \text{ mL}}$$

NaCl: $0.45 \text{ g} : 100 \text{ mL} = x \text{ g} : 500 \text{ mL}$

$$\frac{100x}{100} = \frac{225}{100}$$

$$x = 2.25 \text{ g NaCl}$$

*or*

$$\frac{0.45 \text{ g}}{100 \text{ mL}} = \frac{x \text{ g}}{500 \text{ mL}}$$

## Answer to Critical Thinking Question

Troubleshooting should have been done by the nurses caring for the client. If the client's pain was not being relieved the device should have been checked for possible malfunctioning and to determine whether the machine had been set up properly. It is mandatory that all programming be double-checked by nurses and the pump be monitored frequently to ensure that it is functioning. The client's continual complaint of severe pain with no relief should have been a key to the nurses caring for the client.

## Answers to Chapter Review

1. B
2. C
3. A
4. D
5. pain
6. push *or* bolus
7. intravenous piggyback
8. higher

9. 25 g dextrose : 1.125 g NaCl

Equivalent: 1 L = 1,000 mL

Therefore 0.5 L = 500 mL

Dextrose:

5 g : 100 mL = $x$ g : 500 mL

$$\frac{100x}{100} = \frac{2,500}{100}$$

$x$ = 25 g dextrose

*or*

$$\frac{5\ g}{100\ mL} = \frac{x\ g}{500\ mL}$$

NaCl:

0.225 g : 100 mL = $x$ g : 500 mL

$$\frac{100x}{100} = \frac{1,12.5}{100}$$

$x$ = 1.125 g NaCl

*or*

$$\frac{0.225\ g}{100\ mL} = \frac{x\ g}{500\ mL}$$

10. 37.5 g dextrose : 3.375 g NaCl

Dextrose:

5 g : 100 mL = $x$ g : 750 mL

$$\frac{100x}{100} = \frac{3,750}{100}$$

$x$ = 37.5 g of dextrose

*or*

$$\frac{5\ g}{100\ mL} = \frac{x\ g}{750\ mL}$$

NaCl:

0.45 g : 100 mL = $x$ g : 750 mL

$$\frac{100x}{100} = \frac{337.5}{100}$$

$x$ = 3.375 g NaCl

*or*

$$\frac{0.45\ g}{100\ mL} = \frac{x\ g}{750\ mL}$$

## CHAPTER 22

### Answers to Practice Problems

1. $x$ mL/hr = $\dfrac{1,800\ mL}{24\ hr}$; $x$ = 75 mL/hr

2. $x$ mL/hr = $\dfrac{2,000\ mL}{24\ hr}$; $x$ = 83.3 = 83 mL/hr

3. $x$ mL/hr = $\dfrac{500\ mL}{12\ hr}$; $x$ = 41.6 = 42 mL/hr

4. *Remember:* When infusion time is less than an hour, use a ratio and proportion to determine the rate in mL/hr.

100 mL : 45 min = $x$ mL : 60 min

$$\frac{45x}{45} = \frac{6,000}{45}; x = 133.3; x = 133\ mL/hr$$

5. $x$ mL/hr = $\dfrac{1,500\ mL}{24\ hr}$; $x$ = 62.5 = 63 mL/hr

6. $x$ mL/hr = $\dfrac{750\ mL}{16\ hr}$; $x$ = 46.8 = 47 mL/hr

7. *Remember:* When infusion time is less than an hour, use a ratio and proportion to determine the rate in mL/hr.

30 mL : 20 min = $x$ mL : 60 min

$$\frac{20x}{20} = \frac{1,800}{20} = 90; x = 90\ mL/hr$$

8. 10 gtt/mL, macrodrop

9. 60 gtt/mL, microdrop

10. 20 gtt/mL, macrodrop

11. 15 gtt/mL, macrodrop

12. $x$ gtt/min = $\dfrac{75\ mL \times 10\ gtt/mL}{60\ min}$ =

$$\frac{75 \times 10}{60} = \frac{75 \times 1}{6} = \frac{75}{6}$$

$x = \dfrac{75}{6}$; $x$ = 12.5 = 13 gtt/min

Answer: 13 gtt/min; 13 macrogtt/min

13. $x$ gtt/min = $\dfrac{30\ mL \times 60\ gtt/mL}{60\ min}$ =

$$\frac{30 \times 60}{60} = \frac{30 \times 1}{1} = \frac{30}{1}$$

$x = \dfrac{30}{1}$; $x$ = 30 gtt/min

Answer: 30 gtt/min; 30 microgtt/min

14. $x$ gtt/min = $\dfrac{125\ mL \times 15\ gtt/mL}{60\ min}$ =

$$\frac{125 \times 15}{60} = \frac{125 \times 1}{4} = \frac{125}{4}$$

$x = \dfrac{125}{4}$; $x$ = 31.2 = 31 gtt/min

Answer: 31 gtt/min; 31 macrogtt/min

15. Step 1: Calculate mL/hr.

$$x \text{ mL/hr} = \frac{1{,}000 \text{ mL}}{6 \text{ hr}}; x = 166.6 = 167 \text{ mL/hr}$$

Step 2: Calculate gtt/min

$$x \text{ gtt/min} = \frac{167 \text{ mL} \times 15 \text{ gtt/mL}}{60 \text{ min}} =$$

$$\frac{167 \times 15}{60} = \frac{167 \times 1}{4} = \frac{167}{4}$$

$$x = \frac{167}{4}; x = 41.7 = 42 \text{ gtt/min}$$

Answer: 42 gtt/min; 42 macrogtt/min

16. $x \text{ gtt/min} = \dfrac{60 \text{ mL} \times 60 \text{ gtt/mL}}{45 \text{ min}} =$

$$\frac{60 \times 60}{45} = \frac{60 \times 4}{3} = \frac{240}{3}$$

$$x = \frac{240}{3}; x = 80 \text{ gtt/min}$$

Answer: 80 gtt/min; 80 microgtt/min

**NOTE**

These problems could also be done by first determining rate in mL/min to be administered and then calculating rate in gtt/min or by using dimensional analysis.

17. Step 1: Calculate mL/hr.

$$x \text{ mL/hr} = \frac{1{,}000 \text{ mL}}{16 \text{ hr}}; x = 62.5 = 63 \text{ mL/hr}$$

Step 2: Calculate gtt/min.

$$x \text{ gtt/min} = \frac{63 \text{ mL} \times 15 \text{ gtt/mL}}{60 \text{ min}} =$$

$$\frac{63 \times 15}{60} = \frac{63 \times 1}{4} = \frac{63}{4}$$

$$x = \frac{63}{4}; x = 15.7 = 16 \text{ gtt/min}$$

Answer: 16 gtt/min; 16 macrogtt/min

18. Step 1: Calculate mL/hr.

$$x \text{ mL/hr} = \frac{150 \text{ mL}}{2 \text{ hr}}; x = 75 \text{ mL/hr}$$

Step 2: Calculate gtt/min.

$$x \text{ gtt/min} = \frac{75 \text{ mL} \times 20 \text{ gtt/mL}}{60 \text{ min}} =$$

$$\frac{75 \times 20}{60} = \frac{75 \times 1}{3} = \frac{75}{3}$$

$$x = \frac{75}{3}; x = 25 \text{ gtt/min}$$

Answer: 25 gtt/min; 25 macrogtt/min

19. Step 1: Calculate mL/hr.

$$x \text{ mL/hr} = \frac{3{,}000 \text{ mL}}{24 \text{ hr}}; x = 125 \text{ mL/hr}$$

Step 2: Calculate gtt/min.

$$x \text{ gtt/min} = \frac{125 \text{ mL} \times 10 \text{ gtt/mL}}{60 \text{ min}} =$$

$$\frac{125 \times 10}{60} = \frac{125 \times 1}{6} = \frac{125}{6}$$

$$x = \frac{125}{6}; x = 20.8 = 21 \text{ gtt/min}$$

Answer: 21 gtt/min; 21 macrogtt/min

20. Step 1: Calculate mL/hr.

$$x \text{ mL/hr} = \frac{2{,}000 \text{ mL}}{12 \text{ hr}}; x = 166.6 = 167 \text{ mL/hr}$$

Step 2: Calculate gtt/min.

$$x \text{ gtt/min} = \frac{167 \text{ mL} \times 15 \text{ gtt/mL}}{60 \text{ min}} =$$

$$\frac{167 \times 15}{60} = \frac{167 \times 1}{4} = \frac{167}{4}$$

$$x = \frac{167}{4}; x = 41.7 = 42 \text{ gtt/min}$$

Answer: 42 gtt/min; 42 macrogtt/min

21. $x \text{ gtt/min} = \dfrac{60 \text{ mL} \times 60 \text{ gtt/mL}}{30 \text{ min}} =$

$$\frac{60 \times 60}{30} = \frac{60 \times 2}{1} = \frac{120}{1}$$

$$x = \frac{120}{1}; x = 120 \text{ gtt/min}$$

Answer: 120 gtt/min; 120 microgtt/min

**NOTE**

Practice problems could also have been done by first determining the rate in mL/min and then calculating the rate in gtt/min.

22. 20 gtt/mL

$$\frac{60}{20}$$

Answer: 3

23. 10 gtt/mL

$$\frac{60}{10}$$

Answer: 6

24. 60 gtt/mL

$$\frac{60}{60}$$

Answer: 1

25. Step 1: Determine the drop factor constant.
$$60 \div 10 = 6$$
Step 2: Calculate gtt/min.
$$x \text{ gtt/min} = \frac{200 \text{ mL/hr}}{6}; x = 33.3 = 33 \text{ gtt/min}$$
Answer: 33 gtt/min; 33 macrogtt/min

26. Step 1: Determine the drop factor constant.
$$60 \div 15 = 4$$
Step 2: Calculate gtt/min.
$$x \text{ gtt/min} = \frac{50 \text{ mL/hr}}{4}; x = 12.5 = 13 \text{ gtt/min}$$
Answer: 13 gtt/min; 13 macrogtt/min

27. Step 1: Determine the drop factor constant.
$$60 \div 60 = 1$$
Step 2: Calculate gtt/min.
$$x \text{ gtt/min} = \frac{80 \text{ mL/hr}}{1}; x = 80 \text{ gtt/min}$$
Answer: 80 gtt/min; 80 microgtt/min

28. Step 1: Determine the drop factor constant.
$$60 \div 20 = 3$$
Step 2: Calculate gtt/min.
$$x \text{ gtt/min} = \frac{140 \text{ mL/hr}}{3}; x = 46.6 = 47 \text{ gtt/min}$$
Answer: 47 gtt/min; 47 macrogtt/min

29. Step 1: Determine mL/hr.
$$x \text{ mL/hr} = \frac{1,000 \text{ mL}}{10 \text{ hr}}; x = 100 \text{ mL/hr}$$
Step 2: Determine the drop factor constant.
$$60 \div 10 = 6$$
Step 3: Calculate gtt/min.
$$x \text{ gtt/min} = \frac{100 \text{ mL/hr}}{6}; x = 16.6 = 17 \text{ gtt/min}$$
Answer: 17 gtt/min; 17 macrogtt/min

30. Step 1: Determine mL/hr.
$$x \text{ mL/hr} = \frac{1,500 \text{ mL}}{12 \text{ hr}}; x = 125 \text{ mL/hr}$$
Step 2: Determine the drop factor constant.
$$60 \div 15 = 4$$
Step 3: Calculate gtt/min.
$$x \text{ gtt/min} = \frac{125 \text{ mL/hr}}{4}; x = 31.2 = 31 \text{ gtt/min}$$
Answer: 31 gtt/min; 31 macrogtt/min

31. Remember that small volumes are multiplied and expressed in mL/hr.
Step 1: Determine mL/hr.
$$40 \text{ mL/20 min} = 40 \times 3 \ (3 \times 20 \text{ min})$$
$$= 120 \text{ mL/hr}$$
Step 2: Determine the drop factor constant.
$$60 \div 10 = 6$$
Step 3: Calculate gtt/min.
$$x \text{ gtt/min} = \frac{120 \text{ mL/hr}}{6}; x = 20 \text{ gtt/min}$$
Answer: 20 gtt/min; 20 macrogtt/min

32. $$x \text{ gtt/min} = \frac{125 \text{ mL} \times 15 \text{ gtt/mL}}{60 \text{ min}} =$$
$$\frac{125 \times 15}{60} = \frac{125 \times 1}{4} = \frac{125}{4}$$
$$x = \frac{125}{4}; x = 31.2 = 31 \text{ gtt/min}$$
Answer: 31 gtt/min; 31 macrogtt/min

33. Step 1: Determine mL/hr.
$$x \text{ mL/hr} = \frac{2,500 \text{ mL}}{16 \text{ hr}}; x = 156.2 = 156 \text{ mL/hr}$$
Step 2: Calculate gtt/min.
$$x \text{ gtt/min} = \frac{156 \text{ mL} \times 10 \text{ gtt/mL}}{60 \text{ min}} =$$
$$\frac{156 \times 10}{60} = \frac{156 \times 1}{6} = \frac{156}{6}$$
$$x = \frac{156}{6}; x = 26 \text{ gtt/min}$$
Answer: 26 gtt/min; 26 macrogtt/min

34. $$x \text{ gtt/min} = \frac{100 \text{ mL} \times 60 \text{ gtt/mL}}{60 \text{ min}} =$$
$$\frac{100 \times 60}{60} = \frac{100 \times 1}{1} = \frac{100}{1}$$
$$x = \frac{100}{1}; x = 100 \text{ gtt/min}$$
Answer: 100 gtt/min; 100 microgtt/min

35. 1 L = 1,000 mL
2 L = 2,000 mL
Step 1: Determine mL/hr.
$$x \text{ mL/hr} = \frac{2,000 \text{ mL}}{10 \text{ hr}}; x = 200 \text{ mL/hr}$$
Step 2: Calculate gtt/min.
$$x \text{ gtt/min} = \frac{200 \text{ mL} \times 15 \text{ gtt/mL}}{60 \text{ min}} =$$
$$\frac{200 \times 15}{60} = \frac{200 \times 1}{4} = \frac{200}{4}$$
$$x = \frac{200}{4}; x = 50 \text{ gtt/min}$$
Answer: 50 gtt/min; 50 macrogtt/min

**NOTE**

Practice problems 32-35 could also have been done by using the shortcut method (determining drop factor constant and then calculating gtt/min). This method would give the same answers.

36. $x$ gtt/min $= \dfrac{130 \text{ mL} \times 15 \text{ gtt/mL}}{60 \text{ min}} =$

$\dfrac{130 \times 15}{60} = \dfrac{130 \times 1}{4} = \dfrac{130}{4}$

$x = \dfrac{130}{4}; x = 32.5 = 33$ gtt/min

Answer: 33 gtt/min; 33 macrogtt/min

37. $x$ gtt/min $= \dfrac{250 \text{ mL} \times 10 \text{ gtt/min}}{60 \text{ min}} =$

$\dfrac{250 \times 10}{60} = \dfrac{250 \times 1}{6} = \dfrac{250}{6}$

$x = \dfrac{250}{6}; x = 41.6 = 42$ gtt/min

Answer: 42 gtt/min; 42 macrogtt/min

38. a. 1 g : 10 mL = 1 g : $x$ mL

*or*

$\dfrac{1 \text{ g}}{1 \text{ g}} \times 10 \text{ mL} = x \text{ mL}$

Answer: 10 mL. The dosage ordered is contained in a volume of 10 mL. 10 mL of medication is added to the 50 mL of IV solution to give a total of 60 mL.

b. $x$ gtt/min $= \dfrac{60 \text{ mL} \times 10 \text{ gtt/mL}}{45 \text{ min}} =$

$\dfrac{60 \times 10}{45} = \dfrac{60 \times 2}{9} = \dfrac{120}{9}$

$x = \dfrac{120}{9}; x = 13.3 = 13$ gtt/min

Answer: 13 gtt/min; 13 macrogtt/min

39. a. 150 mg : 1 mL = 900 mg : $x$ mL

*or*

$\dfrac{900 \text{ mg}}{150 \text{ mg}} \times 1 \text{ mL} = x \text{ mL}$

Answer: 6 mL. The dosage ordered is more than the available strength; therefore more than 1 mL is needed to administer the dosage ordered.

b. $x$ gtt/min $= \dfrac{75 \text{ mL} \times 10 \text{ gtt/mL}}{30 \text{ min}} =$

$\dfrac{75 \times 10}{30} = \dfrac{75 \times 1}{3} = \dfrac{75}{3}$

$x = \dfrac{75}{3}; x = 25$ gtt/min

Answer: 25 gtt/min; 25 macrogtt/min

40. a. 300 mg : 2 mL = 300 mg : $x$ mL

*or*

$\dfrac{300 \text{ mg}}{300 \text{ mg}} \times 2 \text{ mL} = x \text{ mL}$

Answer: 2 mL. The dosage ordered is contained in a volume of 2 mL. Label indicates 300 mg per 2 mL.

b. $x$ gtt/min $= \dfrac{50 \text{ mL} \times 10 \text{ gtt/mL}}{30 \text{ min}} =$

$\dfrac{50 \times 10}{30} = \dfrac{50 \times 1}{3} = \dfrac{50}{3}$

$x = \dfrac{50}{3}; x = 16.6 = 17$ gtt/min

Answer: 17 gtt/min; 17 macrogtt/min

41. a. 50 mg : 1 mL = 500 mg : $x$ mL

*or*

$\dfrac{500 \text{ mg}}{50 \text{ mg}} \times 1 \text{ mL} = x \text{ mL}$

Answer: 10 mL. The dosage ordered is greater than the available strength; therefore you will need more than 1 mL to administer the ordered dosage. The volume of medication is added to the 100 mL of IV solution to get a total of 110 mL.

b. $x$ gtt/min $= \dfrac{110 \text{ mL} \times 15 \text{ gtt/mL}}{60 \text{ min}} =$

$\dfrac{110 \times 15}{60} = \dfrac{110 \times 1}{4} = \dfrac{110}{4}$

$x = \dfrac{110}{4}; x = 27.5 = 28$ gtt/min

Answer: 28 gtt/min; 28 macrogtt/min

42. a. 50 mg : 10 mL = 20 mg : $x$ mL

*or*

$\dfrac{20 \text{ mg}}{50 \text{ mg}} \times 10 \text{ mL} = x \text{ mL}$

Answer: 4 mL. The dosage ordered is less than the available strength; therefore you will need less than 10 mL to administer the ordered dosage.

Step 1: Calculate mL/hr.

$x$ mL/hr $= \dfrac{300 \text{ mL}}{6 \text{ hr}}; x = 50$ mL/hr

Step 2: Calculate gtt/min.

b. $x$ gtt/min $= \dfrac{50 \text{ mL} \times 60 \text{ gtt/mL}}{60 \text{ min}} =$

$\dfrac{50 \times 60}{60} = \dfrac{50 \times 1}{1} = \dfrac{50}{1}$

$x = \dfrac{50}{1}; x = 50$ gtt/min

Answer: 50 gtt/min; 50 microgtt/min

43. a.    16 mg : 1 mL = 300 mg : $x$ mL

*or*

$$\frac{300 \text{ mg}}{16 \text{ mg}} \times 1 \text{ mL} = x \text{ mL}$$

Answer: 18.8 mL (18.75 mL rounded to the nearest tenth). The dosage ordered is more than the available strength; therefore you will need more than 1 mL to administer the ordered dosage.

Alternate method for calculating dosage:

320 mg : 20 mL = 300 mg : $x$ mL

*or*

$$\frac{300 \text{ mg}}{320 \text{ mg}} \times 20 \text{ mL} = x \text{ mL}$$

Answer: 18.8 mL (18.75 mL rounded to nearest tenth)

b.  $x$ gtt/min = $\dfrac{300 \text{ mL} \times 10 \text{ gtt/mL}}{60 \text{ min}}$ =

$$\frac{300 \times 10}{60} = \frac{300 \times 1}{6} = \frac{300}{6}$$

$$x = \frac{300}{6}; x = 50 \text{ gtt/min}$$

Answer: 50 gtt/min; 50 macrogtt/min

44. The label indicates each milliliter contains 10 mg of the medication. To administer the ordered dose, you will need to add 10 mL of medication to the IV volume. 100 mL of IV fluid and medication volume gives a total of 110 mL.

$$x \text{ gtt/min} = \frac{110 \text{ mL} \times 10 \text{ gtt/mL}}{60 \text{ min}} =$$

$$\frac{110 \times 10}{60} = \frac{110 \times 1}{6} = \frac{110}{6}$$

$$x = \frac{110}{6}; x = 18.3 = 18 \text{ gtt/min}$$

Answer: 18 gtt/min; 18 macrogtt/min

45.  15 mEq : 1,000 mL = 4 mEq : $x$ mL

$$\frac{15x}{15} = \frac{4,000}{15}$$

$$x = 266.6 = 267 \text{ mL/hr}$$

*or*

$$\frac{15 \text{ mEq}}{1,000 \text{ mL}} = \frac{4 \text{ mEq}}{x \text{ mL}}$$

Answer: 267 mL/hr to deliver 4 mEq of potassium chloride

46.  50 units : 250 mL = 10 units : $x$ mL

$$\frac{50x}{50} = \frac{2,500}{50}$$

$$x = 50 \text{ mL/hr}$$

*or*

$$\frac{50 \text{ units}}{250 \text{ mL}} = \frac{10 \text{ units}}{x \text{ mL}}$$

Answer: 50 mL/hr must be administered for the client to receive 10 units/hr.

47.  40 units : 250 mL = 15 units : $x$ mL

$$\frac{40x}{40} = \frac{3,750}{40}$$

$$x = 93.7 = 94 \text{ mL/hr}$$

*or*

$$\frac{40 \text{ units}}{250 \text{ mL}} = \frac{15 \text{ units}}{x \text{ mL}}$$

Answer: 94 mL/hr must be administered for the client to receive 15 units/hr.

## NOTE

Problem 48 asks for time in hours so minutes are changed to parts of hours.

48.  60 microgtt/min = $\dfrac{150 \text{ mL} \times 60 \text{ gtt/mL}}{x \text{ min}}$

$$60 = \frac{150 \times 60}{x}$$

$$60 = \frac{9,000}{x}$$

$$\frac{60x}{60} = \frac{9,000}{60}$$

$$x = 150 \text{ minutes}$$

60 min = 1 hr; 150 min ÷ 60 = 2.5 hr

Answer: 2 ½ hr

## NOTE

Because the formula is time in minutes, 5 hours was changed to minutes by multiplying 5 × 60 (60 min = 1 hr).

49.  35 macrogtt/min = $\dfrac{x \text{ mL} \times 15 \text{ gtt/mL}}{300 \text{ min}}$

$$35 = x \times \frac{\cancel{15}^{1}}{\cancel{300}_{20}}$$

$$35 = \frac{x}{20}$$

$$x = 35 \times 20 = 700$$

$$x = 700 \text{ mL}$$

**NOTE**

Problem 50 asks for time in hours so minutes are changed to parts of hours.

50. $45 \text{ macrogtt/min} = \dfrac{180 \text{ mL} \times 15 \text{ gtt/mL}}{x \text{ min}}$

$$45 = \dfrac{180 \times 15}{x}$$

$$45 = \dfrac{2,700}{x}$$

$$\dfrac{45x}{45} = \dfrac{2,700}{45}$$

$$x = 60 \text{ min}$$

60 min = 1 hr; 60 min ÷ 60 = 1 hr

Answer: 1 hr

**NOTE**

Formula is in minutes; therefore 8 hr × 60 = 480 min.

51. $45 \text{ macrogtt/min} = \dfrac{x \text{ mL} \times 15 \text{ gtt/mL}}{480 \text{ min}}$

$$45 = x \, (\times) \, \dfrac{\cancel{15}^{\,1}}{\cancel{480}_{\,32}}$$

$$45 = \dfrac{x}{32}$$

$$x = 45 \times 32 = 1,440$$

$$x = 1,440 \text{ mL}$$

Answer: 1,440 mL

**NOTE**

Problem 52 asks for time in hours so minutes are changed to parts of hours.

52. $60 \text{ microgtt/min} = \dfrac{90 \text{ mL} \times 60 \text{ gtt/mL}}{x \text{ min}}$

$$60 = \dfrac{90 \times 60}{x}$$

$$60 = \dfrac{5,400}{x}$$

$$\dfrac{60x}{60} = \dfrac{5,400}{60}$$

$$x = 90 \text{ min}$$

60 min = 1 hr; 90 min ÷ 60 = 1.5 hr

Answer: $1\frac{1}{2}$ hr

53. Step 1: Determine mL/hr for the remaining solution.

$$x \text{ mL/hr} = \dfrac{250 \text{ mL}}{3 \text{ hr}}; x = 83.3 = 83 \text{ mL/hr}$$

Step 2: Calculate gtt/min.

$$x \text{ gtt/min} = \dfrac{83 \text{ mL} \times 15 \text{ gtt/mL}}{60 \text{ min}} =$$

$$\dfrac{83 \times 15}{60} = \dfrac{83 \times 1}{4} = \dfrac{83}{4}$$

$$x = \dfrac{83}{4}; x = 20.7 = 21 \text{ gtt/min}$$

a. Answer: 21 gtt/min; 21 macrogtt/min

b. Determine the percentage of change.

$$\dfrac{21 - 16}{16} = \dfrac{5}{16} = 0.312 = 31\%$$

c. Percentage of change is greater than 25%. Assess client. Consult prescriber; order may need to be revised.

54. Step 1: Determine mL/hr for the remaining solution.

$$x \text{ mL/hr} = \dfrac{200 \text{ mL}}{1.5 \text{ hr}}; x = 133.3 = 133 \text{ mL/hr}$$

Step 2: Calculate gtt/min.

$$x \text{ gtt/min} = \dfrac{133 \text{ mL} \times 15 \text{ gtt/mL}}{60 \text{ min}} =$$

$$\dfrac{133 \times 15}{60} = \dfrac{133 \times 1}{4} = \dfrac{133}{4}$$

$$x = \dfrac{133}{4}; x = 33.2 = 33 \text{ gtt/min}$$

a. Answer: 33 gtt/min; 33 macrogtt/min

b. Determine the percentage of change.

$$\dfrac{33 - 21}{21} = \dfrac{12}{21} = 0.571 = 57\%$$

c. Percentage of change is greater than 25%. Assess client. Consult prescriber; order may need to be revised.

55. Step 1: Determine mL/hr for the remaining solution.

$$x \text{ mL/hr} = \dfrac{850 \text{ mL}}{6 \text{ hr}}; x = 141.6 = 142 \text{ mL/hr}$$

Step 2: Calculate gtt/min.

$$x \text{ gtt/min} = \dfrac{142 \text{ mL} \times 20 \text{ gtt/mL}}{60 \text{ min}} =$$

$$\dfrac{142 \times 20}{60} = \dfrac{142 \times 1}{3} = \dfrac{142}{3}$$

$$x = \dfrac{142}{3}; x = 47.3 = 47 \text{ gtt/min}$$

a.  Answer: 47 gtt/min; 47 macrogtt/min

b.  Determine the percentage of change.
$$\frac{47-42}{42}=\frac{5}{42}=0.119=12\%$$

c.  This is an acceptable increase. Assess if client can tolerate adjustment in rate. Check hospital policy.

56.  Step 1:  Determine mL/hr for the remaining solution.
$$x \text{ mL/hr}=\frac{750 \text{ mL}}{8 \text{ hr}}; x=93.7=94 \text{ mL/hr}$$

Step 2:  Calculate gtt/min.
$$x \text{ gtt/min}=\frac{94 \text{ mL}\times 20 \text{ gtt/mL}}{60 \text{ min}}=$$
$$\frac{94\times 20}{60}=\frac{94\times 1}{3}=\frac{94}{3}$$
$$x=\frac{94}{3}; x=31.3=31 \text{ gtt/min}$$

a.  Answer:  31 gtt/min; 31 macrogtt/min

b.  Determine the percentage of change.
$$\frac{31-28}{28}=\frac{3}{28}=0.107=11\%$$

c.  The percentage of change is 11%. This is an acceptable increase. Assess if client can tolerate adjustment in rate. Check if allowed by institution policy.

57.  Step 1:  Determine mL/hr for remaining solution.
$$x \text{ mL/hr}=\frac{250 \text{ mL}}{3 \text{ hr}}; x=83.3=83 \text{ mL/hr}$$

Step 2:  Calculate gtt/min.
$$x \text{ gtt/min}=\frac{83 \text{ mL}\times 60 \text{ gtt/mL}}{60 \text{ min}}=$$
$$\frac{83\times 60}{60}=\frac{83\times 1}{1}=\frac{83}{1}$$
$$x=83 \text{ gtt/min}$$

a.  Answer: 83 gtt/min; 83 microgtt/min

b.  Determine the percentage of change.
$$\frac{83-100}{100}=\frac{-17}{100}=-0.17=17\%$$

c.  The percentage of change is −17%. This is an acceptable decrease. Assess client to see if able to tolerate adjustment in rate. Check if allowed by institution policy.

58.  $$\frac{500 \text{ mL}}{60 \text{ mL/hr}}=8.33 \text{ hr}$$

$0.33\times 60=19.8=20$ min

a.  Answer: 8 hr + 20 min = infusion time

b.  Answer: 6:20 AM (10:00 PM + 8 hr + 20 min); military time: 0620

59.  $$\frac{250 \text{ mL}}{80 \text{ mL/hr}}=3.12 \text{ hr}$$

$0.12\times 60=7.2=7$ min

a.  Answer: 3 hr + 7 min = infusion time

b.  Answer: 5:07 AM (2:00 AM + 3 hr + 7 min); military time: 0507

60.  $$\frac{1,000 \text{ mL}}{40 \text{ mL/hr}}=25 \text{ hr}$$

a.  Answer: 25 hr = infusion time

b.  Answer: 3:10 PM August 27 (2:10 PM on August 26 + 25 hr); military time: 1510

(Most IV solutions are not considered sterile after 24 hr; therefore it should be changed after 24 hr.)

61.  $$\frac{1,000 \text{ mL}}{60 \text{ mL/hr}}=16.66 \text{ hr}$$

$0.66\times 60=39.6=40$ min

a.  Answer: 16 hr + 40 min = infusion time

b.  Answer: 10:40 PM (6:00 AM + 16 hr + 40 min); military time: 2240

62.  $$\frac{500 \text{ mL}}{75 \text{ mL/hr}}=6.66 \text{ hr}$$

$0.66\times 60=39.6=40$ min

a.  Answer: 6 hr + 40 minutes = infusion time

b.  Answer: 8:40 PM (2:00 PM + 6 hr + 40 min); military time: 2040

63.  Step 1:  60 gtt : 1 mL = 25 gtt : $x$ mL
$$\frac{60x}{60}=\frac{25}{60}$$
$$x=25\div 60=0.41 \text{ mL/min}$$
Step 2: 0.41 mL/min × 60 min = 24.6 = 25 mL/hr
Step 3:  $$\frac{1,000 \text{ mL}}{25 \text{ mL/hr}}=40 \text{ hr}$$
Answer: 40 hr = infusion time

64.  Step 1:  15 gtt : 1 mL = 17 gtt : $x$ mL
$$\frac{15x}{15}=\frac{17}{15}$$
$$x=17\div 15=1.13=1.1 \text{ mL/min}$$
Step 2: 1.1 mL/min × 60 min = 66 mL/hr
Step 3:  $$\frac{250 \text{ mL}}{66 \text{ mL/hr}}=3.78 \text{ hr}$$
$60\times 0.78=46.8=47$ min
Answer: 3 hr + 47 min = infusion time

65.  Step 1:  20 gtt : 1 mL = 30 gtt : $x$ mL
$$\frac{20x}{20}=\frac{30}{20}$$
$$x=30\div 20=1.5 \text{ mL/min}$$

Step 2: $1.5 \text{ mL/min} \times 60 \text{ min} = 90 \text{ mL/hr}$

Step 3: $\dfrac{1{,}000 \text{ mL}}{90 \text{ mL/hr}} = 11.11 \text{ hr}$

$60 \times 0.11 = 6.6 = 7 \text{ min}$

Answer: $11 \text{ hr} + 7 \text{ min} = \text{infusion time}$

66. Step 1: $10 \text{ gtt} : 1 \text{ mL} = 20 \text{ gtt} : x \text{ mL}$

$\dfrac{10x}{10} = \dfrac{20}{10}$

$x = 2 \text{ mL/min}$

Step 2: $2 \text{ mL/min} \times 60 \text{ min} = 120 \text{ mL/hr}$

Step 3: $\dfrac{1{,}000 \text{ mL}}{120 \text{ mL/hr}} = 8.33 \text{ hr}$

$60 \times 0.33 = 19.8 = 20 \text{ min}$

Answer: $8 \text{ hr} + 20 \text{ min} = \text{infusion time}$

67. Step 1: $15 \text{ gtt} : 1 \text{ mL} = 10 \text{ gtt} : x \text{ mL}$

$\dfrac{15x}{15} = \dfrac{10}{15}$

$x = 0.666 = 0.67 \text{ mL/min}$

Step 2: $0.67 \text{ mL/min} \times 60 \text{ min} = 40.2 \text{ mL/hr} = 40 \text{ mL/hr}$

Step 3: $\dfrac{100 \text{ mL}}{40 \text{ mL/hr}} = 2.5 \text{ hr}$

Answer: $2 \text{ hr} + 30 \text{ min} = \text{infusion time}$

68. Step 1: $15 \text{ gtt} : 1 \text{ mL} = 30 \text{ gtt} : x \text{ mL}$

$\dfrac{15x}{15} = \dfrac{30}{15}$

$x = 2 \text{ mL/min}$

Step 2: $35 \text{ mL} \div 2 \text{ mL/min} = 17.5 = 18 \text{ min}$

Answer: $18 \text{ min} = \text{infusion time}$

69. Step 1: $60 \text{ gtt} : 1 \text{ mL} = 35 \text{ gtt} : x \text{ mL}$

$\dfrac{60x}{60} = \dfrac{35}{60}$

$x = 0.58 \text{ mL/min}$

Step 2: $20 \text{ mL} \div 0.58 \text{ mL/min} = 34.4 = 34 \text{ min}$

Answer: $34 \text{ min} = \text{infusion time}$

70. a. $5 \text{ mg} : 1 \text{ mL} = 20 \text{ mg} : x \text{ mL}$

$\dfrac{5x}{5} = \dfrac{20}{5}$

$x = 4 \text{ mL}$

Answer: 4 mL. The dosage ordered is greater than the available strength; therefore more than 1 mL is needed to administer the dosage ordered.

*or*

$\dfrac{20 \text{ mg}}{5 \text{ mg}} \times 1 \text{ mL} = x \text{ mL}$

$x \text{ mL} = \dfrac{1 \text{ mL}}{5 \text{ mg}} \times \dfrac{20 \text{ mg}}{1}$

b. $5 \text{ mg} : 1 \text{ min} = 20 \text{ mg} : x \text{ min}$

$\dfrac{5x}{5} = \dfrac{20}{5}$

$x = 4 \text{ min}$

c. $5 \text{ mg} : 60 \text{ sec} = x \text{ mg} : 15 \text{ sec}$

$\dfrac{60x}{60} = \dfrac{15}{60}$

$x = 1.25 \text{ mg per 15 sec}$

71. a. $250 \text{ mg} : 5 \text{ mL} = 150 \text{ mg} : x \text{ mL}$

$\dfrac{250x}{250} = \dfrac{750}{250}$

$x = 3 \text{ mL}$

*or*

$\dfrac{150 \text{ mg}}{250 \text{ mg}} \times 5 \text{ mL} = x \text{ mL}$

Answer: 3 mL. The dosage ordered is less than the available strength; therefore you would need less than 5 mL to administer the dosage ordered.

b. $50 \text{ mg} : 1 \text{ min} = 150 \text{ mg} : x \text{ min}$

$\dfrac{50x}{50} = \dfrac{150}{50}$

$x = 3 \text{ min}$

72. a. 10 mL diluent

b. $1 \text{ mg} : 60 \text{ sec} = x \text{ mg} : 30 \text{ sec}$

$\dfrac{60x}{60} = \dfrac{30}{60}$

$x = 0.5 \text{ mg/30 sec}$

## Answers to Critical Thinking Questions

a. The nurse was accustomed to using 20 gtt/mL and calculated the IV rate using 20 gtt/mL. The tubing used at the institution delivered 10 gtt/mL, and the nurse did not check the drop factor on the IV set package. Failure to check the drop factor of the IV tubing resulted in an incorrect IV rate.

b. Because of the excessive IV rate, the client developed signs of fluid overload and could have developed congestive heart failure.

c. The nurse should never assume what the drop factor for IV tubing is for macrodrop administration sets because they can vary. The nurse should have checked the IV tubing package for the drop factor, which is printed on the package.

## Answers to Chapter Review

**NOTE**

Many of the IV problems involving gtt/min could also be done by using the shortcut method or dimensional analysis.

**NOTE**

Some answers in the Chapter Review reflect the number of drops rounded to the nearest whole number and the rate in mL/hr.

1.  a.  Determine mL/hr.

$$x \text{ mL/hr} = \frac{1,000 \text{ mL}}{8 \text{ hr}}; x = 125 \text{ mL/hr}$$

   b.  Calculate gtt/min.

$$x \text{ gtt/min} = \frac{125 \text{ mL} \times 20 \text{ gtt/mL}}{60 \text{ min}}$$

   $x = 42$ gtt/min; 42 macrogtt/min

2.  a.  Determine mL/hr.

$$x \text{ mL/hr} = \frac{2,500 \text{ mL}}{24 \text{ hr}}; x = 104 \text{ mL/hr}$$

   b.  Calculate gtt/min.

$$x \text{ gtt/min} = \frac{104 \text{ mL} \times 10 \text{ gtt/mL}}{60 \text{ min}}$$

   $x = 17$ gtt/min; 17 macrogtt/min

3.  a.  Determine mL/hr.

$$x \text{ mL/hr} = \frac{500 \text{ mL}}{4 \text{ hr}}; x = 125 \text{ mL/hr}$$

   b.  Calculate gtt/min.

$$x \text{ gtt/min} = \frac{125 \text{ mL} \times 15 \text{ gtt/mL}}{60 \text{ min}}$$

   $x = 31$ gtt/min; 31 macrogtt/min

4.  a.  Determine mL/hr.

$$x \text{ mL/hr} = \frac{300 \text{ mL}}{6 \text{ hr}}; x = 50 \text{ mL/hr}$$

   b.  Calculate gtt/min.

$$x \text{ gtt/min} = \frac{50 \text{ mL} \times 60 \text{ gtt/mL}}{60 \text{ min}}$$

   $x = 50$ gtt/min; 50 microgtt/min

5.  a.  Determine mL/hr.

$$x \text{ mL/hr} = \frac{1,000 \text{ mL}}{24 \text{ hr}}; x = 41.6 = 42 \text{ mL/hr}$$

   b.  Calculate gtt/min.

$$x \text{ gtt/min} = \frac{42 \text{ mL} \times 60 \text{ gtt/mL}}{60 \text{ min}}$$

   $x = 42$ gtt/min; 42 microgtt/min

6.  a.  Determine mL/hr.

$$x \text{ mL/hr} = \frac{500 \text{ mL}}{12 \text{ hr}}; x = 41.6 = 42 \text{ mL/hr}$$

   b.  Calculate gtt/min.

$$x \text{ gtt/min} = \frac{42 \text{ mL} \times 20 \text{ gtt/mL}}{60 \text{ min}}$$

   $x = 14$ gtt/min; 14 macrogtt/min

7.  a.  Determine mL/hr.

$$x \text{ mL/hr} = \frac{1,000 \text{ mL}}{10 \text{ hr}}; x = 100 \text{ mL/hr}$$

   b.  Calculate gtt/min.

$$x \text{ gtt/min} = \frac{100 \text{ mL} \times 20 \text{ gtt/mL}}{60 \text{ min}}$$

   $x = 33$ gtt/min; 33 macrogtt/min

8.  a.  Determine mL/hr.

$$x \text{ mL/hr} = \frac{1,500 \text{ mL}}{12 \text{ hr}}; x = 125 \text{ mL/hr}$$

   b.  Calculate gtt/min.

$$x \text{ gtt/min} = \frac{125 \text{ mL} \times 10 \text{ gtt/mL}}{60 \text{ min}}$$

   $x = 21$ gtt/min; 21 macrogtt/min

9.  a.  Determine mL/hr.

$$x \text{ mL/hr} = \frac{500 \text{ mL}}{4 \text{ hr}}; x = 125 \text{ mL/hr}$$

   b.  Calculate gtt/min.

$$x \text{ gtt/min} = \frac{125 \text{ mL} \times 20 \text{ gtt/mL}}{60 \text{ min}}$$

   $x = 42$ gtt/min; 42 macrogtt/min

10. a.  Determine mL/hr.

$$x \text{ mL/hr} = \frac{250 \text{ mL}}{4 \text{ hr}}; x = 63 \text{ mL/hr}$$

   b.  Calculate gtt/min.

$$x \text{ gtt/min} = \frac{63 \text{ mL} \times 20 \text{ gtt/mL}}{60 \text{ min}}$$

   $x = 21$ gtt/min; 21 macrogtt/min

11. a.  Determine mL/hr.

$$x \text{ mL/hr} = \frac{1,500 \text{ mL}}{8 \text{ hr}}; x = 188 \text{ mL/hr}$$

   b.  Calculate gtt/min.

$$x \text{ gtt/min} = \frac{188 \text{ mL} \times 20 \text{ gtt/mL}}{60 \text{ min}}$$

   $x = 63$ gtt/min; 63 macrogtt/min

12. a. Determine mL/hr.

$$x \text{ mL/hr} = \frac{3,000 \text{ mL}}{24 \text{ hr}}; x = 125 \text{ mL/hr}$$

  b. Calculate gtt/min.

$$x \text{ gtt/min} = \frac{125 \text{ mL} \times 15 \text{ gtt/mL}}{60 \text{ min}}$$

$$x = 31 \text{ gtt/min}; 31 \text{ macrogtt/min}$$

13. 1 L = 1,000 mL

   2 L = 2,000 mL

  a. Determine mL/hr.

$$x \text{ mL/hr} = \frac{2,000 \text{ mL}}{24 \text{ hr}}; x = 83 \text{ mL/hr}$$

  b. Calculate gtt/min.

$$x \text{ gtt/min} = \frac{83 \text{ mL} \times 15 \text{ gtt/mL}}{60 \text{ min}}$$

$$x = 21 \text{ gtt/min}; 21 \text{ macrogtt/min}$$

14. a. Determine mL/hr.

$$x \text{ mL/hr} = \frac{500 \text{ mL}}{4 \text{ hr}}; x = 125 \text{ mL/hr}$$

  b. Calculate gtt/min.

$$x \text{ gtt/min} = \frac{125 \text{ mL} \times 60 \text{ gtt/mL}}{60 \text{ min}}$$

$$x = 125 \text{ gtt/min}; 125 \text{ microgtt/min}$$

15. a. Determine mL/hr.

$$x \text{ mL/hr} = \frac{1,000 \text{ mL}}{6 \text{ hr}}; x = 167 \text{ mL/hr}$$

  b. Calculate gtt/min.

$$x \text{ gtt/min} = \frac{167 \text{ mL} \times 20 \text{ gtt/mL}}{60 \text{ min}}$$

$$x = 56 \text{ gtt/min}; 56 \text{ macrogtt/min}$$

16. a. Determine mL/hr.

$$x \text{ mL/hr} = \frac{250 \text{ mL}}{8 \text{ hr}}; x = 31 \text{ mL/hr}$$

  b. Calculate gtt/min.

$$x \text{ gtt/min} = \frac{31 \text{ mL} \times 60 \text{ gtt/mL}}{60 \text{ min}}$$

$$x = 31 \text{ gtt/min}; 31 \text{ microgtt/min}$$

17. $x \text{ gtt/min} = \dfrac{50 \text{ mL} \times 60 \text{ gtt/mL}}{60 \text{ min}}$

   $x = 50 \text{ gtt/min}; 50 \text{ microgtt/min}$

18. $x \text{ gtt/min} = \dfrac{150 \text{ mL} \times 15 \text{ gtt/mL}}{60 \text{ min}}$

   $x = 38 \text{ gtt/min}; 38 \text{ macrogtt/min}$

19. a. Determine mL/hr.

$$x \text{ mL/hr} = \frac{500 \text{ mL}}{6 \text{ hr}}; x = 83 \text{ mL/hr}$$

  b. Calculate gtt/min.

$$x \text{ gtt/min} = \frac{83 \text{ mL} \times 15 \text{ gtt/mL}}{60 \text{ min}}$$

$$x = 21 \text{ gtt/min}; 21 \text{ macrogtt/min}$$

20. a. Determine mL/hr.

$$x \text{ mL/hr} = \frac{1,500 \text{ mL}}{12 \text{ hr}}; x = 125 \text{ mL/hr}$$

  b. Calculate gtt/min.

$$x \text{ gtt/min} = \frac{125 \text{ mL} \times 10 \text{ gtt/mL}}{60 \text{ min}}$$

$$x = 21 \text{ gtt/min}; 21 \text{ macrogtt/min}$$

21. a. Determine mL/hr.

$$x \text{ mL/hr} = \frac{1,500 \text{ mL}}{24 \text{ hr}}; x = 63 \text{ mL/hr}$$

  b. Calculate gtt/min.

$$x \text{ gtt/min} = \frac{63 \text{ mL} \times 15 \text{ gtt/mL}}{60 \text{ min}}$$

$$x = 16 \text{ gtt/min}; 16 \text{ macrogtt/min}$$

22. a. Determine mL/hr.

$$x \text{ mL/hr} = \frac{2,000 \text{ mL}}{16 \text{ hr}}; x = 125 \text{ mL/hr}$$

  b. Calculate gtt/min.

$$x \text{ gtt/min} = \frac{125 \text{ mL} \times 20 \text{ gtt/mL}}{60 \text{ min}}$$

$$x = 42 \text{ gtt/min}; 42 \text{ macrogtt/min}$$

23. a. Determine mL/hr.

$$x \text{ mL/hr} = \frac{500 \text{ mL}}{8 \text{ hr}}; x = 63 \text{ mL/hr}$$

  b. Calculate gtt/min.

$$x \text{ gtt/min} = \frac{63 \text{ mL} \times 15 \text{ gtt/mL}}{60 \text{ min}}$$

$$x = 16 \text{ gtt/min}; 16 \text{ macrogtt/min}$$

24. a. Determine mL/hr.

$$x \text{ mL/hr} = \frac{250 \text{ mL}}{10 \text{ hr}}; x = 25 \text{ mL/hr}$$

  b. Calculate gtt/min.

$$x \text{ gtt/min} = \frac{25 \text{ mL} \times 60 \text{ gtt/mL}}{60 \text{ min}}$$

$$x = 25 \text{ gtt/min}; 25 \text{ microgtt/min}$$

25. $x \text{ gtt/min} = \dfrac{75 \text{ mL} \times 60 \text{ gtt/mL}}{60 \text{ min}}$

   $x = 75 \text{ gtt/min}; 75 \text{ microgtt/min}$

26. $x \text{ gtt/min} = \dfrac{125 \text{ mL} \times 20 \text{ gtt/mL}}{60 \text{ min}}$

   $x = 42 \text{ gtt/min}; 42 \text{ macrogtt/min}$

27. $x \text{ gtt/min} = \dfrac{40 \text{ mL} \times 60 \text{ gtt/mL}}{60 \text{ min}}$

    $x = 40 \text{ gtt/min}; 40 \text{ microgtt/min}$

28. $x \text{ gtt/min} = \dfrac{50 \text{ mL} \times 60 \text{ gtt/mL}}{45 \text{ min}}$

    $x = 67 \text{ gtt/min}; 67 \text{ microgtt/min}$

29. $x \text{ gtt/min} = \dfrac{90 \text{ mL} \times 15 \text{ gtt/mL}}{60 \text{ min}}$

    $x = 23 \text{ gtt/min}; 23 \text{ macrogtt/min}$

30. $x \text{ gtt/min} = \dfrac{150 \text{ mL} \times 10 \text{ gtt/mL}}{60 \text{ min}}$

    $x = 25 \text{ gtt/min}; 25 \text{ macrogtt/min}$

31. a. Determine mL/hr.

    $x \text{ mL/hr} = \dfrac{2,500 \text{ mL}}{24 \text{ hr}}; x = 104 \text{ mL/hr}$

    b. Calculate gtt/min.

    $x \text{ gtt/min} = \dfrac{104 \text{ mL} \times 15 \text{ gtt/mL}}{60 \text{ min}}$

    $x = 26 \text{ gtt/min}; 26 \text{ macrogtt/min}$

32. $x \text{ gtt/min} = \dfrac{50 \text{ mL} \times 10 \text{ gtt/mL}}{40 \text{ min}}$

    $x = 13 \text{ gtt/min}; 13 \text{ macrogtt/min}$

33. $x \text{ gtt/min} = \dfrac{100 \text{ mL} \times 20 \text{ gtt/mL}}{30 \text{ min}}$

    $x = 67 \text{ gtt/min}; 67 \text{ macrogtt/min}$

34. a. Determine mL/hr.

    $x \text{ mL/hr} = \dfrac{250 \text{ mL}}{5 \text{ hr}}; x = 50 \text{ mL/hr}$

    b. Calculate gtt/min.

    $x \text{ gtt/min} = \dfrac{50 \text{ mL} \times 20 \text{ gtt/mL}}{60 \text{ min}}$

    $x = 17 \text{ gtt/min}; 17 \text{ macrogtt/min}$

35. $x \text{ gtt/min} = \dfrac{80 \text{ mL} \times 20 \text{ gtt/mL}}{60 \text{ min}}$

    $x = 27 \text{ gtt/min}; 27 \text{ macrogtt/min}$

36. $x \text{ gtt/min} = \dfrac{150 \text{ mL} \times 10 \text{ gtt/mL}}{30 \text{ min}}$

    $x = 50 \text{ gtt/min}; 50 \text{ macrogtt/min}$

37. $x \text{ gtt/min} = \dfrac{50 \text{ mL} \times 60 \text{ gtt/mL}}{30 \text{ min}}$

    $x = 100 \text{ gtt/min}; 100 \text{ microgtt/min}$

38. a. Determine mL/hr.

    $x \text{ mL/hr} = \dfrac{500 \text{ mL}}{3 \text{ hr}}; x = 167 \text{ mL/hr}$

    b. Calculate gtt/min.

    $x \text{ gtt/min} = \dfrac{167 \text{ mL} \times 10 \text{ gtt/mL}}{60 \text{ min}}$

    $x = 28 \text{ gtt/min}; 28 \text{ macrogtt/min}$

39. a. Determine mL/hr.

    $x \text{ mL/hr} = \dfrac{250 \text{ mL}}{2 \text{ hr}}; x = 125 \text{ mL/hr}$

    b. Calculate gtt/min.

    $x \text{ gtt/min} = \dfrac{125 \text{ mL} \times 15 \text{ gtt/mL}}{60 \text{ min}}$

    $x = 31 \text{ gtt/min}; 31 \text{ macrogtt/min}$

40. a. Determine mL/hr.

    $x \text{ mL/hr} = \dfrac{1,750 \text{ mL}}{24 \text{ hr}}; x = 73 \text{ mL/hr}$

    b. Calculate gtt/min.

    $x \text{ gtt/min} = \dfrac{73 \text{ mL} \times 10 \text{ gtt/mL}}{60 \text{ min}}$

    $x = 12 \text{ gtt/min}; 12 \text{ macrogtt/min}$

41. a. Determine mL/hr.

    $x \text{ mL/hr} = \dfrac{150 \text{ mL}}{1.5 \text{ hr}}; x = 100 \text{ mL/hr}$

    b. Calculate gtt/min.

    $x \text{ gtt/min} = \dfrac{100 \text{ mL} \times 60 \text{ gtt/mL}}{60 \text{ min}}$

    $x = 100 \text{ gtt/min}; 100 \text{ microgtt/min}$

42. $1 \text{ L} = 1,000 \text{ mL}$

    $2 \text{ L} = 2,000 \text{ mL}$

    $x \text{ mL/hr} = \dfrac{2,000 \text{ mL}}{16 \text{ hr}}; x = 125 \text{ mL/hr}$

43. $x \text{ mL/hr} = \dfrac{500 \text{ mL}}{4 \text{ hr}}; x = 125 \text{ mL/hr}$

44. $x \text{ mL/hr} = \dfrac{200 \text{ mL}}{2 \text{ hr}}; x = 100 \text{ mL/hr}$

45. $x \text{ mL/hr} = \dfrac{500 \text{ mL}}{8 \text{ hr}}; x = 63 \text{ mL/hr}$

46. Determine mL/hr.

    $x \text{ mL/hr} = \dfrac{1,100 \text{ mL}}{12 \text{ hr}}; x = 92 \text{ mL/hr}$

47. a. Determine mL/hr.

    $x \text{ mL/hr} = \dfrac{500 \text{ mL}}{6 \text{ hr}}; x = 83 \text{ mL/hr}$

    b. Calculate gtt/min.

    $x \text{ gtt/min} = \dfrac{83 \text{ mL} \times 10 \text{ gtt/mL}}{60 \text{ min}}$

    $x = 14 \text{ gtt/min}; 14 \text{ macrogtt/min}$

48. a. Determine mL/hr.

$$x \text{ mL/hr} = \frac{3,000 \text{ mL}}{20 \text{ hr}}; x = 150 \text{ mL/hr}$$

   b. Calculate gtt/min.

$$x \text{ gtt/min} = \frac{150 \text{ mL} \times 20 \text{ gtt/mL}}{60 \text{ min}}$$

   $x = 50$ gtt/min; 50 macrogtt/min

49. a. Determine mL/hr.

$$x \text{ mL/hr} = \frac{500 \text{ mL}}{6 \text{ hr}}; x = 83 \text{ mL/hr}$$

   b. Calculate gtt/min.

$$x \text{ gtt/min} = \frac{83 \text{ mL} \times 15 \text{ gtt/mL}}{60 \text{ min}}$$

   $x = 21$ gtt/min; 21 macrogtt/min

50. Time remaining = 7 hr

    Volume remaining = 300 mL

   a. Determine mL/hr for remaining solution.

$$x \text{ mL/hr} = \frac{300 \text{ mL}}{7 \text{ hr}}; x = 43 \text{ mL/hr}$$

   b. Determine gtt/min (recalculated rate).

$$x \text{ gtt/min} = \frac{43 \text{ mL} \times 15 \text{ gtt/mL}}{60 \text{ min}}$$

   $x = 11$ gtt/min

   Answer: 11 macrogtt/min; 11 gtt/min

   c. Determine the percentage change.

$$\frac{11 - 13}{13} = \frac{-2}{13} = -0.153 = -15\%$$

   The $-15\%$ is within the acceptable 25% variation. Assess if client can tolerate adjustment in rate.

   Negative percentage of variation ($-15\%$) indicates the adjusted rate will be decreased. Assess client, check institution policy, and continue to assess client during rate change.

51. Time remaining = 4 hr

    Volume remaining = 600 mL

   a. Determine mL/hr for remaining solution.

$$x \text{ mL/hr} = \frac{600 \text{ mL}}{4 \text{ hr}}; x = 150 \text{ mL/hr}$$

   b. Determine gtt/min (recalculated rate).

$$x \text{ gtt/min} = \frac{150 \text{ mL} \times 20 \text{ gtt/mL}}{60 \text{ min}}$$

   $x = 50$ gtt/min

   Answer: 50 gtt/min; 50 macrogtt/min

   c. Determine the percentage change.

$$\frac{50 - 42}{42} = \frac{8}{42} = 0.190 = 19\%$$

   The percentage of change is 19%. This is an acceptable increase. Assess if client can tolerate the adjustment in rate (42 gtt/min to 50 gtt/min). Check if allowed by institution policy. Assess client during rate change.

52. Time remaining = 4 hr

    Volume remaining = 400 mL

   a. Determine mL/hr for remaining solution.

$$x \text{ mL/hr} = \frac{400 \text{ mL}}{4 \text{ hr}}; x = 100 \text{ mL/hr}$$

   After determining mL/hr, gtt/min is recalculated.

   b. Determine gtt/min (recalculated rate).

$$x \text{ gtt/min} = \frac{100 \text{ mL} \times 15 \text{ gtt/mL}}{60 \text{ min}}$$

   $x = 25$ gtt/min

   Answer: 25 gtt/min; 25 macrogtt/min

   c. The IV was ahead. The original IV order was 125 mL/hr = 31 gtt/min (31 macrogtt/min). The IV would have to be decreased from 31 gtt/min (31 macrogtt/min) to 25 gtt/min (25 macrogtt/min). Determine the percentage change.

$$\frac{25 - 31}{31} = \frac{-6}{31} = -0.193 = -19\%$$

   The $-19\%$ is within acceptable 25% variation. Assess if client can tolerate the adjustment in rate. Negative percentage of variation ($-19\%$) indicates the adjusted rate will be decreased. Check institution policy. Assess client during rate change.

53. Time remaining = 5 hr

    Volume remaining = 250 mL

   a. Determine mL/hr for remaining solution.

$$x \text{ mL/hr} = \frac{250 \text{ mL}}{5 \text{ hr}}; x = 50 \text{ mL/hr}$$

   b. Determine gtt/min (recalculated rate).

$$x \text{ gtt/min} = \frac{50 \text{ mL} \times 10 \text{ gtt/mL}}{60 \text{ min}}$$

   $x = 8$ gtt/min

   Answer: 8 gtt/min; 8 macrogtt/min

c. The IV is ahead. The IV rate would need to be decreased from 14 gtt/min (14 macrogtt/min) to 8 gtt/min (8 macrogtt/min). Determine the percentage change.

$$\frac{8 - 14}{14} = \frac{-6}{14} = -0.428 = -43\%$$

The percentage of change is less than 25%. Assess client. Check with prescriber; order may need to be revised, even though a negative variation indicates IV will be decreased. (Do not decrease.)

54. Time remaining = 4 hr

Volume remaining = 600 mL

a. Determine mL/hr for remaining solution.

$$x \text{ mL/hr} = \frac{600 \text{ mL}}{4 \text{ hr}}; x = 150 \text{ mL/hr}$$

b. Determine gtt/min (recalculated rate).

$$x \text{ gtt/min} = \frac{150 \text{ mL} \times 15 \text{ gtt/mL}}{60 \text{ min}} = 38 \text{ gtt/min}$$

Answer: 38 gtt/min; 38 macrogtt/min

c. IV is not on schedule. The IV will have to be increased from 25 gtt/min (25 macrogtt/min) to 38 gtt/min (38 macrogtt/min). Determine the percentage of increase.

$$\frac{38 - 25}{25} = \frac{13}{25} = 52\%$$

The percentage of change is greater than 25%. Assess client. Check with prescriber; order may need to be revised. (Do not increase.)

55. 80 macrogtt/min (80 gtt/min) =

$$\frac{900 \text{ mL} \times 15 \text{ gtt/mL}}{x \text{ min}}$$

$$80 = \frac{900 \times 15}{x}$$

$$\frac{80x}{80} = \frac{13,500}{80}$$

$$x = 168.75 \text{ minutes}$$

60 min = 1 hr; 168.75 ÷ 60 = 2.81 hr

Time: 2.81 hr. Since 0.81 represents a fraction of an additional hour (0.81 × 60 = 48.6 = 49 min), convert it to minutes—multiply by 60 minutes.

Answer: 2 hr and 49 min

56. $\dfrac{1,000 \text{ mL}}{100 \text{ mL/hr}} = 10 \text{ hr}$

57. 20 macrogtt/min (20 gtt/min) =

$$\frac{1,000 \text{ mL} \times 10 \text{ gtt/mL}}{x \text{ min}}$$

$$20 = \frac{1,000 \times 10}{x}$$

$$\frac{20x}{20} = \frac{10,000}{20}$$

$$x = 500 \text{ min}$$

60 min = 1 hr; 500 ÷ 60 = 8.33 hr

Time: 8.33 hr

$$0.33 \times 60 = 19.8 = 20 \text{ min}$$

Answer: 8 hr and 20 min

58. 25 macrogtt/min (25 gtt/min) =

$$\frac{450 \text{ mL} \times 20 \text{ gtt/mL}}{x \text{ min}}$$

$$25 = \frac{450 \times 20}{x}$$

$$\frac{25x}{25} = \frac{9,000}{25}$$

$$x = 360 \text{ min}$$

60 min = 1 hr; 360 ÷ 60 = 6 hr

Answer: 6 hr

59. 10 macrogtt/min (10 gtt/min) =

$$\frac{100 \text{ mL} \times 15 \text{ gtt/mL}}{x \text{ min}}$$

$$10 = \frac{100 \times 15}{x}$$

$$\frac{10x}{10} = \frac{1,500}{10}$$

$$x = 150 \text{ min}$$

60 min = 1 hr; 150 ÷ 60 = 2.5 = 2 1/2 hr

Answer: 2 1/2 hr

60. 25 macrogtt/min (25 gtt/min) =

$$\frac{x \text{ mL} \times 15 \text{ gtt/mL}}{480 \text{ min}}$$

$$25 = \frac{x \times 15}{480}$$

$$25 = \frac{15x}{480}$$

$$\frac{15x}{15} = \frac{25 \times 480}{15}$$

$$\frac{15x}{15} = \frac{12,000}{15}$$

$$x = 800 \text{ mL}$$

**NOTE**

Formula, time expressed in minutes; therefore hours are expressed as minutes. 10 hr = 600 min (60 min = 1 hr).

61. 40 microgtt/min (40 gtt/min) = $\dfrac{x \text{ mL} \times 60 \text{ gtt/mL}}{600 \text{ min}}$

$$40 = \frac{x \times 60}{600}$$

$$40 = \frac{60x}{600}$$

$$\frac{60x}{60} = \frac{40 \times 600}{60}$$

$$\frac{60x}{60} = \frac{24,000}{60}$$

$$x = 400 \text{ mL}$$

**NOTE**

Formula, time expressed in minutes; therefore hours are expressed as minutes. 5 hr = 300 min (60 min = 1 hr).

62. 30 macrogtt/min (30 gtt/min) = $\dfrac{x \text{ mL} \times 15 \text{ gtt/mL}}{300 \text{ min}}$

$$30 = \frac{x \times 15}{300}$$

$$30 = \frac{15x}{300}$$

$$\frac{15x}{15} = \frac{30 \times 300}{15}$$

$$\frac{15x}{15} = \frac{9,000}{5}$$

$$x = 600 \text{ mL}$$

**NOTE**

For problems 63-67 a ratio and proportion could be set up in a format other than the one shown in the problems.

63. 10 mEq : 500 mL = 2 mEq : $x$ mL

$$10x = 500 \times 2$$

$$\frac{10x}{10} = \frac{1,000}{10}$$

$$x = 100 \text{ mL}$$

Answer: 100 mL of fluid would be needed to administer 2 mEq of potassium chloride.

64. 30 mEq : 1,000 mL = 4 mEq : $x$ mL

$$\frac{30x}{30} = \frac{4,000}{30} = 133.3$$

133 mL would deliver 4 mEq of potassium chloride.

65. 50 units : 250 mL = 7 units : $x$ mL

$$\frac{50x}{50} = \frac{1,750}{50}; x = 35 \text{ mL/hr}$$

Answer: 35 mL/hr

66. 100 units : 250 mL = 18 units : $x$ mL

$$\frac{100x}{100} = \frac{4,500}{100}; x = 45 \text{ mL/hr}$$

Answer: 45 mL/hr

67. 100 units : 100 mL = 11 units : $x$ mL

$$\frac{100x}{100} = \frac{1,100}{100}; x = 11 \text{ mL/hr}$$

Answer: 11 mL/hr

68. $x$ gtt/min = $\dfrac{150 \text{ mL} \times 10 \text{ gtt/mL}}{60 \text{ min}}$

$$x = 25 \text{ gtt/min}$$

Answer: 25 gtt/min; 25 macrogtt/min

69. $x$ gtt/min = $\dfrac{40 \text{ mL} \times 60 \text{ gtt/mL}}{40 \text{ min}}$

$$x = 60 \text{ gtt/min}$$

Answer: 60 gtt/min; 60 microgtt/min

70. $x$ gtt/min = $\dfrac{35 \text{ mL} \times 60 \text{ gtt/mL}}{30 \text{ min}}$

$$x = 70 \text{ gtt/min}$$

Answer: 70 gtt/min; 70 microgtt/min

71. $x$ gtt/min = $\dfrac{80 \text{ mL} \times 15 \text{ gtt/mL}}{40 \text{ min}}$

$$x = 30 \text{ gtt/min}$$

Answer: 30 gtt/min; 30 macrogtt/min

72. $x$ gtt/min = $\dfrac{50 \text{ mL} \times 10 \text{ gtt/mL}}{25 \text{ min}}$

$$x = 20 \text{ gtt/min}$$

Answer: 20 gtt/min; 20 macrogtt/min

73. $x$ gtt/min = $\dfrac{65 \text{ mL} \times 15 \text{ gtt/mL}}{60 \text{ min}}$

$$x = 16 \text{ gtt/min}$$

Answer: 16 gtt/min; 16 macrogtt/min

74. Step 1: 60 gtt : 1 mL = 50 gtt : $x$ mL

$$\frac{60x}{60} = \frac{50}{60}$$

$$x = 50 \div 60; x = 0.83 \text{ mL/min}$$

Step 2: 0.83 mL × 60 min = 49.8 = 50 mL/hr

Step 3: $\dfrac{50 \text{ mL}}{50 \text{ mL/hr}} = 1 \text{ hr}$

Answer: 1 hr = infusion time

75. Step 1: $\dfrac{500 \text{ mL}}{80 \text{ mL/hr}} = 6.25 \text{ hr}$

    Step 2: $60 \times 0.25 = 15 \text{ min}$

         6 hr and 15 min = infusion time

    Step 3: (7:00 PM + 6 hr + 15 min)

    Answer: 1:15 AM; military time: 0115

76. $\dfrac{150 \text{ mL}}{25 \text{ mL/hr}} = 6 \text{ hr}$

    a. 6 hr = infusion time

    b. (3:10 AM + 6 hr = 9:10 AM). IV will be completed at 9:10 AM; military time: 0910.

77. Conversion is required. Equivalent:

    1 L = 1,000 mL

    Therefore 2.5 L = 2,500 mL

    Step 1: $\dfrac{2,500 \text{ mL}}{150 \text{ mL/hr}} = 16.66 \text{ hr}$

    Step 2: $60 \times 0.66 = 39.6 = 40 \text{ min}$

    16 hr and 40 min = infusion time

78. a. 10 mg : 1 mL = 120 mg : $x$ mL

       $\dfrac{10x}{10} = \dfrac{120}{10}$; $x = 12 \text{ mL}$

            *or*

       $\dfrac{120 \text{ mg}}{10 \text{ mg}} \times 1 \text{ mL} = x \text{ mL}$

       Answer: 12 mL. The dosage ordered is more than the available strength; therefore more than 1 mL would be required to administer the dosage ordered.

    b. 40 mg : 1 min = 120 mg : $x$ min

       $\dfrac{40x}{40} = \dfrac{120}{40}$; $x = 3 \text{ min}$

       Answer: 3 min

79. a. 100 mg : 20 mL = 60 mg : $x$ mL

       $\dfrac{100x}{100} = \dfrac{1,200}{100}$; $x = 12 \text{ mL}$

            *or*

       $\dfrac{60 \text{ mg}}{100 \text{ mg}} \times 20 \text{ mL} = x \text{ mL}$

       Answer: 12 mL. The dosage ordered is less than the available strength; therefore you will need less than 20 mL to administer the dosage ordered.

    b. $\dfrac{12 \text{ mL}}{2 \text{ min}} = 6 \text{ mL/min}$

80. $x$ gtt/min $= \dfrac{100 \text{ mL} \times 10 \text{ gtt/mL}}{60 \text{ min}}$;

    $x = 16.6 = 17 \text{ gtt/min}$

    Answer: 17 gtt/min; 17 macrogtt/min

81. $x$ gtt/min $= \dfrac{100 \text{ mL} \times 60 \text{ gtt/mL}}{30 \text{ min}}$; $x = 200 \text{ gtt/min}$

    Answer: 200 gtt/min; 200 microdrop/min

82. 30,000 units : 500 mL = 1,500 units : $x$ mL

    $\dfrac{30,000x}{30,000} = \dfrac{750,000}{30,000}$

    $x = \dfrac{750,000}{30,000}$; $x = 25 \text{ mL/hr}$

    Answer: 25 mL/hr

83. 100 units : 500 mL = 20 units : $x$ mL

    $\dfrac{100x}{100} = \dfrac{10,000}{100}$; $x = 100 \text{ mL/hr}$

    Answer: 100 mL/hr

84. 100 units : 250 mL = 15 units : $x$ mL

    $\dfrac{100x}{100} = \dfrac{3,750}{100}$; $x = 37.5 = 38 \text{ mL/hr}$

    Answer: 38 mL/hr

## CHAPTER 23

### Answers to Practice Problems

1. 25,000 units : 1,000 mL = 1,000 units : $x$ mL

              *or*

      $\dfrac{25,000 \text{ units}}{1,000 \text{ mL}} = \dfrac{1,000 \text{ units}}{x \text{ mL}}$

          $25,000x = 1,000 \times 1,000$

          $\dfrac{25,000x}{25,000} = \dfrac{1,000,000}{25,000}$

             $x = 40 \text{ mL/hr}$

    Answer: 40 mL/hr. To infuse 1,000 units/hr from a solution of 25,000 units in D5 0.9% NS, the flow rate would be 40 mL/hr.

2. 25,000 units : 1,000 mL = $x$ units : 35 mL

          $\dfrac{1,000x}{1,000} = \dfrac{875,000}{1,000}$

            $x = 875 \text{ units/hr}$

3. 30,000 units : 750 mL = $x$ units : 25 mL

          $\dfrac{750x}{750} = \dfrac{750,000}{750}$

           $x = 1,000 \text{ units/hr}$

    Answer: 1,000 units/hr

4. Calculate units/hr infusing.

1,000 mL : 25,000 units = 100 mL : *x* units

$$\frac{1,000x}{1,000} = \frac{2,500,000}{1,000}$$

$$x = 2,500 \text{ units/hr}$$

Answer: 2,500 units/hr

5. Convert the weight to kilograms.

Conversion factor: 2.2 lb = 1 kg

176 lb ÷ 2.2 = 80 kg

a. Calculate the heparin bolus dosage.

80 units/k̸g̸ × 80 k̸g̸ = 6,400 units

Answer: 6,400 units

b. Calculate the infusion rate for the IV drip (initial).

18 units/k̸g̸/hr × 80 k̸g̸ = 1,440 units/hr

c. Determine the rate in mL/hr at which to set the infusion rate.

1,000 mL : 20,000 units = *x* mL : 1,440 units

$$\frac{20,000x}{20,000} = \frac{1,440,000}{20,000}$$

$$x = 72 \text{ mL/hr}$$

Answer: 72 mL/hr

## Answers to Critical Thinking Questions

a. The nurse used the incorrect concentration of heparin to prepare the IV solution. Heparin concentration of 100 units per mL is used for maintaining the patency of a line and for flushing.

b. The nurse should have read the label carefully because heparin comes in a variety of concentrations. Heparin IV flushes are available in 10 units per mL and 100 units per mL. Heparin for IV flush is never used interchangeably with heparin for injection.

## Answers to Chapter Review

1. 10,000 units : 1 mL = 3,500 units : *x* mL

*or*

$$\frac{3,500 \text{ units}}{10,000 \text{ units}} \times 1 \text{ mL} = x \text{ mL}$$

*x* = 0.35 mL. The dosage ordered is less than the available strength; therefore you will need less than 1 mL to administer the dosage.

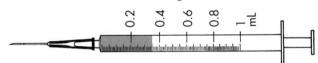

2. 20,000 units : 1 mL = 16,000 units : *x* mL

*or*

$$\frac{16,000 \text{ units}}{20,000 \text{ units}} \times 1 \text{ mL} = x \text{ mL}$$

Answer: 0.8 mL. The dosage ordered is less than the available strength; therefore you will need less than 1 mL to administer the dosage.

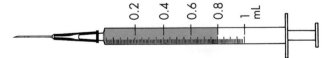

3. 2,500 units : 1 mL = 2,000 units : *x* mL

*or*

$$\frac{2,000 \text{ units}}{2,500 \text{ units}} \times 1 \text{ mL} = x \text{ mL}$$

Answer: 0.8 mL. The dosage ordered is less than the available strength; therefore you will need less than 1 mL to administer the dosage.

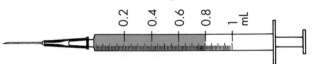

4. 5,000 units : 1 mL = 2,000 units : *x* mL

*or*

$$\frac{2,000 \text{ units}}{5,000 \text{ units}} \times 1 \text{ mL} = x \text{ mL}$$

Answer: 0.4 mL. The dosage ordered is less than the available strength; therefore you will need less than 1 mL to administer the dosage.

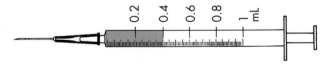

5. 1,000 units : 1 mL = 500 units : $x$ mL

*or*

$$\frac{500\ units}{1,000\ units} \times 1\ mL = x\ mL$$

Answer: 0.5 mL. The dosage ordered is less than the available strength; therefore you will need less than 1 mL to administer the dosage.

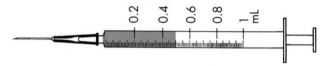

6. 10 units : 1 mL = 10 units : $x$ mL

*or*

$$\frac{10\ units}{10\ units} \times 1\ mL = x\ mL$$

1 mL contains 10 units so you will need 1 mL to flush the heparin lock.

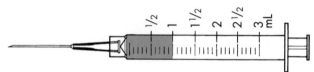

7. 10,000 units : 1 mL = 50,000 units : $x$ mL

*or*

$$\frac{50,000\ units}{10,000\ units} \times 1\ mL = x\ mL$$

Answer: 5 mL would be needed to administer the dosage. The dosage ordered is more than the available strength; therefore you will need more than 1 mL to administer the dosage.

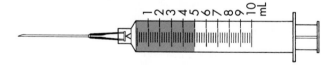

8. 20,000 units : 1 mL = 15,000 units : $x$ mL

*or*

$$\frac{15,000\ units}{20,000\ units} \times 1\ mL = x\ mL$$

Answer: 0.75 mL. The dosage ordered is less than the available strength; therefore you will need less than 1 mL to administer the dosage.

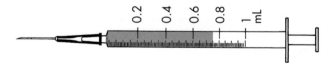

9. 2,500 units : 1 mL = 3,000 units : $x$ mL

*or*

$$\frac{3,000\ units}{2,500\ units} \times 1\ mL = x\ mL$$

Answer: 1.2 mL. The dosage ordered is more than the available strength; therefore you will need more than 1 mL to administer the dosage.

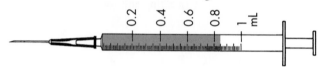

10. 20,000 units : 1 mL = 17,000 units : $x$ mL

*or*

$$\frac{17,000\ units}{20,000\ units} \times 1\ mL = x\ mL$$

Answer: 0.85 mL. The dosage ordered is less than the available strength; therefore you will need less than 1 mL to administer the dosage.

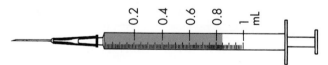

11. 10,000 units : 1 mL = 8,500 units : $x$ mL

*or*

$$\frac{8,500\ units}{10,000\ units} \times 1\ mL = x\ mL$$

Answer: 0.85 mL. The dosage ordered is less than the available strength; therefore you will need less than 1 mL to administer the dosage.

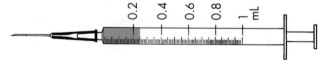

12. 10,000 units : 1 mL = 2,500 units : $x$ mL

*or*

$$\frac{2,500\ units}{10,000\ units} \times 1\ mL = x\ mL$$

Answer: 0.25 mL. The dosage ordered is less than the available strength; therefore you will need less than 1 mL to administer the dosage.

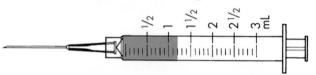

13. 25,000 units : 1,000 mL = 2,000 units : $x$ mL

$$\frac{25,000x}{25,000} = \frac{2,000,000}{25,000}$$

$x = 80$ mL/hr. To administer 2,000 units of heparin per hour, 80 mL/hr must be given.

14. 25,000 units : 500 mL = 1,500 units : $x$ mL

$$\frac{25,000x}{25,000} = \frac{750,000}{25,000}$$

$$x = \frac{750,000}{25,000}$$

$x = 30$ mL/hr. To administer 1,500 units of heparin per hour, 30 mL/hr must be given.

15. 25,000 units : 250 mL = 1,800 units : $x$ mL

$$\frac{25,000x}{25,000} = \frac{450,000}{25,000}$$

$x = 18$ mL/hr. To administer 1,800 units of heparin per hour, 18 mL/hr must be given.

16. 40,000 units : 1,000 mL = $x$ units : 25 mL

$$\frac{1,000x}{1,000} = \frac{1,000,000}{1,000}$$

$$x = \frac{1,000,000}{1,000}$$

$$x = 1,000 \text{ units/hr}$$

17. 25,000 units : 250 mL = $x$ units : 11 mL

$$\frac{250x}{250} = \frac{275,000}{250}$$

$$x = 1,100 \text{ units/hr}$$

18. 40,000 units : 500 mL = $x$ units : 30 mL

$$\frac{500x}{500} = \frac{1,200,000}{500}$$

$$x = 2,400 \text{ units/hr}$$

19. 20,000 units : 500 mL = $x$ units : 12 mL

$$\frac{500x}{500} = \frac{240,000}{500}$$

$$x = 480 \text{ units/hr}$$

20. 25,000 units : 500 mL = $x$ units : 15 mL

$$\frac{500x}{500} = \frac{375,000}{500}$$

$$x = 750 \text{ units/hr}$$

21. 1 L = 1,000 mL

a. Calculate mL/hr.

$$\frac{1,000 \text{ mL}}{24 \text{ hr}} = 41.6 = 42 \text{ mL/hr}$$

b. Calculate units/hr.

40,000 units : 1,000 mL = $x$ units : 42 mL

$$\frac{1,000x}{1,000} = \frac{1,680,000}{1,000}$$

$$x = \frac{1,680,000}{1,000}$$

$$x = 1,680 \text{ units/hr}$$

22. 1 L = 1,000 mL

a. Calculate mL/hr.

$$\frac{1,000 \text{ mL}}{10 \text{ hr}} = 100 \text{ mL/hr}$$

b. Calculate units/hr.

15,000 units : 1,000 mL = $x$ units: 100 mL

$$\frac{1,000x}{1,000} = \frac{1,500,000}{1,000}$$

$$x = \frac{1,500,000}{1,000}$$

$$x = 1,500 \text{ units/hr}$$

23. 1 L = 1,000 mL

35,000 units : 1,000 mL = $x$ units : 20 mL

$$\frac{1,000x}{1,000} = \frac{700,000}{1,000}$$

$$x = \frac{700,000}{1,000}$$

$$x = 700 \text{ units/hr}$$

24. 10,000 units : 500 mL = $x$ units : 120 mL

$$\frac{500x}{500} = \frac{1,200,000}{500}$$

$$x = \frac{1,200,000}{500}$$

$$x = 2,400 \text{ units/hr}$$

25. 25,000 units : 500 mL = $x$ units : 25 mL

$$\frac{500x}{500} = \frac{625,000}{500}$$

$$x = 1,250 \text{ units/hr}$$

26. 20,000 units : 500 mL = $x$ units : 40 mL

$$\frac{500x}{500} = \frac{800,000}{500}$$

$$x = 1,600 \text{ units/hr}$$

27. Calculate mL/hr to be administered.

40,000 units : 1,000 mL = 1,400 units : $x$ mL

$$\frac{40,000x}{40,000} = \frac{1,400,000}{40,000}$$

$$x = 35 \text{ mL/hr}$$

28. 1 L = 1,000 mL

    40,000 units : 1,000 mL = 1,000 units : $x$ mL

$$\frac{40,000x}{40,000} = \frac{1,000,000}{40,000}$$

$$x = \frac{1,000,000}{40,000}$$

$$x = 25 \text{ mL/hr}$$

29. 1 L = 1,000 mL

    25,000 units : 1,000 mL = 2,000 units : $x$ mL

$$\frac{25,000x}{25,000} = \frac{2,000,000}{25,000}$$

$$x = \frac{2,000,000}{25,000}$$

$$x = 80 \text{ mL/hr}$$

30. 50,000 units : 1,000 mL = $x$ units : 60 mL

$$\frac{1,000x}{1,000} = \frac{3,000,000}{1,000}$$

$$x = \frac{3,000,000}{1,000}$$

$$x = 3,000 \text{ units/hr}$$

31. 25,000 units : 500 mL = $x$ units : 120 mL

$$\frac{500x}{500} = \frac{500,000}{500}$$

$$x = \frac{5,000,000}{500}$$

$$x = 1,000 \text{ units/hr}$$

32. 20,000 units : 500 mL = $x$ units : 20 mL

$$\frac{500x}{500} = \frac{400,000}{500}$$

$$x = \frac{400,000}{500}$$

$$x = 800 \text{ units/hr}$$

33. 1 L = 1,000 mL

    25,000 units : 1,000 mL = $x$ units : 56 mL

$$\frac{1,000x}{1,000} = \frac{1,400,000}{1,000}$$

$$x = \frac{1,400,000}{1,000}$$

$$x = 1,400 \text{ units/hr}$$

34. 20,000 units : 1,000 mL = $x$ units : 45 mL

$$\frac{1,000x}{1,000} = \frac{900,000}{1,000}$$

$$x = \frac{900,000}{1,000}$$

$$x = 900 \text{ units/hr}$$

35. 30,000 units : 500 mL = $x$ units : 25 mL

$$\frac{500x}{500} = \frac{750,000}{500}$$

$$x = \frac{750,000}{500}$$

$$x = 1,500 \text{ units/hr}$$

36. 1 L = 1,000 mL

    20,000 units : 1,000 mL = $x$ units : 40 mL

$$\frac{1,000x}{1,000} = \frac{800,000}{1,000}$$

$$x = \frac{800,000}{1,000}$$

$$x = 800 \text{ units/hr}$$

37. 40,000 units : 500 mL = $x$ units : 25 mL

$$\frac{500x}{500} = \frac{1,000,000}{500}$$

$$x = \frac{1,000,000}{500}$$

$$x = 2,000 \text{ units/hr}$$

38. 1 L = 1,000 mL

    35,000 units : 1,000 mL = $x$ units : 20 mL

$$\frac{1,000x}{1,000} = \frac{700,000}{1,000}$$

$$x = \frac{700,000}{1,000}$$

$$x = 700 \text{ units/hr}$$

39. 1 L = 1,000 mL

    25,000 units : 1,000 mL = $x$ units: 30 mL

$$\frac{1,000x}{1,000} = \frac{750,000}{1,000}$$

$$x = \frac{750,000}{1,000}$$

$$x = 750 \text{ units/hr}$$

40. 1 L = 1,000 mL

    40,000 units : 1,000 mL = $x$ units: 30 mL

$$\frac{1,000x}{1,000} = \frac{1,200,000}{1,000}$$

$$x = 1,200 \text{ units/hr}$$

41. 1 L = 1,000 mL

    20,000 units : 1,000 mL = $x$ units : 80 mL

$$\frac{1,000x}{1,000} = \frac{1,600,000}{1,000}$$

$$x = 1,600 \text{ units/hr}$$

42. $1 \text{ L} = 1,000 \text{ mL}$

50,000 units : 1,000 mL $= x$ units : 10 mL

$$\frac{1,000x}{1,000} = \frac{500,000}{1,000}$$

$$x = 500 \text{ units/hr}$$

43. $1 \text{ L} = 1,000 \text{ mL}$

20,000 units : 500 mL $= x$ units : 30 mL

$$\frac{500x}{500} = \frac{600,000}{500}$$

$$x = 1,200 \text{ units/hr}$$

44. $1 \text{ L} = 1,000 \text{ mL}$

30,000 units : 1,000 mL $= x$ units : 25 mL

$$\frac{1,000x}{1,000} = \frac{750,000}{1,000}$$

$$x = 750 \text{ units/hr}$$

45. 100 units per mL is appropriate for flush. Heparin for injection cannot be interchanged with heparin lock solution. Check order with prescriber.

46. a. First determine units/kg the client should receive.

18 units/k̶g̶ × 80 k̶g̶ = 1,440 units

b. 1,000 mL : 25,000 units $= x$ mL : 1,440 units

$$\frac{25,000x}{25,000} = \frac{1,440,000}{25,000}$$

$$x = 57.6 = 58 \text{ mL/hr}$$

Answer: 58 mL/hr

47. a. Convert the weight to kilograms.

Conversion factor: 2.2 lb = 1 kg

200 lb ÷ 2.2 = 90.9 kg

b. Calculate the heparin bolus dosage.

80 units/k̶g̶ × 90.9 k̶g̶ = 7,272 units

Answer: 7,272 units

48. a. Convert the weight to kilograms.

Conversion factor: 2.2 lb = 1 kg

210 lb ÷ 2.2 = 95.45 kg = 95.5 kg

Calculate the heparin bolus dosage.

80 units/k̶g̶ × 95.5 k̶g̶ = 7,640 units

Answer: 7,640 units

b. Calculate the infusion rate for the heparin drip.

18 units/k̶g̶/hr × 95.5 k̶g̶ = 1,719 units/hr

c. Calculate the infusion rate in mL/hr.

1,000 mL : 25,000 units $= x$ mL : 1,719 units/hr

$$\frac{25,000x}{25,000} = \frac{1,719,000}{25,000}$$

$$x = 68.7 = 69 \text{ mL/hr}$$

Answer: 69 mL/hr

49. a. Convert the weight to kilograms.

110 lb ÷ 2.2 = 50 kg

b. 18 units k̶g̶/hr × 50 k̶g̶ = 900 units

Answer: 900 units/hr

50. a. Convert the weight to kilograms.

154 lb ÷ 2.2 = 70 kg

Calculate the heparin bolus dosage.

80 units/k̶g̶ × 70 k̶g̶ = 5,600 units

Answer: 5,600 units

b. Calculate the infusion rate for the heparin drip.

14 units/k̶g̶/hr × 70 k̶g̶ = 980 units/hr

Answer: 980 units/hr

c. Calculate the infusion rate in mL/hr.

1,000 mL : 20,000 units $= x$ mL : 980 units

$$\frac{20,000x}{20,000} = \frac{980,000}{20,000}$$

$$x = 49 \text{ mL/hr}$$

## CHAPTER 24

### Answers to Practice Problems

1. a. Step 1: Conversion: Equivalent: 1,000 mcg = 1 mg.

Therefore 250 mg = 250,000 mcg.

Step 2: 250,000 mcg : 500 mL $= x$ mcg : 1 mL

$$\frac{500x}{500} = \frac{250,000}{500} ; x = 500 \text{ mcg/mL}$$

Concentration of solution is 500 mcg/mL.

Step 3: Calculate dosage range.

Lower dosage:

2.5 mcg/k̶g̶/min × 50 k̶g̶ = 125 mcg/min

Upper dosage:

5 mcg/k̶g̶/min × 50 k̶g̶ = 250 mcg/min

Step 4: Convert dosage range to mL/min.

Lower dosage:

500 mcg : 1 mL = 125 mcg : $x$ mL

$$\frac{500x}{500} = \frac{125}{500}$$

$$x = 0.25 \text{ mL/min}$$

Upper dosage:

500 mcg : 1 mL = 250 mcg : $x$ mL

$$\frac{500x}{500} = \frac{250}{500}$$

$$x = 0.5 \text{ mL/min}$$

Step 5: Convert mL/min to mL/hr.

Lower dosage: 0.25 mL × 60 min =
$\qquad\qquad$ 15 mL/hr (gtt/min)

Upper dosage: 0.5 mL × 60 min =
$\qquad\qquad$ 30 mL/hr (gtt/min)

A dosage range of 2.5-5 mcg/kg/min is equal to a flow rate of 15-30 mL/hr (gtt/min).

b. Determine dosage infusing per minute at 25 mL/hr:

$$500 \text{ mcg} : 1 \text{ mL} = x \text{ mcg} : 25 \text{ mL}$$
$$x = 12{,}500 \text{ mcg/hr}$$

12,500 mcg ÷ 60 min = 208.3 mcg/min

2.  a.  $2 \text{ mg} : 250 \text{ mL} = x \text{ mg} : 30 \text{ mL}$

$$\frac{250x}{250} = \frac{60}{250}$$
$$x = 0.24 \text{ mg/hr}$$

b. Convert milligrams to micrograms (1,000 mcg = 1 mg).

0.24 mg = 240 mcg/hr

c. Convert mcg/hr to mcg/min.

240 mcg/hr ÷ 60 min = 4 mcg/min

3.  a.  Change grams to milligrams. (Note that you were asked to calculate mg/hr.)

$$0.25 \text{ g} = 250 \text{ mg} \ (1 \text{ g} = 1{,}000 \text{ mg})$$

b. Calculate mg/hr.

$$250 \text{ mg} : 500 \text{ mL} = 20 \text{ mL} : x \text{ mL}$$
$$\frac{250x}{250} = \frac{10{,}000}{250}$$
$$x = 40 \text{ mg/hr}$$

4.  *Note:* Calculate units per hour only.

Step 1: 60 gtt : 1 mL = 15 gtt : x mL

$$\frac{60x}{60} = \frac{15}{60}$$
$$x = 0.25 \text{ mL/min}$$

Step 2: 0.25 mL/min × 60 min = 15 mL/hr

Step 3: 10 units : 1,000 mL = x units : 15 mL

$$\frac{1{,}000x}{1{,}000} = \frac{150}{1{,}000}; x = 0.15 \text{ units/hr}$$

5.  Step 1: Determine the dosage per minute.

$$60 \text{ kg} \times 3 \text{ mcg/kg/min} = 180 \text{ mcg/min}$$

Step 2: Convert to dosage per hour.

$$180 \text{ mcg/min} \times 60 \text{ min} = 10{,}800 \text{ mcg/hr}$$

Step 3: Convert to like units (1,000 mcg = 1 mg).

$$10{,}800 \text{ mcg} = 10.8 \text{ mg}$$

Calculate flow rate (mL/hr).

$$50 \text{ mg} : 250 \text{ mL} = 10.8 \text{ mg} : x \text{ mL}$$
$$50x = 250 \times 10.8$$
$$\frac{50x}{50} = \frac{2{,}700}{50}$$
$$x = 54 \text{ mL/hr}$$

6.  a.  $50 \text{ mg} : 250 \text{ mL} = x \text{ mg} : 3 \text{ mL}$

$$\frac{250x}{250} = \frac{150}{250}$$
$$x = 0.6 \text{ mg/hr}$$

Convert to micrograms (1,000 mcg = 1 mg).

$$0.6 \text{ mg} = 600 \text{ mcg/hr}$$

b. Convert mcg/hr to mcg/min.

$$600 \text{ mcg/hr} \div 60 \text{ min} = 10 \text{ mcg/min}$$

## Answers to Critical Thinking Questions

a. The nurse made the error in the second step (converting 180 mcg to mg to match the units in the solution strength). This led to the error in the mL/hr rate.

$$180 \text{ mcg} = 0.18 \text{ mg} \ (1{,}000 \text{ mcg} = 1 \text{ mg})$$
$$180 \div 1{,}000 = 0.18 \text{ mg}$$

b. The error would result in an incorrect IV rate in mL/hr; the answer obtained is used to determine the rate in mL/hr. Use of 0.018 mg would net an incorrect answer.

$$1 \text{ mg} : 250 \text{ mL} = 0.018 \text{ mg} : x \text{ mL}$$
$$x = 250 \times 0.018$$
$$x = 4.5 = 5 \text{ mL/hr}$$

c. The rate in mL/hr should be 45 mL/hr and not 5 mL/hr.

$$1 \text{ mg} : 250 \text{ mL} = 0.18 \text{ mg} : x \text{ mL}$$
$$x = 250 \times 0.18$$
$$x = 45 \text{ mL/hr}$$

d. The nurse should have double-checked the math at each step. In addition, having another nurse check the calculation may have helped in recognizing the error in calculation.

## Answers to Chapter Review

1.  a.  Calculate the dosage per hr.

    $2 \text{ mg} : 250 \text{ mL} = x \text{ mg} : 30 \text{ mL}$

    $$\frac{250x}{250} = \frac{60}{250}$$

    $$x = \frac{60}{250}$$

    $$x = 0.24 \text{ mg/hr}$$

    b.  Convert milligrams to micrograms ($1,000 \text{ mcg} = 1 \text{ mg}$).

    $1,000 \times 0.24 \text{ mg/hr} = 240 \text{ mcg/hr}$

    c.  Convert mcg/hr to mcg/min.

    $240 \text{ mcg/hr} \div 60 \text{ min} = 4 \text{ mcg/min}$

2.  a.  Calculate dosage per hr.

    $4 \text{ mg} : 500 \text{ mL} = x \text{ mg} : 40 \text{ mL}$

    $$\frac{500x}{500} = \frac{160}{500}$$

    $$x = \frac{160}{500}$$

    $$x = 0.32 \text{ mg/hr}$$

    b.  Convert to micrograms ($1,000 \text{ mcg} = 1 \text{ mg}$).

    $1,000 \times 0.32 \text{ mg/hr} = 320 \text{ mcg/hr}$

    c.  Convert mcg/hr to mcg/min.

    $320 \text{ mcg/hr} \div 60 \text{ min} = 5.33 = 5.3 \text{ mcg/min}$

3.  Step 1: Determine dosage per hour.

    $800 \text{ mg} : 500 \text{ mL} = x \text{ mg} : 30 \text{ mL}$

    $$\frac{500x}{500} = \frac{24,000}{500}$$

    $$x = \frac{24,000}{500}$$

    $$x = 48 \text{ mg/hr}$$

    a.  Step 2: Convert milligrams to micrograms ($1,000 \text{ mcg} = 1 \text{ mg}$).

    $48 \text{ mg/hr} \times 1,000 = 48,000 \text{ mcg/hr}$

    b.  Step 3: Convert mcg/hr to mcg/min.

    $48,000 \text{ mcg/hr} \div 60 \text{ min} = 800 \text{ mcg/min}$

    c.  $200 \text{ mg} : 5 \text{ mL} = 800 \text{ mg} : x \text{ mL}$

    *or*

    $$\frac{800 \text{ mg}}{200 \text{ mg}} \times 5 \text{ mL} = x \text{ mL}$$

    Answer: 20 mL. The dosage ordered is greater than what is available. Therefore you will need more than 5 mL to administer the dosage.

4.  a.  Determine dosage per hour.

    $50 \text{ mg} : 250 \text{ mL} = x \text{ mg} : 30 \text{ mL}$

    $$\frac{250x}{250} = \frac{1,500}{250}$$

    $$x = \frac{1,500}{250}$$

    $$x = 6 \text{ mg/hr}$$

    Convert milligrams to micrograms ($1,000 \text{ mcg} = 1 \text{ mg}$).

    $6 \text{ mg/hr} \times 1,000 = 6,000 \text{ mcg/hr}$

    b.  Convert mcg/hr to mcg/min.

    $6,000 \text{ mcg/hr} \div 60 \text{ min} = 100 \text{ mcg/min}$

    c.  $50 \text{ mg} : 2 \text{ mL} = 50 \text{ mL} : x \text{ mL}$

    $$\frac{50 \text{ mg}}{50 \text{ mg}} \times 2 \text{ mL} = x \text{ mL}$$

    Answer: 2 mL. The dosage ordered is contained in a volume of 2 mL.

    Alternate solution: $25 \text{ mg} : 1 \text{ mL} = 50 \text{ mg} : x \text{ mL}$

    *or*

    $$\frac{50 \text{ mg}}{25 \text{ mg}} \times 1 \text{ mL} = x \text{ mL}$$

5.  a.  Calculate mg/hr.

    $100 \text{ mg} : 250 \text{ mL} = x \text{ mg} : 25 \text{ mL}$

    $$\frac{250x}{250} = \frac{2,500}{250}$$

    $$x = \frac{2,500}{250}$$

    $$x = 10 \text{ mg/hr}$$

    Convert milligrams to micrograms ($1,000 \text{ mcg} = 1 \text{ mg}$).

    $10 \text{ mg} = 10,000 \text{ mcg/hr}$

    b.  Convert mcg/hr to mcg/min.

    $10,000 \text{ mcg/hr} \div 60 \text{ min} = 166.66 = 166.7 \text{ mcg/min}$

6.  a.  Convert metric weight to the same as answer requested. Convert grams to milligrams.

    $1 \text{ g} = 1,000 \text{ mg}$; therefore $2 \text{ g} = 2,000 \text{ mg}$

    $2,000 \text{ mg} : 250 \text{ mL} = x \text{ mg} : 60 \text{ mL}$

    $$\frac{250x}{250} = \frac{120,000x}{250}$$

    $$x = \frac{120,000}{250}$$

    $$x = 480 \text{ mg/hr}$$

    b.  Convert mg/hr to mg/min.

    $480 \text{ mg/hr} \div 60 \text{ min} = 8 \text{ mg/min}$

7. a. Step 1: Convert grams to milligrams
   (1,000 mg = 1 g).

   $$0.25 \text{ g} = 250 \text{ mg}$$

   Step 2: Calculate mg/hr.

   $$250 \text{ mg} : 6 \text{ hr} = x \text{ mg} : 1 \text{ hr}$$

   $$\frac{6x}{6} = \frac{250}{6}$$

   $$x = \frac{250}{6}$$

   $$x = 41.66 = 41.7 \text{ mg/hr}$$

   b. $500 \text{ mg} : 20 \text{ mL} = 250 \text{ mg} : x \text{ mL}$

   *or*

   $$\frac{250 \text{ mg}}{500 \text{ mg}} \times 20 \text{ mL} = x \text{ mL}$$

   Answer: 10 mL. The dosage ordered is less than the available strength; therefore you will need less than 20 mL to administer the dosage.

8. a. Convert grams to milligrams (1,000 mg = 1 g).

   $$2 \text{ g} = 2,000 \text{ mg}$$

   Calculate mg/hr.

   $$2,000 \text{ mg} : 250 \text{ mL} = x \text{ mg} : 30 \text{ mL}$$

   $$\frac{250x}{250} = \frac{60,000}{250}$$

   $$x = \frac{60,000}{250}$$

   $$x = 240 \text{ mg/hr}$$

   b. Convert mg/hr to mg/min.

   $$240 \text{ mg} \div 60 \text{ min} = 4 \text{ mg/min}$$

9. a. Step 1: Calculate gtt/min to mL/min.

   $$60 \text{ gtt} : 1 \text{ mL} = 45 \text{ gtt} : x \text{ mL}$$

   $$\frac{60x}{60} = \frac{45}{60}$$

   $$x = \frac{45}{60}$$

   $$x = 0.75 \text{ mL/min}$$

   Step 2: Calculate units/min.

   $$20 \text{ units} : 1,000 \text{ mL} = x \text{ units} : 0.75 \text{ mL}$$

   $$\frac{1,000x}{1,000} = \frac{15}{1,000}$$

   $$x = \frac{15}{1,000}$$

   $$x = 0.015 \text{ units/min}$$

   b. Calculate units/hr.

   $$0.015 \text{ units/min} \times 60 \text{ min} = 0.9 \text{ units/hr}$$

10. $30 \text{ units} : 1,000 \text{ mL} = x \text{ units} : 40 \text{ mL}$

    $$\frac{1,000x}{1,000} = \frac{1,200}{1,000}$$

    $$x = \frac{1,200}{1,000}$$

    $$x = 1.2 \text{ units/hr}$$

11. $30 \text{ units} : 500 \text{ mL} = x \text{ units} : 45 \text{ mL}$

    $$\frac{500x}{500} = \frac{1,350}{500}$$

    $$x = \frac{1,350}{500}$$

    $$x = 2.7 \text{ units/hr}$$

12. a. Change metric measures to same as question.
    1 g = 1,000 mg; therefore 2 g = 2,000 mg.

    Calculate mg/hr.

    $$2,000 \text{ mg} : 500 \text{ mL} = x \text{ mg} : 30 \text{ mL}$$

    $$\frac{500x}{500} = \frac{60,000}{500}$$

    $$x = \frac{60,000}{500}$$

    $$x = 120 \text{ mg/hr}$$

    b. Change mg/hr to mg/min.

    $$120 \text{ mg/hr} \div 60 \text{ min} = 2 \text{ mg/min}$$

13. a. Change metric measures to same as question.

    $$2 \text{ g} = 2,000 \text{ mg} (1 \text{ g} = 1,000 \text{ mg})$$

    Calculate mg/hr.

    $$2000 \text{ mg} : 500 \text{ mL} = x \text{ mg} : 45 \text{ mL}$$

    $$\frac{500x}{500} = \frac{90,000}{500}$$

    $$x = \frac{90,000}{500}$$

    $$x = 180 \text{ mg/hr}$$

    b. Change mg/hr to mg/min

    $$180 \text{ mg/hr} \div 60 \text{ min} = 3 \text{ mg/min}$$

14. Determine dosage per hour.

    $$500 \text{ mcg/min} \times 60 \text{ min} = 30,000 \text{ mcg/hr}$$

    Convert micrograms to milligrams.

    $$1,000 \text{ mcg} = 1 \text{ mg}$$

    $$30,000 \text{ mcg/hr} = 30 \text{ mg/hr}$$

    Calculate flow rate in mL/hr.

    $$50 \text{ mg} : 250 \text{ mL} = 30 \text{ mg} : x \text{ mL}$$

    $$\frac{50x}{50} = \frac{7,500}{50}$$

    $$x = 150 \text{ mL/hr}$$

    Set at 150 mL/hr to deliver 30 mg/hr.

15. $400 \text{ mg} : 500 \text{ mL} = x \text{ mg} : 35 \text{ mL}$

$$\frac{500x}{500} = \frac{14,000}{500}$$

$$x = 28 \text{ mg/hr}$$

16. a. Calculate mg/hr.

$2 \text{ mg} : 250 \text{ mL} = x \text{ mg} : 45 \text{ mL}$

$$\frac{250x}{250} = \frac{90}{250}$$

$$x = \frac{90}{250}$$

$$x = 0.36 \text{ mg/hr}$$

  b. Convert milligrams to micrograms (1,000 mcg = 1 mg).

$0.36 \text{ mg} \times 1,000 = 360 \text{ mcg/hr}$

  c. Convert mcg/hr to mcg/min.

$360 \text{ mcg} \div 60 \text{ min} = 6 \text{ mcg/min}$

17. Convert metric weight to same as question.

$1,000 \text{ mg} = 1 \text{ g}$

Calculate mg/hr.

$1,000 \text{ mg} : 10 \text{ hr} = x \text{ mg} : 1 \text{ hr}$

$$\frac{10x}{10} = \frac{1,000}{10}$$

$$x = 100 \text{ mg/hr}$$

18. a. Convert grams to milligrams.

$2 \text{ g} = 2,000 \text{ mg} (1,000 \text{ mg} = 1 \text{ g})$

$2000 \text{ mg} : 250 \text{ mL} = x \text{ mg} : 22 \text{ mL}$

$$\frac{250x}{250} = \frac{44,000}{250}$$

$$x = \frac{44,000}{250}$$

$$x = 176 \text{ mg/hr}$$

  b. Change mg/hr to mg/min.

$176 \text{ mg/hr} \div 60 \text{ min} = 2.93 = 2.9 \text{ mg/min}$

19. Calculate dosage per hour.

$4 \text{ mg} : 250 \text{ mL} = x \text{ mg} : 8 \text{ mL}$

$$\frac{250x}{250} = \frac{32}{250}$$

$$x = \frac{32}{250}$$

$$x = 0.128 \text{ mg/hr}$$

Convert milligrams to micrograms (1,000 mcg = 1 mg).

$0.128 \text{ mg/hr} \times 1,000 = 128 \text{ mcg/hr}$

20. Convert g to mg.

$2.5 \text{ g} = 2,500 \text{ mg} (1 \text{ g} = 1,000 \text{ mg})$

  a. $250 \text{ mL} : 2,500 \text{ mg} = 30 \text{ mL} : x \text{ mg}$

$$\frac{250x}{250} = \frac{75,000}{250}$$

$$x = \frac{75,000}{250}$$

$$x = 300 \text{ mg/hr}$$

  b. Convert mg/hr to mg/min.

$300 \text{ mg/hr} \div 60 \text{ min} = 5 \text{ mg/min}$

21. a. Calculate mg/hr.

$500 \text{ mg} : 500 \text{ mL} = x \text{ mg} : 30 \text{ mL}$

$$\frac{500x}{500} = \frac{15,000}{500}$$

$$x = \frac{15,000}{500}$$

$$x = 30 \text{ mg/hr}$$

Convert milligrams to micrograms (1,000 mcg = 1 mg).

$30 \text{ mg} = 30,000 \text{ mcg/hr}$

  b. Convert mcg/hr to mcg/min.

$30,000 \text{ mcg/hr} \div 60 \text{ min} = 500 \text{ mcg/min}$

22. $25 \text{ g} : 300 \text{ mL} = 2 \text{ g} : x \text{ mL}$

$$\frac{25x}{25} = \frac{600}{25}$$

$$x = \frac{600}{25}$$

$$x = 24 \text{ mL/hr; would administer 2 g}$$

23. Determine dosage per hour.

$200 \text{ mcg/min} \times 60 \text{ min} = 12,000 \text{ mcg/hr}$

Convert micrograms to milligrams (1,000 mcg = 1 mg).

$12,000 \text{ mcg} \div 1,000 = 12 \text{ mg/hr}$

Calculate the mL/hr.

$400 \text{ mg} : 500 \text{ mL} = 12 \text{ mg} : x \text{ mL}$

$$\frac{400x}{400} = \frac{6,000}{400}$$

$$x = 15 \text{ mL/hr}$$

24. $25 \text{ g} : 300 \text{ mL} = 3 \text{ g} : x \text{ mL}$

$$\frac{25x}{25} = \frac{900}{25}$$

$$x = \frac{900}{25}$$

$$x = 36 \text{ mL/hr; would administer 3 g}$$

25. Convert dosage per minute to dosage per hour.

$$10 \text{ mcg/min} \times 60 \text{ min} = 600 \text{ mcg/hr}$$

   a. Convert measures to like units of measurement (mcg to mg; 1,000 mcg = 1 mg).

$$600 \text{ mcg} = 600 \div 1,000 = 0.6 \text{ mg}$$

   b. Calculate mL/hr.

$$50 \text{ mg} : 250 \text{ mL} = 0.6 \text{ mg} : x \text{ mL}$$

$$\frac{50x}{50} = \frac{150}{50}$$

$$x = 3 \text{ mL/hr}$$

   c. Calculate the flow rate in gtt/min.

$$x \text{ gtt/min} = \frac{3 \text{ mL} \times 60 \text{ gtt/mL}}{60 \text{ min}}$$

$$x = 3 \text{ gtt/min}; 3 \text{ microgtt/min}$$

   To deliver 10 mcg/min, the IV is to infuse at 3 gtt/min (3 microgtt/min).

26. Convert weight in pounds to kilograms (2.2 lb = 1 kg).

$$120 \text{ lb} = 54.54 = 54.5 \text{ kg}$$

   Calculate dosage per minute.

$$54.5 \text{ kg} \times 2 \text{ mcg/kg/min} = 109 \text{ mcg/min}$$

27. No conversion of weight is required.

$$80 \text{ kg} \times 3 \text{ mcg/kg/min} = 240 \text{ mcg/min}$$

28. No conversion of weight is required.

$$73.5 \text{ kg} \times 0.7 \text{ mg/kg/hr} = 51.45 \text{ mg/hr}$$

29. a. Convert weight in pounds to kilograms (2.2 lb = 1 kg).

$$110 \text{ lb} \div 2.2 = 50 \text{ kg}$$

   Calculate the dosage per hour.

$$50 \text{ kg} \times 0.7 \text{ mg/kg/hr} = 35 \text{ mg/hr}$$

   b. Calculate the dosage per minute.

$$35 \text{ mg/hr} \div 60 \text{ min} = 0.58 \text{ mg/min} = 0.6 \text{ mg/min}$$

   c. The dosage is safe; it falls within the safe range.

30. Step 1: Convert to like units.

   Equivalent: 1,000 mcg = 1 mg

   Therefore 2 mg = 2,000 mcg

   Step 2: Calculate the concentration of solution in mcg per mL.

$$2,000 \text{ mcg} : 500 \text{ mL} = x \text{ mcg} : 1 \text{ mL}$$

$$\frac{500x}{500} = \frac{2,000}{500}$$

$$x = 4 \text{ mcg per mL}$$

   Lower dosage: 4 mcg : 1 mL = 2 mcg : x mL

$$\frac{4x}{4} = \frac{2}{4}$$

$$x = 0.5 \text{ mL/min}$$

Upper dosage: 4 mcg : 1 mL = 6 mcg : x mL

$$\frac{4x}{4} = \frac{6}{4}$$

$$x = 1.5 \text{ mL/min}$$

Step 3: Convert mL/min to mL/hr.

   Lower dosage: 0.5 mL × 60 min =

$$30 \text{ mL/hr (gtt/min)}$$

   Upper dosage: 1.5 mL × 60 min =

$$90 \text{ mL/hr (gtt/min)}$$

   A dosage range of 2-6 mcg/min is equal to a flow rate of 30-90 mL/hr (gtt/min).

31. Step 1: Convert to like units of measurement.

   Equivalent: 1,000 mcg = 1 mg

   Therefore 5,000 mg = 5,000,000 mcg

   Step 2: Calculate the concentration of solution in mcg per mL.

$$5,000,000 \text{ mcg} : 500 \text{ mL} = x \text{ mcg} : 1 \text{ mL}$$

$$\frac{500x}{500} = \frac{5,000,000}{500}$$

$$x = 10,000 \text{ mcg per mL}$$

   The concentration of solution is 10,000 mcg per mL.

   Step 3: Calculate the dosage range.

   Lower dosage: 50 mcg/kg/min × 60 kg =

$$3,000 \text{ mcg/min}$$

   Upper dosage: 75 mcg/kg/min × 60 kg =

$$4,500 \text{ mcg/min}$$

   Step 4: Convert the dosage range to mL/min.

$$10,000 \text{ mcg} : 1 \text{ mL} = 1,000 \text{ mcg} : x \text{ mL}$$

   Lower dosage: 10,000 mcg : 1 mL =

$$3,000 \text{ mcg} : x \text{ mL}$$

$$\frac{10,000x}{10,000} = \frac{3,000}{10,000}$$

$$x = 0.3 \text{ mL/min}$$

   Upper dosage: 10,000 mcg : 1 mL =

$$4,500 \text{ mcg} : x \text{ mL}$$

$$\frac{10,000x}{10,000} = \frac{4,500}{10,000}$$

$$x = 0.45 \text{ mL/min}$$

Step 5: Convert mL/min to mL/hr.

   Lower dosage: 0.3 mL × 60 min =

$$18 \text{ mL/hr (gtt/min)}$$

   Upper dosage: 0.45 mL × 60 min =

$$27 \text{ mL/hr (gtt/min)}$$

   a. A dosage range of 50-75 mcg is equal to a flow rate of 18-27 mL/hr (gtt/min).

   b. Determine the dosage per minute infusing at 24 mL/hr.

$$10,000 \text{ mcg} : 1 \text{ mL} = x \text{ mcg} : 24 \text{ mL}$$

$$x = 10,000 \times 24 = 240,000 \text{ mcg/hr}$$

$$240,000 \text{ mcg/hr} \div 60 \text{ min} = 4,000 \text{ mcg/min}$$

32. Calculate the dosage per minute for the client.

$$65 \text{ k\!\!/g} \times 10 \text{ mcg/k\!\!/g/min} = 650 \text{ mcg/min}$$

Determine the dosage per hour.

$$650 \text{ mcg/m\!\!/in} \times 60 \text{ m\!\!/in} = 39,000 \text{ mcg/hr}$$

Convert to like units.

$$1,000 \text{ mcg} = 1 \text{ mg}$$
$$39,000 \text{ mcg/hr} = 39 \text{ mg/hr}$$

Calculate mL/hr flow rate.

$$500 \text{ mg} : 250 \text{ mL} = 39 \text{ mg} : x \text{ mL}$$
$$x = 19.5 = 20 \text{ mL/hr}$$

Answer: To deliver a dosage of 10 mcg/kg, set the flow rate at 20 mL/hr (gtt/min).

33. Convert grams to milligrams.

$$1,000 \text{ mg} = 1 \text{ g}$$
$$0.25 \text{ g} = 250 \text{ mg}$$

Calculate mg/hr.

$$250 \text{ mg} \div 6 = 41.6 = 42 \text{ mg/hr}$$

Answer: The client is receiving 42 mg of aminophylline per hour.

34. a. Convert grams to milligrams.

$$1 \text{ g} = 1,000 \text{ mg}$$

Calculate mg/hr.

$$1,000 \text{ mg} : 500 \text{ mL} = x \text{ mg} : 20 \text{ mL}$$
$$\frac{500x}{500} = \frac{20,000}{500}$$
$$x = \frac{20,000}{500}$$
$$x = 40 \text{ mg/hr}$$

b. Convert mg/hr to mg/min.

$$40 \text{ mg/hr} \div 60 \text{ min} = 0.66 \text{ mg/min} = 0.7 \text{ mg}$$

Answer: At the rate of 20 mL/hr, the client is receiving a dosage of 40 mg/hr or 0.7 mg/min.

35. a. Convert gtt/min to mL/min.

$$60 \text{ gtt} : 1 \text{ mL} = 15 \text{ gtt} : x \text{ mL}$$
$$x = 0.25 = 0.3 \text{ mL/min}$$

Determine mg/min.

$$300 \text{ mg} : 500 \text{ mL} = x \text{ mg} : 0.3 \text{ mL}$$
$$x = 0.18 = 0.2 \text{ mg/min}$$

b. Calculate mg/hr.

$$0.2 \text{ mg/m\!\!/in} \times 60 \text{ m\!\!/in} = 12 \text{ mg/hr}$$

Answer: At 15 gtt/min, the client is receiving a dosage of 0.2 mg/min and 12 mg/hr.

36. a. 10,240 mcg/min
    b. 102 mL/hr

Calculate the dosage per minute.

$$100 \text{ mcg/k\!\!/g/min} \times 102.4 \text{ k\!\!/g} = 10,240 \text{ mcg/min}$$

Convert mcg/min to mg/min.

$$10,240 \text{ mcg} \div 1,000 = 10.24 = 10.2 \text{ mg/min}$$

Convert mg/min to mg/hr.

$$10.2 \text{ mg/m\!\!/in} \times 60 \text{ m\!\!/in} = 612 \text{ mg/hr}$$

Calculate flow rate.

$$1 \text{ g} = 1,000 \text{ mg}; 1.5 \text{ g} = 1,500 \text{ mg}$$
$$1,500 \text{ mg} : 250 \text{ mL} = 612 \text{ mg} : x \text{ mL}$$
$$1,500 x = 250 \times 612$$
$$\frac{1,500x}{1,500} = \frac{153,000}{1,500}$$
$$x = 102 \text{ mL/hr}$$

*or*

$$\frac{1,500 \text{ mg}}{250 \text{ mL}} = \frac{612 \text{ mg}}{x \text{ mL}}$$

37. a. 0.27 mg/min
    b. 270 mcg/min

Calculate mg/hr infusing.

$$500 \text{ mL} : 400 \text{ mg} = 20 \text{ mL} : x \text{ mg}$$

*or*

$$\frac{500 \text{ mL}}{400 \text{ mg}} = \frac{20 \text{ mL}}{x \text{ mg}}$$
$$500x = 400 \times 20$$
$$\frac{500x}{500} = \frac{8,000}{500}$$
$$x = 16 \text{ mg/hr}$$

Calculate the mg/min infusing.

$$16 \text{ mg/hr} \div 60 \text{ min} = 0.266 = 0.27 \text{ mg/min}$$
$$0.27 \text{ mg/min} = 270 \text{ mcg/min}$$

38. 11 mL/hr

Calculate dosage per minute.

$$3 \text{ mcg/k\!\!/g/min} \times 59.1 \text{ k\!\!/g} = 177.3 \text{ mcg/min}$$

Convert mcg/min to mcg/hr.

$$177.3 \text{ mcg/m\!\!/in} \times 60 \text{ m\!\!/in} = 10,638 \text{ mcg/hr}$$

Convert mcg/hr to mg/hr.

$$10,638 \text{ mcg/hr} = 10.63 = 10.6 \text{ mg/hr}$$

Calculate the flow rate.

$$250 \text{ mg} : 250 \text{ mL} = 10.6 \text{ mg} : x \text{ mL}$$

*or*

$$\frac{250 \text{ mg}}{250 \text{ mL}} = \frac{10.6 \text{ mg}}{x \text{ mL}}$$
$$250x = 250 \times 10.6$$
$$\frac{250x}{250} = \frac{2,650}{250}$$
$$x = 10.6 = 11 \text{ mL/hr}$$

39.  a. 375 mcg/min

  b. 22,500 mcg/hr

  c. 23 mL/hr

    Convert client's weight to kilograms
    (2.2 lb = 1 kg).

$$165 \text{ lb} \div 2.2 = 75 \text{ kg}$$

    Calculate dosage per minute.

$$5 \text{ mcg/kg/min} \times 75 \text{ kg} = 375 \text{ mcg/min}$$

    Convert mcg/min to mcg/hr.

$$375 \text{ mcg/min} \times 60 \text{ min} = 22,500 \text{ mcg/hr}$$

    Convert mcg/hr to mg/hr.

$$22,500 \text{ mcg/hr} = 22.5 \text{ mg/hr}$$

    Calculate flow rate.

$$250 \text{ mg} : 250 \text{ mL} = 22.5 \text{ mg} : x \text{ mL}$$

*or*

$$\frac{250 \text{ mg}}{250 \text{ mL}} = \frac{22.5 \text{ mg}}{x \text{ mL}}$$

$$250x = 250 \times 22.5$$

$$\frac{250x}{250} = \frac{5,625}{250}$$

$$x = 22.5 = 23 \text{ mL/hr}$$

40.  a.  $5 \text{ mg} : 1 \text{ mL} = 125 \text{ mg} : x \text{ mL}$

*or*

$$\frac{125 \text{ mg}}{5 \text{ mg}} \times 1 \text{ mL} = x \text{ mL}$$

    Answer: 25 mL. The dosage ordered is more than
    the available strength. Therefore you will need more
    than 5 mL to administer the dosage.

  b.  $125 \text{ mg} : 125 \text{ mL} = 20 \text{ mg} : x \text{ mL}$

$$125x = 125 \times 20$$

$$\frac{125x}{125} = \frac{2,500}{125}$$

$$x = 20 \text{ mL/hr}$$

41.  Calculate the dosage per hour.

$$2 \text{ mg/min} \times 60 \text{ min} = 120 \text{ mg/hr}$$

    Convert grams to milligrams.

$$1,000 \text{ mg} = 1 \text{ g}; 2 \text{ g} = 2,000 \text{ mg}$$

    Calculate mL/hr.

$$2,000 \text{ mg} : 500 \text{ mL} = 120 \text{ mg} : x \text{ mL}$$

$$2,000x = 500 \times 120$$

$$\frac{2,000x}{2,000} = \frac{60,000}{2,000}$$

$$x = 30 \text{ mL/hr}$$

# CHAPTER 25

## Answers to Practice Problems

1. 6.8 kg
2. 30.9 kg
3. 14.1 kg
4. 23.6 kg
5. 32.3 kg

6. 60.5 kg
7. 3.8 kg
8. 2.6 kg
9. 46.9 lb

10. 38.9 lb
11. 48.4 lb
12. 33 lb
13. 74.8 lb

14. 157.1 lb
15. 160.6 lb
16. 216.3 lb
17. 4 kg

18. 1.5 kg
19. 2.9 kg
20. 3.6 kg
21. 1.9 kg

**NOTE**

Any of the methods presented in Chapter 25 can be used
to calculate dosages; not all are shown in the Answer Key.

22.  a. 25 to 50 mg/kg/day

  b. Convert weight first (2.2 lb = 1 kg).

$$35 \div 2.2 = 15.9 \text{ kg}$$

$$\frac{25 \text{ mg}}{x \text{ mg}} = \frac{1 \text{ kg}}{15.9 \text{ kg}} \quad x = 397.5 \text{ mg/day}$$

$$\frac{50 \text{ mg}}{x \text{ mg}} = \frac{1 \text{ kg}}{15.9 \text{ kg}} \quad x = 795 \text{ mg/day}$$

*or*

$$25 \text{ mg/kg/day} \times 15.9 \text{ kg} = 397.5 \text{ mg/day}$$

$$50 \text{ mg/kg/day} \times 15.9 \text{ kg} = 795 \text{ mg/day}$$

  c. Dosage range is 397.5 to 795 mg/day.

  d. The dosage ordered falls within the range that is
     safe (150 mg × 4 = 600 mg). 600 mg/day falls
     within the 397.5 to 795 mg/day range.

  e.  $125 \text{ mg} : 5 \text{ mL} = 150 \text{ mg} : x \text{ mL}$

*or*

$$\frac{150 \text{ mg}}{125 \text{ mg}} \times 5 \text{ mL} = x \text{ mL}$$

$$x = 6 \text{ mL}$$

23.  a.  $\dfrac{15 \text{ mg}}{x \text{ mg}} = \dfrac{1 \text{ kg}}{35 \text{ kg}} \quad x = 525 \text{ mg/day}$

    525 mg—maximum dosage for 24 hr

*or*

$$35 \text{ kg} \times 15 \text{ mg/kg/day} = 525 \text{ mg/day}$$

b. $\dfrac{525 \text{ mg}}{3} = 175$ mg q8h

c. No, not safe. 200 mg × 3 = 600 mg/day. It also exceeds the dosage that should be given q8h. This is greater than the maximum dosage. Check order with the prescriber.

24. a. $\dfrac{8 \text{ mg}}{x \text{ mg}} = \dfrac{1 \text{ kg}}{40 \text{ kg}}$    $x = 320$ mg/day

*or*

8 mg/kg/day × 40 kg = 320 mg/day

$\dfrac{25 \text{ mg}}{x \text{ mg}} = \dfrac{1 \text{ kg}}{40 \text{ kg}}$    $x = 1{,}000$ mg

*or*

25 mg/kg/day × 40 kg = 1,000 mg/day

Answer: 1,000 mg is maximum dosage.

b. four divided dosages

320 mg ÷ 4 = 80 mg/dose

1,000 mg ÷ 4 = 250 mg/dose

Answer: 80-250 mg/dose divided dosage range (250 mg/dose is maximum divided dosage)

25. a. Weight conversion (2.2 lb = 1 kg)

9 ÷ 2.2 = 4.1 kg

b. $\dfrac{3 \text{ mg}}{x \text{ mg}} = \dfrac{1 \text{ kg}}{4.1 \text{ kg}}$    $x = 12.3$ mg/day

*or*

3 mg/kg/day × 4.1 kg = 12.3 mg/day

$\dfrac{5 \text{ mg}}{x \text{ mg}} = \dfrac{1 \text{ kg}}{4.1 \text{ kg}}$    $x = 20.5$ mg/day

*or*

5 mg/kg/day × 4.1 kg = 20.5 mg/day

Safe dosage range for the child for a day is 12.3-20.5 mg/day

c. The dosage ordered is safe.

10 mg × 2 = 20 mg/day. The maximum dosage per day is 20.5 mg.

d. 20 mg : 5 mL = 10 mg : $x$ mL

*or*

$\dfrac{10 \text{ mg}}{20 \text{ mg}} \times 5 \text{ mL} = x$ mL

$x = 2.5$ mL

You need to give 2.5 mL to administer the ordered dosage of 10 mg.

26. a. Convert weight to kilograms (2.2 lb = 1 kg).

84 lb ÷ 2.2 = 38.2 kg

$\dfrac{0.1 \text{ mg}}{x \text{ mg}} = \dfrac{1 \text{ kg}}{38.2 \text{ kg}}$    $x = 3.8$ mg/dose

*or*

38.2 kg × 0.1 mg/kg/dose = 3.82 mg = 3.8 mg/dose

*or*

$\dfrac{0.2 \text{ mg}}{x \text{ mg}} = \dfrac{1 \text{ kg}}{38.2 \text{ kg}} = 7.6$ mg/dose

38.2 kg × 0.2 mg/kg/dose = 7.64 mg = 7.6 mg/dose

b. 3.8-7.6 mg/dosage

c. The dosage ordered is safe. 7.5 mg is less than 7.6 mg.

d. You would administer 0.5 mL.

15 mg : 1 mL = 7.5 mg : $x$ mL

*or*

$\dfrac{7.5 \text{ mg}}{15 \text{ mg}} \times 1 \text{ mL} = x$ mL

$x = 0.5$ mL

27. Convert weight to kilograms (2.2 lb = 1 kg).

a. 11 lb ÷ 2.2 = 5 kg

$\dfrac{4 \text{ mg}}{x \text{ mg}} = \dfrac{1 \text{ kg}}{5 \text{ kg}}$    $x = 20$ mg/day

*or*

4 mg/kg/day × 5 kg = 20 mg/day

$\dfrac{8 \text{ mg}}{x \text{ mg}} = \dfrac{1 \text{ kg}}{5 \text{ kg}}$    $x = 40$ mg/day

*or*

8 mg/kg/day × 5 kg = 40 mg/day

b. 20 to 40 mg/day

c. The dosage that is ordered is safe. It falls within the safe range. 15 mg × 2 = 30 mg/day.

d. 125 mg : 5 mL = 15 mg : $x$ mL

*or*

$\dfrac{15 \text{ mg}}{125 \text{ mg}} \times 5 \text{ mL} = x$ mL

You would administer 0.6 mL.

28. Convert the child's weight to kilograms (2.2 lb = 1 kg).

a. 44 lb ÷ 2.2 = 20 kg

$\dfrac{2.5 \text{ mg}}{x \text{ mg}} = \dfrac{1 \text{ kg}}{20 \text{ kg}}$    $x = 50$ mg/day

*or*

20 kg × 2.5 mg/kg/day = 50 mg/day

b. 50 mg/day

29. a. Convert weight (2.2 lb = 1 kg).

38 lb ÷ 2.2 = 17.3 kg

b. $\dfrac{40 \text{ mg}}{x \text{ mg}} = \dfrac{1 \text{ kg}}{17.3 \text{ kg}}$    $x = 692$ mg/day

*or*

40 mg/k̶g̶/day × 17.3 k̶g̶ = 692 mg/day

c. $\dfrac{692 \text{ mg}}{4} = 173$ mg/dose

d. The dosage ordered is not safe. 200 mg × 4 = 800 mg/day. 800 mg is greater than 692 mg/day. It also exceeds the dose that should be given q6h. Check with prescriber.

30. a. 20-40 mg/kg/day

b. Convert weight (2.2 lb = 1 kg).

16 lb ÷ 2.2 = 7.27 = 7.3 kg

$\dfrac{20 \text{ mg}}{x \text{ mg}} = \dfrac{1 \text{ kg}}{7.3 \text{ kg}}$    $x = 146$ mg/day

*or*

20 mg/k̶g̶/day × 7.3 k̶g̶ = 146 mg/day

$\dfrac{40 \text{ mg}}{x \text{ mg}} = \dfrac{1 \text{ kg}}{7.3 \text{ kg}}$    $x = 292$ mg/day

*or*

40 mg/k̶g̶/day × 7.3 k̶g̶ = 292 mg/day

c. Safe dosage range for the child is 146-292 mg/day.

d. The dosage ordered is not safe.
125 mg × 3 = 375 mg/day. 375 mg/day is greater than 146-292 mg/day; check with prescriber.

31. Convert weight (2.2 lb = 1 kg).

a. 44 lb ÷ 2.2 = 20 kg

$\dfrac{30 \text{ mg}}{x \text{ mg}} = \dfrac{1 \text{ kg}}{20 \text{ kg}}$    $x = 600$ mg/day

*or*

30 mg/k̶g̶/day × 20 k̶g̶ = 600 mg/day

$\dfrac{50 \text{ mg}}{x \text{ mg}} = \dfrac{1 \text{ kg}}{20 \text{ kg}}; x = 1,000$ mg

*or*

50 mg/k̶g̶/day × 20 k̶g̶ = 1,000 mg/day

b. 600-1,000 mg/day

c. The dosage ordered is safe.
250 mg × 4 = 1,000 mg. 1,000 mg falls within the safe range.

32. No weight conversion is required.

$\dfrac{0.25 \text{ mg}}{x \text{ mg}} = \dfrac{1 \text{ kg}}{66.3 \text{ kg}}$    $x = 16.57 = 16.6$ mg

*or*

0.25 mg/k̶g̶ × 66.3 k̶g̶ = 16.57 = 16.6 mg

Answer: 16.6 mg is the dosage for the adult.

33. Weight conversion is required (2.2 lb = 1 kg).

a. 200 lb ÷ 2.2 = 90.9 kg

$\dfrac{150 \text{ mg}}{x \text{ mg}} = \dfrac{1 \text{ kg}}{90.9 \text{ kg}}$    $x = 13,635$ mg/day

*or*

150 mg/k̶g̶/day × 90.9 k̶g̶ = 13,635 mg/day

$\dfrac{200 \text{ mg}}{x \text{ mg}} = \dfrac{1 \text{ kg}}{90.9 \text{ kg}}$    $x = 18,180$ mg/day

*or*

200 mg/k̶g̶/day × 90.9 k̶g̶ = 18,180 mg/day

To determine the number of grams, convert the milligrams obtained to grams (1,000 mg = 1 g).

13,635 mg ÷ 1,000 = 13.63 g

(13.6 g to nearest tenth)

18,180 mg ÷ 1,000 = 18.18 g

(18.2 g to nearest tenth)

b. The daily dosage range in grams is 13.6-18.2 g/day.

34. Convert weight (2.2. lb = 1 kg, 16 oz = 1 lb).

6 oz ÷ 16 = 0.37 lb = 0.4 lb (to nearest tenth)

Total weight in pounds = 12.4 lb

a. 12.4 lb ÷ 2.2 = 5.63 kg (5.6 to nearest tenth)

$\dfrac{15 \text{ mg}}{x \text{ mg}} = \dfrac{1 \text{ kg}}{5.6 \text{ kg}}$    $x = 84$ mg/day

*or*

15 mg/k̶g̶/day × 5.6 k̶g̶ = 84 mg/day

$\dfrac{50 \text{ mg}}{x \text{ mg}} = \dfrac{1 \text{ kg}}{5.6 \text{ kg}}$    $x = 280$ mg/day

*or*

50 mg/k̶g̶/day × 5.6 k̶g̶ = 280 mg/day

b. The safe dosage range is 84-280 mg/day.

35. 0.6 m$^2$

36. 0.78 m$^2$

37. 0.9 m$^2$

38. 0.8 m$^2$

39. 0.28 m$^2$

40. 0.44 m$^2$

41. 0.8 m$^2$

42. 0.28 m$^2$

43. 0.52 m$^2$

44. 0.45 m$^2$

45. 0.9 m$^2$

46. 0.3 m$^2$

47. 0.58 m$^2$

48. 0.51 m$^2$

49. 0.68 m$^2$

50. 0.18 m$^2$

51. $\sqrt{\dfrac{95.5\ (\text{kg}) \times 180\ (\text{cm})}{3{,}600}}$

$\sqrt{4.775} = 2.185 = 2.19\ \text{m}^2$

Answer: $2.19\ \text{m}^2$

52. $\sqrt{\dfrac{10\ (\text{kg}) \times 70\ (\text{cm})}{3{,}600}}$

$\sqrt{0.194} = 0.44\ \text{m}^2$

Answer: $0.44\ \text{m}^2$

53. $\sqrt{\dfrac{4.8\ (\text{lb}) \times 21\ (\text{in})}{3{,}131}}$

$\sqrt{0.032} = 0.178 = 0.18\ \text{m}^2$

Answer: $0.18\ \text{m}^2$

54. $\sqrt{\dfrac{170\ (\text{lb}) \times 67\ (\text{in})}{3{,}131}}$

$\sqrt{3.637} = 1.907 = 1.91\ \text{m}^2$

Answer: $1.91\ \text{m}^2$

55. $\sqrt{\dfrac{92\ (\text{lb}) \times 35\ (\text{in})}{3{,}131}}$

$\sqrt{1.028} = 1.014 = 1.01\ \text{m}^2$

Answer: $1.01\ \text{m}^2$

56. $\sqrt{\dfrac{24\ (\text{kg}) \times 92\ (\text{cm})}{3{,}600}}$

$\sqrt{0.613} = 0.783 = 0.78\ \text{m}^2$

Answer: $0.78\ \text{m}^2$

57. a. $0.52\ \text{m}^2$

b. $\dfrac{0.52\ \text{m}^2}{1.7\ (\text{m}^2)} \times 25\ \text{mg} = \dfrac{0.52 \times 25}{1.7} = \dfrac{13}{1.7} = 7.64$

Answer: $7.6\ \text{mg}$

58. a. $0.52\ \text{m}^2$

b. $\dfrac{0.52\ \text{m}^2}{1.7\ (\text{m}^2)} \times 200\ \text{mg} = \dfrac{0.52 \times 200}{1.7} = \dfrac{104}{1.7}$

$\dfrac{104}{1.7} = 61.17 = 61.2\ \text{mg}$

$\dfrac{0.52\ \text{m}^2}{1.7\ (\text{m}^2)} \times 400\ \text{mg} = \dfrac{208}{1.7} = 122.35$

$122.35\ \text{mg} = 122.4\ \text{mg}$

Answer: The child's dosage range is 61.2-122.4 mg.

59. $\dfrac{1.5\ \text{m}^2}{1.7\ (\text{m}^2)} \times 5\ \text{mg} = \dfrac{1.5 \times 5}{1.7} = \dfrac{7.5}{1.7}$

$\dfrac{7.5}{1.7} = 4.41\ \text{mg} = 4.4\ \text{mg}$

$\dfrac{1.5\ \text{m}^2}{1.7\ (\text{m}^2)} \times 15\ \text{mg} = \dfrac{22.5}{1.7} = 13.23$

$13.23\ \text{mg} = 13.2\ \text{mg}$

Answer: 4.4-13.2 mg

60. $\dfrac{0.8\ \text{m}^2}{1.7\ (\text{m}^2)} \times 20\ \text{mg} = \dfrac{0.8 \times 20}{1.7} = \dfrac{16}{1.7}$

$\dfrac{16}{1.7} = 9.41\ \text{mg} = 9.4\ \text{mg}$

Answer: The dosage is incorrect. The correct dosage is 9.4 mg.

61. $\dfrac{0.9\ \text{m}^2}{1.7\ (\text{m}^2)} \times 25\ \text{mg} = \dfrac{0.9 \times 25}{1.7} = \dfrac{22.5}{1.7}$

$\dfrac{22.5}{1.7} = 13.23\ \text{mg} = 13.2\ \text{mg}$

Answer: The dosage is incorrect. The correct dosage is 13.2 mg.

62. $\dfrac{1.5\ \text{m}^2}{1.7\ (\text{m}^2)} \times 250\ \text{mg} = \dfrac{1.5 \times 250}{1.7} = \dfrac{375}{1.7}$

$\dfrac{375}{1.7} = 220.58\ \text{mg}$

Answer: The child's dosage is 220.6 mg.

63. $\dfrac{0.74\ \text{m}^2}{1.7\ (\text{m}^2)} \times 20\ \text{mg} = \dfrac{0.74 \times 20}{1.7} = \dfrac{22.2}{1.7}$

$\dfrac{14.8}{1.7} = 8.70 = 8.7\ \text{mg}$

$\dfrac{0.74\ \text{m}^2}{1.7\ (\text{m}^2)} \times 30\ \text{mg} = \dfrac{0.74 \times 30}{1.7} = \dfrac{22.2}{1.7}$

$\dfrac{22.2}{1.7} = 13.05 = 13.1\ \text{mg}$

Answer: The child's dosage range is 8.7-13.1 mg.

64. $\dfrac{0.67\ \text{m}^2}{1.7\ (\text{m}^2)} \times 20\ \text{mg} = \dfrac{13.4}{1.7} = 7.88\ \text{mg} = 7.9\ \text{mg}.$

The dosage is correct.

65. $\dfrac{0.94\ \text{m}^2}{1.7\ (\text{m}^2)} \times 10\ \text{mg} = 5.5\ \text{mg}$

$\dfrac{0.94\ \text{m}^2}{1.7\ (\text{m}^2)} \times 20\ \text{mg} = 11.1\ \text{mg}$

Answer: The child's dosage range is 5.5-11.1 mg.

66. a. $0.45\ \text{m}^2$

b. $\dfrac{0.45\ \text{m}^2}{1.7\ (\text{m}^2)} \times 500\ \text{mg} = \dfrac{225}{1.7} = 132.35$

Answer: The child's dosage is 132.4 mg.

67. $\dfrac{1.3\ \text{m}^2}{1.7\ (\text{m}^2)} \times 500\ \text{mg} = \dfrac{1.3 \times 500}{1.7} = \dfrac{650}{1.7} = 382.35$

Answer: The child's dosage is 382.4 mg.

68. a. $0.55\ \text{m}^2$

b. $\dfrac{0.55\ \text{m}^2}{1.7\ (\text{m}^2)} \times 25\ \text{mg} = \dfrac{0.55 \times 25}{1.7} = \dfrac{13.75}{1.7}$

$\dfrac{13.75}{1.7} = 8.08$

Answer: The child's dosage is 8.1 mg.

69. $\dfrac{0.52 \; m^2}{1.7 \; (m^2)} \times 15 \text{ mg} = \dfrac{0.52 \times 15}{1.7} = \dfrac{7.8}{1.7} = 4.58$

Answer: The child's dosage is 4.6 mg.

70. $\dfrac{1.1 \; m^2}{1.7 \; (m^2)} \times 150 \text{ mg} = \dfrac{1.1 \times 150}{1.7} = \dfrac{165}{1.7} = 97.05$

Answer: The child's dosage is 97.1 mg.

71. a. Dilution volume: 27 mL

b. $x \text{ gtt/min} = \dfrac{30 \text{ mL (diluted medication)} \times 60 \text{ gtt/mL}}{50 \text{ min}}$

$x = \dfrac{30 \times 60}{50} = \dfrac{1800}{50} = 36 \text{ gtt/min}$

*or*

Use a ratio and proportion to determine mL/hr first. Remember that with a burette when a pump or controller is not used, mL/hr = gtt/min.

$30 \text{ mL} : 50 \text{ min} = x \text{ mL} : 60 \text{ min}$

*or*

$\dfrac{30 \text{ mL}}{50 \text{ min}} = \dfrac{x \text{ mL}}{60 \text{ min}}$

Answer: $x = 36$ gtt/min; 36 microgtt/min

c. 36 mL/hr

72. a. Dilution volume: 13 mL

b. $x \text{ gtt/min} = \dfrac{15 \text{ mL (diluted medication)} \times 60 \text{ gtt/mL}}{45 \text{ min}}$

$x = \dfrac{15 \times 60}{45} = \dfrac{900}{45} = 20 \text{ gtt/min}$

*or*

Use a ratio and proportion and determine mL/hr first.

$15 \text{ mL} : 45 \text{ min} = x \text{ mL} : 60 \text{ min}$

*or*

$\dfrac{15 \text{ mL}}{45 \text{ min}} = \dfrac{x \text{ mL}}{60 \text{ min}}$

Answer: $x = 20$ gtt/min; 20 microgtt/min

c. 20 mL/hr

73. Step 1: Determine the dosage range per hour.

10 units/kg/hr × 17 kg = 170 units/hr

25 units/kg/hr × 17 kg = 425 units/hr

Step 2: Determine dosage infusing per hour.

2,500 units : 250 mL = x units : 50 mL

$250x = 2,500 \times 50$

$\dfrac{250x}{250} = \dfrac{125,000}{250} = 500$

$x = 500 \text{ units/hr}$

Step 3: Compare the dosage ordered to see if it is within the safe range.

The IV is infusing at 50 mL/hr, which is 500 units/hr. The normal dosage range is 170-425 units/hr. 500 units/hr is greater than the dosage range. Check with the prescriber before administering.

74. Step 1: Determine the dosage range.

0.75 m² × 100 mg/m²/day = 75 mg/day

0.75 m² × 250 mg/m²/day = 187.5 mg/day

The dosage range is 75-187.5 mg per day.

Step 2: Determine the dosage the child is receiving.

84 mg q12h (2 dosages)

84 mg × 2 = 168 mg/day

Step 3: Determine if dosage is within safe range. The 84 mg q12h (84 mg × 2 = 168 mg/day) is within the safe range of 75-187.5 mg/day, so administer the medication.

## Answers to Critical Thinking Questions

Scenario: According to the *Harriet Lane Handbook* the recommended dosage for a child for ibuprofen as an antipyretic is 5-10 mg/kg/dose q6-8h p.o. The 7-month-old weighs 18½ lb. The prescriber ordered 20 mg p.o. q6h for a temperature above 102° F.

a. 42-84 mg/dose

b. Contact the prescriber; the dosage is too low. The dose is not safe because it is below the recommended therapeutic dose to decrease the child's temperature.

c. The nurse should have notified the prescriber immediately so that the order could be revised. The child's temperature indicates an underdosage that is not safe. Do not assume it is safe because the dosage is lower than the recommended dosage.

## Answers to Chapter Review

**NOTE**

Alternate ways of doing problems 1-13 in the Chapter Review are possible, such as a ratio and proportion, or dimensional analysis. These methods are shown in the examples in Chapter 25. Refer to them if necessary.

1. Convert weight (2.2 lb = 1 kg).

    $$22 \text{ lb} = 22 \div 2.2 = 10 \text{ kg}$$
    $$1 \text{ mg/kg} \times 10 \text{ kg} = 10 \text{ mg}$$

    The dosage ordered for this child is safe.

2. Convert weight (2.2 lb = 1 kg).

    a. $23 \text{ lb} = 23 \div 22 = 10.5 \text{ kg}$

    b. $20 \text{ mg/kg/day} \times 10.5 \text{ kg} = 210 \text{ mg/day}$
       $40 \text{ mg/kg/day} \times 10.5 \text{ kg} = 420 \text{ mg/day}$

       The safe range for this 10.5-kg child is 210-420 mg/day.

    c. The drug is given in divided dosages q8h.

       $$q8h = 24 \div 8 = 3 \text{ doses per day}$$
       $$210 \text{ mg} \div 3 = 70 \text{ mg per dosage}$$
       $$420 \text{ mg} \div 3 = 140 \text{ mg per dosage}$$

       The dosage range is 70-140 mg per dosage q8h.

    d. The dosage ordered is not safe; 150 mg × 3 = 450 mg/day. 450 mg/day is greater than 420 mg/day. Also the dose being given q8h exceeds the dose recommended.

       Notify the prescriber, and question the order.

3. Convert child's weight in kilograms to pounds. The recommended dosage is stated in pounds.

    $$2.2 \text{ lb} = 1 \text{ kg}$$

    a. $17 \text{ kg} = 17 \times 2.2 = 37.4 \text{ lb}$

       The dosage range is stated as 2.2-3.2 mg/lb/day.
       $2.2 \text{ mg/lb/day} \times 37.4 \text{ lb} = 82.28 \text{ mg} = 82.3 \text{ mg/day}$
       $3.2 \text{ mg/lb/day} \times 37.4 \text{ lb} = 119.68 \text{ mg} = 119.7 \text{ mg/day}$

    b. The dosage range is 82.3-119.7 mg/day.

       $$q6h = 4 \text{ dosages}$$
       $82.3 \text{ mg} \div 4 = 20.57 \text{ mg} = 20.6 \text{ mg per dose}$
       $119.7 \text{ mg} \div 4 = 29.92 \text{ mg} = 29.9 \text{ mg per dose}$

       The divided dosage range is 20.6-29.9 mg per dose.

       The dosage ordered is 25 mg q6h.

    c. This dosage is safe because 25 mg × 4 = 100 mg/day. It falls in the safe dosage range.

    d. $5 \text{ mg} : 1 \text{ mL} = 25 \text{ mg} : x \text{ mL}$

       *or*

       $$\frac{25 \text{ mg}}{5 \text{ mg}} \times 1 \text{ mL} = x \text{ mL}$$

       $$x = 5 \text{ mL}$$

Answer: Give 5 mL per dose. The dosage ordered is greater than the available strength; therefore you need more than 1 mL to administer the dosage.

4. No conversion of weight is required. The child's weight is in kilograms, and the recommended dosage is expressed in kilograms (12.5 mg/kg).

    $$12.5 \text{ mg/kg/day} \times 35 \text{ kg} = 437.5 \text{ mg/day}$$
    $$q6h = 4 \text{ dosages}$$
    $$437.5 \text{ mg} \div 4 =$$
    $$109.37 = 109.4 \text{ mg per dosage}$$

    Dosage ordered is not safe because 100 mg × 4 = 400 mg/day. 400 mg/day is less than 437.5 mg/day. Check with prescriber; dosage may be too low to be effective.

5. No conversion of weight is required. The child's weight is in pounds, and the recommended dosage is expressed in pounds (2 mg/lb).

    $$2 \text{ mg/lb/day} \times 30 \text{ lb} = 60 \text{ mg/day}$$
    $$q12 = 2 \text{ dosages}$$
    $$60 \text{ mg} \div 2 = 30 \text{ mg per dosage}$$

    75 mg × 2 = 150 mg/day. This dosage is too high; notify the prescriber. 150 mg/day is greater than 60 mg/day.

6. Convert the child's weight in pounds to kilograms. The recommended dosage is expressed in kilograms (50 mg/kg/day).

    $$42 \text{ lb} = 42 \div 2.2 = 19.1 \text{ kg}$$
    $$50 \text{ mg/kg/day} \times 19.1 \text{ kg} = 955 \text{ mg/day}$$
    $$955 \text{ mg} \div 4 = 238.8 \text{ mg per dosage}$$

    The dosage ordered is not safe because 250 mg × 4 = 1,000 mg/day. 1,000 mg/day is greater than 955 mg/day. Also the dose being administered q6h exceeds the recommended dose. Notify the prescriber.

7. Convert the child's weight in pounds to kilograms. The recommended dosage is stated in kilograms (10 to 25 mg/kg/24 hr).

    $$36 \text{ lb} = 36 \div 2.2 = 16.4 \text{ kg}$$
    $$10 \text{ mg/kg/day} \times 16.4 \text{ kg} = 164 \text{ mg/day}$$
    $$25 \text{ mg/kg/day} \times 16.4 \text{ kg} = 410 \text{ mg/day}$$

The medication is given q6-8h. The dosage in this problem is ordered q8h.

$$24 \div 8 = 3 \text{ dosages}$$
$$164 \text{ mg} \div 3 = 54.7 \text{ mg/dosage}$$
$$410 \text{ mg} \div 3 = 136.7 \text{ mg/dosage}$$

The dosage ordered is 150 mg q8h.

$$150 \text{ mg} \times 3 = 450 \text{ mg/day}$$

Notify the prescriber; the dosage is high (not safe). 450 mg/day is greater than the dosage range of 164-410 mg/day.

8. a. Convert the child's weight in pounds to kilograms. The recommended dosage is expressed in kilograms (25-50 mg/kg).

$$66 \text{ lb} = 66 \div 2.2 = 30 \text{ kg}$$
$$25 \text{ mg/kg/day} \times 30 \text{ kg} = 750 \text{ mg/day}$$
$$50 \text{ mg/kg/day} \times 30 \text{ kg} = 1,500 \text{ mg/day}$$

The safe range is 750-1,500 mg/day.

The medication is given in divided dosages (4).

The dosage ordered is q6h.

$$24 \div 6 = 4 \text{ dosages}$$
$$750 \text{ mg} \div 4 = 187.5 \text{ mg/per dosage}$$
$$1,500 \text{ mg} \div 4 = 375 \text{ mg/per dosage}$$

The dosage range is 187.5-375 mg per dose q6h. 250 mg × 4 = 1000 mg/day. This is a safe dosage because the total dosage falls within the safe range for 24 hr, and the divided dosage also falls within the safe range.

   b. You would give 10 mL for one dosage.

$$125 \text{ mg} : 5 \text{ mL} = 250 \text{ mg} : x \text{ mL}$$

*or*

$$\frac{250 \text{ mg}}{125 \text{ mg}} \times 5 \text{ mL} = x \text{ mL}$$

$$x = 10 \text{ mL}$$

The dosage ordered is greater than the available strength; therefore you will need more than 5 mL to administer the dosage.

9. a. No conversion of weight is required. The child's weight is stated in kilograms, and the recommended dosage is 20-40 mg/kg/day.

$$20 \text{ mg/kg/day} \times 35 \text{ kg} = 700 \text{ mg/day}$$
$$40 \text{ mg/kg/day} \times 35 \text{ kg} = 1,400 \text{ mg/day}$$

The safe range is 700-1,400 mg/day.

The drug is given in divided dosages q12h.

$$24 \div 12 = 2 \text{ dosages}$$
$$700 \text{ mg} \div 2 = 350 \text{ mg}$$
$$1,400 \text{ mg} \div 2 = 700 \text{ mg}$$

350-700 mg per dosage is safe.

The prescriber ordered 400 mg IM q12h. This dosage is safe. 400 mg × 2 = 800 mg/day. The total dosage falls within the safe range for 24 hr.

   b. Administer 1 mL.

$$400 \text{ mg} : 1 \text{ mL} = 400 \text{ mg} : x \text{ mL}$$

*or*

$$\frac{400 \text{ mg}}{400 \text{ mg}} \times 1 \text{ mL} = x \text{ mL}$$

$$x = 1 \text{ mL}$$

The dosage ordered is contained in 1 mL.

10. Convert the child's weight in pounds to kilograms. The recommended dosage is expressed in kilograms (120 mg/kg).

$$46 \text{ lb} = 46 \div 2.2 = 20.9 \text{ kg}$$
$$120 \text{ mg/kg/day} \times 20.9 \text{ kg} = 2,508 \text{ mg/day}$$

The drug is given in four equally divided dosages.

The dosage for this child is ordered q6h.

$$24 \div 6 = 4 \text{ dosages.}$$
$$2,508 \text{ mg} \div 4 = 627 \text{ mg per dosage}$$
$$250 \text{ mg} \times 4 = 1,000 \text{ mg/day}$$

The dosage ordered is too low. Notify the prescriber. 250 mg for each dosage is less than 627 mg, and 1,000 mg/day is less than 2,508 mg/day. The dosage ordered is not safe, so it may not be effective.

11. Convert the neonate's weight in grams to kilograms (1,000 g = 1 kg).

   a. 3,500 g = 3.5 kg

   b. $30 \text{ mg/kg} \times 3.5 \text{ kg} = 105 \text{ mg}$

The safe dosage for the neonate is 105 mg q12h.

12. No weight conversion is required. The child's weight is in kilograms, and the recommended dosage is expressed in kilograms (50-100 mg/kg/day).

   a. $50 \text{ mg/kg/day} \times 14 \text{ kg} = 700 \text{ mg/day}$
      $100 \text{ mg/kg/day} \times 14 \text{ kg} = 1,400 \text{ mg/day}$
      700-1,400 mg/day

   b. $24 \div 6 = 4 \text{ dosages}$
      $700 \text{ mg} \div 4 = 175 \text{ mg per dose}$
      $1,400 \text{ mg} \div 4 = 350 \text{ mg per dose}$

Divided dosage range is 175-350 mg per dosage.

   c. $250 \text{ mg} \times 4 = 1,000 \text{ mg/day}$

The dosage ordered is safe. 1,000 mg/day falls within range of 700-1,400 mg/day; it does not exceed the dosage allowed for the day or per dose.

13. Weight conversion is required (2.2 lb = 1 kg).

    a. 190 lb ÷ 2.2 = 86.4 kg

    b. 86.4 kg × 25 mcg/kg = 2,160 mcg

    86.4 kg × 30 mcg/kg = 2,592 mcg

    To determine the number of milligrams, convert the micrograms obtained to milligrams (1,000 mcg = 1 mg).

    2,160 mcg ÷ 1,000 = 2.16 mg (2.2 mg, to the nearest tenth)

    2,592 mcg ÷ 1,000 = 2.59 (2.6 mg to the nearest tenth)

    The daily dosage range in milligrams is 2.2-2.6.

14. a. 0.45 m²

    b. $\dfrac{0.45 \text{ m}^2}{1.7 \text{ (m}^2)} \times 500 \text{ mg} = 132.35 = 132.4 \text{ mg}$

15. a. 0.54 m²

    b. $\dfrac{0.54 \text{ m}^2}{1.7 \text{ (m}^2)} \times 25 \text{ mg} = 7.9 \text{ mg}$

16. a. 1.2 m²

    b. $\dfrac{1.2 \text{ m}^2}{1.7 \text{ (m}^2)} \times 250 \text{ mg} = 176.5 \text{ mg}$

17. a. 1.1 m²

    b. $\dfrac{1.1 \text{ m}^2}{1.7 \text{ (m}^2)} \times 30 \text{ mg} = 19.4 \text{ mg}$

18. a. 1.05 m²

    b. $\dfrac{1.05 \text{ m}^2}{1.7 \text{ (m}^2)} \times 150 \text{ mg} = 92.6 \text{ mg}$

19. $\dfrac{0.7 \text{ m}^2}{1.7 \text{ (m}^2)} \times 50 \text{ mg} = 20.6 \text{ mg}$

20. $\dfrac{0.66 \text{ m}^2}{1.7 \text{ (m}^2)} \times 10 \text{ mg} = 3.9 \text{ mg}$

    $\dfrac{0.66 \text{ m}^2}{1.7 \text{ (m}^2)} \times 20 \text{ mg} = 7.8 \text{ mg}$

    The dosage range is 3.9-7.8 mg.

21. $\dfrac{0.55 \text{ m}^2}{1.7 \text{ (m}^2)} \times 2,000 \text{ units} = 647.1 \text{ units}$

22. $\dfrac{0.55 \text{ m}^2}{1.7 \text{ (m}^2)} \times 200 \text{ mg} = 64.7 \text{ mg}$

    $\dfrac{0.55 \text{ m}^2}{1.7 \text{ (m}^2)} \times 250 \text{ mg} = 80.9 \text{ mg}$

    The dosage range is 64.7-80.9 mg.

23. $\dfrac{0.22 \text{ m}^2}{1.7 \text{ (m}^2)} \times 150 \text{ mg} = 19.4 \text{ mg}$

24. Dosage is incorrect; the child's dosage is 17.3 mg.

    $\dfrac{0.49 \text{ m}^2}{1.7 \text{ (m}^2)} \times 60 \text{ mg} = 17.3 \text{ mg}$

    The dosage of 25 mg is too high.

25. $\dfrac{0.32 \text{ m}^2}{1.7 \text{ (m}^2)} \times 10 \text{ mg} = 1.9 \text{ mg}$

    The dosage of 4 mg is too high.

26. Dosage is correct.

    $\dfrac{0.68 \text{ m}^2}{1.7 \text{ (m}^2)} \times 125 \text{ mg} = 50 \text{ mg}$

    $\dfrac{0.68 \text{ m}^2}{1.7 \text{ (m}^2)} \times 150 \text{ mg} = 60 \text{ mg}$

    The dosage of 50 mg falls within the range of 50-60 mg.

27. Dosage is incorrect.

    $\dfrac{0.55 \text{ m}^2}{1.7 \text{ (m}^2)} \times 25 \text{ mg} = 8.1 \text{ mg}$

    The dosage of 5 mg is too low.

28. The dosage is correct.

    $\dfrac{1.2 \text{ m}^2}{1.7 \text{ (m}^2)} \times 75 \text{ mg} = 52.9 \text{ mg}$

    $\dfrac{1.2 \text{ m}^2}{1.7 \text{ (m}^2)} \times 100 \text{ mg} = 70.6 \text{ mg}$

    The dosage ordered is 60 mg and falls within the dosage range of 52.9-70.6 mg.

29. $\sqrt{\dfrac{100 \text{ (lb)} \times 55 \text{ (in)}}{3,131}} = \sqrt{\dfrac{5,500}{3,131}} = \sqrt{1.756}$

    $\sqrt{1.756} = 1.325$

    Answer: 1.33 m²

30. $\sqrt{\dfrac{60.9 \text{ (kg)} \times 130 \text{ (cm)}}{3,600}} = \sqrt{\dfrac{7,917}{3,600}} = \sqrt{2.199}$

    $\sqrt{2.199} = 1.482$

    Answer: 1.48 m²

31. $\sqrt{\dfrac{55 \text{ (lb)} \times 45 \text{ (in)}}{3,131}} = \sqrt{\dfrac{2,475}{3,131}} = \sqrt{0.790}$

    $\sqrt{0.790} = 0.888$

    Answer: 0.89 m²

32. $\sqrt{\dfrac{60 \text{ (lb)} \times 35 \text{ (in)}}{3,131}} = \sqrt{\dfrac{2,100}{3,131}} = \sqrt{0.670}$

    $\sqrt{0.670} = 0.818$

    Answer: 0.82 m²

33. $\sqrt{\dfrac{65 \text{ (kg)} \times 132 \text{ (cm)}}{3,600}} = \sqrt{\dfrac{8,580}{3,600}} = \sqrt{2.383}$

    $\sqrt{2.383} = 1.543$

    Answer: 1.54 m²

34. $\sqrt{\dfrac{24 \text{ (lb)} \times 28 \text{ (in)}}{3,131}} = \sqrt{\dfrac{672}{3,131}} = \sqrt{0.214}$

    $\sqrt{0.214} = 0.462$

    Answer: 0.46 m²

35. $\sqrt{\dfrac{6\ (kg) \times 55\ (cm)}{3,600}} = \sqrt{\dfrac{330}{3,600}} = \sqrt{0.091}$

$\sqrt{0.091} = 0.301$

Answer: 0.3 m$^2$

36. $\sqrt{\dfrac{42\ (lb) \times 45\ (in)}{3,131}} = \sqrt{\dfrac{1,890}{3,131}} = \sqrt{0.603}$

$\sqrt{0.603} = 0.776$

Answer: 0.78 m$^2$

37. $\sqrt{\dfrac{8\ (kg) \times 70\ (cm)}{3,600}} = \sqrt{\dfrac{560}{3,600}} = \sqrt{0.155}$

$\sqrt{0.155} = 0.393$

Answer: 0.39 m$^2$

38. $\sqrt{\dfrac{74\ (kg) \times 160\ (cm)}{3,600}} = \sqrt{\dfrac{11,840}{3,600}} = \sqrt{3.288}$

$\sqrt{3.288} = 1.813$

Answer: 1.81 m$^2$

39. $10\ mg : 1\ mL = 7\ mg : x\ mL$

*or*

$\dfrac{7\ mg}{10\ mg} \times 1\ mL = x\ mL$

Answer: 0.7 mL. The dosage ordered is less than the available strength; therefore you will need less than 1 mL to administer the dosage.

40. $10\ mg : 1\ mL = 150\ mg : x\ mL$

*or*

$\dfrac{150\ mg}{10\ mg} \times 1\ mL = x\ mL$

Answer: 15 mL. The dosage ordered is more than the available strength; therefore you will need more than 1 mL to administer the dosage.

41. $0.05\ mg : 1\ mL = 0.1\ mg : x\ mL$

*or*

$\dfrac{0.1\ mg}{0.05\ mg} \times 1\ mL = x\ mL$

Answer: 2 mL. The dosage ordered is more than the available strength; therefore you will need more than 1 mL to administer the dosage.

42. $50\ mg : 5\ mL = 80\ mg : x\ mL$

*or*

$\dfrac{80\ mg}{50\ mg} \times 5\ mL = x\ mL$

Answer: 8 mL. The dosage ordered is greater than the available strength; therefore you will need more than 5 mL to administer the dosage.

43. $125\ mg : 5\ mL = 250\ mg : x\ mL$

*or*

$\dfrac{250\ mg}{125\ mg} \times 5\ mL = x\ mL$

Answer: 10 mL. The dosage ordered is greater than the available strength; therefore you will need more than 5 mL to administer the dosage.

44. Conversion required. Equivalent: 1,000 mg = 1 g. Therefore 0.25 g = 250 mg.

$100\ mg : 5\ mL = 250\ mg : x\ mL$

*or*

$\dfrac{250\ mg}{100\ mg} \times 5\ mL = x\ mL$

Answer: 12.5 mL. The dosage ordered is greater than the available strength; therefore you will need more than 5 mL to administer the dosage.

45. $250\ mg : 5\ mL = 100\ mg : x\ mL$

*or*

$\dfrac{100\ mg}{250\ mg} \times 5\ mL = x\ mL$

Answer: 2 mL. The dosage ordered is less than the available strength; therefore you will need less than 5 mL to administer the dosage.

46. $20\ mg : 2\ mL = 7.3\ mg : x\ mL$

*or*

$\dfrac{7.3\ mg}{20\ mg} \times 2\ mL = x\ mL$

Answer: 0.73 mL. The dosage ordered is less than the available strength; therefore you will need less than 2 mL to administer the dosage.

47. $0.4\ mg : 1\ mL = 0.1\ mg : x\ mL$

*or*

$\dfrac{0.1\ mg}{0.4\ mg} \times 1\ mL = x\ mL$

Answer: 0.25 mL. The dosage ordered is less than the available strength; therefore you will need less than 1 mL to administer the dosage.

48. $250\ mg : 1\ mL = 160\ mg : x\ mL$

*or*

$\dfrac{160\ mg}{250\ mg} \times 1\ mL = x\ mL$

Answer: 0.64 mL. The dosage ordered is less than the available strength; therefore you will need less than 1 mL to administer the dosage.

49. $15\ mg : 1\ mL = 3.5\ mg : x\ mL$

*or*

$\dfrac{3.5\ mg}{15\ mg} \times 1\ mL = x\ mL$

Answer: 0.23 mL. The dosage ordered is less than the available strength; therefore you will need less than 1 mL to administer the dosage.

50. $20 \text{ mg} : 2 \text{ mL} = 60 \text{ mg} : x \text{ mL}$

    *or*

    $$\frac{60 \text{ mg}}{20 \text{ mg}} \times 2 \text{ mL} = x \text{ mL}$$

    Answer: 6 mL. The dosage ordered is more than the available strength; therefore you will need more than 2 mL to administer the dosage.

51. Conversion required. Equivalent: 1,000 mg = 1 g. Therefore 0.4 g = 400 mg.

    $160 \text{ mg} : 5 \text{ mL} = 400 \text{ mg} : x \text{ mL}$

    *or*

    $$\frac{400 \text{ mg}}{160 \text{ mg}} \times 5 \text{ mL} = x \text{ mL}$$

    Answer: 12.5 mL. The dosage ordered is more than the available strength; therefore you will need more than 5 mL to administer the dosage.

52. $25 \text{ mg} : 1 \text{ mL} = 35 \text{ mg} : x \text{ mL}$

    *or*

    $$\frac{35 \text{ mg}}{25 \text{ mg}} \times 1 \text{ mL} = x \text{ mL}$$

    Answer: 1.4 mL. The dosage ordered is more than the available strength; therefore you will need more than 1 mL to administer the dosage.

53. $150 \text{ mg} : 1 \text{ mL} = 100 \text{ mg} : x \text{ mL}$

    *or*

    $$\frac{100 \text{ mg}}{150 \text{ mg}} \times 1 \text{ mL} = x \text{ mL}$$

    Answer: 0.66 = 0.7 mL. The dosage ordered is less than the available strength; therefore you will need less than 1 mL to administer the dosage.

54. $300,000 \text{ units} : 1 \text{ mL} = 150,000 \text{ units} : x \text{ mL}$

    *or*

    $$\frac{150,000 \text{ units}}{300,000 \text{ units}} \times 1 \text{ mL} = x \text{ mL}$$

    Answer: 0.5 mL. The dosage ordered is less than the available strength; therefore you will need less than 1 mL to administer the dosage.

55. $100 \text{ mg} : 2 \text{ mL} = 150 \text{ mg} : x \text{ mL}$

    *or*

    $$\frac{150 \text{ mg}}{100 \text{ mg}} \times 2 \text{ mL} = x \text{ mL}$$

    Answer: 3 mL. The dosage ordered is more than the available strength; therefore you will need more than 2 mL to administer the dosage.

56. $125 \text{ mg} : 5 \text{ mL} = 62.5 \text{ mg} : x \text{ mL}$

    *or*

    $$\frac{62.5 \text{ mg}}{125 \text{ mg}} \times 5 \text{ mL} = x \text{ mL}$$

    Answer: 2.5 mL. The dosage ordered is less than the available strength; therefore you will need less than 5 mL to administer the dosage.

57. $25 \text{ mg} : 1 \text{ mL} = 20 \text{ mg} : x \text{ mL}$

    *or*

    $$\frac{20 \text{ mg}}{25 \text{ mg}} \times 1 \text{ mL} = x \text{ mL}$$

    Answer: 0.8 mL. The dosage ordered is less than the available strength; therefore you will need less than 1 mL to administer the dosage.

58. $200 \text{ mg} : 5 \text{ mL} = 300 \text{ mg} : x \text{ mL}$

    *or*

    $$\frac{300 \text{ mg}}{200 \text{ mg}} \times 5 \text{ mL} = x \text{ mL}$$

    Answer: 7.5 mL. The dosage ordered is more than the available strength; therefore you will need more than 5 mL to administer the dosage.

59. $2 \text{ mg} : 5 \text{ mL} = 3 \text{ mg} : x \text{ mL}$

    *or*

    $$\frac{3 \text{ mg}}{2 \text{ mg}} \times 5 \text{ mL} = x \text{ mL}$$

    Answer: 7.5 mL. The dosage ordered is more than the available strength; therefore you will need more than 5 mL to administer the dosage.

60. $125 \text{ mg} : 5 \text{ mL} = 250 \text{ mg} : x \text{ mL}$

    *or*

    $$\frac{250 \text{ mg}}{125 \text{ mg}} \times 5 \text{ mL} = x \text{ mL}$$

    Answer: 10 mL. The dosage ordered is more than the available strength; therefore you will need more than 5 mL to administer the dosage.

61. $80 \text{ mg} : 15 \text{ mL} = 40 \text{ mg} : x \text{ mL}$

    *or*

    $$\frac{40 \text{ mg}}{80 \text{ mg}} \times 15 \text{ mL} = x \text{ mL}$$

    Answer: 7.5 mL. The dosage ordered is less than the available strength; therefore you will need less than 15 mL to administer the dosage.

62.    15 mg : 0.6 mL = 45 mg : $x$ mL

*or*

$$\frac{45 \text{ mg}}{15 \text{ mg}} \times 0.6 \text{ mL} = x \text{ mL}$$

Answer: 1.8 mL. The dosage ordered is greater than the available strength; therefore you will need more than 0.6 mL to administer the dosage.

63.    40 mg : 1 mL = 14 mg : $x$ mL

*or*

$$\frac{14 \text{ mg}}{40 \text{ mg}} \times 1 \text{ mL} = x \text{ mL}$$

Answer: 0.35 mL = 0.4 rounded to the nearest tenth. The dosage ordered is less than the available strength; therefore you will need less than 1 mL to administer the dosage.

64.    8 mg : 1 mL = 20 mg : $x$ mL

*or*

$$\frac{20 \text{ mg}}{8 \text{ mg}} \times 1 \text{ mL} = x \text{ mL}$$

Answer: 2.5 mL. The dosage ordered is more than the available strength; therefore you will need more than 1 mL to administer the dosage.

65.    10 mg : 1 mL = 75 mg : $x$ mL

*or*

$$\frac{75 \text{ mg}}{10 \text{ mg}} \times 1 \text{ mL} = x \text{ mL}$$

Answer: 7.5 mL. The dosage ordered is greater than the available strength; therefore you will need more than 1 mL to administer the dosage.

66. Convert the child's weight in pounds to kilograms. The recommended dosage is expressed in kilograms (20 mg/kg/day).

10 lb = 10 ÷ 2.2 = 4.5 kg

20 mg/kg/day × 4.5 kg = 90 mg/day

The medication is given in three divided doses. The dosage for the child is ordered q8h.

24 ÷ 8 = 3 doses.

90 mg ÷ 3 = 30 mg per dose

180 mg × 3 = 540 mg/day

Notify the prescriber; the dosage is high (not safe).

540 mg/day is greater than 90 mg/day. In addition, the dose the child is receiving q8h exceeds the dose recommended.

67. Convert the child's weight in pounds to kilograms. The recommended dosage is in kilograms (15 mg/kg/day).

45 lb = 45 ÷ 2.2 = 20.5 kg

15 mg/kg/day × 20.5 kg = 307.5 mg/day

The medication is given in divided doses q12h.

The dosage for the child is ordered q12h.

24 ÷ 12 = 2 doses

307.5 mg ÷ 2 = 153.8 mg per dose

200 mg × 2 = 400 mg/day

Notify the prescriber; the dosage is high (not safe).

400 mg/day is greater than 307.5 mg/day. In addition, the dose the child is receiving q12h is higher than the dose recommended.

68. Convert the child's weight in pounds to kilograms. The recommended dosage is in kilograms (22.5 mg/kg).

66 lb = 66 ÷ 2.2 = 30 kg

22.5 mg/kg × 30 kg = 675 mg/dose

The medication is given up to three times a day. The dosage for the child is ordered tid. The dosage ordered is not safe. The child is receiving 650 mg/dose, which is less than the recommended dosage and may not be effective. Notify the prescriber.

69. a. Convert the child's weight in pounds to kilograms. The recommended dosage is in kilograms (4 mg/kg).

65 lb = 65 ÷ 2.2 = 29.5 kg

4 mg/kg × 29.5 kg = 118 mg/dose

The safe dosage for this child is 118 mg/dosage.

b. The dosage for the child is ordered twice a day. Dosage is not safe; 120 mg × 2 = 240 mg/day.

This is greater than 118 mg per dosage (118 mg × 2 = 236 mg/day).

Notify the prescriber.

70. Convert the child's weight in pounds to kilograms. The recommended dosage is in kilograms (0.25-1 mg/kg).

31 lb = 31 ÷ 2.2 = 14.1 kg

0.25 mg/kg/day × 14.1 kg = 3.5 mg/day

1 mg/kg/day × 14.1 kg = 14.1 mg/day

The safe dosage range for this child is 3.5-14.1 mg/day.

71. $0.8 \text{ m}^2 \times \dfrac{2 \text{ mg}}{\text{m}^2} = 1.6 \text{ mg}$

72. $0.82 \text{ m}^2 \times \dfrac{250 \text{ mg}}{\text{m}^2} = 205 \text{ mg}$

73. $1.83 \text{ m}^2 \times \dfrac{10 \text{ units}}{\text{m}^2} = 18.3 \text{ units}$

$1.83 \text{ m}^2 \times \dfrac{20 \text{ units}}{\text{m}^2} = 36.6 \text{ units}$

Dosage range is 18.3 to 36.6 units

## NOTE

For problems 74-76, a ratio and proportion could be set up and mL/hr determined first, which, when a burette is used without a pump or controller, is the same as gtt/min. If gtt/min is determined first, remember that it is the same as mL/hr.

74. $x \text{ gtt/min} = \dfrac{30 \text{ mL} \times 60 \text{ gtt/mL}}{20 \text{ min}}$

$x = \dfrac{1,800}{20}; x = 90 \text{ gtt/min}$

*or*

mL/hr determined with ratio and proportion

$30 \text{ mL} : 20 \text{ min} = x \text{ mL} : 60 \text{ min}$

*or*

$\dfrac{30 \text{ mL}}{20 \text{ min}} = \dfrac{x \text{ mL}}{60 \text{ min}}$

  a. 90 gtt/min; 90 microgtt/min

  b. 90 mL/hr

75. $x \text{ gtt/min} = \dfrac{80 \text{ mL} \times 60 \text{ gtt/mL}}{60 \text{ min}}$

$x = \dfrac{4,800}{60}; x = 80 \text{ gtt/min}$

*or*

Determine mL/hr

$80 \text{ mL} : 60 \text{ min} = x \text{ mL} : 60 \text{ min}$

$\dfrac{80 \text{ mL}}{60 \text{ min}} = \dfrac{x \text{ mL}}{60 \text{ min}}$

  a. 80 gtt/min; 80 microgtt/min

  b. 80 mL/hr

76. $x \text{ gtt/min} = \dfrac{40 \text{ mL} \times 60 \text{ gtt/mL}}{45 \text{ min}}$

$\dfrac{2,400}{45} = 53 \text{ gtt/min}$

*or*

Determine mL/hr

$40 \text{ mL} : 45 \text{ min} = x \text{ mL} : 60 \text{ min}$

$\dfrac{40 \text{ mL}}{45 \text{ min}} = \dfrac{x \text{ mL}}{60 \text{ min}}$

  a. 53 gtt/min; 53 microgtt/min

  b. 53 mL/hr

77. Step 1: Calculate the safe dosage range for child.
          $23 \text{ kg} \times 40 \text{ mg/kg} = 920 \text{ mg}$
          $23 \text{ kg} \times 50 \text{ mg/kg} = 1,150 \text{ mg}$

    Step 2: Calculate the dosage the child receives in 24 hours.
          500 mg q12hr (2 dosages) $500 \times 2 = 1,000 \text{ mg}$

    Step 3: Compare dosage ordered with safe range.
          The dosage ordered is 1,000 mg; it is within the safe range of 920-1,150 mg/day. Calculate the dosage to administer.

78. Step 1: Calculate the safe dosage range for the child.
          $20 \text{ kg} \times 0.05 \text{ mg/kg} = 1 \text{ mg}$

    Step 2: Child receives 2 mg of medication at 10 AM.

    Step 3: The dosage ordered is 2 mg. 1 mg is the safe dosage; consult with the prescriber before administering (2 mg is more than 1 mg).

79. Step 1: Determine the safe dosage range for the child.
          $15 \text{ kg} \times 6 \text{ mcg/kg/day} = 90 \text{ mcg/day}$
          $15 \text{ kg} \times 8 \text{ mcg/kg/day} = 120 \text{ mcg/day}$

    Step 2: 55 mcg q12h (2 dosages);
          $55 \text{ mcg} \times 2 = 110 \text{ mcg/day}$

    Step 3: The dosage ordered is 110 mcg; it is within the safe range of 90-120 mcg/day. Calculate the dosage to administer.

## ANSWERS TO COMPREHENSIVE POST-TEST

### NOTE

Calculations may be performed using formula method, ratio and proportion, or dimensional analysis.

1.  $200 \text{ mg} : 5 \text{ mL} = 300 \text{ mg} : x \text{ mL}$

    *or*

    $$\frac{300 \text{ mg}}{200 \text{ mg}} \times 5 \text{ mL} = x \text{ mL}$$

    Answer: 7.5 mL

2.  Conversion is required.

    Equivalent: 1,000 mg = 1 g

    $500 \text{ mg} : 1 \text{ tab} = 1,000 \text{ mg} : x \text{ tab}$

    *or*

    $$\frac{1000 \text{ mg}}{500 \text{ mg}} \times 1 \text{ tab} = x \text{ tab}$$

    Answer: 2 tabs

3.  $0.1 \text{ mg} : 1 \text{ cap} = 0.2 \text{ mg} : x \text{ cap}$

    *or*

    $$\frac{0.2 \text{ mg}}{0.1 \text{ mg}} \times 1 \text{ cap} = x \text{ cap}$$

    Answer: 2 caps

4.  a. Tablets B: Septra DS.

    b. The prescriber's order indicates DS, which means double strength; therefore the client should be given the tabs that are labeled DS.

5.  $0.1 \text{ mg} : 1 \text{ mL} = 1 \text{ mg} : x \text{ mL}$

    *or*

    $$\frac{1 \text{ mg}}{0.1 \text{ mg}} \times 1 \text{ mL} = x \text{ mL}$$

    Answer: 10 mL

6.  $10,000 \text{ units} : 1 \text{ mL} = 6,500 \text{ units} : x \text{ mL}$

    *or*

    $$\frac{6500 \text{ units}}{10,000 \text{ units}} \times 1 \text{ mL} = x \text{ mL}$$

    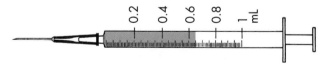

    Answer: 0.65 mL

7.  Conversion is required. Equivalent: 1,000 mg = 1 g

    Therefore 0.75 g = 750 mg

    $1,200 \text{ mg} : 120 \text{ mL} = 750 \text{ mg} : x \text{ mL}$

    *or*

    $$\frac{750 \text{ mg}}{1,200 \text{ mg}} \times 120 \text{ mL} = x \text{ mL}$$

    Answer: 75 mL

8.  a.  $50 \text{ mg} : 10 \text{ mL} = 75 \text{ mg} : x \text{ mL}$

    *or*

    $$\frac{75 \text{ mg}}{50 \text{ mg}} \times 10 \text{ mL} = x \text{ mL}$$

    Answer: 15 mL

    b.  1.  Determine mL/hr.

        $$x \text{ mL/hr} = \frac{1,000 \text{ mL}}{6 \text{ hr}}; x = 166.6 = 167 \text{ mL/hr}$$

        2.  Use formula and determine gtt/min.

        $$x \text{ gtt/min} = \frac{167 \text{ mL} \times 10 \text{ gtt/mL}}{60 \text{ min}};$$

        $x = 27.8 = 28 \text{ gtt/min}; 28 \text{ macrogtt/min}$

### NOTE

Problem 8 could also be done by using the shortcut method illustrated in Chapter 22.

9.  Convert weight in pounds to kilograms. Equivalent: 2.2 lb = 1 kg

    Therefore 110 lb ÷ 2.2 = 50 kg

    $50 \text{ k\!\!/g} \times 1 \text{ mg/k\!\!/g} = 50 \text{ mg}$

    Answer: 50 mg

10. Conversion is required. Equivalent: 1,000 mg = 1 g

    Therefore 0.3 g = 300 mg

    $150 \text{ mg} : 1 \text{ tab} = 300 \text{ mg} : x \text{ tab}$

    *or*

    $$\frac{300 \text{ mg}}{150 \text{ mg}} \times 1 \text{ tab} = x \text{ tab}$$

    Answer: 2 tabs

11. a.  95 mg per mL (Vial is 1 g.)

    b.  Conversion is required. 1,000 mg = 1 g

    Therefore 0.25 g = 250 mg

    $95 \text{ mg} : 1 \text{ mL} = 250 \text{ mg} : x \text{ mL}$

    *or*

    $$\frac{250 \text{ mg}}{95 \text{ mg}} \times 1 \text{ mL} = x \text{ mL}$$

    Answer: 2.63 mL = 2.6 mL to nearest tenth

    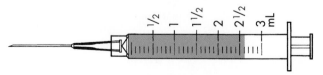

12. Answer: 2 tabs (one 50-mg tab and one 25-mg tab)

 Total = 75 mg (50-mg tab + 25-mg tab)

 Administer the least number of tablets to client.

13. Step 1: Determine mL/hr.

$$x \text{ mL/hr} = \frac{250 \text{ mL}}{3 \text{ hr}}; x = 83.3 = 83 \text{ mL/hr}$$

 Step 2: Calculate gtt/min.

$$x \text{ gtt/min} = \frac{83 \text{ mL} \times 20 \text{ gtt/mL}}{60 \text{ min}}$$

$$x = 27.6 = 28 \text{ gtt/min}$$

 Answer: 28 macrogtt/min; 28 gtt/min

 The shortcut method could also have been used to do the problem.

14. $$x \text{ gtt/min} = \frac{80 \text{ mL} \times 15 \text{ gtt/mL}}{60 \text{ min}}$$

$$x = 20 \text{ gtt/min}$$

 Answer: 20 macrogtt/min; 20 gtt/min

15. $$x \text{ gtt/min} = \frac{100 \text{ mL} \times 10 \text{ gtt/mL}}{45 \text{ min}}$$

$$x = 22.2 = 22 \text{ gtt/min}$$

 Answer: 22 macrogtt/min; 22 gtt/min

16. $$\frac{1,000 \text{ mL}}{60 \text{ mL/hr}} = 16.66$$

$$60 \times 0.66 = 39.6 = 40 \text{ min}$$

 Answer: 16 hr + 40 min

17. $6 \text{ mg/kg/day} \times 12 \text{ kg} = 72 \text{ mg/day}$

 $12 \text{ mg/kg/day} \times 12 \text{ kg} = 144 \text{ mg/day}$

 Divided dosage: $72 \text{ mg/day} \div 2 = 36 \text{ mg q12h}$

 $144 \text{ mg/day} \div 2 = 72 \text{ mg q12h}$

 The safe dosage range is 72-144 mg/day.

 The divided dosage is 36-72 mg q12h.

 Answer: The prescriber ordered 60 mg q12h. The dosage is safe (60 mg × 2 = 120 mg); it falls within the safe dosage range.

18. $$\frac{100 \text{ mL}}{50 \text{ mL/hr}} = 2 \text{ hr}$$

 a. 2 hr

 b. 12 noon or 12 PM (10:00 AM and 2 hours); military time: 1200

19. Determine the dosage per hour.

 $10 \text{ mcg/min} \times 60 \text{ min} = 600 \text{ mcg/hr}$

 Convert to like units of measurement.

 1,000 mcg = 1 mg, therefore

 600 mcg = 0.6 mg

Calculate mL/hr.

 $50 \text{ mg} : 250 \text{ mL} = 0.6 \text{ mg} : x \text{ mL}$

*or*

$$\frac{50 \text{ mg}}{250 \text{ mL}} = \frac{0.6 \text{ mg}}{x \text{ mL}}$$

$$x = 3 \text{ mL/hr}$$

 Answer: To deliver 10 mcg/min, set the flow rate at 3 mL/hr (gtt/min).

20. 22 units

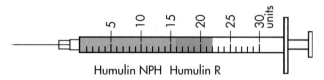

 Humulin NPH   Humulin R

21. a. 52 mL

 b. $$x \text{ gtt/min} = \frac{55 \text{ mL} \times 60 \text{ gtt/mL}}{50 \text{ min}}$$

$$x = 66 \text{ gtt/min}$$

 Answer: 66 microgtt/min; 66 gtt/min. The short-cut method could also have been used to do this problem.

 c. 66 mL/hr (gtt/min with a microdrop = mL/hr)

22. Administer two 20-mg tablets. The client should receive the least number of tabs. If 10-mg tabs are used, the client would require 4 tabs. Generally the maximum number of tablets that should be administered is three. Remember to question any order requiring more than this.

 $$\begin{array}{r} 1 \text{ 20-mg tab} \\ + 1 \text{ 20-mg tab} \\ \hline 40 \text{ mg} \end{array}$$

23. $$\sqrt{\frac{102 \text{ (lb)} \times 51 \text{ (in)}}{3,131}} = \sqrt{1.66} = 1.288 = 1.29 \text{ m}^2$$

 Answer: 1.29 m²

24. a. $$\sqrt{\frac{13.6 \text{ (kg)} \times 60 \text{ cm}}{3,600}} = \sqrt{0.226} = 0.475$$

$$= 0.48 \text{ m}^2$$

 Answer: 0.48 m².

 b. $0.48 \text{ m}^2 \times 500 \text{ mg/m}^2 = 240 \text{ mg}$

 Answer: 240 mg

 c. $50 \text{ mg} : 1 \text{ mL} = 240 \text{ mg} : x \text{ mL}$

*or*

$$\frac{240 \text{ mg}}{50 \text{ mg}} \times 1 \text{ mL} = x \text{ mL}$$

 Answer: 4.8 mL. The dosage ordered is greater than the available strength; therefore you will need more than 1 mL to administer the dosage.

25. a.  $25 \text{ mg} : 1 \text{ tab} = 50 \text{ mg} : x \text{ tab}$

    *or*

    $\dfrac{50 \text{ mg}}{25 \text{ mg}} \times 1 \text{ tab} = x \text{ tab}$

    Answer: 2 tabs

  b.  Hold the medication because the systolic BP (top number) is less than 100 and notify the prescriber.

26.  $\dfrac{2}{5} \times 250 \text{ mL} = x \text{ mL}$

    $\dfrac{500}{5} = x$

    $x = 100 \text{ mL of Ensure Plus}$

    $250 \text{ mL} - 100 \text{ mL} = 150 \text{ mL (water)}$

    Therefore you would add 150 mL of water to 100 mL of Ensure Plus to make 250 mL 2/5-strength Ensure Plus.

27.  $x \text{ mL/hr} = \dfrac{400 \text{ mL}}{6 \text{ hr}}$

    $x = 66.6 = 67 \text{ mL/hr}$

    Answer: 67 mL/hr

28.  $x \text{ gtt/min} = \dfrac{70 \text{ mL} \times 60 \text{ gtt/mL}}{50 \text{ min}}$

    $x = 84 \text{ gtt/min}$

  a.  84 microgtt/min; 84 gtt/min. The shortcut method could also have been used to do this problem.

  b.  84 mL/hr (gtt/min with a microdrop = mL/hr)

29.  Step 1:  Calculate the normal daily dosage range.

    $40 \text{ mg/kg/day} \times 21.4 \text{ kg} = 856 \text{ mg}$
    $50 \text{ mg/kg/day} \times 21.4 \text{ kg} = 1,070 \text{ mg}$

    The safe dosage range is 856-1,070 mg/day.

    Step 2:  Calculate the dosage infusing in 24 hr.

    500 mg q12h = (2 dosages)
    $500 \text{ mg} \times 2 = 1,000 \text{ mg in 24 hr}$

    Step 3:  Assess the accuracy of dosage ordered.

    500 mg q12h (1,000 mg) falls within the 856-1,070 mg/day dosage range. Administer the medication as ordered.

30.  $1 \text{ L} = 1,000 \text{ mL}$; therefore $2 \text{ L} = 2,000 \text{ mL}$

  a.  Dextrose:  $5 \text{ g} : 100 \text{ mL} = x \text{ g} : 2,000 \text{ mL}$

    $\dfrac{100x}{100} = \dfrac{10,000}{100}$

    *or*

    $\dfrac{5 \text{ g}}{100 \text{ mL}} = \dfrac{x \text{ g}}{2,000 \text{ mL}}$

    $x = 100 \text{ g dextrose}$

  b.  NaCl:  $0.225 \text{ g} : 100 \text{ mL} = x \text{ g} : 2,000 \text{ mL}$

    $\dfrac{100x}{100} = \dfrac{450}{100}$

    *or*

    $\dfrac{0.225 \text{ g}}{100 \text{ mL}} = \dfrac{x \text{ g}}{2,000 \text{ mL}}$

    $x = 4.5 \text{ g NaCl}$

## NOTE

Remember, ¼ NS (sodium chloride) is written as 0.225.

31.  Time remaining:  $3 \text{ hr} - 1.5 \text{ hr} = 1.5 \text{ hr} (1\frac{1}{2})$

    Volume remaining:  $500 \text{ mL} - 175 \text{ mL} = 325 \text{ mL}$

  a.  Step 1:  Calculate mL/hr.

    $325 \text{ mL} \div 1.5 \text{ hr} = 216.6 = 217 \text{ mL/hr}$

    Step 2:  Calculate the gtt/min.

    $x \text{ gtt/min} = \dfrac{217 \text{ mL} \times 10 \text{ gtt/mL}}{60 \text{ min}}$

    $x = \dfrac{217 \times 1}{6} = \dfrac{217}{6}$

    $x = 36 \text{ gtt/min}; 36 \text{ macrogtt/min}$

    The IV rate would have to be changed to 36 gtt/min (36 macrogtt/min).

  b.  Step 3:  Determine the percentage of change.

    $\dfrac{36 - 28}{28} = \dfrac{8}{28} = 0.285 = 29\%$

  c.  Course of action: Assess the client, and notify the prescriber. This increase is greater than 25%.

32.  Time remaining:  $8 \text{ hr} - 4 \text{ hr} = 4 \text{ hr}$

    Volume remaining:  $1,000 \text{ mL} - 600 \text{ mL} = 400 \text{ mL}$

  a.  Step 1:  Calculate mL/hr.

    $400 \text{ mL} \div 4 \text{ hr} = 100 \text{ mL/hr}$

    Step 2:  Calculate the gtt/min.

    $x \text{ gtt/min} = \dfrac{100 \text{ mL} \times 15 \text{ gtt/mL}}{60 \text{ min}}$

    $x = \dfrac{100 \times 1}{4} = \dfrac{100}{4}$

    $x = 25 \text{ gtt/min}; 25 \text{ macrogtt/min}$

    The IV rate would have to be changed to 25 gtt/min (25 macrogtt/min).

  b.  Step 3:  Determine the percentage of change.

    $\dfrac{25 - 31}{31} = \dfrac{-6}{31} = -0.193 = -19\%$

  c.  Course of action: Assess the client and lower the IV rate to 25 gtt/min (25 macrogtt/min). This is an acceptable decrease ($-19\%$); it is within the acceptable 25% variation. Also check the institution's policy and continue observation of the client.

**NOTE**

In problems 31 and 32, in addition to determining mL/hr, another shortcut method could be used to determine the drop factor constant and then gtt/min calculated using the drop factor constant.

33. Calculate the units/hr infusing.

$$500 \text{ mL} : 20,000 \text{ units} = 25 \text{ mL} : x \text{ units}$$

$$\frac{500x}{500} = \frac{500,000}{500}$$

$$x = 1,000 \text{ units/hr}$$

An IV of 500 mL containing 20,000 units of heparin infusing at 25 mL/hr is administering 1,000 units /hr.

34. a.  $50 \text{ mg} : 1 \text{ mL} = 25 \text{ mg} : x \text{ mL}$

*or*

$$\frac{25 \text{ mg}}{50 \text{ mg}} \times 1 \text{ mL} = x \text{ mL}$$

$$x = 0.5 \text{ mL}$$

b.  $25 \text{ mg} : 1 \text{ min} = 25 \text{ mg} : x \text{ min}$

$$\frac{25x}{25} = \frac{25}{25} = 1$$

$$x = 1 \text{ min}$$

35. $80 \text{ mg} : 250 \text{ mL} = x \text{ mg} : 20 \text{ mL}$

$$\frac{250x}{250} = \frac{1600}{250} = 6.4$$

$$x = 6.4 \text{ mg/hr}$$

36. a.  $5 \text{ mg} : 1 \text{ mL} = 25 \text{ mg} : x \text{ mL}$

$$\frac{25 \text{ mg}}{5 \text{ mg}} \times 1 \text{ mL} = x \text{ mL}$$

$$x = 5 \text{ mL}$$

b.  $\dfrac{5 \text{ mL}}{2 \text{ min}} = 2.5 \text{ mL/min}$

37. $1,000 \text{ mg} = 1 \text{ g}$

$0.75 \text{ g} = 750 \text{ mg}$

Answer: 90 tabs (3 tabs per dosage × 3 = 9 tabs; 9 tabs × 10 days = 90 tabs)

38. $1,000 \text{ mcg} = 1 \text{ mg}$       $0.375 \text{ mg} = 375 \text{ mcg}$

a. Give the client one 250-mcg tab and one 125-mcg tab.

250-mcg tab

+125-mcg tab
_____

375 mcg

b. 2 tabs (one 250-mcg tab and one 125-mcg tab) Give the least number of tablets without scoring.

39.    $15 \text{ mcg} : 0.5 \text{ mL} = 12 \text{ mcg} : x \text{ mL}$

*or*

$$\frac{12 \text{ mcg}}{15 \text{ mcg}} \times 0.5 \text{ mL} = x \text{ mL}$$

$$x = 0.4 \text{ mL}$$

40. a.    $50,000 \text{ units} : 1 \text{ mL} = 125,000 \text{ units} : x \text{ mL}$

$$\frac{50,000x}{50,000} = \frac{125,000}{50,000} = 2.5$$

$$x = 2.5 \text{ mL}$$

*or*

$$\frac{125,000 \text{ units}}{50,000 \text{ units}} \times 1 \text{ mL} = x \text{ mL}$$

b.

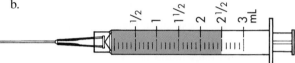

Alternate solution:

$$250,000 \text{ unit} : 5 \text{ mL} = 125,000 \text{ units} : x \text{ mL}$$

*or*

$$\frac{125,000 \text{ units}}{250,000 \text{ units}} \times 5 \text{ mL} = x \text{ mL}$$

41. Convert weight: 2.2 lb = 1 kg

$242 \text{ lb} \div 2.2 = 110 \text{ kg}$

a. $80 \text{ units/kg} \times 110 \text{ kg} = 8,800 \text{ units}$

b. $14 \text{ units/kg/hr} \times 110 \text{ kg} = 1,540 \text{ units/hr}$

42. $20 \text{ units/kg/hr} \times 88 \text{ kg} = 1,760 \text{ units/hr}$

43. Convert weight: 2.2 lb = 1 kg

$184 \text{ lb} \div 2.2 = 83.63 = 83.6 \text{ kg}$

$25 \text{ units/kg/hr} \times 83.6 \text{ kg} = 2,090 \text{ units/hr}$

44. a.    $0.25 \text{ mg} : 1 \text{ mL} = 0.375 \text{ mg} : x \text{ mL}$

*or*

$$\frac{0.375 \text{ mg}}{0.25 \text{ mg}} \times 1 \text{ mL} = x \text{ mL}$$

Answer: 1.5 mL

b. $1.5 \text{ mL} : 5 \text{ min} = x \text{ mL} : 1 \text{ min}$

$5x = 1.5$

$x = 0.3 \text{ mL/min}$

45. a.    $10 \text{ mg} : 1 \text{ mL} = 8 \text{ mg} : x \text{ mL}$

*or*

$$\frac{8 \text{ mg}}{10 \text{ mg}} \times 1 \text{ mL} = x \text{ mL}$$

Answer: 0.8 mL

b. $10 \text{ mg} : 4 \text{ min} = 8 \text{ mg} : x \text{ min}$

$$\frac{10x}{10} = \frac{32}{10}$$

$$x = 3.2 \text{ min}$$

# Bibliography

Administration on Aging: *A profile of older Americans: 2007.* Retrieved from http://www.aoa.gov/AoAroot/Aging_Statistics/Profile/2007/docs/2007profile.pdf. Accessed April 7, 2008.

Clayton BD, Stock, YN, Harroun RD: *Basic pharmacology for nurses,* ed 14, St. Louis, 2007, Mosby.

Cohen MR (ed): *Medication errors,* ed 2, Washington, DC, 2007, American Pharmacists Association.

Elkin MK, Perry AG, Potter PA: *Nursing interventions and clinical skills,* ed 4, St. Louis, 2007, Mosby.

Grissinger M, Globus NJ: How technology affects your risk of medication errors. *Nurs2004* 34 (1):36-41, 2004.

Harkreader H, Hogan MA: *Fundamentals of nursing: caring and clinical judgment,* ed. 3, St. Louis, 2007, Saunders.

Hidle A: Implementing technology to improve medication safety in health care facilities: a literature review. *J N Y State Nurses Assoc,* 38 (2):4-9, 2007 Fall-2008 Winter.

Institute for Safe Medication Practices: *ISMP's list of error-prone abbreviations and symbols, and dose designations.* Retrieved from http://www.ismp.org/Tools/errorproneabbreviations.pdf. Accessed April 20, 2008.

Institute of Medicine: *Preventing medication errors,* Washington, DC, 2006, National Academies Press.

Johns Hopkins Hospital: *The Harriet Lane handbook,* ed 17, St. Louis, 2005, Mosby.

The Joint Commission: *Official "Do Not Use" list.* Retrieved from http://www.jointcommission.org/NR/rdonlyres/2329F8F5-6EC5-4E21-B932-54B2B7D53F00/0/dnu_list.pdf. Accessed on April 20, 2008.

Kaplan JM, Ancheta R, Jacobs BR, Clinical Informatics Outcomes Research Group: Inpatient verbal orders and the impact of computerized provider order entry. J Pediatr 149:461-474, 2006

Potter PA, Perry AG: *Fundamentals of nursing,* ed 7, St. Louis, 2009, Mosby.

Skidmore-Roth L. *Mosby's 2008 nursing drug reference,* ed 21, St. Louis, 2008, Mosby.

Snyderman N: Study: One in fifteen kids hurt in hospital. *The Today Show,* April 7, 2008.

Wong DL, Hockenberry MJ: *Wong's nursing care of infants and children,* ed 8, St. Louis, 2007, Mosby.

# Index

## A

Abbreviations
  in apothecary system, 71, 72
  commonly used, 127*t*
  on "Do Not Use" List, 128*t*, 133*t*
  for form of medication, 163, 163*f*
  ISMP's error-prone, 133*t*–136*t*
  for IV solutions, 433, 433*b*
  on labels, 163, 163*f*, 167
  on medication order, 126, 126*t*
    for insulin, 415
  on medication record, 143
  in metric system, 62, 62*b*
  for routes of administration, 130
  in scheduling of medication, 154*t*
Access device, intermittent venous, 444–445, 444*f*
Acronyms
  on "Do Not Use" List, 128*t*, 133*t*
  ISMP's error-prone, 133*t*–136*t*
Activated partial thromboplastin time (APTT), heparin dosage calculation and, 509, 509*f*
ADC. *See* Automated dispensing cabinet (ADC)
Addition
  of decimals, 26–27
  of fractions, 13–14
ADD-Vantage system, 442, 443*f*
Administration. *See* Medication administration
Adrenalin label, 162
Amoxicillin label, 165*f*
Ampicillin, dosage calculation for, 261–262
Ampule, 310–311, 311*f*
Analgesia, patient-controlled, 446–447, 447*f*
Anticoagulants, 505, 505*f*. *See Also* Heparin
Apidra, 405, 408
Apothecary system, 70–73, 71*f*
  chapter review for, 76
  household equivalents, 74*b*, 78*t*
  metric equivalents, 72, 72*f*, 74*b*, 78*t*
  metric system *versus*, 60
  points to remember regarding, 75
  practice problems for, 75–76
  Roman numerals in, 4
Approximately, symbol for, 126*t*
APTT. *See* Activated partial thromboplastin time (APTT), heparin dosage calculation and
Arabic numbers
  in apothecary system, 71
  in metric system, 63
  Roman numeral equivalents for, 5*b*
Aspart, 405, 408
Atropine
  dosage calculation of, 335–336
  labeling of, 159, 160*f*
Automated dispensing cabinet (ADC), 151, 151*f*

## B

Balloon infusion device, 448, 448*f*
Bar-code
  on labels, 164
  in medication delivery, 151, 152, 152*f*
Barrel of syringe, 313, 313*f*
Baxter Mini-Bag Plus, 442, 443*f*
BD SafetyGlide needle, 314*f*
Blood and blood products administration, 440, 440*f*
Body surface area (BSA)
  burn assessment and, 45, 46*f*
  dose calculations based on, 537, 558–566
    in pediatric intravenous therapy, 570–572

Body temperature on Celsius *versus* Fahrenheit scales, 95, 95*f*
Body weight. *See Also* Weight
  adult dosage calculations based on, 551
  critical care solution administration based on, 525–526
  pediatric dosage calculations based on, 537, 538–551
    grams to kilograms conversion in, 543–544
    for heparin, 509–510, 509*f*
    kilograms to pounds conversion in, 541–542
    points to remember regarding, 557–558
    pounds to kilograms conversion in, 538–540
    practice problems for, 552–557
Boiling point of water on Celsius *versus* Fahrenheit scale, 94–95, 95*f*
Bolus
  heparin, 509
  intravenous, 445, 491–494
Brand name. *See* Trade name
Breaking of scored tablet, 254–255, 255*f*
BSA. *See* Body surface area (BSA)
Buccal medication, administration of, 117
Burette, pediatric intravenous therapy with, 566, 566*f*, 567–570
Burn, percentages in assessment of, 45, 46*f*

## C

Cabinet, unit-dose, 151*f*
Calan SR. *See* Verapamil hydrochloride
Calibrated burette in pediatric intravenous therapy, 566, 566*f*, 567–570
Calibrated dropper, 119, 119*f*
  measurement of oral liquids in, 278, 278*f*
Caplet, 254
Capsule, 256–257, 257*f*
  dosage calculations for, 258–266
    practice problems for, 266–277
  maximum number of for single dose, 259
  medication labeling and, 164, 165
  ratio and proportion for representation of weight of, 41
Cardizem CD. *See* Diltiazem HCl
Carpuject, 312, 313*f*
Cartridge, parenteral medication in, 312, 313*f*
Ceftazidime, pediatric dosage calculation for, 550
Celsius, Fahrenheit conversion to, 94–97, 95*f*, 103
Centi-, 61, 61*t*
Centimeter, 97
  in body surface area calculation, 561
  cubic, 65
  equivalents
    household, 78*t*
    metric, 64*b*
Central line for intravenous therapy, 441
  of parenteral nutrition, 439–440
Change, symbol for, 126*t*
Charting. *See* Documentation
Child, 536–587
  chapter review for, 573–587
  critical thinking questions associated with, 573
  dosage calculations for, 536–587
    based on body surface area, 558–566
    based on body weight, 538–551
    grams to kilograms conversion in, 543–544
    kilograms to pounds conversion in, 541–542
    points to remember regarding, 557–558, 566
    pounds to kilograms conversion in, 538–540

Child *(Continued)*
    practice problems for, 540, 542, 544, 552–557, 562, 564–565
    principles relating to, 537–538
    safe daily dosage in, 546
  equipment for oral administration to, 120, 121*f*
  intravenous therapy for, 566–570, 567*f*
    determining safety of, 570–572
    points to remember regarding, 572
  medication error in, 109
  oral and parenteral medications for, 572
Cipro label, 129*f*
Cisplatin, dosage calculation based on body surface area, 562
Client
  full name of on medication order, 128
  refusal of medication by, 114–115
  six rights of medication administration and, 113–114, 113*b*
  teaching of, 116
    elderly patients and, 112
Clock
  conversion, 72, 72*f*
  showing traditional and military time, 101*f*
Combined medications, labels for, 168–170, 168*f*, 169*f*
Completion times in intravenous therapy, 102–103, 486
Complex fraction, 10
Computers
  advantages and disadvantages of, 153
  for medication dispension, 151, 151*f*
  in medication administration, 147–148
  in medication orders, 125, 132
Computer-based drug administration software, 152
Computerized physician order entry (CPOE), 125, 148
  errors in, 153
Containers, medication, 112, 112*f*
Continuous intravenous infusion, 432
Continuous subcutaneous insulin infusion pump (CSII pump), 410
Controlled substance, labeling of, 168
Control number on medication label, 167
Conversions, 77–93
  between Celsius and Fahrenheit, 94–97, 95*f*
  chapter reviews for, 91–93, 104–106
  in completion times calculations, 102–103
  grains to milligrams, 262–263
  grams to kilograms, 543–544
  grams to milligrams, 261–262
  in intake and output calculations, 86–90, 86*f*, 88*f*, 89*f*
  kilograms to pounds, 541–542
  methods of, 78–81
    decimal point movement, 78–79
    dimensional analysis, 239
    ratio and proportion, 80–81
  metric, apothecary, and household system equivalents and, 77, 78*t*
  to military time, 100–102, 101*f*
  points to remember regarding, 91, 103–104
  pounds to kilograms, 538–540
  practice problems for, 79, 83, 90, 96–97, 102, 103
  relating to length, 97–98, 97*b*
  relating to weight, 98–100
  within same system, 81–83
    metric, 65–66, 65*f*
  between systems, 83–85

---

Page numbers followed by *b, t,* and *f* indicate boxes, tables, and figures, respectively.